PROLOG

Personal Review of Learning in Obstetrics and Gynecology

Obstetrics

NINTH EDITION

Critique Book

ONLINE ASSESSMENT

See instructions on the inside front cover.

ACOG

American College of Obstetricians & Gynecologists

Library of Congress Cataloging-in-Publication Data

American College of Obstetricians and Gynecologists
PROLOG. Obstetrics, Ninth Edition
Washington, DC : American College of Obstetricians and Gynecologists, [2023]
Identifiers: LCCN 2022038981 | ISBN 9781948258661 (paperback) |
ISBN 9781948258678 (ebook)
Classification: LCC RG532 .P76 2023 | DDC 618.20076—dc23/eng/20221110
LC record available at https://lccn.loc.gov/2022038981

Printed in the United States of America

45/765

American College of Obstetricians and Gynecologists
409 12th Street SW
Washington, DC 20024-2188

Contributors

PROLOG Editorial and Advisory Committee

CHAIR

Donna D. Johnson, MD
Lawrence L. Hester Endowed Chair
Professor and Chair
Department of Obstetrics and Gynecology
Division of Maternal–Fetal Medicine
Medical University of South Carolina
Charleston, South Carolina

MEMBERS

Daniel R. Grow, MD
Professor, Department of Obstetrics and Gynecology
Division and Fellowship Director, Reproductive Endocrinology and Infertility
University of Connecticut Health Center
Farmington, Connecticut

Amy M. Johnson, MD
Professor, Department of Obstetrics and Gynecology
Residency Program Director
University of Connecticut School of Medicine
Hartford HealthCare
Farmington, Connecticut

Heather Z. Sankey, MD
Ronald T. Burkman Endowed Chair of Obstetrics and Gynecology
Baystate Health
Professor and Chair
University of Massachusetts Chan Medical School–Baystate
Springfield, Massachusetts

PROLOG Task Force for *Obstetrics,* Ninth Edition

CO-CHAIRS

Keith H. Nelson, MD
Professor and Program Director
Department of Obstetrics and Gynecology
East Carolina University Brody School of Medicine
Greenville, North Carolina

Deborah M. Feldman, MD
Associate Professor, Department of Obstetrics and Gynecology
University of Connecticut School of Medicine
Division Director, Maternal–Fetal Medicine
Hartford HealthCare
Hartford, Connecticut

MEMBERS

Carrie L. Bell, MD
Associate Clinical Professor
Fellowship Director, Women's Health Fellowship
Department of Obstetrics and Gynecology
University of Michigan
Ann Arbor, Michigan

Kimberly B. Fortner, MD
Professor and Maternal–Fetal Medicine Fellowship Program Director
Department of Obstetrics and Gynecology
Vice Chair of Obstetrics Quality and Service
Vice President of Women and Infants Center of Excellence
University of Tennessee Medical Center
Knoxville, Tennessee

Christina A. Herrera, MD, MSCI
Department of Obstetrics and Gynecology
Division of Maternal–Fetal Medicine
Winnie Palmer Hospital for Women & Babies
Orlando Health
Orlando, Florida

Jason Hildebrand, MD
Assistant Professor
Associate Program Director
Department of Obstetrics and Gynecology
East Carolina University Brody School of Medicine
Greenville, North Carolina

Melissa I. March, MD
Medical Director, High Risk Obstetrics
Department of Obstetrics and Gynecology
Division of Maternal–Fetal Medicine
University Hospitals Cleveland Medical Center
Assistant Professor
Case Western Reserve University School of Medicine
Cleveland, Ohio

Sara Dawn O'Dell, DO
General Obstetrics and Gynecology
Washington Permanente Medical Group
Clinical Instructor
University of Washington
Seattle, Washington

Ruth Anne Queenan, MD, MBA
Luminis Health
Anne Arundel Hospital
Center for Maternal–Fetal Medicine
Annapolis, Maryland

(continued on next page)

Corina Schoen, MD
Assistant Professor of Obstetrics and Gynecology
Division of Maternal–Fetal Medicine
Department of Obstetrics and Gynecology
University of Massachusetts Chan Medical School–Baystate
Springfield, Massachusetts

Linda M. Szymanski, MD, PhD
Associate Professor
Maternal Section Head
Division of Maternal–Fetal Medicine
Department of Obstetrics and Gynecology
Mayo Clinic
Rochester, Minnesota

Lorene Atkins Temming, MD, MSCI
Medical Director, Labor and Delivery
Wake Forest School of Medicine, Charlotte Campus, Third-Year Ob-Gyn Clerkship Director
Assistant Professor, Maternal–Fetal Medicine
Department of Obstetrics and Gynecology
Atrium Health, Carolinas Medical Center
Charlotte, North Carolina

ACOG STAFF

DISCLOSURE STATEMENT

The Accreditation Council for Continuing Medical Education (ACCME) requires that all faculty and planning committee members disclose any financial interests relative to topics within this edition of PROLOG. This information will be obtained in advance by staff via the American College of Obstetricians and Gynecologists' (ACOG) online disclosure system. There must be ample time for resolution of all potential conflicts of interest. This information (with resolution of any conflicts of interest) should be on file before honoraria are paid.

DISCLOSURE OF FACULTY AND INDUSTRY RELATIONSHIPS

In accordance with ACOG's policy, all faculty and planning committee members have signed a conflict of interest statement in which they have disclosed any financial interests or other relationships with industry relative to topics in this edition of PROLOG. Such disclosure allows for better evaluation of the objectivity of the information presented.

CONFLICT OF INTEREST DISCLOSURE

This PROLOG unit was developed under the direction of the PROLOG Advisory Committee and Task Force for *Obstetrics*, Ninth Edition. PROLOG is planned and produced in accordance with the Standards for Commercial Support of the ACCME. Any discussion of unapproved use of products is clearly cited in the appropriate critique.

Current guidelines state that continuing medical education (CME) health care professionals must ensure that CME activities are free from the control of any commercial interest. The task force and advisory committee members declare that neither they nor any business associate nor any member of their immediate families has material interest, financial interest, or other relationships with any company manufacturing commercial products relative to the topics included in this publication or with any provider of commercial services discussed in the unit. All potential conflicts have been resolved through ACOG's mechanism for resolving potential and real conflicts of interest.

Preface

Purpose

PROLOG (Personal Review of Learning in Obstetrics and Gynecology) is a voluntary, strictly confidential self-evaluation program. PROLOG was developed specifically as a personal study resource for the practicing obstetrician–gynecologist. It is presented as a self-assessment mechanism that, with its accompanying performance information, should assist the physician in designing a personal, self-directed, lifelong learning program. It may be used as a valuable study tool, a reference guide, and a means of attaining up-to-date information in the specialty. The content is carefully selected and presented in multiple-choice questions that are clinically oriented. The questions are designed to stimulate and challenge physicians in areas of medical care that they confront in their practices or when they work as consultant obstetrician–gynecologists.

Process

The PROLOG series offers the most current information available in five areas of the specialty: 1) obstetrics; 2) gynecology and surgery; 3) reproductive endocrinology and infertility; 4) gynecologic oncology and critical care; and 5) patient management in the office. The series includes a sixth volume for the subspecialty of female pelvic medicine and reconstructive surgery. A new PROLOG edition is produced annually, addressing one of these subject areas. *Obstetrics*, Ninth Edition, is the first unit in the ninth 5-year PROLOG series.

Each unit of PROLOG represents the efforts of a task force of subject matter experts under the supervision of an advisory committee. PROLOG sets forth current information as viewed by recognized authorities in the field of women's health. This educational resource does not define a standard of care, nor is it intended to dictate an exclusive course of management. It presents recognized methods and techniques of clinical practice for consideration by obstetrician–gynecologists to incorporate in their practices. Variations of practice that take into account the needs of the individual patient, resources, and the limitations that are special to the institution or type of practice may be appropriate.

Each unit of PROLOG is presented as a two-part book, with performance information and cognate credit available to those who choose to submit their assessment for confidential scoring. The first part of this PROLOG edition is the Critique Book, which contains a discussion or critique of each question. Each critique provides the rationale for correct and incorrect options for each multiple-choice question. Current, accessible references are listed with each critique.

The second part of this PROLOG edition is the Assessment Book, which contains educational objectives for the unit and questions. The questions can be completed by taking an online assessment. Participants can work through the unit at their own pace, choosing to use PROLOG as a closed-book or open-book assessment. Submitting the online assessment is voluntary but encouraged. Participants can earn continuing medical education (CME) credits only by submitting and passing the online assessment.

Continuing Medical Education Credit

ACCME ACCREDITATION

The American College of Obstetricians and Gynecologists is accredited by the Accreditation Council for Continuing Medical Education (ACCME) to provide continuing medical education for physicians.

AMA PRA CATEGORY 1 CREDIT(S)™

The American College of Obstetricians and Gynecologists designates this enduring material for a maximum of 25 *AMA PRA Category 1 Credits*™. Physicians should claim only the credit commensurate with the extent of their participation in the activity.

ACOG COGNATE CREDIT(S)

The American College of Obstetricians and Gynecologists designates this enduring material for a maximum of 25 Category 1 College Cognate Credits. The American College of Obstetricians and Gynecologists has a reciprocity agreement with the American Medical Association that allows *AMA PRA Category 1 Credits*™ to be equivalent to College Cognate Credits.

Participants who submit their assessment for scoring and receive a passing of 80% will be credited with 25 CME credits for this unit. Those who complete the assessment for CME credit will receive a performance report that provides a comparison of their scores with the scores of a sample group of physicians who have taken the unit as an examination. An individual may request credit only once for each edition. Participants receive CME verification immediately after they pass the online assessment. **Paper answer sheets are NOT available for this edition.**

Credit for PROLOG *Obstetrics*, Ninth Edition, is initially available through December 2025. During that year, the unit will be reevaluated. If the content remains current, credit is extended for an additional 3 years, with credit for the unit automatically withdrawn after December 2028.

Electronic Assessment for CME Credit

To receive the CME credits for this edition, participants must complete an online assessment. Assessment results must be 80% or higher to achieve a passing score and attain CME credit. To access the online assessment, please visit https://prolog.acog.org. Test results and the CME certificate will be available upon completion of the examination.

If you purchased a print book, use the key code located on the inside front cover of the Critique Book and follow the directions provided. If you purchased an eBook, please follow the instructions online through https://prolog.acog.org to purchase and access the assessment. **Paper answer sheets are NOT available for this edition.**

Conclusion

PROLOG was developed specifically as a personal study resource for the practicing obstetrician–gynecologist. It is presented as a self-assessment mechanism that, with its accompanying performance information, should assist the physician in designing a personal, self-directed learning program. The many quality resources developed by ACOG, as detailed each year in ACOG's *Publications and Educational Materials Catalog*, are available to help fulfill the educational interests and needs that have been identified. PROLOG is not intended as a substitute for the certification or recertification programs of the American Board of Obstetrics and Gynecology.

PROLOG CME Schedule	
Gynecologic Oncology and Critical Care, Eighth Edition	Credit through 2026
Patient Management in the Office, Eighth Edition	Credit through 2027
Obstetrics, Ninth Edition	Credit through 2027
Gynecology and Surgery, Ninth Edition	Credit through 2027
Reproductive Endocrinology and Infertility, Ninth Edition	Credit through 2027
Urogynecology and Reconstructive Pelvic Surgery, Second Edition	Credit through June 2028

PROLOG Objectives

PROLOG is a voluntary, strictly confidential, personal continuing education resource that is designed to be stimulating and enjoyable. By participating in PROLOG, obstetrician–gynecologists will be able to

- review and update clinical knowledge
- recognize areas of knowledge and practice in which they excel, be stimulated to explore other areas of the specialty, and identify areas requiring further study
- plan continuing education activities in light of identified strengths and deficiencies
- compare and relate present knowledge and skills with those of other participants
- obtain continuing medical education credit, if desired
- have complete personal control of the setting and of the pace of the experience

The obstetrician–gynecologist who completes *Obstetrics*, Ninth Edition, will be able to

- demonstrate an understanding of maternal and fetal physiology and pathophysiology and the effects on normal and complicated pregnancies
- identify components of antepartum care that optimize maternal and perinatal outcomes in uncomplicated pregnancies, including education regarding normal pregnancy
- diagnose and plan efficacious and cost-effective management of medical and obstetric conditions encountered during the antepartum period
- identify the risks and prognosis of selected complications of pregnancy and in the neonate
- describe antenatal genetic screening and diagnostic tests and identify the indications, risks, and predictive value for each
- diagnose problems and manage obstetric emergencies
- select appropriate management strategies for intrapartum care and delivery
- consider medical–legal principles, risk management, and office management guidelines in obstetric practice

Obstetrics, Ninth Edition, includes the following topics (item numbers appear in parentheses):

Counseling

Evaluation of fetal death (8)
Exercise in pregnancy (19)
Migraine (64)
Obesity in a pregnant patient (2)
Peripartum cardiomyopathy (43)
Preterm prelabor rupture of membranes (172–175)
Smoking cessation (36)
Timing of classical cesarean birth (10)

Epidemiology and Biostatistics

Anticoagulation for use postpartum and during breastfeeding (24)
Barriers to breastfeeding (4)
Electronic fetal monitoring (44)
Human immunodeficiency virus testing in a pregnant patient (13)
Neonatal encephalopathy (71)
Obstetric anesthesia (51)
Perinatal survival (70)
Teratogenic drugs (120–124)

Ethical and Legal Issues

Informed consent and shared decision making (197–200)
Maternal levels of care (157–161)
Neonatal levels of care (14)
Periviable birth (48)
Substance use disorder (21)
Vaginal birth after multiple cesarean births (40)

Medical Management

Anemia (73)
Antepartum fetal surveillance (91)
Anticoagulation (201–204)
Asthma medications (27)
Brachial plexus injury (47)
Breast cancer screening (45)
Breastfeeding challenges (106)
Cerebral palsy (86)
Cervical insufficiency (11)
Contraception in a breastfeeding patient (116–119)
Delayed cord clamping (15)
Enhanced recovery after surgery (68)
Evaluation for thyroid disorders in pregnancy (72)
Fetal death in a patient with a previous cesarean birth (74)
Fetal growth restriction (62)
Group B streptococci (139–143)
Hemolysis, elevated liver enzymes, and low platelet count syndrome (9)
High risk for open neural tube defects and recommendation of dosing (22)
Hypertension in pregnancy (38)
Hyperthyroidism (46)
Immunization in pregnancy (79)
Induction in a patient undergoing a trial of labor after cesarean birth (34)
Induction of labor (92)

Physiology

Prevention and Population Health

Screening and Diagnosis

Surgical Management

A complete subject matter index is included at the end of the Critique Book.

1 Ultrasound features of placenta accreta

A 36-year-old gravida 3, para 2, presents for the initiation of prenatal care in the third trimester. She has a history of a term cesarean birth followed by a term vaginal birth. She has no other surgical history and has no medical problems. On physical examination, she has a fundal height of 36 cm. She undergoes an obstetric ultrasonographic examination. The gestational age is estimated at 36 5/7 weeks of gestation by fetal biometry. She has an anterior placenta previa. Placental lacunae are identified along with loss of the retroplacental hypoechoic zone. The retroplacental myometrium is measured at 1 mm. Excessive color Doppler flow is present in the retroplacental space. The sonographic feature exhibited in this patient's examination that has the strongest association with a placenta accreta is the

(A) excessive color Doppler flow in the retroplacental space
(B) loss of the retroplacental hypoechoic zone
(C) placental lacunae
* (D) placenta previa
(E) thin retroplacental myometrium

The placenta accreta spectrum represents a range of abnormal placental attachment to the uterine myometrium during pregnancy. A *placenta accreta* is defined as the attachment of the chorionic villi beyond the decidua basalis and to the underlying myometrium. A *placenta increta* is represented by trophoblastic invasion into the myometrium, and a *placenta percreta* (Fig. 1-1) demonstrates invasion through the uterine serosa and potentially into surrounding organs, most commonly the bladder. The basic mechanism for the abnormal attachment or invasion of the trophoblasts is a failure of normal decidualization, usually due to uterine scarring.

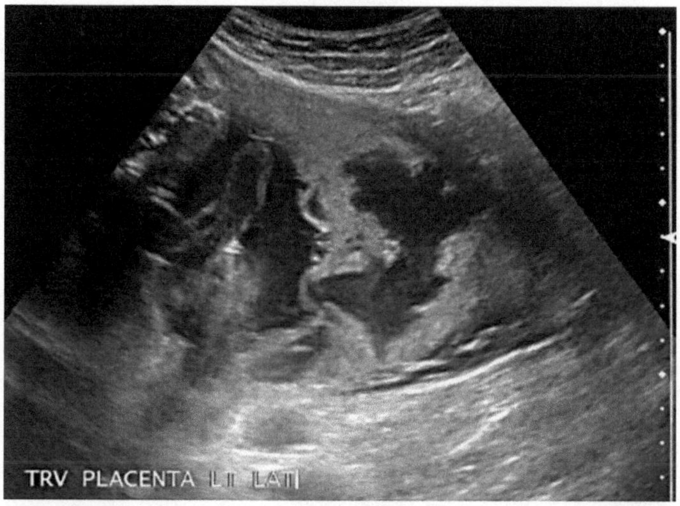

FIGURE 1-1. Transabdominal sonogram of placenta percreta shows multiple and massive placental "lakes" or "lacunae." (Reproduced with permission from Dr. Martha Rac in Cunningham FG. Placenta previa and morbidly adherent placenta. In: Yeomans ER, Hoffman BL, Gilstrap LC III, Cunningham FG, editors. Cunningham and Gilstrap's operative obstetrics. McGraw Hill; 2017. p. 435–53.)

Risk factors for placenta accreta spectrum include previous uterine surgery, advanced maternal age, multiparity, and a placenta previa. Cesarean birth is the most common uterine surgery and the most common risk factor for placenta accreta spectrum. The incidence of placenta accreta spectrum has increased steadily with the increasing rate of cesarean births. A 2016 study using national inpatient sample data noted 1 in 272 hospital discharges associated with delivery were complicated by placenta accreta spectrum. With one previous cesarean birth, the risk of placenta accreta spectrum in the next gestation is 0.3%. With five or more cesarean births, the risk increases to 6.74%. Placenta previa is an independent risk factor for placenta accreta spectrum with a 3% rate of accreta in affected pregnancies. The highest a priori risk of placenta accreta spectrum is in patients with a history of cesarean birth and a persistent placenta previa. There is an 11% risk of placenta accreta spectrum during the second cesarean birth if there is a current placenta previa, increasing to 40%, 61%, and 67% for the third, fourth, and fifth cesarean births, respectively.

The maternal morbidity and mortality linked with placenta accreta spectrum is associated with the risk of massive hemorrhage and the sequelae of these events. The fetal risks are mainly related to preterm birth. These risks can be mitigated with early recognition of placenta accreta spectrum during the antenatal period. The primary diagnostic tool for antenatal detection of placenta accreta spectrum is ultrasonography. Typically, obstetric practice includes obtaining a dating ultrasonography early in pregnancy and a fetal anatomic survey examination in the second trimester. Ultrasonographic findings associated with placenta accreta disorder can be noted as early as the first trimester. Those patients with the highest a priori risk of placenta accreta spectrum should be referred to centers with expertise in high-risk obstetrics and with experience in the detection and management of these disorders. Implantation of

*Indicates correct answer.
Note: See Appendix A for a table of normal values for laboratory tests.

the gestational sac within or near the previous uterine cesarean scar is associated with subsequent placenta accreta syndrome in many cases. One systematic review found that 82.4% of confirmed placenta accreta syndromes had demonstrated implantation in the lower uterine segment, within or near the previous scar in the first trimester.

Second- and third-trimester ultrasonographic findings associated with placenta accreta spectrum include a persistent placenta previa, vascular lacunae in the placenta, loss of the normal hypoechoic zone between the placenta and the myometrium, thinned retroplacental myometrium, an abnormal uterovesical interface, placental bulging or exophytic extension, and abnormalities of color Doppler flow. The ultrasound marker with the strongest association with placenta accreta disorder in a patient with a previous cesarean birth is a persistent placenta previa. Of placenta accreta spectrum cases, 80% are associated with a persistent placenta previa. Vascular lacunae are large, irregular echolucencies found in the placenta parenchyma, usually in large numbers when associated with placenta accreta spectrum. This finding has the greatest sensitivity of all two-dimensional grayscale sonographic markers besides a placenta previa. The absence of placental lacunae has a negative predictive value of 88–100% for placenta accreta spectrum. Loss of the normal hypoechoic zone between the placenta and myometrium represents an absence of the normal decidual layer. This finding has been associated with placenta accreta spectrum with a sensitivity reported as high as 84.3%. *Thinning of the retroplacental myometrium* commonly is defined as less than 1 mm. Undue pressure with the ultrasound transducer could falsely diagnose a thinned myometrium or exaggerate the measurement. Abnormalities at the uterovesical interface include bladder wall disruption and bridging vessels with hypervascularity on color Doppler flow. *Placental bulging* is defined as placental tissue distorting the normal uterine contour. The absence of a bulge has an 88% specificity for excluding placenta accreta spectrum. An exophytic mass of placental tissue outside the uterus is diagnostic for a placenta percreta. Other color Doppler flow findings associated with placenta accreta spectrum include turbulent lacunar blood flow, increased subplacental vascularity, gaps in myometrial blood flow, and bridging vessels from the placenta to the myometrium (Fig. 1-2).

The reported accuracy of ultrasonography in the detection of placenta accreta spectrum is biased by the patient selection in most studies. The patients with the highest a priori risk are being included in the studies, and they receive the most extensive ultrasonographic evaluations. With that in mind, one large systematic review from the United States included 23 studies and 3,707 patients with placenta accreta spectrum. This study found ultrasonography was 90.7% sensitive and 96.9% specific for placenta accreta spectrum. Most ultrasound markers mentioned also are commonly noted in patients without placenta accreta spectrum and without risks for it, and the absence of ultrasound markers does not preclude the existence of abnormal placentation; thus, clinical risk factors remain important considerations.

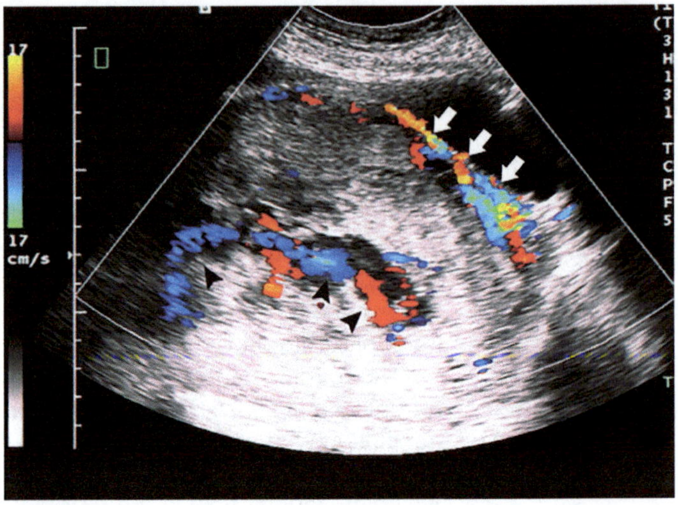

FIGURE 1-2. Transvaginal sonogram of placental invasion with a morbidly adherent placenta. (Reprinted from Cunningham FG, Leveno KJ, Bloom SL, Dashe JS, Hoffman BL, Casey BM, et al. Williams obstetrics. 25th ed. McGraw-Hill Education; 2018.)

Magnetic resonance imaging (MRI) is not recommended as the primary diagnostic imaging modality in patients at high risk of placenta accreta spectrum but can be considered in certain cases in which ultrasonography performs suboptimally. Overall, MRI is more expensive and at best has comparable sensitivity (94.4%) and specificity (84%) to obstetric ultrasonography for the placenta accreta spectrum. Studies investigating MRI detection of placenta accreta spectrum are again biased by patient selection, with only the highest a priori risk cases advancing to MRI evaluation. Examples of cohorts in which MRI may be an appropriate adjunct examination include patients with high body mass indices, those with posterior placentas, and those for whom depth of invasion needs to be assessed.

Early suspicion for placenta accreta spectrum can decrease maternal and fetal morbidity and mortality. These patients should receive obstetric care from centers with experience in the care of placenta accreta spectrum. Delivery is planned between 34 0/7 and 35 6/7 weeks of gestation, before the onset of labor. Corticosteroids should be administered before delivery, but assessment of fetal lung maturity is not necessary. Of patients with placenta accreta spectrum, 50% will experience hemorrhage and require emergency delivery if they proceed beyond 36 weeks of gestation. Delivery should occur at a Level 3 or 4 maternal care center. The cesarean birth should be attended by a multidisciplinary team with experience and expertise in the care of placenta accreta spectrum and complex pelvic surgery. Hemorrhage preparation should be meticulously planned before surgery. Cesarean hysterectomy, leaving the placenta in situ, should be the rule in cases of placenta accreta spectrum. Attempts at uterine preservation, whether with placental removal and defect repair or expectant management with placental retention, should be rare. Attempts at conservative and expectant management require extensive counseling, observation, and follow-up. The risks of expectant management with placenta accreta syndrome include hemorrhage and infection, both of which can be severe.

D'Antonio F, Iacovella C, Bhide A. Prenatal identification of invasive placentation using ultrasound: systematic review and meta-analysis. Ultrasound Obstet Gynecol 2013;42:509–17. doi: 10.1002/uog.13194 https://obgyn.onlinelibrary.wiley.com/doi/10.1002/uog.13194

Placenta accreta spectrum. Obstetric Care Consensus No. 7. American College of Obstetricians and Gynecologists. Obstet Gynecol 2018;132:e259–75. doi: 10.1097/AOG.0000000000002983 https://journals.lww.com/greenjournal/Fulltext/2018/12000/Obstetric_Care_Consensus_No__7__Placenta_Accreta.50.aspx

Shainker SA, Coleman B, Timor-Tritsch IE, Bhide A, Bromley B, Cahill AG, et al. Special Report of the Society for Maternal-Fetal Medicine Placenta Accreta Spectrum Ultrasound Marker Task Force: consensus on definition of markers and approach to the ultrasound examination in pregnancies at risk for placenta accreta spectrum. Society for Maternal-Fetal Medicine [published erratum appears in Am J Obstet Gynecol 2021;225:91]. Am J Obstet Gynecol 2021;224:B2–14. doi: 10.1016/j.ajog.2020.09.001 https://www.ajog.org/article/S0002-9378(20)31053-X/fulltext

2 Obesity in a pregnant patient

A 31-year-old gravida 3, para 1, is admitted in labor at 38 weeks of gestation. Her body mass index (BMI) is 51. Her obstetric history is notable for a previous cesarean birth, and she elects to undergo a trial of labor. During labor she is diagnosed with intra-amniotic infection. Two hours later, the fetal heart rate shows tachycardia with persistent late decelerations, and cesarean birth is performed. In addition to the use of pneumatic compression devices, the best pharmacologic management to reduce the risk of venous thromboembolism (VTE) in this patient is to initiate

(A) direct oral anticoagulant
* (B) low-molecular-weight heparin (LMWH)
(C) unfractionated subcutaneous heparin
(D) warfarin

The prevalence of obesity has increased during the past several decades. Based on the 2017–2018 National Health and Nutrition Examination Survey, the prevalence of obesity in women aged 20–39 years is 39.7%, with a significant proportion of women having class II (BMI 35 or greater) or class III (BMI 40 or greater) obesity. Patients with obesity are at increased risk of pregnancy complications during all stages of pregnancy. The intrapartum complications include cesarean birth, unsuccessful trial of labor, endometritis, wound complications (including dehiscence), and VTE.

Venous thromboembolism is a major cause of maternal morbidity and mortality, especially in the postpartum period, with a higher risk in the setting of obesity and cesarean birth. Professional organizations that have developed guidelines defining risk factors for VTE include the American College of Chest Surgeons, the Royal College of Obstetricians and Gynaecologists, and the National Partnership for Maternal Safety. Recommendations from these professional organizations conflict regarding the prophylaxis of VTE in the postpartum period. Much of the variation in these recommendations is related to the paucity of high-grade evidence, with reliance on observational data, rather than adequately powered clinical trials. Estimates of the risk of VTE vary widely between these professional organizations. Weighing the potential benefit of pharmacologic prophylaxis against the potential adverse outcomes associated with pharmacologic prophylaxis has led to conflicting recommendations.

Over the last several years, individual institutions have been encouraged to develop and incorporate safety bundles into institutional practice guidelines for VTE prophylaxis for women who undergo cesarean birth. Such guidelines should consider the basis for the recommendations from various professional organizations. Checklists are helpful in the implementation of these guidelines.

All women undergoing cesarean birth should have pneumatic compression devices placed preoperatively and continued until the patient is fully ambulatory. In very high-risk groups, pharmacologic prophylaxis for VTE should be considered in addition to mechanical prophylaxis. Factors that increase the risk of VTE and characterize patients as very high-risk include class III obesity, immobility, preeclampsia, fetal growth restriction, infection, and emergency cesarean birth.

Pharmacologic thromboprophylaxis with LMWH should be considered for very high-risk patients after cesarean birth and should be continued until the patient is fully ambulatory. Weight-based dosing is preferred to BMI-stratified dosing, because weight-based dosing is associated with higher levels of anti-factor Xa. Low-molecular-weight heparin can be continued for 10 days to 6 weeks in the setting of ongoing risk factors. In the described patient with several risk factors but without a prior VTE or acquired thrombophilia, LMWH is recommended for prophylaxis.

Low-molecular-weight heparin is preferred to unfractionated heparin as first-line pharmacologic agent for VTE prophylaxis because it has a longer half-life, more predictable anticoagulation effect, fewer bleeding risks, and a lower risk of heparin-induced thrombocytopenia.

Postpartum treatment with warfarin is an option in patients with a history of prior VTE or in patients with an inherited or acquired thrombophilia. In these patients, either LMWH or warfarin is a reasonable choice.

Direct oral anticoagulant use has become standard in the treatment of thromboembolism in nonpregnant patients. These agents inhibit thrombin or factor Xa, but they have not been studied during pregnancy and lactation, and they demonstrate transplacental transfer and are detected in breast milk. Currently, these agents are not recommended during pregnancy and the postpartum period, especially in lactating women.

Obesity in pregnancy. ACOG Practice Bulletin No. 230. American College of Obstetricians and Gynecologists. Obstet Gynecol 2021;137:e128–44. doi: 10.1097/AOG.0000000000004395 https://journals.lww.com/greenjournal/Fulltext/2021/06000/Obesity_in_Pregnancy__ACOG_Practice_Bulletin,.38.aspx

Society for Maternal–Fetal Medicine Consult Series #51: thromboembolism prophylaxis for cesarean delivery. Am J Obstet Gynecol 2020;223:B11–7. doi: 10.1016/j.ajog.2020.04.032 https://www.ajog.org/article/S0002-9378(20)30518-4/fulltext

Thromboembolism in pregnancy. ACOG Practice Bulletin No. 196. American College of Obstetricians and Gynecologists [published erratum appears in Obstet Gynecol 2018;132:1068]. Obstet Gynecol 2018;132:e1–e17. doi: 10.1097/AOG.0000000000002706 https://journals.lww.com/greenjournal/Fulltext/2018/07000/ACOG_Practice_Bulletin_No__196__Thromboembolism_in.54.aspx

3 Reverse cascade testing for syphilis

A 32-year-old multiparous patient at 14 weeks of gestation has a positive treponemal-specific chemiluminescent immunoassay test. She reports feeling well. Human immunodeficiency virus and other sexually transmitted infection screenings are negative. She reports a penicillin allergy as a child. The best next step in the management of the positive treponemal test is

(A) ceftriaxone
(B) penicillin desensitization
(C) penicillin skin testing
* (D) quantitative nontreponemal test
(E) repeat treponemal testing in 2 weeks

Before treatment is initiated, this patient needs a confirmatory test for syphilis.

All pregnant patients should be tested for syphilis as early as possible in their prenatal care. The Centers for Disease Control and Prevention (CDC), American Academy of Pediatrics, and the American College of Obstetricians and Gynecologists endorse screening at pregnancy registration, early in the third trimester, and again at delivery. Screening for syphilis infection in pregnant patients reduces the incidence of congenital syphilis and adverse pregnancy outcomes associated with maternal infection. The challenging component of syphilis screening is the risk of a false-positive result that requires further clinical evaluation and may provoke anxiety.

Syphilis is caused by the bacterial spirochete *Treponema pallidum*. The current screening test for syphilis relies on detection of antibodies to the infection rather than direct detection of the bacteria. Because of the high rate of false-positive results among antibody tests, screening for syphilis infection requires a two-step algorithm when a positive result is encountered. Two methods for syphilis screening are currently in use: 1) traditional algorithm and 2) reverse sequence algorithm (Fig. 3-1). Traditional screening involves an initial nontreponemal antibody test, such as a venereal disease research laboratory (VDRL) test or rapid plasma reagin (RPR) test, followed by a confirmatory treponemal antibody test, such as fluorescent treponemal antibody absorption or *T pallidum* particle agglutination (TPPA) test. The reverse sequence screening algorithm starts with an automated treponemal test, such as an enzyme-linked chemiluminescence test or multiplex flow immunoassay. If that test result is positive, a quantitative nontreponemal test (RPR or VDRL) will be administered, as in the described patient. If the test results of the reverse sequence algorithm are discordant, a second treponemal test (preferably using a different treponemal antibody, as in TPPA test) is performed.

The reverse sequence algorithm was developed because nontreponemal tests (RPR and VDRL) are cumbersome and difficult, requiring repetitive pipette motions as well as the expense of time and reagents. Biologic false-positive nontreponemal and treponemal tests are relatively common in pregnant women, further emphasizing the need for confirmatory testing with either a traditional or reverse sequence algorithm. A false-positive nontreponemal test result can be related to acute febrile illness or recent immunizations, and these abnormalities typically are transitory, lasting for less than 6 months.

Accuracy of the screening test does not necessarily change with repeated assessments, especially with the same test, as in the example above (enzyme-linked chemiluminescence test). The actual diagnosis of syphilis must be confirmed using an alternate testing modality, such as RPR or VDRL, as delineated in Figure 3-1.

Maternal infection with syphilis occurs through sexual transmission when the spirochete passes from an open lesion across intact mucous membranes or abraded skin into the new host. Syphilis infections are staged based on history and physical examination. A primary syphilis diagnosis includes finding a painless macular lesion producing the classic chancre. Primary syphilis can be unrecognized in women if the lesion is in the vagina or on the cervix.

Secondary syphilis is a disseminated process occurring around 6 weeks to 6 months after primary syphilis. Some patients will have a generalized macular papular rash involving the skin of the palms and soles of the feet as well as mucous membranes. Secondary syphilis also may be notable for generalized lymphadenopathy, fever, weight loss, and condylomata lata.

Latent syphilis by definition is asymptomatic and is divided into the early latent or late latent period. Women with latent syphilis can transmit the infection to their fetus and to sexual partners.

Tertiary syphilis is infrequently diagnosed. It includes clinical manifestations, such as formation of gummatous disease and cardiovascular disease, and generally manifests 5–20 years after the disease has become latent.

Maternal syphilis infection is associated with higher rates of adverse obstetric outcomes, including fetal growth restriction, preterm birth, stillbirth, and congenital syphilis. Mother-to-child transmission of syphilis can occur during all stages of maternal infection, with the highest risk in primary and secondary syphilis infections. Congenital syphilis symptoms include rash, hemorrhagic rhinitis, hepatosplenomegaly, skeletal anomalies, and meningitis.

When syphilis is diagnosed in pregnancy, a penicillin regimen is recommended according to the stage of infection. The CDC recommends intravenous benzathine penicillin G for the treatment of syphilis in all pregnant women, given limited data on the efficacy and or safety of alternative antibiotic regimens. *T pallidum* is a slow growing organism, and penicillin is active against the dividing microorganism. Prolonged and continuous doses are required for eradication, especially among tissues that sequester *T pallidum.* To date, no clinically relevant penicillin-resistant strains have been identified. Parenteral (intramuscular or intravenous) penicillin G is the only therapy with documented safety and efficacy for treatment of infection for the patient and the fetus during pregnancy. If the stage of

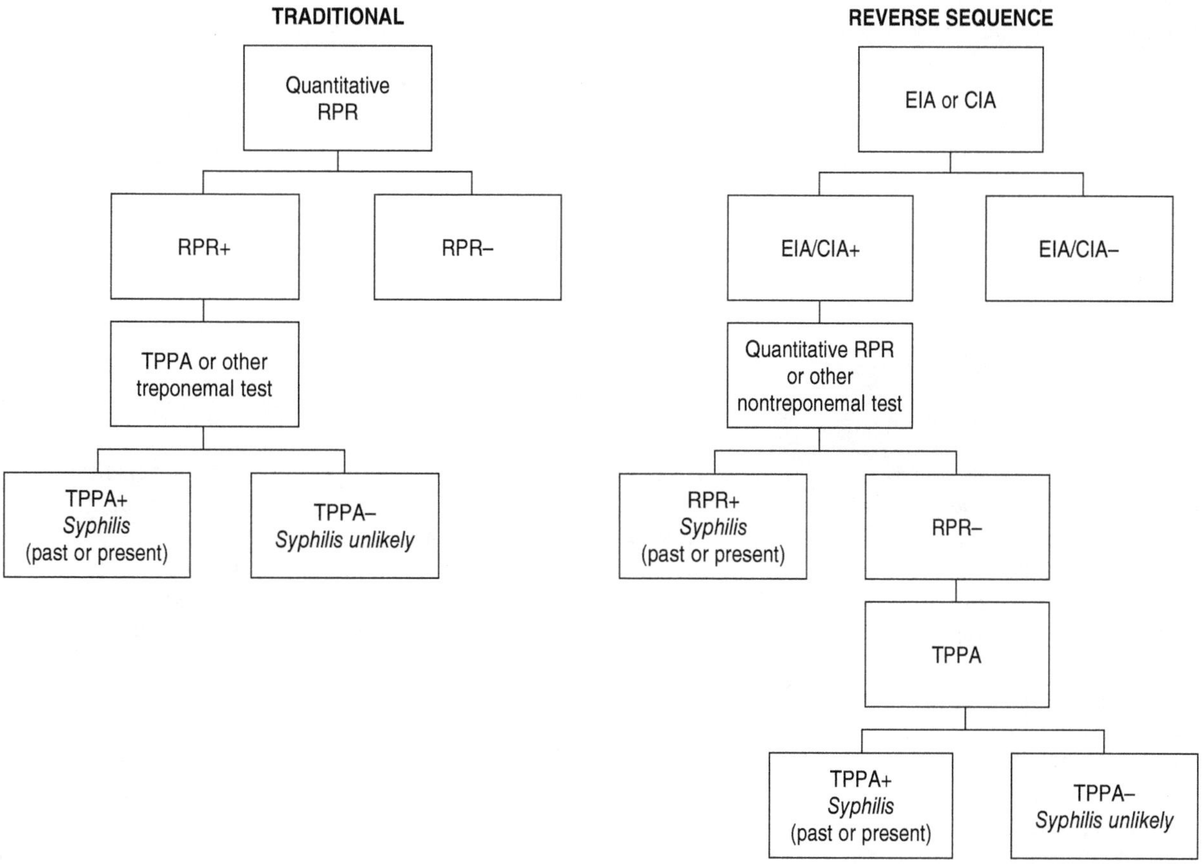

FIGURE 3-1. Syphilis serologic screening algorithms. Abbreviations: CIA/EIA, chemiluminescence and enzyme immunoassays; RPR, rapid plasma reagin; TPPA, *Treponema pallidum* particle agglutination. (Reprinted from Lin JS, Eder M, Bean S. Screening for syphilis infection in pregnant women: a reaffirmation evidence update for the U.S. Preventive Services Task Force. In: Evidence Synthesis, No. 167. Agency for Healthcare Research and Quality; 2018. Accessed April 21, 2022. https://www.ncbi.nlm.nih.gov/books/NBK525910/ *and* adapted from Centers for Disease Control and Prevention [CDC]. Discordant results from reverse sequence syphilis screening—five laboratories, United States, 2006–2010. Centers for Disease Control and Prevention. MMWR Morb Mortal Wkly Rep 2011;60:133–7. https://www.cdc.gov/mmwr/preview/mmwrhtml/mm6005a1.htm)

syphilis is unknown, the penicillin dosage should follow the late-latent or tertiary stage treatment, which is penicillin G benzathine intramuscularly once weekly for 3 weeks. Women who have sexual contacts with individuals known or suspected to have syphilis can be presumptively treated with a single dose of penicillin G benzathine intramuscularly.

Women who report a penicillin allergy should be evaluated and, if they have a severe penicillin allergy, desensitized and treated with penicillin. For penicillin-allergic individuals with unknown reactions, skin testing is a safe, rapid, and sensitive way to assess the reaction to penicillin. Skin testing uses a bioassay and involves pricking the skin and administering minor (benzylpenicilloate, benzylpenilloate, or benzylpenicilline) and major isomers (penicilloyl-polylysine) to evaluate for immunoglobulin E (IgE)-mediated response. The skin test alone identifies 90–99% of patients with IgE-mediated penicillin allergy. Following negative skin testing, a penicillin-allergic patient then takes an oral challenge with amoxicillin and is observed for 1 hour. With a negative skin test and a negative oral challenge, the risk of IgE-mediated anaphylaxis to penicillin approaches zero.

For pregnant women with confirmed immediate-type allergic reactions to penicillin, the only appropriate treatment for confirmed syphilis infection is desensitization followed by penicillin therapy. Penicillin desensitization usually requires admission to a critical care unit and collaborative care, specifically with allergy specialists. Desensitization yields temporary tolerance to penicillin and remains effective only as long as the patient is receiving the medication.

Treatment with alternate antibiotics, such as with amoxicillin or cephalosporins, has not been shown to effectively reduce the risk of congenital syphilis. Doxycycline and tetracycline, additional alternate agents, are contraindicated in pregnancy. Finally, erythromycin and azithromycin are not recommended to treat syphilis in pregnancy because they do not cross the placental barrier sufficiently to result in eradication of the spirochete in the fetus. In areas where desensitization is not possible, use of alternative agents such as erythromycin, azithromycin, or ceftriaxone may be considered for use with treatment of the newborn after delivery, per the World Health Organization.

Centers for Disease Control and Prevention. Managing persons who have a history of penicillin allergy. In: Sexually transmitted infections treatment guidelines, 2021. CDC; 2021. Accessed February 11, 2022. https://www.cdc.gov/std/treatment-guidelines/penicillin-allergy.htm

Curry SJ, Krist AH, Owens DK, Barry MJ, Caughey AB, Davidson KW, et al. Screening for syphilis infection in pregnant women: US Preventive Services Task Force Reaffirmation Recommendation Statement. US Preventive Services Task Force. JAMA 2018;320:911–7. doi: 10.1001/jama.2018.11785 https://jamanetwork.com/journals/jama/fullarticle/2698933

Lin JS, Eder M, Bean S. Screening for syphilis infection in pregnant women: a reaffirmation evidence update for the U.S. Preventive Services Task Force. In: Evidence Synthesis, No. 167. Agency for Healthcare Research and Quality; 2018. Accessed April 21, 2022. https://www.ncbi.nlm.nih.gov/books/NBK525910/

Macy E, Contreras R. Health care use and serious infection prevalence associated with penicillin "allergy" in hospitalized patients: a cohort study. J Allergy Clin Immunol 2014;133:790–6. doi: 10.1016/j.jaci.2013.09.021 https://www.jacionline.org/article/S0091-6749(13)01467-X/fulltext

4 Barriers to breastfeeding

A 30-year-old transgender woman is in the process of adopting a neonate and is interested in chestfeeding. She wants to start immediately after delivery. She has done her own research and is following a lactation induction program available on the internet. In addition to taking higher doses of estrogen and progesterone, she has started using a breast pump several times daily. She also has continued androgen suppression medication because she has not yet had an orchiectomy. The most appropriate U.S. Food and Drug Administration (FDA)-approved medication to recommend to this patient in support of her chestfeeding goal is

(A) cabergoline
(B) domperidone
(C) droperidol
* (D) metoclopramide
(E) spironolactone

Successful lactation induction can occur in the absence of pregnancy. It is sometimes experienced by partners in same-sex relationships or in families involving a gestational carrier or adoption. Inducing lactation in transgender individuals can be more challenging, but successful case reports have been published. With the growth of nontraditional families, obstetricians need to be aware of resources for lesbian, gay, bisexual, transgender, and queer patients who wish to breastfeed or chestfeed. *Chestfeeding* is a term used by transmasculine and nonbinary parents to describe feeding their infant from their body.

There is limited published information on inducing lactation, and there is no standard guidance for individuals who are interested in pursuing this option. However, resources are available to assist individuals who are interested in breastfeeding without experiencing a pregnancy (Box 4-1).

BOX 4-1

Breastfeeding Resources for Lesbian, Gay, Bisexual, Transgender, and Queer Individuals

Academy of Breastfeeding Medicine
https://www.bfmed.org/

Institute for the Advancement of Breastfeeding & Lactation Education
https://lacted.org/questions/0195-lgbtq-breastfeeding/

La Leche League International
https://www.llli.org/

United States Breastfeeding Committee
http://www.usbreastfeeding.org/page/lgbtqia

In general, lactation induction involves three components: 1) hormonal priming of the mammary tissue, 2) prolactin promotion, and 3) hormone withdrawal with expression. Hormonal priming involves increasing doses of estrogen and progesterone in an attempt to mimic the hormonal changes that occur during pregnancy. Estrogen and progesterone doses are gradually increased over at least a 3- to 6-month period with subsequent reductions in doses as delivery approaches. In transgender women, an androgen blocker, such as spironolactone, is continued during lactation induction if they have not had a bilateral orchiectomy.

Prolactin promotion is achieved by adding a galactogogue to the regimen. Galactogogues are medications or supplements that induce, maintain, or augment the milk supply. Metoclopramide and domperidone, dopamine antagonists that increase prolactin secretion, are the most commonly used pharmaceutical galactogogues. Data are inconclusive on their effectiveness, and no specific galactogogue is recommended by the Academy of Breastfeeding Medicine. Metoclopramide, a medication that is approved by the FDA, often is prescribed off-label to induce or augment lactation. Therefore, this is the correct answer in this scenario. Although evidence may be strongest for domperidone as a galactogogue, it is not approved for use by the FDA and is not available in the United States because of concerns that it may trigger fatal cardiac arrhythmias, cardiac arrest, and sudden death. Domperidone is available in Canada and other countries. Herbal galactogogues also are options.

The expression component involves increased hand expression and pumping as delivery approaches. It is important to remember that inducing lactation can be a difficult and time-consuming process.

Cabergoline is a dopamine agonist that inhibits prolactin secretion and, therefore, is not indicated in this scenario. It is prescribed to treat hyperprolactinemia. Droperidol may be a dopamine antagonist, but it is most commonly used as an antiemetic. Spironolactone, an androgen blocker, is frequently prescribed as a component of feminizing hormone therapy in addition to supplemental estrogen and progesterone. This patient already is taking androgen suppression therapy, which is likely spironolactone, because she has not yet undergone gender-affirming surgery. Orchiectomy, the surgical removal of one or both testicles, stops the production of testosterone and sperm, eliminating the need for long-term androgen suppression therapy.

Transgender men who become pregnant and deliver a baby may choose to chestfeed their babies. It may be more difficult if they have undergone chest reduction surgery, but it is still possible. Obstetricians should be aware that these individuals may decide not to lactate secondary to body dysphoria and the desire to resume testosterone treatment after pregnancy.

Barriers to breastfeeding: supporting initiation and continuation of breastfeeding. ACOG Committee Opinion No. 821. American College of Obstetrician and Gynecologists. Obstet Gynecol 2021;137:e54–62. doi: 10.1097/AOG.0000000000004249 https://journals.lww.com/greenjournal/Fulltext/2021/02000/Barriers_to_Breastfeeding__Supporting_Initiation.47.aspx

Breastfeeding challenges. ACOG Committee Opinion No. 820. American College of Obstetricians and Gynecologists. Obstet Gynecol 2021;137:e42–53. doi: 10.1097/AOG.0000000000004253 https://journals.lww.com/greenjournal/Fulltext/2021/02000/Breastfeeding_Challenges__ACOG_Committee_Opinion,.46.aspx

Brodribb W. ABM clinical protocol #9: use of galactogogues in initiating or augmenting maternal milk production, second revision 2018. Breastfeed Med 2018;13:307–14. doi: 10.1089/bfm.2018.29092.wjb https://www.liebertpub.com/doi/10.1089/bfm.2018.29092.wjb

Farrow A. Lactation support and the LGBTQI community. J Hum Lact 2015;31:26–8. doi: 10.1177/0890334414554928 https://journals.sagepub.com/doi/10.1177/0890334414554928

Ferri RL, Rosen-Carole CB, Jackson J, Carreno-Rijo E, Greenberg KB. ABM Clinical Protocol #33: lactation care for lesbian, gay, bisexual, transgender, queer, questioning, plus patients. Academy of Breastfeeding Medicine. Breastfeed Med 2020;15:284–93. doi: 10.1089/bfm.2020.29152.rlf https://www.liebertpub.com/doi/10.1089/bfm.2020.29152.rlf

García-Acosta JM, San Juan-Valdivia RM, Fernández-Martínez AD, Lorenzo-Rocha ND, Castro-Peraza ME. Trans* pregnancy and lactation: a literature review from a nursing perspective. Int J Environ Res Public Health 2019;17:44. doi: 10.3390/ijerph17010044. doi: 10.3390/ijerph17010044 https://www.mdpi.com/1660-4601/17/1/44

La Leche League International. Support for transgender and non-binary parents. LLLI; 2022. Accessed March 21, 2022. https://www.llli.org/breastfeeding-info/transgender-non-binary-parents/

Optimizing support for breastfeeding as part of obstetric practice. Committee Opinion No. 658. American College of Obstetricians and Gynecologists. Obstet Gynecol 2016;127:e86–92. doi: 10.1097/AOG.0000000000001318 https://journals.lww.com/greenjournal/Fulltext/2016/02000/Committee_Opinion_No__658__Optimizing_Support_for.57.aspx

Reisman T, Goldstein Z. Case report: induced lactation in a transgender woman. Transgend Health 2018;3:24–6. doi: 10.1089/trgh.2017.0044 https://www.liebertpub.com/doi/full/10.1089/trgh.2017.0044

Wamboldt R, Shuster S, Sidhu BS. Lactation induction in a transgender woman wanting to breastfeed: case report. J Clin Endocrinol Metab 2021;106:e2047–52. doi: 10.1210/clinem/dgaa976 https://academic.oup.com/jcem/article-abstract/106/5/e2047/6123860?redirectedFrom=fulltext&login=false

5 Vitamin D deficiency

A 32-year-old gravida 1 presents for her initial prenatal visit at 8 weeks of gestation. She is a vegan and has a body mass index of 36. She currently takes a vitamin B_{12} supplement and is concerned about other nutritional deficiencies. In addition to routine prenatal laboratory tests, the best additional test to screen for nutritional deficiencies is

(A) folate level
(B) iron level
* (C) 25-hydroxy vitamin D level
(D) zinc level

Obstetricians should consider screening for certain vitamin deficiencies in pregnant patients with various risk factors. Vegan patients are at risk of multiple vitamin deficiencies because of the exclusion of animal products from the diet. Low vitamin D is the most common nutrient deficiency among vegans, so screening for deficiency is appropriate in these patients.

Vitamin D is a fat-soluble vitamin obtained from consuming fortified milk, fish oils, fish, and dietary supplements. Vitamin D is also produced endogenously in the skin with exposure to sunlight. Vitamin D deficiency is one of the most common nutritional deficiencies affecting pregnant women and is associated with adverse outcomes in the neonate. It is important that pregnant patients with risk factors be screened.

Vitamin D deficiency is common during pregnancy, particularly in high-risk groups. Because vitamin D is found naturally in highest quantities in animal products such as shellfish and cod liver oil, and often found in fortified animal products such as milk, vegetarians and vegans are at particular risk of vitamin D deficiency. Women with limited sun exposure, including those who live in colder climates or in higher latitudes and those who work inside or wear protective clothing, are at risk. In addition, races and ethnicities with darker skin are more at risk of vitamin D deficiency due to decreased endogenous production from sunlight.

Severe vitamin D deficiency increases risks of disordered skeletal homeostasis leading to congenital rickets and fractures in the newborn. Vitamin D deficiency also increases risk of osteoporosis and osteopenia, can cause osteomalacia and muscle weakness, and can increase the risk of fracture in adults. Less severe vitamin D deficiency has been implicated in cases of preeclampsia, diabetes mellitus, and preterm birth, although the data are mixed, in part because of the highly heterogeneous nature of studies done on vitamin D. There are some studies that suggest decreased rates of preeclampsia when vitamin D deficiency is corrected, although this evidence is not sufficient to recommend vitamin D supplementation for the prevention of preeclampsia. Additionally, in the nonpregnant population, studies have shown that vitamin D supplementation may decrease the risk of cardiovascular disease, autoimmune disease, infectious diseases, and some forms of cancer.

It is recommended that pregnant women with risk factors be screened for vitamin D deficiency. There is not sufficient evidence to recommend screening all pregnant women at this time. The serum 25-hydroxy vitamin D concentration is the best indicator of nutritional vitamin D status. Although an optimal level in pregnancy has not been determined, most experts suggest that circulating 25-hydroxy vitamin D of less than 32 ng/mL be treated. When vitamin D deficiency is identified, vitamin D daily is safe for supplementing pregnant women. High-dose regimens typically used in the nonpregnant person have not been studied extensively in pregnancy, but doses of up to 2,000–4,000 international units daily are commonly used. Reaching adequate levels of vitamin D for vegans may be difficult because few plant foods are fortified with this vitamin. For this reason, supplementation seems to be the most effective way to replenish vitamin D in vegan patients.

In addition to vitamin D deficiency, vegan pregnant patients also are at risk of deficiencies in vitamin B_{12}, omega-3 fatty acids, zinc, and iron because of dietary exclusion of animal products. These can be supplemented by eating plant foods fortified with B_{12}, chia seeds or walnuts for omega-3 fatty acids, grains and beans for zinc, and leafy green vegetables for iron. Additionally, vegetarian and vegan pregnant patients should strive for good protein intake, increasing by up to 25 g of protein per day and aiming to reach 1.1 g/kg per day. Vegan pregnant patients also should consume one to two servings of dark green vegetables, three to four servings of bean and soy products, at least six servings of whole grains, and four to five servings of other vegetables and fruits in addition to nuts, seeds, and wheat germ daily.

Regarding the vegan patient in this scenario, there is no recommendation to screen for zinc, folate, or iron deficiency. All pregnant women should be screened for anemia with a complete blood count in the first trimester and again at 24–28 weeks of gestation. If they are anemic, iron deficiency should be evaluated. If the patient has microcytic anemia, iron deficiency should be evaluated. If they have macrocytic anemia, screening for folate deficiency may be appropriate. For the patient in question, screening for vitamin D deficiency because of her vegan diet is the best answer.

Anemia in pregnancy. ACOG Practice Bulletin No. 233. American College of Obstetricians and Gynecologists. Obstet Gynecol 2021;138:e55–64. doi: 10.1097/AOG.0000000000004477 https://journals.lww.com/greenjournal/Fulltext/2021/08000/Anemia_in_Pregnancy__ACOG_Practice_Bulletin,.34.aspx

De-Regil LM, Palacios C, Lombardo LK, Peña-Rosas JP. Vitamin D supplementation for women during pregnancy. Cochrane Database of Systematic Reviews 2016, Issue 1. Art. No.: CD008873. doi: 10.1002/14651858.CD008873.pub3 https://www.cochranelibrary.com/cdsr/doi/10.1002/14651858.CD008873.pub3/full

Pilz S, Zittermann A, Obeid R, Hahn A, Pludowski P, Trummer C, et al. The role of vitamin D in fertility and during pregnancy and lactation: a review of clinical data. Int J Environ Res Public Health 2018;15:2241. doi: 10.3390/ijerph15102241 https://www.mdpi.com/1660-4601/15/10/2241

Sebastiani G, Herranz Barbero A, Borrás-Novell C, Alsina Casanova M, Aldecoa-Bilbao V, Andreu-Fernández V, et al. The effects of vegetarian and vegan diet during pregnancy on the health of mothers and offspring. Nutrients 2019;11:557. doi: 10.3390/nu11030557. doi: 10.3390/nu11030557 https://www.mdpi.com/2072-6643/11/3/557

Vitamin D: screening and supplementation during pregnancy. ACOG Committee Opinion No. 495. American College of Obstetricians and Gynecologists. Obstet Gynecol 2011;118:197–8. doi: 10.1097/AOG.0b013e318227f06b https://journals.lww.com/greenjournal/Citation/2011/07000/Committee_Opinion_No__495__Vitamin_D__Screening.32.aspx

6 Prophylaxis for a pregnant patient with potential exposure to human immunodeficiency virus

A 29-year-old transgender patient at 12 weeks of gestation presents for a scheduled obstetric visit. The patient's partner recently tested positive for human immunodeficiency virus (HIV) and has started antiretroviral therapy. Previously, the couple was not using condoms but started to use them after this test result. The patient's routine prenatal screening included a negative HIV screening test 2 weeks ago. In addition to repeat HIV testing, the best next step to reduce this patient's risk of contracting HIV is to initiate

(A) dolutegravir
(B) enfuvirtide
(C) fostemsavir
(D) lamivudine and abacavir
* (E) tenofovir and emtricitabine

Identification of HIV in pregnancy is important for the pregnant person and the fetus. After exposure, conversion to HIV positivity can occur within 2–4 weeks or up to 6 months later. There is a higher rate of vertical transmission if the initial exposure occurs during pregnancy or lactation compared with transmission rates in individuals currently being treated for HIV who become pregnant.

The combination of two nucleoside (and nucleotide) reverse transcriptase inhibitors plus a third agent is the mainstay of HIV treatment. Strategies to reduce perinatal transmission and improve health include identification of acute infection through opt-out screening in the first and third trimesters, additional screening in at-risk individuals, preexposure prophylaxis (PrEP) for at-risk pregnant patients, and treatment of HIV-positive pregnant patients.

The opt-out screening for every pregnant person identifies HIV-positive individuals. Preexposure prophylaxis is indicated for persons who are HIV negative and at high risk of exposure. Shared decision making can be used by reproductive-aged individuals at risk of HIV—those who would benefit most from PrEP in pregnancy (Fig. 6-1). The described patient potentially has had multiple exposures already and likely will continue to be exposed during pregnancy; therefore, PrEP should be initiated as soon as possible with tenofovir disoproxil fumarate plus emtricitabine once daily. In the United States, for persons assigned female sex at birth, the number of individuals with PrEP indications in 2019 was 227,010 with only 20,856 (9.2%) of them being prescribed PrEP.

Preexposure prophylaxis is recommended over postexposure prophylaxis (PEP) when a person will have multiple high-risk exposures. The use of PrEP has been shown to be safe in the prevention of HIV in nonpregnant people whose partners are HIV positive. PrEP also has been used in pregnancy in at-risk individuals. For transfeminine persons taking gender-affirming hormones (exogenous estrogen and androgen blockers), hormone-induced changes to drug metabolism can reduce the available amount of tenofovir and its metabolites by approximately 30%, reducing protection from PrEP.

The Antiretroviral Pregnancy Registry is a voluntary, confidential registry that enrolls approximately 25% of individuals with HIV delivering newborns annually in the United States. The registry has enough registrants to detect a twofold increase in birth defects from all of the antiretroviral therapies, and thus far an increase has not been identified. Prenatal exposure to tenofovir has been associated with decreased bone mineral content in infants and a decrease of 0.5 cm in infant height and head circumference at 1 year. In breast milk, tenofovir was not detected in 94% of infant serum samples in a cohort of HIV-negative breastfeeding individuals taking tenofovir and emtricitabine.

Before starting PrEP, baseline testing should be completed. This testing includes combined HIV antibody and antigen

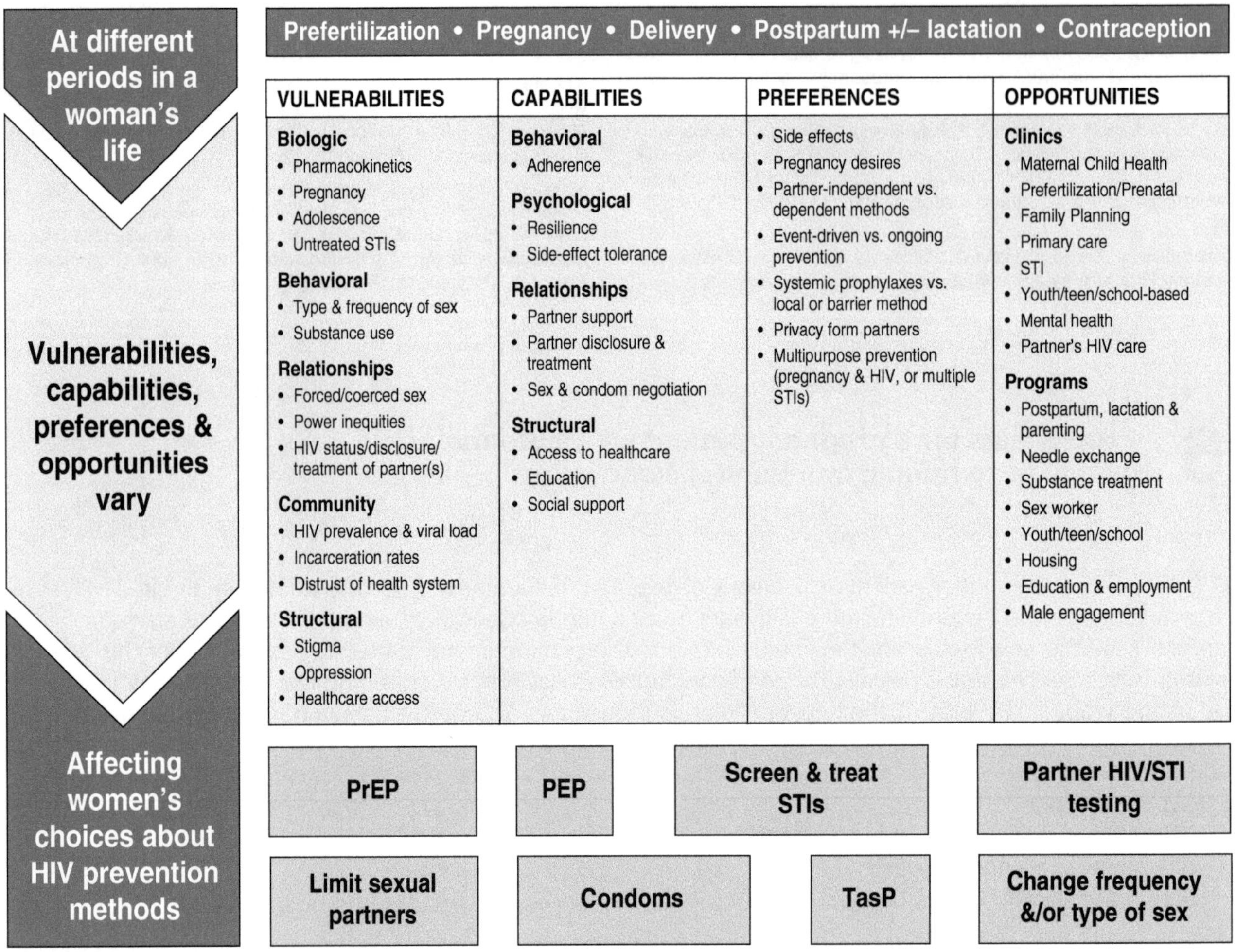

FIGURE 6-1. Applying shared decision making to HIV prevention strategies for reproductive-aged women. A woman's vulnerabilities to HIV, capabilities, preferences and opportunities vary over time and may change before pregnancy, during pregnancy and postpartum. Shared decision making can be used during each of these periods to elicit a woman's vulnerabilities, capabilities and preferences, facilitating a women's choice of HIV prevention method(s) that best meet her current needs. Clinics and programmes provide opportunities to use shared decision making to offer HIV prevention and support a women's chosen method. Abbreviations: PEP, postexposure prophylaxis; PrEP, preexposure prophylaxis; STIs, sexually transmitted infections; TasP, treatment as prevention of a partner living with HIV. (Reprinted from Seidman DL, Weber S, Cohan D. Offering pre-exposure prophylaxis for HIV prevention to pregnant and postpartum women: a clinical approach. J Int AIDS Soc 2017;20:21295. doi: 10.7448/IAS.20.2.21295 https://onlinelibrary.wiley.com/doi/full/10.7448/IAS.20.2.21295)

testing, serum creatinine, hepatitis B surface antigen, hepatitis C immunoglobulin G (IgG) antibody, hepatitis A IgG (for men who have sex with men or those using intravenous drugs), and genital and nongenital chlamydia and gonorrhea screening by nucleic acid amplification. The combined HIV antibody and antigen test is recommended 1 month into treatment and every 3 months thereafter. Additionally, every 3 months, a creatinine clearance and gonorrhea, chlamydia, and syphilis testing are recommended. Hepatitis C IgG antibody is recommended annually (more often in cases of intravenous drug use or men having sex with men). Individuals taking PrEP are seen every 90 days to support this screening and to refill medications. Assessment of risk factors and risk reduction counseling are recommended at every visit. If PrEP is discontinued for 7 days for any reason, retesting combined HIV antibody and antigen is recommended before restarting PrEP. Nonadherence to PrEP can result in seroconversion to a wild type of HIV. If this happens, then a regimen with a base of dolutegravir, bictegravir, or darunavir, boosted with ritonavir or cobicistat, is added to the tenofovir and emtricitabine. The next step is completing resistance testing to determine the ideal drug combination.

When comparing PrEP-exposed pregnancies with unexposed pregnancies, no difference was found in preterm live births, pregnancy loss, or congenital anomalies. Daily tenofovir and emtricitabine significantly reduced the rate of new infection by up to 75%. Despite the benefit of PrEP, the cost of the medication, adverse effects, change in relationship status, lack of or inadequate health insurance coverage, and lack of or limited access to health care contribute to a significant discontinuation rate. Postexposure prophylaxis is indicated to prevent acute HIV infection in a seronegative individual after a single high-risk exposure. The described patient will have continued exposure to HIV and PEP is not indicated. Fostemsavir is an attachment inhibitor and enfuvirtide is a fusion inhibitor. Both drugs are used in patients with multidrug-resistant HIV. The patient in this scenario is treatment-naive, and the use of agents for multidrug-resistant disease is not appropriate.

Centers for Disease Control and Prevention. Core indicators for monitoring the Ending the HIV Epidemic initiative (preliminary data): National HIV Surveillance System data reported through September 2021; and preexposure prophylaxis (PrEP) data reported through June 2021. HIV Surveillance Data Tables 2021;2(5). Accessed February 4, 2022. https://www.cdc.gov/hiv/library/reports/surveillance-data-tables/vol-2-no-5/index.html

Heffron R, Mugo N, Hong T, Celum C, Marzinke MA, Ngure K, et al. Pregnancy outcomes and infant growth among babies with in-utero exposure to tenofovir-based preexposure prophylaxis for HIV prevention. Partners Demonstration Project and the Partners PrEP Study Teams. AIDS 2018;32:1707–13. doi: 10.1097/QAD.0000000000001867 https://journals.lww.com/aidsonline/Fulltext/2018/07310/Pregnancy_outcomes_and_infant_growth_among_babies.17.aspx

Preexposure prophylaxis for the prevention of human immunodeficiency virus. Committee Opinion No. 595. American College of Obstetricians and Gynecologists. Obstet Gynecol 2014;123:1133–6. doi: 10.1097/01.AOG.0000446855.78026.21 https://journals.lww.com/greenjournal/Fulltext/2014/05000/Committee_Opinion_No_595__Preexposure_Prophylaxis.41.aspx

Saag MS, Gandhi RT, Hoy JF, Landovitz RJ, Thompson MA, Sax PE, et al. Antiretroviral drugs for treatment and prevention of HIV infection in adults: 2020 recommendations of the International Antiviral Society-USA Panel. JAMA 2020;324:1651–69. doi: 10.1001/jama.2020.17025 https://jamanetwork.com/journals/jama/fullarticle/2771873

7 Ultrasonography to estimate due date

A 15-year-old presents for an initial prenatal visit at 16 weeks of gestation, measured by her last menstrual period. She has a copy of her report from her ultrasonography performed 1 week ago demonstrating a crown-rump length of 87 mm. On examination today, her fundal height measures 22 cm and ultrasound biometry is consistent with 18 2/7 weeks of gestation. For the described patient, the most appropriate measurement to establish gestational age is

(A) average of both ultrasound measurements
(B) crown-rump length performed last week
(C) fundal height measurement
(D) last menstrual period
* (E) ultrasound biometry performed today

An accurately assigned estimated due date (EDD) is important for the individual patient as well as for research aimed at improving pregnancy outcomes. The EDD should be determined, discussed with the patient, and documented clearly in the patient's medical record. Accuracy of the EDD decreases with advancing gestational age, and an EDD assigned after 22 weeks of gestation is considered suboptimal.

Estimated due date is conventionally assigned by adding 280 days to the first day of the last menstrual period. However, this method of dating is accurate only when a patient has a regular, 28-day menstrual cycle and ovulates on the 14th day of that cycle. It does not account for irregularities in cycle length and timing of ovulation. Studies demonstrate that approximately one half of women accurately recall their last menstrual period. In a randomized controlled trial, 41.3% of women randomized to first-trimester ultrasonography for dating had their due dates changed based on that examination.

In the first trimester (through 13 6/7 weeks of gestation), ultrasound measurement of crown–rump length is the most accurate method to confirm or establish EDD. When the crown–rump length is greater than 84 mm (which corresponds to 14 0/7 weeks of gestation), crown–rump length becomes less accurate and second-trimester biometric measurements should be used for dating. In the first trimester, when the patient is at less than 14 0/7 weeks of gestation and the crown–rump length is less than 84 mm, the EDD should be changed to correspond to the ultrasound findings if the ultrasound dating differs by more than 7 days from last menstrual period dating. The American College of Obstetricians and Gynecologists refines this guideline further as shown in Table 7-1.

After 14 0/7 weeks of gestation, biometric measurements of the biparietal diameter, head circumference, abdominal circumference, and femur length should be combined using regression formulas to generate gestational age. As gestational age advances, ultrasound measurements become less accurate because of expected individual variation in growth, and a wider range of discrepancy is needed to justify reassigning gestational age of the pregnancy (Table 7-1). Assessment of gestational age by ultrasonography after 28 weeks of gestation is the least reliable method. In the third trimester, there is a risk that rather than dates being incorrect, a small fetus may be growth restricted or a large fetus may have macrosomia. For this reason, management decisions should be made based on consideration of the entire clinical picture and interval growth.

In the described patient, there are several pieces of information on which to base EDD. These are last menstrual period, which indicates a gestational age of 16 weeks of gestation, crown–rump length of 87 mm, fundal height of 22 cm, and

TABLE 7-1. Guidelines for Redating Based on Ultrasonography

GESTATIONAL AGE RANGE*	METHOD OF MEASUREMENT	DISCREPANCY BETWEEN ULTRASOUND DATING AND LMP DATING THAT SUPPORTS REDATING
13 6/7 or less wk	CRL	
8 6/7 or less wk		More than 5 d
9 0/7 to 13 6/7 wk		More than 7 d
14 0/7 to 15 6/7 wk	BPD, HC, AC, FL	More than 7 d
16 0/7 to 21 6/7 wk	BPD, HC, AC, FL	More than 10 d
22 0/7 to 27 6/7 wk	BPD, HC, AC, FL	More than 14 d
28 0/7 wk and beyond†	BPD, HC, AC, FL	More than 21 d

Abbreviations: AC, abdominal circumference; BPD, biparietal diameter; CRL, crown–rump length; FL, femur length; HC, head circumference; LMP, last menstrual period.

*Based on LMP.

†Because of the risk of redating a small fetus that may be growth restricted, management decisions based on third-trimester ultrasonography alone are especially problematic and need to be guided by careful consideration of the entire clinical picture and close surveillance.

Reprinted from Methods for estimating the due date. Committee Opinion No. 700. American College of Obstetricians and Gynecologists. Obstet Gynecol 2017;129:e150–4. doi: 10.1097/AOG.0000000000002046 https://journals.lww.com/greenjournal/pages/articleviewer.aspx?year=2017&issue=05000&article=00050&type=Fulltext

complete biometry of 18 2/7 weeks of gestation. Because the crown–rump length measurement is greater than 84 mm and would correspond to greater than 14 weeks of gestation, it is less accurate. Because there is a discrepancy of 16 days (greater than 10 days) from the patient's last menstrual period dating, complete biometry of 18 2/7 weeks is the most accurate for assigning EDD.

Kaelin Agten A, Xia J, Servante JA, Thornton JG, Jones NW. Routine ultrasound for fetal assessment before 24 weeks' gestation. Cochrane Database of Systematic Reviews 2021, Issue 8. Art. No.: CD014698. doi: 10.1002/14651858.CD014698 https://www.cochranelibrary.com/cdsr/doi/10.1002/14651858.CD014698/full

Methods for estimating the due date. Committee Opinion No. 700. American College of Obstetricians and Gynecologists. Obstet Gynecol 2017;129:e150–4. doi: 10.1097/AOG.0000000000002046. https://journals.lww.com/greenjournal/pages/articleviewer.aspx?year=2017&issue=05000&article=00050&type=Fulltext

8 Evaluation of fetal death

A 30-year-old gravida 1, para 0, at 30 weeks of gestation presents to the labor and delivery unit with a fetal death. She has no significant medical, surgical, or social history. She undergoes an uncomplicated induction of labor and vaginal delivery. The fetal weight is in the 1st percentile for gestational age, and gross physical examination of the fetus is unremarkable. The patient requests an autopsy evaluation. A cytogenetic specimen of placenta is sent for chromosomal microarray analysis, and the remaining placenta is sent for pathologic examination. In addition to this placental evaluation, the next most appropriate test to determine the cause of the fetal death is

* (A) antiphospholipid antibodies
(B) factor V Leiden
(C) hemoglobin A_{1c}
(D) parvovirus immunoglobulin G (IgG) or M (IgM)
(E) toxicology screen

Antiphospholipid syndrome (APS) testing is recommended in the evaluation of most stillbirth cases (Fig. 8-1). Antiphospholipid antibody testing has the highest yield in cases of stillbirth involving fetal growth restriction, preeclampsia, or placental insufficiency. In a large, secondary analysis of 512 stillbirths enrolled in the Stillbirth Collaborative Research Network, antiphospholipid antibody testing was found to be useful in determining potential causes of stillbirth in 11% of cases. Other useful tests include autopsy, genetic evaluation, and placental pathology (Fig. 8-2). Antiphospholipid antibody testing is recommended in this scenario because the fetus is growth restricted.

Antiphospholipid antibodies include anticardiolipin, β_2-glycoprotein, and lupus anticoagulant. Criteria for test positivity include anticardiolipin IgG/IgM in moderate to high titer (greater than 40 or greater than the 99th percentile), β_2-glycoprotein IgG or IgM in moderate to high titer (greater than the 99th percentile), or positive lupus anticoagulant (ideally performed while a patient is not being treated with anticoagulants). A positive test must be confirmed with repeat testing at least 12 weeks later. Persistence of test positivity is confirmatory.

Antiphospholipid syndrome is diagnosed by evidence of one positive clinical criterion and one positive laboratory criterion. Clinical criteria include vascular thromboses or pregnancy morbidity, with one or more unexplained fetal deaths occurring after 10 weeks of gestation, one or more preterm births occurring before 34 weeks of gestation due to preeclampsia or placental insufficiency or both, or three or more unexplained consecutive spontaneous pregnancy losses before 10 weeks of gestation.

Factor V Leiden is the most common heritable thrombophilia and is inherited in an autosomal dominant fashion. Factor V Leiden increases the risk of venous thromboembolism in pregnancy and is associated with more than 40% of these cases. Inherited thrombophilias have not been shown to be associated with stillbirth, and, therefore, screening for inherited thrombophilias in the evaluation of stillbirth is not recommended.

Diabetes mellitus is associated with an increased risk of stillbirth with an estimated rate of 6–10 stillbirths per 1,000 total births (live and stillbirths). Well-controlled diabetes reduces but does not eliminate the risk of stillbirth. Many women already will have been screened during pregnancy. Testing for diabetes might be considered in selected situations, such as for an infant who is large for gestational age or for maternal history of poorly controlled diabetes.

Infections are associated with approximately 10–20% of stillbirths. Viral infections account for the highest risk. Viruses

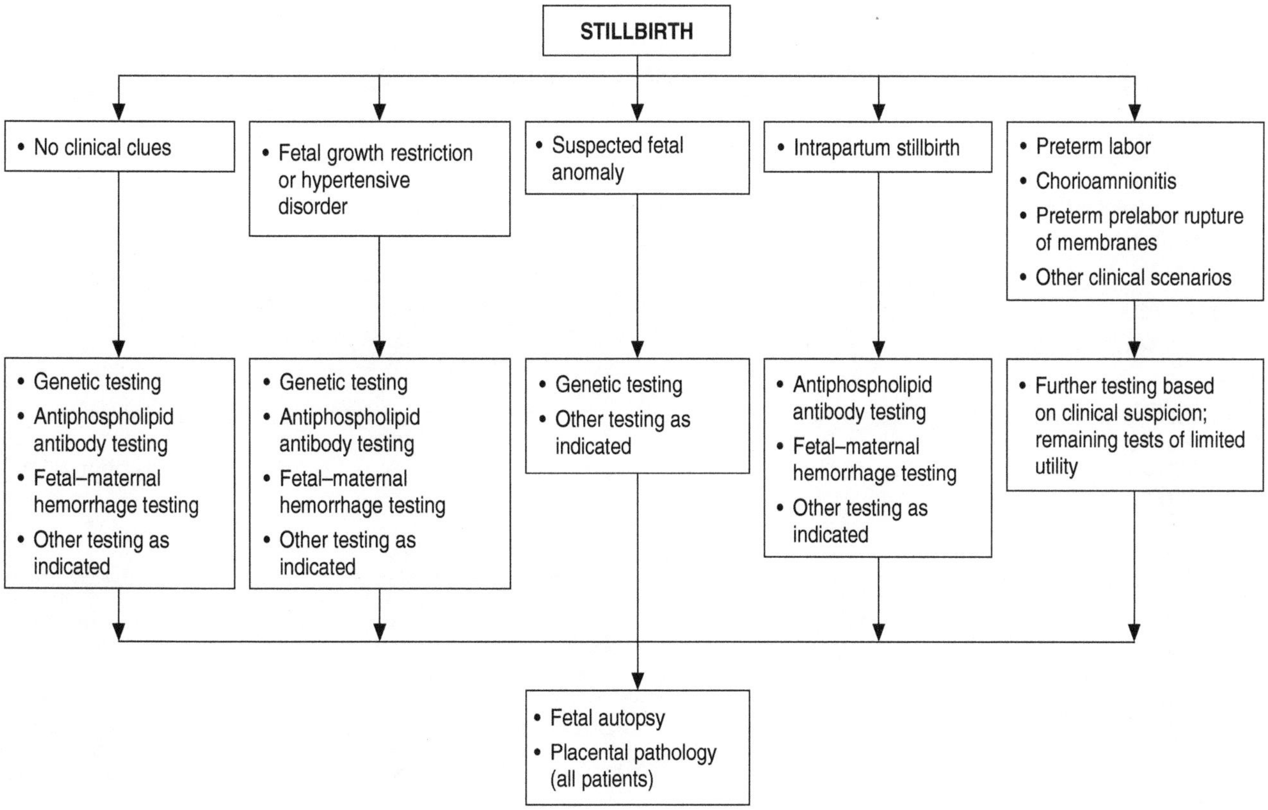

FIGURE 8-1. Evaluation of stillbirth based on test utility in a variety of clinical scenarios. (Adapted from Page JM, Christiansen-Lindquist L, Thorsten V, Parker CB, Reddy UM, Dudley DJ, et al. Diagnostic tests for evaluation of stillbirth: results from the stillbirth collaborative research network. Obstet Gynecol 2017;129:699–706. doi: 10.1097/AOG.0000000000001937. https://journals.lww.com/greenjournal/Fulltext/2017/04000/Diagnostic_Tests_for_Evaluation_of_Stillbirth_.16.aspx)

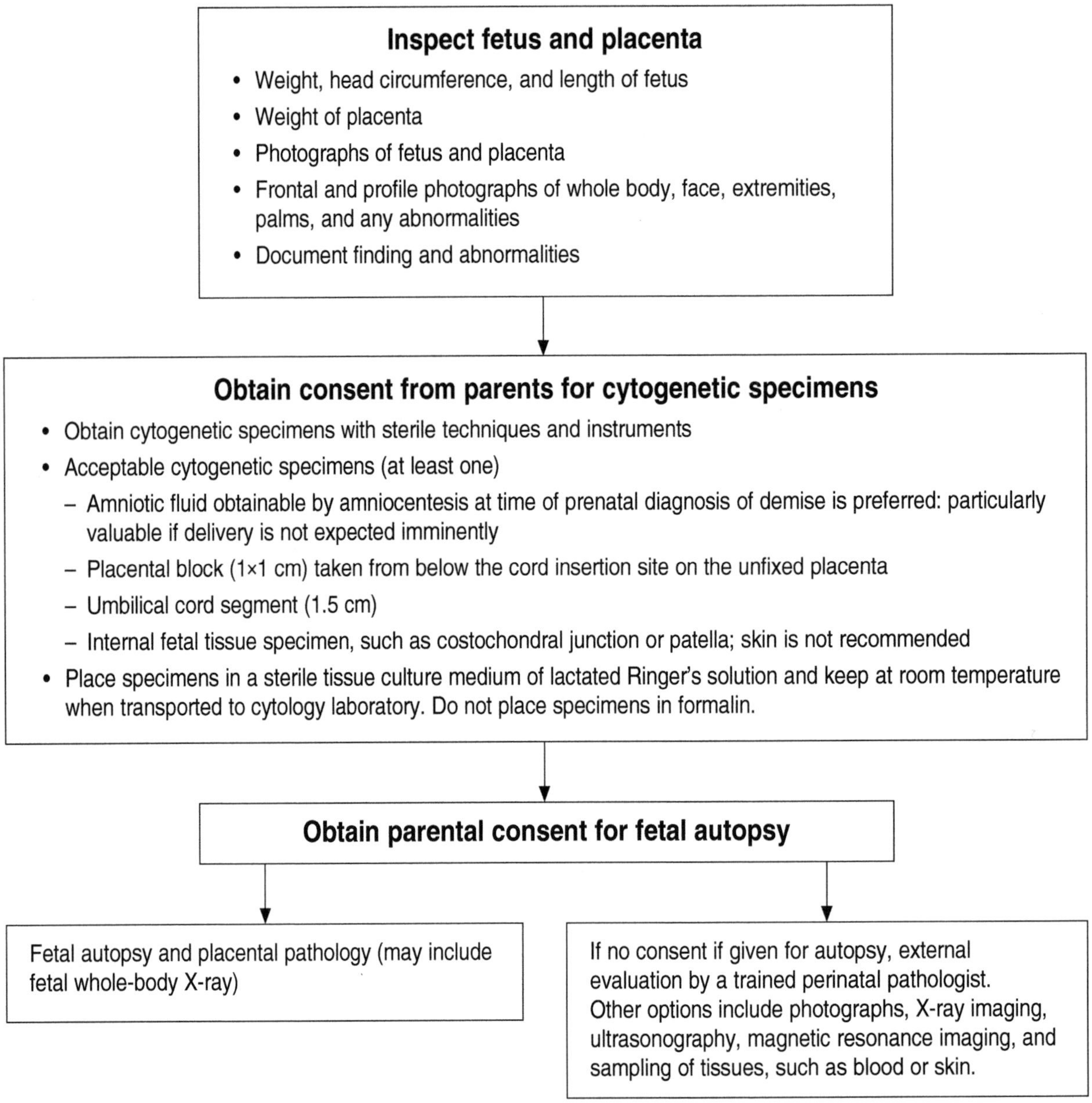

FIGURE 8-2. Fetal and placental evaluation. (Reprinted from Management of stillbirth. ACOG Obstetric Care Consensus No. 10. American College of Obstetricians and Gynecologists. Obstet Gynecol 2020;135:e110–32. doi: 10.1097/AOG.0000000000003719. https://journals.lww.com/greenjournal/Fulltext/2020/03000/Management_of_Stillbirth__Obstetric_Care_Consensus.49.aspx)

associated with an increased risk of stillbirth include cytomegalovirus, parvovirus, and Zika virus. In the aforementioned Stillbirth Collaboration Research Network study, parvovirus testing was found to be useful in 0.4% of cases. Although parvovirus testing might be considered in selected cases such as fetal hydrops, it would not be the most appropriate next test in this case.

Toxicology screening may be considered in selected cases of fetal death but would not be the highest yield test in this case. A toxicology screen may be useful in cases of unexplained placental abruption or concern for maternal illicit substance use.

Management of stillbirth. ACOG Obstetric Care Consensus No. 10. American College of Obstetricians and Gynecologists. Obstet Gynecol 2020;135:e110–32. doi: 10.1097/AOG.0000000000003719. https://journals.lww.com/greenjournal/Fulltext/2020/03000/Management_of_Stillbirth__Obstetric_Care_Consensus.49.aspx

Page JM, Christiansen-Lindquist L, Thorsten V, Parker CB, Reddy UM, Dudley DJ, et al. Diagnostic tests for evaluation of stillbirth: results from the stillbirth collaborative research network. Obstet Gynecol 2017;129:699–706. doi: 10.1097/AOG.0000000000001937. https://journals.lww.com/greenjournal/Fulltext/2017/04000/Diagnostic_Tests_for_Evaluation_of_Stillbirth_.16.aspx

Silver RM, Parker CB, Reddy UM, Goldenberg R, Coustan D, Dudley DJ, et al. Antiphospholipid antibodies in stillbirth. Obstet Gynecol 2013;122:641–57. doi: 10.1097/AOG.0b013e3182a1060e. https://journals.lww.com/greenjournal/Fulltext/2013/09000/Antiphospholipid_Antibodies_in_Stillbirth.22.aspx

9 Hemolysis, elevated liver enzymes, and low platelet count syndrome

A 17-year-old gravida 1, para 0, at 31 weeks of gestation was admitted to the hospital with fatigue, vomiting, and right upper quadrant pain. Her blood pressure on admission was 148/96 mm Hg, and a urine dipstick was negative for protein. Laboratory evaluation revealed the following: alanine aminotransferase, 1,038 units/L; aspartate aminotransferase, 966 units/L; creatinine, 0.6 mg/dL; platelet count, 72,000/mm^3; hemoglobin, 12.2 g/dL; hematocrit, 36%; and lactate dehydrogenase, 854 units/L. Delivery was recommended, and the patient underwent cesarean birth due to a breech presentation, with a quantitative blood loss of 1,200 mL. On the first postoperative day the patient reports minimal bleeding. Her vital signs are within normal limits, her abdomen is soft and nondistended, and the incision is dry and intact. Postoperative hemoglobin is 8.2 g/dL, and platelets are 44,000/mm^3. The best next step in the management of her postoperative laboratory findings is

(A) dexamethasone
(B) hematology consultation
(C) intravenous immunoglobulin
(D) platelet transfusion
* (E) serial complete blood counts

The patient in this scenario has HELLP (hemolysis, elevated liver enzymes, and low platelet count) syndrome. The diagnostic criteria for HELLP include elevated lactate dehydrogenase (as a marker of hemolysis), aspartate aminotransferase more than twice the upper limit of normal, and platelet count less than 100,000/mm^3. Up to 15% of patients with HELLP syndrome lack hypertension or proteinuria (as in the described patient). The most common clinical symptoms include right upper quadrant or epigastric pain, nausea, vomiting, and malaise.

Hemolysis, elevated liver enzymes, and low platelet count syndrome represents one of the most serious forms of the preeclampsia spectrum and carries a higher risk of severe maternal morbidity and mortality. Complications include severe hypertension, abruptio placentae, eclampsia, subcapsular liver hematoma, stroke, perinatal death, and maternal death. For this reason, delivery is recommended in the setting of HELLP syndrome, and expectant management is contraindicated. In some cases, a course of antenatal corticosteroids for fetal lung maturity may be considered depending on the severity of disease and the gestational age.

Hemolysis, elevated liver enzymes, and low platelet count syndrome requires very close monitoring including frequent laboratory assessment. Aspartate aminotransferase concentrations greater than 2,000 IU/L or lactate dehydrogenase concentrations greater than 3,000 IU/L suggest an increased risk of mortality. During the acute phase of the disease, platelet counts may decrease by approximately 40% per day. The nadir of the platelet count occurs at approximately 23 hours after delivery. If the platelet count continues to decrease after 4 days postpartum, other diagnoses should be considered. The management for low platelets in the described postpartum patient is expectant, and laboratory evaluation should be repeated in 12 hours. Most patients will have a platelet count above 100,000/mm^3 by 7 days postpartum. In many patients, a rebound thrombocytosis may occur.

Although corticosteroids may be recommended for fetal lung maturity, they would not be recommended for treatment of thrombocytopenia. Corticosteroids (dexamethasone) have been shown to improve some of the proinflammatory markers of preeclampsia and can increase the platelet count (standardized mean difference, 0.67; 95% CI, 0.24–1.10). However, corticosteroids given after delivery for treatment of persistent thrombocytopenia have not been shown to decrease the risk of severe maternal morbidity or mortality. Thus, the clinical benefit is questionable, and there is insufficient evidence for recommending corticosteroids in this setting.

A hematology consultation might be indicated if improvement is not seen after 4 days or the platelet count continues to decrease. At this time, supportive care is indicated.

Intravenous immunoglobulin to increase the platelet count is a therapy that might be considered for a patient with immune thrombocytopenia. The described patient does not appear to have immune-mediated thrombocytopenia.

A platelet transfusion could be considered for a patient with a severely low platelet count and increased risk of bleeding or signs of active bleeding. The risk of bleeding increases with a platelet count of less than 50,000/mm^3. Although the described patient is at an increased risk of bleeding, she currently is not bleeding and a transfusion is not indicated. Furthermore, in the setting of HELLP syndrome, the effect of a platelet transfusion is transient, because platelets are quickly consumed when the disease is active.

Barton JR, Sibai BM. Diagnosis and management of hemolysis, elevated liver enzymes, and low platelets syndrome. Clin Perinatol 2004;31:807–33, vii. doi: 10.1016/j.clp.2004.06.008. https://www.sciencedirect.com/science/article/abs/pii/S0095510804000703

Gestational hypertension and preeclampsia. ACOG Practice Bulletin No. 222. American College of Obstetricians and Gynecologists. Obstet Gynecol 2020;135:e237–60. doi: 10.1097/AOG.0000000000003891. https://journals.lww.com/greenjournal/Fulltext/2020/06000/Gestational_Hypertension_and_Preeclampsia__ACOG.46.aspx

Sibai BM. Evaluation and management of severe preeclampsia before 34 weeks' gestation. Publications Committee, Society for Maternal-Fetal Medicine. Am J Obstet Gynecol 2011;205:191–8. doi: 10.1016/j.ajog.2011.07.017. https://www.ajog.org/article/S0002-9378(11)00918-5/fulltext

10 Timing of classical cesarean birth

A 28-year-old gravida 3, para 1, at 24 weeks of gestation presents to establish prenatal care. She reports no complications with this pregnancy. She has no contributing medical problems. Her first pregnancy was an emergency cesarean birth with low transverse hysterotomy at 27 weeks of gestation due to bradycardia after a motor vehicle collision. Her second pregnancy was an emergency cesarean birth at 37 weeks of gestation when she presented in labor and experienced a uterine rupture. Her prenatal laboratory tests are normal, and her physical examination is unremarkable. An obstetric ultrasonography examination confirms her gestational age and a fundal placenta. The most appropriate gestational age for a planned repeat cesarean birth for this patient is

(A) 30 weeks
(B) 32 weeks
(C) 34 weeks
* (D) 36 weeks
(E) 38 weeks

A trial of labor after a previous cesarean birth is an option for most patients in subsequent pregnancies. The maternal benefits of a vaginal birth after cesarean (VBAC) versus a repeat cesarean birth are well established, including lower maternal morbidity in terms of hemorrhage, infection, and venous thromboembolic events. A successful VBAC also propagates these benefits to subsequent pregnancies. There are risks to the woman and fetus with a trial of labor after a previous cesarean birth, most of which are incurred when labor is unsuccessful and the need for a cesarean birth arises or when a uterine rupture has occurred.

One of the main considerations when assessing a patient for a trial of labor after a previous cesarean birth is the location of the previous hysterotomy. One previous cesarean birth with a low transverse incision carries a 0.5–0.9% risk of uterine rupture in a subsequent obstetric labor. A *low transverse hysterotomy* is defined as an incision into the noncontractile myometrium of the gravid uterus. There is no universal landmark to demarcate this area, but the majority of transverse hysterotomies in the third trimester will be in the noncontractile myometrium. With no other contraindications to a vaginal birth and with appropriate counseling, these patients are candidates for a trial of labor after a previous cesarean birth. Similarly, a patient with a history of a low vertical incision, in the noncontractile portion of the myometrium, has a similar success rate with VBAC and no consistent evidence of increased maternal or neonatal morbidity. These patients also are candidates for labor.

For patients with more than one previous low transverse hysterotomy, the risk of uterine rupture in a subsequent pregnancy is 0.9–3.7%. Although the rate of uterine rupture is higher, there are limited data demonstrating a slight increase in morbidity. For this reason, women with two previous low transverse hysterotomies can safely consider a trial of labor in future pregnancies.

For patients who have had a previous hysterotomy in the contractile myometrium, the risk of uterine rupture in a subsequent labor is substantially higher. For a patient with a previous classical hysterotomy, the uterine rupture risk is 2–9%. For those who had a T-shaped hysterotomy, the risk is 4–9%. Similarly, those without a previous cesarean birth but with a previous transmural myomectomy have variably increased risks of uterine rupture in subsequent labors based on the extent of their previous surgery. The highest risk of uterine rupture during labor exists in patients with a history of a uterine rupture in a preceding pregnancy. According to small case series, the recurrence risk of uterine rupture is 6% for previous lower segment defects and 15–32% for upper uterine segment ruptures.

In a case in which the type of previous hysterotomy cannot be established, the clinical context of the previous delivery should be assessed. An unknown type of previous hysterotomy is not a contraindication to a trial of labor in a subsequent pregnancy if the clinical suspicion for a previous classical hysterotomy is low.

For those patients who have increased risk of uterine rupture because of previous hysterotomy, those with a previous classical or T-shaped hysterotomy, and those with histories of transmural myomectomies or with a history of uterine rupture, a trial of labor after cesarean birth is contraindicated. Late-preterm or early-term delivery is medically indicated in these cases with the goal of achieving a cesarean birth before the onset of labor. The recommended delivery window for patients with previous classical and T-shaped hysterotomies and those with previous uterine ruptures is 36 0/7 to 37 0/7 weeks of gestation. In patients with previous transmural myomectomies, the window is 37 0/7 to 38 6/7 weeks of gestation based on the extent of the previous surgery but can be performed even earlier to be more consistent with a previous classical hysterotomy in patients with the most extensive myomectomies.

Cunningham FG, Leveno KJ, Bloom SL, Dashe JS, Hoffman BL, Casey BM, et al. Williams obstetrics. 25th ed. McGraw-Hill Education; 2018.

Medically indicated late-preterm and early-term deliveries. ACOG Committee Opinion No. 831. American College of Obstetricians and Gynecologists. Obstet Gynecol 2021;138:e35–9. doi: 10.1097/AOG.0000000000004447. https://journals.lww.com/greenjournal/Fulltext/2021/07000/Medically_Indicated_Late_Preterm_and_Early_Term.38.aspx

Vaginal birth after cesarean delivery. ACOG Practice Bulletin No. 205. American College of Obstetricians and Gynecologists. Obstet Gynecol 2019;133:e110–27. doi: 10.1097/AOG.0000000000003078. https://journals.lww.com/greenjournal/Fulltext/2019/02000/ACOG_Practice_Bulletin_No__205__Vaginal_Birth.40.aspx

11 Cervical insufficiency

A 36-year-old gravida 3, para 1, presents for prenatal care at 8 weeks of gestation. Her obstetric history is complicated by the second-trimester loss of her first pregnancy with painless cervical dilation and a 26-week delivery in her second pregnancy, in which she had a history-indicated cerclage placed at 13 weeks of gestation. To prevent preterm birth in this pregnancy, the best next step is progesterone supplementation and

(A) cervical pessary
(B) serial cervical length ultrasonography
(C) transvaginal cerclage
* (D) transabdominal cerclage

Cerclage placement is recommended in women with a history of cervical insufficiency (history indicated), painless cervical dilation in the second trimester (physical examination indicated), or prior spontaneous preterm birth and a short cervical length in the second trimester (ultrasound indicated) (Box 11-1). *Cervical insufficiency* is not always a straightforward diagnosis but is generally defined as painless cervical dilation in the second trimester followed by expulsion of pregnancy in the absence of other clear pathology. Women with a history suspicious for cervical insufficiency may be offered a history-indicated cerclage or serial transvaginal ultrasound examination in the second trimester, with ultrasound-indicated cerclage placement if a short cervix is diagnosed. This strategy may allow cerclage placement in women with true cervical insufficiency and avoid an unnecessary procedure in more than one half of patients. The described patient had a second-trimester loss suspicious for cervical insufficiency followed by an unsuccessful history-indicated transvaginal cerclage, and serial cervical length measurements would not be recommended because she likely has true cervical insufficiency.

The standard cerclage technique is transvaginal, often using modifications of the McDonald (purse string) or Shirodkar techniques (dissection of the vesicocervical epithelium for higher placement). Transabdominal cerclage also has been described in patients with cervical insufficiency in whom a transvaginal cerclage cannot be placed because of anatomical limitations, such as prior trachelectomy, or in women in whom transvaginal cerclage is unsuccessful. Transabdominal cerclage involves more extensive surgery, and it may be performed before or during pregnancy, with a laparoscopic or open approach. The suture is left in place between pregnancies, and cesarean birth always is indicated with this type of cerclage.

A recent multicenter, randomized controlled trial of transabdominal versus low transvaginal (McDonald) versus high transvaginal (Shirodkar) cervical cerclage in women with a previous unsuccessful low transvaginal cerclage showed a significant reduction in the rate of preterm birth at less than 32 weeks of gestation in women who received transabdominal cerclage compared with low transvaginal cerclage, and did not show a benefit to high transvaginal cerclage. In the described patient, who had an unsuccessful transvaginal cerclage with a preterm delivery at 26 weeks of gestation after history-indicated

BOX 11-1

Indications for Cervical Cerclage in Women With Singleton Pregnancies

History

- History of one or more second-trimester pregnancy losses related to painless cervical dilation and in the absence of labor or abruptio placentae
- Prior cerclage due to painless cervical dilation in the second trimester

Physical Examination

- Painless cervical dilation in the second trimester

Ultrasonographic Finding With a History of Prior Preterm Birth

- Current singleton pregnancy, prior spontaneous preterm birth at less than 34 wk of gestation, and short cervical length (less than 25 mm) before 24 wk of gestation

Reprinted from Cerclage for the management of cervical insufficiency. Practice Bulletin No. 142. American College of Obstetricians and Gynecologists. Obstet Gynecol 2014;123:372–9. doi: 10.1097/01.AOG.0000443276.68274.cc. https://journals.lww.com/greenjournal/Fulltext/2014/02000/Practice_Bulletin_No__142__Cerclage_for_the.33.aspx cerclage placement, transabdominal cerclage is indicated and should be offered as the best option to reduce the risk of preterm delivery. Optimally, a transabdominal cerclage would be placed in the prepregnancy period.

During pregnancy with a transabdominal cerclage, patients are at increased risk of preterm labor and complications related to uterine rupture. Patients with transabdominal cerclage may not exhibit cervical dilation as a sign of labor, making usual methods for evaluation of preterm labor difficult. Given risks for uterine rupture with persistent contractions, women should be delivered by prelabor cesarean birth at 36–37 weeks of gestation.

Cervical pessary placement has been studied in women with a short cervix in singleton and twin pregnancies and is not currently recommended outside of research settings in these populations to decrease the risk of preterm birth.

Cerclage for the management of cervical insufficiency. Practice Bulletin No. 142. American College of Obstetricians and Gynecologists. Obstet Gynecol 2014;123:372–9. doi: 10.1097/01.AOG.0000443276.68274.cc. https://journals.lww.com/greenjournal/Fulltext/2014/02000/Practice_Bulletin_No__142__Cerclage_for_the.33.aspx

Resnik R, Lockwood CJ, Moore TR, Greene MF, Copel JA, Silver RM, editors. Creasy & Resnik's maternal–fetal medicine: principles and practice. 8th ed. Elsevier; 2019.

Shennan A, Chandiramani M, Bennett P, David AL, Girling J, Ridout A, et al. MAVRIC: a multicenter randomized controlled trial of transabdominal vs transvaginal cervical cerclage. Am J Obstet Gynecol 2020;222:261.e1,261.e9. doi: 10.1016/j.ajog.2019.09.040. https://www.ajog.org/article/S0002-9378(19)31206-2/fulltext

12 Diagnosis of congenital infection

A 28-year-old gravida 2, para 1, presents for a fetal anatomic assessment at 20 weeks of gestation. On ultrasonography, several abnormalities are noted, including fetal growth restriction, periventricular calcifications, hyperechoic bowel and liver, and a thickened placenta. She reports no recent illnesses. She is a vegetarian, has no pets, occasionally smokes marijuana, and has a young child in daycare. She is up to date on all vaccinations. The most likely fetal diagnosis is

* (A) cytomegalovirus (CMV)
(B) herpes simplex virus
(C) parvovirus
(D) toxoplasmosis
(E) varicella zoster virus

Maternal viral infections in pregnancy may infect the fetus through the placenta or during the intrapartum period. Viral effects on a developing fetus may be minimal or may cause severe morbidity and mortality, depending on the type of virus, prior maternal exposure, and timing of infection during pregnancy. Cytomegalovirus, parvovirus B19, varicella zoster virus, and toxoplasmosis are commonly associated with fetal and neonatal congenital complications.

Cytomegalovirus is the most common congenital infection, occurring in 0.2–2.2% of all newborns. The incidence of primary CMV infection during pregnancy in the United States is estimated to be up to 4%. Secondary infections are more common, occurring in as many as 13.5% of women during pregnancy. With a primary maternal infection, the risk of transmission to the fetus is 30–40% and is greatest in the third trimester. However, the more severe fetal and neonatal complications from infection occur after infection in the first trimester.

Congenital CMV infection in a newborn may be asymptomatic or may manifest as jaundice, petechiae, thrombocytopenia, hepatosplenomegaly, growth restriction, myocarditis, or nonimmune hydrops. Severely infected infants have a high risk of death (30%) and severe neurologic morbidity (65–80%). Cytomegalovirus can be transmitted by direct contact with urine, blood, or saliva and by sexual contact. Adults with CMV infection are usually asymptomatic or may have a mild syndrome with fever, chills, and lymphadenopathy.

Congenital CMV often is suspected after abnormal findings are noted on prenatal ultrasonography. These findings commonly include abdominal calcifications, hepatosplenomegaly, echogenic intra-abdominal organs, ascites, cerebral ventriculomegaly, intracranial calcifications, microcephaly, hydrops fetalis, or growth restriction. Although fetal periventricular calcifications are not always seen in an infected fetus, when present, they are specifically concerning for congenital CMV. The most sensitive test to detect suspected fetal infection is culture or polymerase chain reaction testing of amniotic fluid after amniocentesis. An alternative is to measure maternal serum titers, including immunoglobulin G and M with reflex avidity testing, with high avidity suggesting remote infection and low avidity suggesting recent infection. Given the ultrasound findings, the fetus in the described scenario likely has a CMV infection.

Herpes simplex virus is transmitted through direct contact and causes oral and genital infections. Genital herpes is one of the most common sexually transmitted infections, with approximately 20% of women showing evidence of past infection with herpes simplex virus 2, the most common cause of genital herpes.

Many women who have not been previously infected have partners who carry the virus and may transmit a new infection during pregnancy. Neonatal herpes usually is acquired during delivery from exposure to the maternal genital tract, but rarely may be acquired in utero. Ultrasound findings may include cutaneous, neurologic, and eye abnormalities. Herpes simplex virus is not the most likely diagnosis in the described patient.

Parvovirus B19 generally is spread from respiratory secretions and hand-to-mouth contact. The most common symptoms are rash, fever, and joint pain, and children have a classic "slapped cheek" facial rash. This virus also may cause a transient aplastic crisis with associated fetal anemia, which may affect a fetus in the form of hydrops fetalis. Severe effects are more commonly seen when transmission occurs earlier than 20 weeks of gestation. Fetal parvovirus B19 infection usually does not cause the ultrasound findings described in the patient above, and this is not the most likely diagnosis.

Toxoplasmosis is an infection caused by the parasite *Toxoplasma gondii*, which is present in undercooked food or the feces of infected animals. Most adults who are infected have no symptoms; some individuals will have a mild syndrome with fever, malaise, or hepatosplenomegaly. It is a rare congenital infection, estimated to occur in 150–200 infants per year in the United States. There is up to a 60% chance of congenital transmission to a fetus during pregnancy, and this risk is highest in the third trimester. However, the severity of fetal infection is worse when the infection occurs at earlier gestational ages. Neonatal and childhood sequelae include visual and hearing loss and developmental delay. Ultrasound findings during pregnancy include intracranial calcifications and microcephaly. In the absence of risk factors, toxoplasmosis infection is not the most likely diagnosis for this patient.

Varicella zoster virus is spread by respiratory droplets or close contact and causes chickenpox, with an itchy vesicular rash, fever, and malaise. After the primary infection, it remains dormant in the sensory ganglia and can cause a vesicular skin rash, known as *shingles*, later in life. This infection was much more common before 1995, when a vaccine became available and was widely administered. The incidence of infection during pregnancy is low, and when it occurs, the risk of congenital varicella syndrome is 2% or less. Infection can cause fetal and neonatal skin scarring, limb hypoplasia, chorioretinitis, and microcephaly. This is not the most likely fetal infection in this scenario.

Cytomegalovirus, parvovirus B19, varicella zoster, and toxoplasmosis in pregnancy. Practice Bulletin No. 151. American College of Obstetricians and Gynecologists [published errata appear in Obstet Gynecol 2016;127:405; Obstet Gynecol 2016;127:405]. Obstet Gynecol 2015;125:1510–25. doi: 10.1097/01.AOG.0000466430.19823.53. https://journals.lww.com/greenjournal/Fulltext/2015/06000/Practice_Bulletin_No__151__Cytomegalovirus,.54.aspx

Infection. In: Woodward PJ, Kennedy A, Sohaey R, Byrne JL, Puchalski MD, Shaffer BL, et al, editors. Diagnostic imaging: obstetrics. 4th ed. Elsevier; 2021. p. 1045–63.

Khalil A, Sotiriadis A, Chaoui R, da Silva Costa F, D'Antonio F, Heath PT, et al. ISUOG Practice Guidelines: role of ultrasound in congenital infection. Ultrasound Obstet Gynecol 2020;56:128–51. doi: 10.1002/uog.21991. https://obgyn.onlinelibrary.wiley.com/doi/10.1002/uog.21991

Management of genital herpes in pregnancy. ACOG Practice Bulletin No. 220. American College of Obstetricians and Gynecologists. Obstet Gynecol 2020;136:850–1. doi: 10.1097/AOG.0000000000004115. https://journals.lww.com/greenjournal/Fulltext/2020/05000/Management_of_Genital_Herpes_in_Pregnancy__ACOG.53.aspx

McAlarnen LA, Amin S, Goodman JR. Severe in utero herpes simplex virus infection in a fetus of an asymptomatic mother. Clin Obstet Gynecol Reprod Med 2018;4(6). doi: 10.15761/COGRM.1000237. https://www.oatext.com/severe-in-utero-herpes-simplex-virus-infection-in-a-fetus-of-an-asymptomatic-mother.php

13 Human immunodeficiency virus testing in a pregnant patient

A 36-year-old gravida 1 presents for prenatal care at 8 weeks of gestation. She is currently incarcerated. Her prenatal labs are all negative, including for human immunodeficiency virus (HIV) testing. The best next step for screening for HIV is

(A) no further HIV screening
(B) screening during the second trimester
* (C) screening during the third trimester
(D) screening on admission to labor and delivery

New HIV cases in the United States have decreased during the past several decades, but approximately 40,000 Americans are infected with HIV each year. Since the 1990s, perinatal transmission has decreased significantly because of advances in medication and prevention strategies.

All pregnant women should be screened for HIV in the first trimester to identify patients living with HIV and initiate treatment. The Centers for Disease Control and Prevention currently recommends an opt-out approach to HIV screening in prenatal care. With this approach, patients are notified that they will receive an HIV test as part of their routine prenatal laboratory tests unless they opt out. Research has shown an increased uptake in HIV testing with the opt-out approach.

Patients identified as being at high risk of HIV should be retested in the third trimester. This includes patients who are receiving care in facilities that have an HIV incidence in pregnant women of at least 1 per 1,000 per year, who live in communities with elevated HIV incidence, who are incarcerated, or who have signs and symptoms consistent with acute HIV infection. These include fever, lymphadenopathy, myalgias, headache, elevation of transaminases, leukopenia, or thrombocytopenia. Other factors that put pregnant patients at high risk include diagnosis with another sexually transmitted infection in the past year, using injection drugs or having sex partners who use injection drugs, exchanging sex for money or drugs, having a new sex partner or more than one sex partner during this pregnancy, and having sex partners known to be infected with HIV or at high risk of HIV.

Vertical transmission can occur at any point in pregnancy; however, transmission risk is less than 1–2% in patients on combined antiretroviral therapy with viral loads less than 1,000 copies/mL, regardless of route of delivery. Patients who test positive for HIV should be referred to infectious disease specialists for treatment as soon as possible. They should be started on combined antiretroviral therapy and have viral load testing 2–4 weeks after initiating or changing treatment, monthly until that level is undetectable, and after that, every 3 months until delivery.

Viral load testing in the third trimester will allow appropriate triage for delivery. Patients with a viral load greater than 1,000 copies/mL should be offered scheduled cesarean birth at 38 0/7 weeks of gestation to decrease the risk of vertical transmission at delivery and should receive intravenous zidovudine before delivery. Patients with a viral load less than 1,000 copies/mL can be offered vaginal delivery, because the mode of delivery does not affect vertical transmission in patients with a low or undetectable viral load. Additionally, duration of ruptured membranes is not an independent risk factor for vertical transmission in patients with low or *undetectable viral load* (defined as less than 1,000 copies/mL). It is unclear whether there is benefit to cesarean birth in the setting of prelabor rupture of membranes with a viral load greater than 1,000 copies/mL, and care should be individualized in this setting.

Routine screening on admission is unnecessary in high-risk women with prior negative results in the first and third trimesters, unless there is specific concern for new exposure since their last test. There currently are no recommendations to routinely screen patients at high risk in the second trimester. Patients who have not been otherwise screened should be screened on admission to labor and delivery with a rapid test, and elective procedures should be held until test results are available. For the described patient, HIV screening in the third trimester is the most appropriate screening strategy.

Cunningham FG, Leveno KJ, Bloom SL, Dashe JS, Hoffman BL, Casey BM, et al. Williams obstetrics. 25th ed. McGraw-Hill Education; 2018.

Labor and delivery management of women with human immunodeficiency virus infection. ACOG Committee Opinion No. 751. American College of Obstetricians and Gynecologists. Obstet Gynecol 2018;132:e131–7. doi: 10.1097/AOG.0000000000002820. https://journals.lww.com/greenjournal/Fulltext/2018/09000/ACOG_Committee_Opinion_No__751__Labor_and_Delivery.69.aspx

Prenatal and perinatal human immunodeficiency virus testing. ACOG Committee Opinion No. 752. American College of Obstetricians and Gynecologists. Obstet Gynecol 2018;132:e138–42. doi: 10.1097/AOG.0000000000002825. https://journals.lww.com/greenjournal/Fulltext/2018/09000/ACOG_Committee_Opinion_No__752__Prenatal_and.70.aspx

Prepregnancy counseling. ACOG Committee Opinion No. 762. American College of Obstetricians and Gynecologists. Fertil Steril 2019;111:32–42. doi: 10.1097/AOG.0000000000003013. https://www.fertstert.org/article/S0015-0282(18)32252-0/fulltext

14 Neonatal levels of care

A 39-year-old gravida 4, para 2, presents to labor and delivery at 33 weeks of gestation with contractions. Her history is complicated by prior preterm birth, and she received vaginal progesterone during this pregnancy. She is found to be 4-cm dilated with regular contractions. If she were to deliver in the next week, the minimum level of neonatal care required to care for her newborn is

(A) Level I
* (B) Level II
(C) Level III
(D) Level IV

To improve outcomes for newborns, the American Academy of Pediatrics has standardized the definitions of levels of newborn care. The levels of care are summarized in Table 14-1.

Level 1 centers are considered *well newborn nurseries.* They are staffed by pediatricians, family physicians, and nurse practitioners. These facilities are able to stabilize and care for neonates born at 35–37 weeks of gestation and stabilize neonates born at less than 35 weeks of gestation until they can be transferred to a higher level of care.

The patient in the above scenario has preterm labor at 33 weeks of gestation, and if she delivers, the neonate will require more complex management than a term infant. A Level II center would be appropriate for this delivery, making this the correct answer choice. Level II centers are known as *special care nurseries.* They are staffed by neonatologists, pediatric hospitalists, and nurse practitioners. These centers are able to care for neonates born at more than 32 weeks of gestation and weighing more than 1,500 g who are not expected to need subspecialty care. A Level II center can provide mechanical ventilation for less than 24 hours, as well as continuous positive airway pressure. They are able to stabilize infants born before 32 weeks of gestation before transfer.

Level III centers are designated *neonatal intensive care units* (NICUs). A NICU can provide care for neonates at all gestational ages and has access to pediatric subspecialists and pediatric surgical specialists. These centers can provide respiratory support, including conventional and high-frequency ventilation. Level III centers should have available pediatric ophthalmology services to care for retinopathy of prematurity, as well as pediatric surgeons who can perform major surgeries, either onsite or at a nearby facility. They can perform advanced imaging, such as computed tomography and magnetic resonance imaging.

Level IV centers are *regional NICUs.* They have the same capabilities as Level III centers but are located in facilities with pediatric subspecialists who can care for complex congenital anomalies and diseases. For example, they have the capability to perform pediatric surgery requiring cardiopulmonary bypass or extracorporeal membrane oxygenation.

Current evidence shows that preterm neonates less than 32 weeks of gestation and very low-birth-weight neonates (neonates weighing less than 1,500 g) have improved outcomes when they are born at a facility with a Level III NICU. Very low-birth-weight neonates have a significantly increased rate of neonatal mortality when cared for in low-volume Level III NICU programs and Level I and II centers. Standardization of neonatal levels of care allows obstetricians and pediatricians to arrange for delivery at appropriate locations for the expected neonate or arrange for transfer after delivery if transfer cannot be performed safely before delivery.

TABLE 14-1. Definitions, Capabilities, and Provider Types: Neonatal Levels of Care

LEVEL OF CARE	CAPABILITIES	PROVIDER TYPES*
Level I	• Provide neonatal resuscitation at every delivery	Pediatricians, family physicians, nurse practitioners, and other advanced practice registered nurses
Well newborn nursery	• Evaluate and provide postnatal care to stable term newborn infants • Stabilize and provide care for infants born at 35–37 wk gestation who remain physiologically stable • Stabilize newborn infants who are ill and those born at less than 35 wk gestation until transfer to a higher level of care	
Level II	Level I capabilities plus:	Level I health care professionals plus:
Special care nursery	• Provide care for infants born at 32 or greater wk gestation and weighing 1,500 or more grams who have physiologic immaturity or who are moderately ill with problems that are expected to resolve rapidly and are not anticipated to need subspecialty services on an urgent basis • Provide care for infants convalescing after intensive care • Provide mechanical ventilation for brief duration (less than 24 h) or continuous positive airway pressure or both • Stabilize infants born before 32 wk gestation and weighing less than 1,500 g until transfer to a neonatal intensive care facility	Pediatric hospitalists, neonatologist, and neonatal nurse practitioners
Level III	Level II capabilities plus:	Level II health care professionals plus:
NICU	• Provide sustained life support • Provide comprehensive care for infants born less than 32 wk gestation and weighing less than 1,500 g and infants born at all gestational ages and birth weights with critical illness • Provide prompt and readily available access to a full range of pediatric medical subspecialists, pediatric surgical specialists, pediatric anesthesiologists, and pediatric ophthalmologists • Provide a full range of respiratory support that may include conventional and/or high-frequency ventilation and inhaled nitric oxide • Perform advanced imaging, with interpretation on an urgent basis, including computed tomography, MRI, and echocardiography	Pediatric medical subspecialists,† *pediatric anesthesiologists,*† pediatric surgeons, and pediatric ophthalmologists†
Level IV	Level III capabilities plus:	Level III health care professionals plus:
Regional NICU	• Located within an institution with the capability to provide surgical repair of complex congenital or acquired conditions • Maintain a full range of pediatric medical subspecialists, pediatric surgical subspecialists, and pediatric anesthesiologists at the site • Facilitate transport and provide outreach education	Pediatric surgical subspecialists

Abbreviations: ECMO, extracorporeal membrane oxygenation; NICU, neonatal intensive care unit.

*Includes all providers with relevant experience, training, and demonstrated competence.

†At the site or at a closely related institution by prearranged consultative agreement.

Reprinted from Levels of neonatal care. American Academy of Pediatrics Committee on Fetus and Newborn. Pediatrics 2012;130:587–97. doi: 10.1542/peds.2012-1999 https://publications.aap.org/pediatrics/article/130/3/587/30212/Levels-of-Neonatal-Care

Levels of neonatal care. American Academy of Pediatrics Committee on Fetus and Newborn. Pediatrics 2012;130:587–97. doi: 10.1542/peds.2012-1999 https://publications.aap.org/pediatrics/article/130/3/587/30212/Levels-of-Neonatal-Care

Periviable birth. Obstetric Care Consensus No. 6. American College of Obstetricians and Gynecologists. Obstet Gynecol 2017;130:e187–99. doi: 10.1097/AOG.0000000000002352 https://journals.lww.com/greenjournal/Fulltext/2017/10000/Obstetric_Care_Consensus_No__6__Periviable_Birth.57.aspx

15 Delayed cord clamping

A 37-year-old gravida 3, para 2, is admitted at 41 weeks of gestation for induction of labor. Her second child developed anemia during infancy, and she is concerned about the risk in this neonate. The most appropriate method to increase iron stores in the neonate is

(A) breastfeeding
* (B) delayed cord clamping
(C) early skin-to-skin contact
(D) iron supplementation

Delayed umbilical cord clamping is defined as delay in clamping the umbilical cord for a minimum of 30–60 seconds. This practice is beneficial for term and preterm neonates.

In newborns there is transfer of a significant amount of blood (80–100 mL at term) from the placenta to the newborn within the first minutes of birth, and most of this occurs within the first few breaths. There is also transfer of immunoglobulins and stem cells. Because this transfer occurs so quickly after birth, and because there was a historical lack of recommendations regarding optimum timing of cord clamping, the interval had been shortened to less than 20 seconds.

Over the last several years, universal delay in cord clamping in all neonates (preterm and term) has been recommended by the World Health Organization, the American Academy of Pediatrics, the Royal College of Obstetricians and Gynaecologists, the American College of Nurse Midwives, and the American College of Obstetricians and Gynecologists. However, universal delay in cord clamping raised several concerns. These include risk of delay in resuscitation of the newborn, excessive placental transfusion, and risk of maternal hemorrhage and subsequent anemia.

A Cochrane review published in 2015, which included 15 randomized controlled trials comparing early and late umbilical cord clamping in term infants, addressed these concerns. In the studies reporting Apgar scores, there was no significant difference between early and delayed cord clamping groups. In term neonates, delayed umbilical cord clamping increased hemoglobin levels at birth and improved iron stores in the first several months of life, which may have a favorable effect on developmental outcomes. In term newborns, delayed cord clamping resulted in a small increase in the incidence of jaundice that required phototherapy. All newborns should be monitored for neonatal jaundice, and pediatric care teams should be aware of the slightly increased risk to term newborns in the setting of delayed cord clamping. Delayed umbilical cord clamping does not increase risk of postpartum hemorrhage. There were no significant differences in breastfeeding between early and delayed cord clamping.

In vigorous preterm neonates, delayed umbilical cord clamping is associated with significant neonatal benefits, including improved transitional circulation, better established red blood cell volume, decreased need for blood transfusion, and lower incidence of necrotizing enterocolitis and intraventricular hemorrhage. Cord milking should not be used before 28 weeks of gestation, given an increased risk of intraventricular hemorrhage.

Delaying cord clamping should not interfere with the active management of the third stage of labor. Immediate cord clamping is indicated in the setting of maternal instability, when there is a need for immediate resuscitation of the newborn, and in settings in which the placental circulation is not intact (placental abruption or cord avulsion).

In the described patient, breastfeeding is associated with a higher risk of iron deficiency anemia. Pediatricians often recommend supplemental iron in infants who are breastfed, but not until they are several months of age. Delayed cord clamping is the correct choice to improve iron stores. Immediate skin-to-skin care is appropriate while waiting for umbilical cord clamping and can be done with the infant on the maternal abdomen.

Baker RD, Greer FR. Diagnosis and prevention of iron deficiency and iron-deficiency anemia in infants and young children (0–3 years of age). Committee on Nutrition American Academy of Pediatrics. Pediatrics 2010;126:1040–50. doi: 10.1542/peds.2010-2576. https://publications.aap.org/pediatrics/article/126/5/1040/65343/Diagnosis-and-Prevention-of-Iron-Deficiency-and

Delayed umbilical cord clamping after birth. ACOG Committee Opinion No. 814. American College of Obstetricians and Gynecologists. Obstet Gynecol 2020;136:e100–6. doi: 10.1097/AOG.0000000000004167. https://journals.lww.com/greenjournal/Fulltext/2020/12000/Delayed_Umbilical_Cord_Clamping_After_Birth__ACOG.37.aspx

McDonald SJ, Middleton P, Dowswell T, Morris PS. Effect of timing of umbilical cord clamping of term infants on maternal and neonatal outcomes. Cochrane Database of Systematic Reviews 2013, Issue 7. Art. No.: CD004074. doi: 10.1002/14651858.CD004074.pub3. https://www.cochranelibrary.com/cdsr/doi/10.1002/14651858.CD004074.pub3/full

16 Microcytic anemia

A patient who self-reports Southeast Asian ancestry presents at 20 weeks of gestation for a survey of fetal anatomy. Ultrasonographic findings are shown in Figure 16-1. Laboratory studies are remarkable for hemoglobin of 8.9 g/dL and mean corpuscular volume (MCV) of 74 cubic micrometers. Her noninvasive prenatal testing showed a low risk of aneuploidy. Her hemoglobin electrophoresis is normal, and serum ferritin concentration is 46 micrograms/dL. The patient declines an amniocentesis. The best next maternal test is

* (A) DNA analysis of the α-globin gene
(B) DNA analysis of the β-globin gene
(C) methylenetetrahydrofolate reductase gene testing
(D) parvovirus immunoglobulin G and immunoglobulin M antibodies
(E) total iron binding capacity

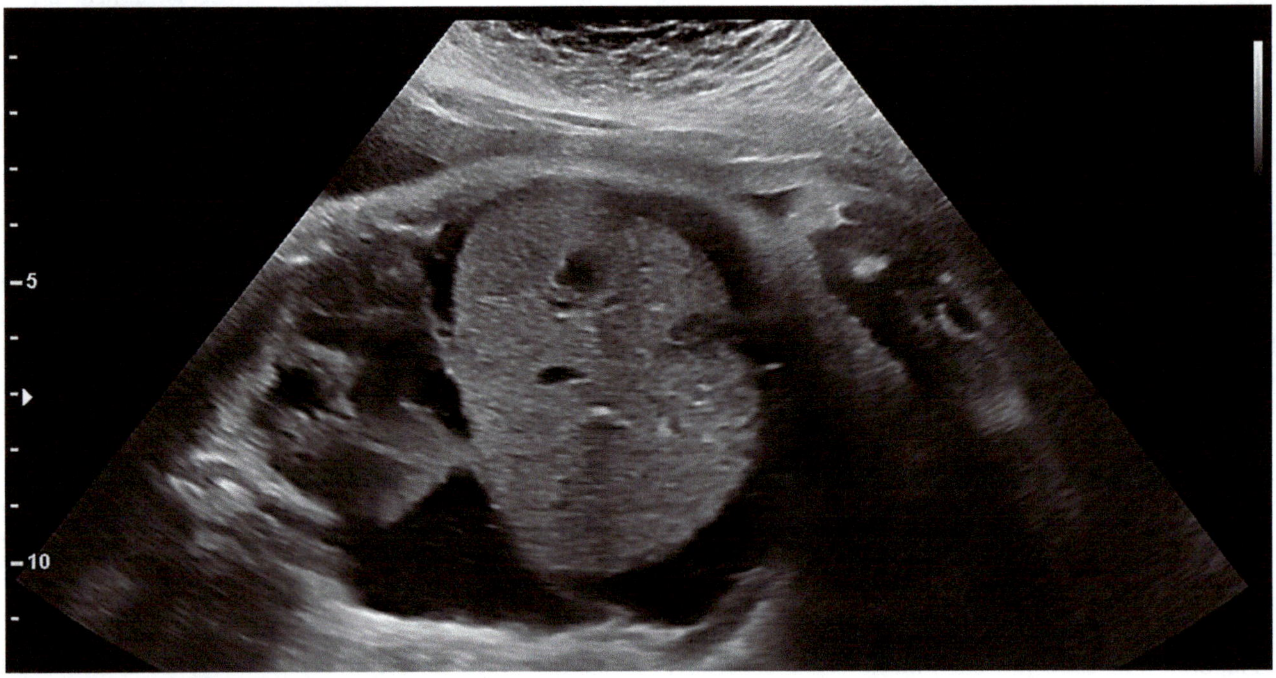

FIGURE 16-1. Described Patient's Fetal Ultrasonography

The prevalence of anemia in pregnant women is 21 in every 1,000, which encompasses all etiologies of low hemoglobin concentration less than 10 g/dL. The etiologies of anemia diagnosed during pregnancy are the same as in nonpregnant individuals, with the exception that pregnancy also may cause a dilutional anemia due to expanded plasma volume. Anemia is categorized based on the MCV and further stratified as microcytic anemia (MCV less than 80 cubic micrometers), normocytic anemia, or macrocytic anemia (MCV greater than 100 cubic micrometers). The most common etiologies for microcytic anemia during pregnancy are iron deficiency and dilutional anemia.

Initial evaluation for microcytic anemia should include iron studies and, in particular, a ferritin concentration. In cases of microcytic anemia with normal iron status, as in the described patient, hemoglobin electrophoresis should be considered, especially in patients who self-report African, Mediterranean, or Southeast Asian ancestry. Hemoglobin electrophoresis will identify hemoglobinopathies that may cause microcytic anemia, including sickle cell disease, sickle trait, sickle hemoglobin C disease, and β-thalassemia (Table 16-1). Hemoglobin electrophoresis cannot detect α-thalassemia because the hemoglobin A2 levels are within normal range. In patients at high risk of α-thalassemia with an otherwise negative evaluation for microcytic anemia, the best next step would be DNA analysis to detect α-globin gene deletions. The different genotypes and phenotypes of α-thalassemia are shown in Table 16-2. One deletion will result in a silent carrier status; however, two

TABLE 16-1. Hemoglobinopathy Features on Electrophoresis

DISORDER	HETEROZYGOUS STATE	HOMOZYGOUS STATE
α^+-Thalassemia	Hb Barts 0–2% (neonatal period)	Hb Barts 5–10% (neonatal period)
α^0-Thalassemia	Hb Barts 5–10% (neonatal period)	Hb Barts (hydrops fetalis)
β^0-Thalassemia	Hb A_2 3.5–7%	Hb F 98%, Hb A_2 2% (major)
β^+-Thalassemia (severe)	Hb A_2 3.5–7%	Hb F 70–95% (major)
β^+-Thalassemia (mild)	Hb A_2 3.5–7%	Hb F 20–40% (intermedia)
Hb S	Hb A, Hb S, Hb A_2	Hb S, Hb F (1–155), Hb A_2

Abbreviation: Hb, hemoglobin.

Modified from Hemoglobinopathies in pregnancy. ACOG Practice Bulletin No. 78. American College of Obstetricians and Gynecologists. Obstet Gynecol 2007;109:229-37. doi: 10.1097/00006250-200701000-00055. https://journals.lww.com/greenjournal/Citation/2007/01000/ACOG_Practice_Bulletin_No__78__Hemoglobinopathies.55.aspx

TABLE 16-2. Genotypes for α-Thalassemia

GENOTYPE	ALLELE ARRANGEMENT	PHENOTYPE
Normal	αα/αα	Normal
α^+-Thalassemia heterozygote	–α/αα αα/–α	Silent carrier
α^+-Thalassemia homozygote	–α/–α	Mild anemia (α-thalassemia minor)
α^0-Thalassemia heterozygote	– –/αα	Mild anemia (α-thalassemia minor)
Compound heterozygous α^0/α^+	– –/–α	Hb H disease, moderate to severe anemia
Homozygous α-thalassemia	– –/– –	Hb Barts disease, hydrops fetalis

Data from Anemia in pregnancy. ACOG Practice Bulletin No. 233. American College of Obstetricians and Gynecologists. Obstet Gynecol 2021;138:e55-64. doi: 10.1097/AOG.0000000000004477. https://journals.lww.com/greenjournal/Fulltext/2021/08000/Anemia_in_Pregnancy__ACOG_Practice_Bulletin,.34.aspx

deletions result in a mild microcytic anemia. Individuals of Asian descent are more likely to carry this mutation on the same allele (*cis* arrangement), making it more likely for a fetus to inherit a nonfunctioning α-globin gene if both parents are of Southeast Asian descent. This results in hemoglobin Barts in the fetus, often resulting in nonimmune hydrops. The fetus in this scenario is presenting with hydrops and microcytic anemia in a patient of Asian ancestry, and the best maternal test is DNA analysis to detect α-thalassemia.

Although β-thalassemia should be considered in at-risk populations with microcytic anemia, DNA analysis of the β-globin gene is not required for diagnosis. Beta-thalassemia is diagnosed by increased hemoglobin F and A2 (greater than 3.5%) on hemoglobin electrophoresis. This patient has a normal electrophoresis. Beta-thalassemia also is not associated with hydrops fetalis.

Parvovirus B19 infection can cause fetal anemia and present with nonimmune fetal hydrops. This patient did not present with symptoms or risk factors for recent parvovirus B19 infection, and fetal anemia due to hemoglobin Barts syndrome is a more likely diagnosis. Although total iron binding capacity can be used to evaluate for iron deficiency anemia, the described patient's ferritin concentration is normal, and iron deficiency anemia can be excluded. Methylenetetrahydrofolate reductase gene testing is not recommended in the diagnosis of nonimmune fetal hydrops or stillbirth.

Cunningham FG, Leveno KJ, Bloom SL, Dashe JS, Hoffman BL, Casey BM, et al. Williams obstetrics. 25th ed. McGraw-Hill Education; 2018.

Hemoglobinopathies in pregnancy. ACOG Practice Bulletin No. 78. American College of Obstetricians and Gynecologists. Obstet Gynecol 2007;109:229–37. doi: 10.1097/00006250-200701000-00055. https://journals.lww.com/greenjournal/Citation/2007/01000/ACOG_Practice_Bulletin_No__78__Hemoglobinopathies.55.aspx

Norton ME, Chauhan SP, Dashe JS. Society for Maternal–Fetal Medicine (SMFM) clinical guideline #7: nonimmune hydrops fetalis. Am J Obstet Gynecol 2015;212:127–39. doi: 10.1016/j.ajog.2014.12.018. https://www.ajog.org/article/S0002-9378(14)02443-0/fulltext

17 Bell palsy

A patient with pregestational diabetes mellitus at 24 weeks of gestation presents with drooping of her left eyelid, increased tearing, and acute-onset decreased taste on the left side of her tongue for 2 days. She reports no other symptoms. Her distal motor examination is unremarkable, and her speech is fluent. There is obvious asymmetry at rest in the forehead and mouth and incomplete closure of the right eye. Her physical appearance is seen in Figure 17-1. Her House–Brackmann facial paralysis score is grade 5. In addition to protecting her left eye with a patch, the best next monotherapy for the patient is

(A) acyclovir
(B) azithromycin
(C) hydroxyzine
(D) immunoglobulin
* (E) prednisone

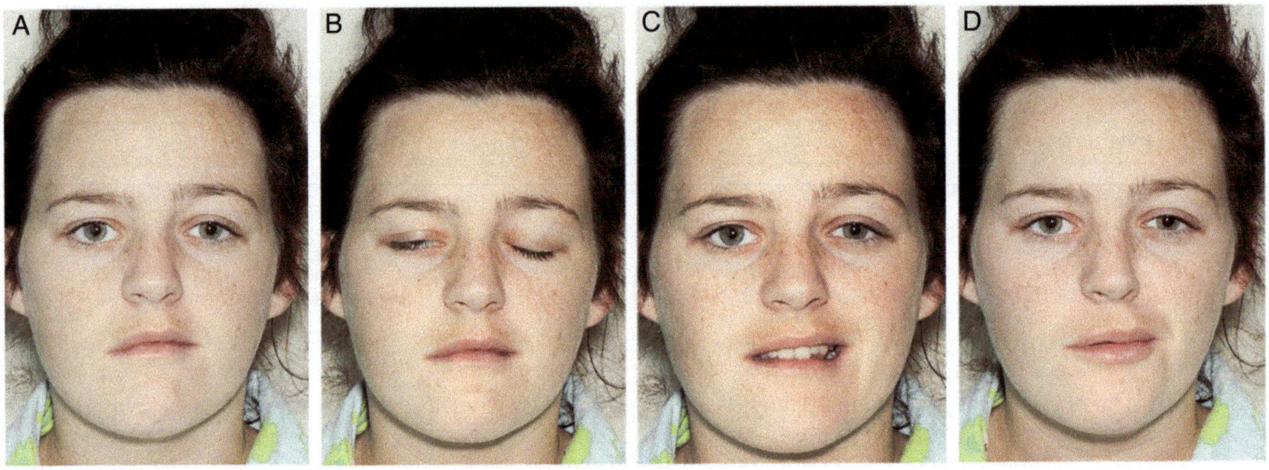

FIGURE 17-1. Described patient's facial examination findings. Patient at rest, closing her eyes, smiling, and whistling. (Reprinted from Fuller G, Morgan C. Bell's palsy syndrome: mimics and chameleons. Pract Neurol 2016;16:439–44. doi: 10.1136/practneurol-2016-001383. https://pn.bmj.com/content/16/6/439.long)

Bell palsy is a relatively uncommon condition, but it is the most common form of facial paralysis and is seen predominantly in women. The incidence is 11–40 cases per 100,000 individuals who are between the ages of 30 and 45 years. Pregnant or postpartum patients are at a twofold to fourfold increased risk of Bell palsy compared with the nonpregnant population. It is characterized by paresis or paralysis in the lower motor neuron of the face. Several risk factors have been associated with Bell palsy, including pregnancy, diabetes mellitus, obesity, hypertension, and upper respiratory infections. Recent viral infection or past infection with herpes simplex virus type 1 or varicella also have been associated with Bell palsy on reactivation.

Bell palsy often has an acute onset of symptoms over the course of a few hours, with the highest severity reached in the first 72 hours. Presentation usually is with acute paresis or paralysis of the facial muscles, but may be accompanied by increased tearing or dry eye (30%), decreased taste (35%), hyperacusis (5%), and pain on the affected side of the face or ear (50% of cases). Synkinesis, a neurologic symptom in which a voluntary muscle movement causes an involuntary contraction in another muscle, may be noted. Severity of the facial paralysis can be graded using the House–Brackmann score (Table 17-1). Alternative diagnoses should be sought if the patient has one or more of the following: severe pain, an unwell appearance, a history of cancer, a previous tick bite with potential Lyme disease, or rash on the external ear or auditory meatus.

A focused patient history will narrow the diagnosis and exclude other causes of facial paralysis. This patient is pregnant and has diabetes, which increases the likelihood that she has Bell palsy. She has no other neurologic involvement or progression in her symptoms that would be consistent with a cerebrovascular accident or thrombus, such as aphasia, distal motor neuron weakness, or headache. She also does not report a recent trauma or surgery that would increase the risk of facial nerve damage.

TABLE 17-1. House–Brackmann Classification of Facial Function

GRADE	CHARACTERISTICS
1	Normal
2	Mild dysfunction, slight weakness or synkinesis, normal symmetry
3	Moderate dysfunction, obvious asymmetry but not disfiguring, noticeable synkinesis, complete eye closure with effort
4	Moderately severe dysfunction, obvious weakness or asymmetry, incomplete eye closure, and mouth asymmetry with maximal effort
5	Barely perceptible motion, asymmetry at rest, slight movement of the mouth
6	No movement

Adapted from House JW, Brackmann DE. Facial nerve grading system. Otolaryngol Head Neck Surg 1985;93:146–7. doi: 10.1177/019459988509300202. https://journals.sagepub.com/doi/10.1177/019459988509300202

When patient history can reliably exclude other causes of facial paresis or paralysis, laboratory tests and diagnostic imaging should not be routinely performed.

All patients with impaired or closed eye should be instructed in methods of eye protection. Seventy percent of Bell palsy patients with full paralysis will fully recover, and 94% of patients with incomplete paralysis will fully recover. Treatment with corticosteroids, if started within the first few days of diagnosis, will increase the likelihood of full recovery. Oral corticosteroids, such as prednisolone, are strongly recommended within the first 72 hours of symptom onset if possible. Monotherapy with antivirals is not recommended because corticosteroids have been shown to be superior for symptom resolution in clinical trials, and the harm caused by the adverse effects of antivirals outweighed their benefits. In a trial of 496 patients, the combination of acyclovir and prednisolone did not improve resolution of symptoms at 9 months compared with placebo (odds ratio, 1.76; 95% CI, 0.75–4.16; P=.2). Prednisolone as monotherapy improved the chance of complete recovery compared to placebo (odds ratio, 3.23; 95% CI, 1.13–9.22; P=.03). Antibiotics, immunoglobulin, and antihistamines are not considered treatments for Bell palsy.

In a pregnant patient, the course of the disease may be more severe with a lower chance of complete recovery compared with nonpregnant patients. The etiology of long-term negative outcomes in pregnant patients is unclear and may be due to a delay in treatment or a more severe underlying nerve palsy. The pathophysiology of the disease in pregnancy is not completely understood. Reactivation of herpes viruses due to relative immunosuppression, hypercoagulability, or hypertension, and increased intravascular volume have all been suggested, as are associations with preeclampsia and obesity. Recurrence in future pregnancies is rare.

Baugh RF, Basura GJ, Ishii LE, Schwartz SR, Drumheller CM, Burkholder R, et al. Clinical practice guideline: Bell's palsy executive summary. Otolaryngol Head Neck Surg 2013;149:656–63. doi: 10.1177/0194599813506835. https://journals.sagepub.com/doi/full/10.1177/0194599813506835

Christensen B. House-Brackmann classification of facial function. 2018. https://emedicine.medscape.com/article/2172449-overview

Evangelista V, Gooding MS, Pereira L. Bell's palsy in pregnancy. Obstet Gynecol Surv 2019;74:674–8. doi: 10.1097/OGX.0000000000000732. https://journals.lww.com/obgynsurvey/Abstract/2019/11000/Bell_s_Palsy_in_Pregnancy.19.aspx

Fuller G, Morgan C. Bell's palsy syndrome: mimics and chameleons. Pract Neurol 2016;16:439–44. doi: 10.1136/practneurol-2016-001383. https://pn.bmj.com/content/16/6/439.long

Gagyor I, Madhok VB, Daly F, Sullivan F. Antiviral treatment for Bell's palsy (idiopathic facial paralysis). Cochrane Database of Systematic Reviews 2019, Issue 9. Art. No.: CD001869. doi: 10.1002/14651858.CD001869.pub9. https://www.cochranelibrary.com/cdsr/doi/10.1002/14651858.CD001869.pub9/full

Loscalzo J, Fauci AS, Kasper DL, Hauser S, Longo D, Jameson JL. Harrison's principles of internal medicine. 21st ed. McGraw-Hill Companies; 2022.

Resnik R, Lockwood CJ, Moore TR, Greene ME, Copel JA, Silver RM, editors. Creasy and Resnik's maternal–fetal medicine: principles and practice. 8th ed. Elsevier; 2018

Sullivan FM, Swan IR, Donnan PT, Morrison JM, Smith BH, McKinstry B, et al. Early treatment with prednisolone or acyclovir in Bell's palsy. N Engl J Med 2007;357:1598–607. doi: 10.1056/NEJMoa072006. https://www.nejm.org/doi/10.1056/NEJMoa072006

18 Low-dose aspirin for reduction of preeclampsia risk

A 33-year-old gravida 5, para 1, with a body mass index (BMI) of 28 presents at 12 weeks of gestation for her first prenatal visit. She has experienced three first-trimester losses and is currently pregnant through intrauterine insemination. Her one live birth was delivered at 36 weeks of gestation because of fetal growth restriction. She takes hydroxychloroquine for systemic lupus erythematosus. She has no other significant health issue. The most appropriate indication for low-dose aspirin administration in this patient is

(A) assisted reproductive technology pregnancy
(B) BMI
(C) history of fetal growth restriction
(D) recurrent pregnancy losses
* (E) systemic lupus erythematosus

Preeclampsia is associated with adverse maternal, fetal, and neonatal outcomes. Hypertension-related disorders remain one of the leading causes of maternal morbidity and mortality in the United States and worldwide. Women diagnosed with preeclampsia also are at increased risk of cardiovascular disease later in life. It is important not only to identify women at risk of developing preeclampsia, but also to offer interventions that may reduce the risk of preeclampsia, particularly because the prevalence of preeclampsia is increasing.

Although a number of interventions have been evaluated, only low-dose aspirin (acetylsalicylic acid) has been shown, both in randomized, controlled studies and multiple meta-analyses, to reduce the risk of preeclampsia in women at increased risk. Various trials have documented beneficial effects on perinatal mortality, preterm birth, fetal growth restriction, and preeclampsia. The size of the risk reduction varies by study because of methodological differences across the trials; however, the risk reduction generally is considered to be 10% or greater. Some studies have shown significantly greater reductions in risk, especially in preterm preeclampsia. Therefore, low-dose aspirin currently is universally recommended in women who are at high risk of preeclampsia because it has been shown to prevent or delay the onset of preeclampsia. Existing data do not demonstrate evidence of harm from daily low-dose aspirin use during pregnancy.

The mechanism responsible for the reduction in preeclampsia risk is not fully understood, but may be related to aspirin's antithrombotic and anti-inflammatory actions. Aspirin interferes with the biosynthesis of thromboxane A_2 (TXA_2), prostacyclin, and other prostaglandins in a dose-dependent fashion. Low-dose aspirin inhibits cyclooxygenase (COX-1), which inhibits platelet generation of TXA_2, reducing both platelet aggregation and vasoconstriction. By reducing other prostaglandins, such as prostaglandin E_2, aspirin provides an anti-inflammatory effect. These actions are thought to play a role in the reduction in preeclampsia risk.

There is no consensus on the ideal dose. Recommendations on when to initiate aspirin also vary. Most trials started aspirin therapy at or after 12 weeks of gestation, and evidence suggests starting before 16 weeks of gestation is more beneficial. The American College of Obstetricians and Gynecologists recommends starting between 12 and 28 weeks of gestation. This extended window is suggested because there may still be some benefit, although not as strong, when initiated after 16 weeks of gestation but before 28 weeks of gestation. In general, women are advised to continue aspirin therapy until delivery rather than discontinuing at 36 weeks of gestation because there is no evidence that continuing throughout pregnancy increases risk of bleeding. Furthermore, low-dose aspirin use is not a contraindication to receiving neuraxial anesthesia.

There are a variety of guidelines for determining who should be prescribed low-dose aspirin. These guidelines have evolved over time to include more women and will likely continue to broaden as more data become available. In general, women with one high-level risk factor and those with more than one moderate-level risk factor will benefit from low-dose aspirin. Box 18-1 outlines ACOG's current recommendations. High-level risk factors include a personal history of preeclampsia, multiple gestation, chronic hypertension, diabetes mellitus, renal disease, and autoimmune disease. Only one high-level risk factor needs to be present to recommend low-dose aspirin. If a woman has two or more moderate risk factors, low-dose aspirin also is recommended. These include nulliparity, a BMI greater than 30, a first-degree relative with preeclampsia, low socioeconomic status, advanced maternal age, or other pregnancy complications, such as small-for-gestational-age neonate, previous adverse outcome, or a pregnancy interval of greater than 10 years.

Using Box 18-1 as a reference, the described patient has autoimmune disease, which is a high-level risk factor for developing preeclampsia. She does not have any of the moderate-level risk factors. Her BMI is less than 30, and at the present time, there is insufficient evidence to recommend low-dose aspirin for women with a history of prior fetal growth restriction or early pregnancy losses. Pregnancy achieved with intrauterine insemination does not meet criteria for low-dose aspirin; however, it has been proposed that in vitro fertilization may need to be considered a moderate risk factor. In the described patient, a history of lupus

BOX 18-1

Low-Dose Aspirin Prophylaxis Recommendations

Pregnant individuals at high risk of preeclampsia with one or more of the following risk factors:

- History of preeclampsia, especially when accompanied by an adverse outcome
- Multifetal gestation
- Chronic hypertension
- Pregestational type 1 or type 2 diabetes mellitus
- Kidney disease
- Autoimmune disease (ie, systemic lupus erythematosus, antiphospholipid syndrome)
- Combinations of multiple moderate risk factors

Pregnant individuals with more than one of several moderate risk factors:

- Nulliparity
- Obesity (ie, body mass index greater than 30)
- Family history of preeclampsia (ie, mother or sister)
- Black race* (as a proxy for underlying racism)
- Lower income
- Age 35 years of older
- Personal history factors (eg, low birth weight or small for gestational age, previous adverse pregnancy outcome, greater than 10-year pregnancy interval)
- In vitro fertilization

*Black race (as a proxy for underlying racism), or lower income. The underlying risk to health is racism and not race. However, there are not yet adequate tools for measuring the known impact of racism on health. Therefore, in this document, Black race serves as a proxy for underlying racism. These factors are associated with increased risk due to environmental social, structural, and historical inequities shaping health exposures, access to health care, and the unequal distribution of resources, not biological propensities.

erythematosus is the most important risk factor for preeclampsia and is an indication for low-dose aspirin.

Baschat AA, Dewberry D, Seravalli V, Miller JL, Block-Abraham D, Blitzer MG. Maternal blood-pressure trends throughout pregnancy and development of pre-eclampsia in women receiving first-trimester aspirin prophylaxis. Ultrasound Obstet Gynecol 2018;52:728–33. doi: 10.1002/uog.18992 https://obgyn.onlinelibrary.wiley.com/doi/10.1002/uog.18992

Henderson JT, Vesco KK, Senger CA. Aspirin use to prevent preeclampsia and related morbidity and mortality. Evidence Synthesis, No. 205. Agency for Healthcare Research and Quality (US); 2021. Accessed March 17, 2022. https://www.ncbi.nlm.nih.gov/books/NBK574449/

Henderson JT, Whitlock EP, O'Conner E, Senger CA, Thompson JH, Rowland MG. Low-dose aspirin for the prevention of morbidity and mortality from preeclampsia: a systematic evidence review for the U.S. Preventive Services Task Force. Evidence Syntheses, No. 112. 2014. Accessed March 17, 2022. https://www.ncbi.nlm.nih.gov/books/NBK196392/

Honigberg MC, Zekavat SM, Aragam K, Klarin D, Bhatt DL, Scott NS, et al. Long-term cardiovascular risk in women with hypertension during pregnancy. J Am Coll Cardiol 2019;74:2743–54. doi: 10.1016/j.jacc.2019.09.052 https://www.jacc.org/doi/10.1016/j.jacc.2019.09.052

LeFevre ML. Low-dose aspirin use for the prevention of morbidity and mortality from preeclampsia: U.S. Preventive Services Task Force recommendation statement. Ann Intern Med 2014;161:819–26. doi: 10.7326/M14-1884 https://www.acpjournals.org/doi/full/10.7326/M14-1884

Low-dose aspirin use during pregnancy. ACOG Committee Opinion No. 743. American College of Obstetricians and Gynecologists. Obstet Gynecol 2018;132:e44–52. doi: 10.1097/AOG.0000000000002708 https://journals.lww.com/greenjournal/Fulltext/2018/07000/ACOG_Committee_Opinion_No__743__Low_Dose_Aspirin.57.aspx

Mallampati D, Grobman W, Rouse DJ, Werner EF. Strategies for prescribing aspirin to prevent preeclampsia: a cost-effectiveness analysis. Obstet Gynecol 2019;134:537–44. doi: 10.1097/AOG.0000000000003413 issue=09000&article=00015&type=Fulltext

Meher S, Duley L, Hunter K, Askie L. Antiplatelet therapy before or after 16 weeks' gestation for preventing preeclampsia: an individual participant data meta-analysis. Am J Obstet Gynecol 2017;216:121–8.e2. doi: 10.1016/j.ajog.2016.10.016 https://www.ajog.org/article/S0002-9378(16)30911-5/fulltext

National Institute for Health and Care Excellence. Hypertension in pregnancy: diagnosis and management. NICE guideline NG133. NICE; 2019. Accessed March 31, 2022. https://www.nice.org.uk/guidance/ng133

19 Exercise in pregnancy

A 22-year-old gravida 1 at 14 weeks of gestation is an athlete who exercises vigorously 5–6 days per week. She wants to continue her exercise regimen during pregnancy. She wears a heart rate monitor during exercise to gauge her intensity level. You advise her that vigorous exercise can be continued during pregnancy. Based on limited data on safety, it is recommended that her intensity level (as determined by percentage of her maximum heart rate) not exceed

(A) 60%
(B) 70%
(C) 80%
* (D) 90%

Regular physical activity is one of the most important steps individuals, including pregnant women, can take to improve their overall health. Pregnancy-specific benefits include less gestational weight gain, reduction in the rates of gestational diabetes mellitus and hypertensive disorders, improvement in mood, a likely reduction in cesarean births, and assistance in maintaining a healthy weight postpartum. Additionally, exercise in women who are overweight or have obesity has been shown to reduce the risk of preterm delivery.

Evidence-based guidelines for physical activity during pregnancy and the postpartum period have been developed that parallel the public health recommendations for all individuals. The American College of Obstetricians and Gynecologists encourages those without obstetric or medical comorbidities to engage in aerobic and strength-conditioning exercises before, during, and after pregnancy. The U.S. Department of Health and Human Services Physical Activity Guidelines for Americans specifies a goal of accumulating at least 150 minutes of moderate-intensity aerobic activity each week. This often is described as 30 minutes of activity 5 days per week. This recommendation also applies to previously physically inactive women. Women who have been performing vigorous-intensity exercise before pregnancy may continue their exercise regimen during pregnancy.

Exercise intensity can be monitored in several ways: target heart rates (calculated using various equations based on aerobic capacity or maximum heart rate), rating of perceived exertion, or MET (metabolic equivalent) levels. Using these monitoring tools, *moderate-intensity* exercise is defined as 40–59% of aerobic capacity reserve, a rating of perceived exertion of 12 or 13–14 on the Borg scale (Table 19-1), and a MET level of 3.0–5.9. The talk test, in which carrying on a conversation (but not singing) is possible while exercising, also can be used to gauge moderate intensity. *Vigorous intensity* is defined as 60–89% of aerobic capacity reserve, rating of perceived exertion of 15–17, and a MET level of 6 or greater. Talking during the activity is difficult if it is vigorous. Most evidence suggests that healthy pregnant women may safely perform vigorous-intensity exercise. However, because of a lack of data, an upper level of exercise intensity in pregnancy that is considered safe has not yet been established. Because limited reports have indicated that intensities exceeding the established upper level of vigorous intensity may compromise fetal well-being, exercising above 90% of maximum heart rate is not recommended in pregnant women. Intensity levels less than 90% of maximum heart rate have not been shown to adversely affect maternal or fetal well-being.

TABLE 19-1. The 15-Grade Scale for Ratings of Perceived Exertion

6	
7	Very, very light
8	
9	Very light
10	
11	Fairly light
12	
13	Somewhat hard
14	
15	Hard
16	
17	Very hard
18	
19	Very, very hard
20	

Reprinted from Borg GA. Psychophysical bases of perceived exertion. Med Sci Sports Exerc 1982;14:377–81. https://journals.lww.com/acsm-msse/Abstract/1982/05000/Psychophysical_bases_of_perceived_exertion.12.aspx

In the absence of data, arbitrary guidelines often are provided to pregnant women (particularly athletes) regarding exercise. Historically, guidance included a recommendation to keep maternal heart rate below 140 beats per minute while exercising; however, this is not evidence-based. Pregnant athletes often are advised to reduce the intensity and duration of their exercise. To improve counseling of pregnant athletes, more data are needed on vigorous exercise during pregnancy, particularly to determine whether an upper limit of exercise intensity exists that, if exceeded, places the fetus at risk. The described patient is young and healthy, and 90% of her maximum heart rate is an appropriate upper limit of intensity.

Liguori G, Feito Y, Fountaine C, Roy BA, editors. ACSM's guidelines for exercise testing and prescription 11th ed. American College of Sports Medicine; 2021.

Perales M, Artal R, Lucia A. Exercise during pregnancy. JAMA 2017;317:1113–4. doi: 10.1001/jama.2017.0593 https://jamanetwork.com/journals/jama/fullarticle/2612623

Syed H, Slayman T, DuChene Thoma K. Physical activity and exercise during pregnancy and the postpartum period. ACOG Committee Opinion No. 804. American College of Obstetricians and Gynecologists. Obstet Gynecol 2021;137:375–6. doi: 10.1097/AOG.0000000000004266 https://journals.lww.com/greenjournal/Fulltext/2021/02000/ACOG_Committee_Opinion_No__804__Physical_Activity.28.aspx

U.S. Department of Health and Human Services. Physical activity guidelines for Americans. 2nd ed. HHS; 2018. Accessed April 21, 2022. https://health.gov/sites/default/files/2019-09/Physical_Activity_Guidelines_2nd_edition.pdf

20 Increased nuchal translucency measurement

A 31-year-old primigravida at 11 weeks of gestation undergoes first-trimester screening and is found to have a nuchal translucency measurement of 6 mm. Chorionic villus sampling returns 46, XY. The most likely fetal anomaly to be found on targeted ultrasonography is

(A) abdominal wall
* (B) cardiac
(C) neural tube
(D) renal
(E) skeletal

Screening with ultrasonography and serum analytes or diagnostic testing for fetal aneuploidy should be offered to all pregnant patients. In the first trimester, ultrasonographic assessment of the nuchal region of the fetus may be performed as part of aneuploidy screening. The "nuchal translucency" refers to the normal fluid-filled hypoechoic space between the back of the neck and the overlying skin. This fluid can be measured between 10 and 14 weeks of gestation and is generally considered abnormal if the fluid measures 3.0 mm or more or above the 99th percentile for the crown–rump length.

It is imperative that nuchal translucency be measured with meticulous technique as undermeasurement by as little as 0.5 mm can significantly reduce test sensitivity. The fetus is examined in the midsagittal plane with the neck in a neutral position, the echogenic tip of the nose and rectangular shape of the palate visible anteriorly, the translucent diencephalon in the center, and the nuchal membrane posteriorly (Fig. 20-1). There are criteria for nuchal translucency measurement put forth by the Fetal Medicine Foundation, the First and Second Trimester Evaluation of Risk (FASTER) research consortium, and the Perinatal Quality Foundation. Nuchal translucency measurement should be performed only by trained and experienced sonographers (Box 20-1).

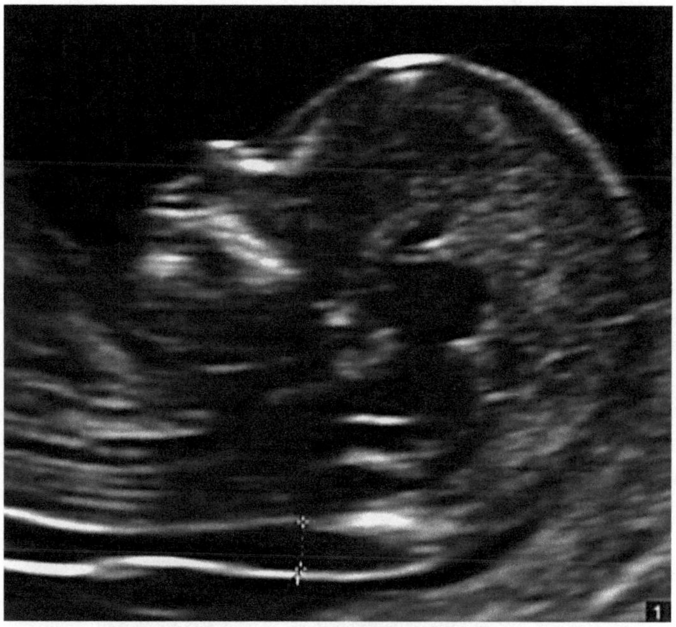

FIGURE 20-1. Nuchal translucency measuring 3.1 mm. (Used with permission of the Perinatal Quality Foundation.)

An enlarged nuchal translucency is independently associated with increased risk of aneuploidy, particularly trisomy 21 and monosomy X, and less commonly, trisomy 13 and 18 and triploidy. The risk of fetal aneuploidy increases with increasing nuchal translucency, with the risk of aneuploidy ranging from 7–75% depending on the nuchal translucency measurement. The FASTER trial showed that nuchal translucency could be combined with maternal serum analytes of β-human chorionic gonadotropin and pregnancy-associated plasma-protein A to increase detection rates for trisomy 21, with a sensitivity of 82–87% at a 5% false-positive rate.

In addition to aneuploidy, fetuses with enlarged nuchal translucency are at increased risk of structural abnormalities, including cardiac, diaphragmatic, renal, and abdominal wall defects. As with aneuploidy, the rate of structural defects increases with increasing nuchal translucency. Although renal, abdominal wall, and skeletal abnormalities may be seen with increased nuchal translucency, cardiac malformations are the most commonly associated structural abnormality and, therefore, cardiac anomaly is the correct answer in the above-described scenario. Major cardiac defects occur in approximately 4–5% of fetuses with enlarged nuchal translucency and normal karyotype. A wide range of cardiac anomalies have been reported in the setting of increased nuchal translucency measurements, with septal defects being the most common. Open neural tube defects typically are not associated with increased nuchal translucency.

Patients who are found to have increased nuchal translucency on first-trimester ultrasonography should be offered genetic counseling and diagnostic testing with either chorionic villus sampling or amniocentesis. They may also be offered noninvasive screening with cell-free DNA. Additionally, patients should undergo detailed ultrasonography at 18–20 weeks of gestation. Fetal echocardiography should be offered at 22–24 weeks of gestation to evaluate for fetal cardiac anomalies. In a small percentage of cases, increased nuchal translucency persists into the second trimester and may be seen on detailed ultrasonography at 18–20 weeks. When nuchal translucency persists, there is a risk of progression to fetal hydrops and close follow-up is recommended.

BOX 20-1

Nuchal Translucency Measurement Criteria

1. Fetus occupies majority of image:
   a. The fetal head, neck, and upper thorax should fill the majority of the image.
   b. The fetus should occupy greater than 50% of the image space.
   c. The image should NOT show the entire fetus or crown–rump length. A second fetus of the same magnitude would not fit in the surrounding space.
2. Margins of NT edges clear:
   a. The ultrasound image should be clear with thin NT membranes (lines). The angle of insonation should be perpendicular to the NT space.
3. Fetus in midsagittal plane:
   a. Midsagittal view of fetal spine seen in cervical and thoracic region
   b. Tip of nose and rectangular-shaped palate seen
   c. Third and fourth ventricle seen in fetal CNS
   d. Should NOT see zygoma, ribs, stomach, or heart
4. Fetal head in neutral position:
   a. The fetal head must be neutral without hyperflexion or hyperextension.
5. Fetus observed away from the amnion:
   a. The amnion should be seen as a separate line from the nuchal membrane in the area of the NT measurement.
6. Correct caliper placement:
   a. Measure the NT at the widest translucent space.
   b. The horizontal crossbars of the calipers must be placed on the echogenic inner borders of the nuchal membranes with none of the horizontal crossbars protruding into the translucent NT space. A vertical line connecting the two calipers should be perpendicular to the long axis of the fetus.
7. ALARA
   a. The ODS, which consists of MI and TI, must be left on each image submitted.
   b. Thermal index for bone should be displayed at this gestational age and its value should be less than or equal to 0.7.
8. Measure the NT three times and report the largest of three acceptable measurements.

Abbreviations: ALARA, as low as reasonably achievable; CNS, central nervous system; ODS, output display standard; MI, mechanical index; NT, nuchal translucency; TI, thermal index.

Modified from Nuchal Translucency Quality Review Program. NT measurement criteria. Perinatal Quality Foundation; 2019. Accessed March 31, 2022. http://ntqr.perinatalquality.org/MyFTP/Documents/NTCriteria.pdf

AIUM practice parameter for the performance of fetal echocardiography. J Ultrasound Med 2020;39:E5–16. doi: 10.1002/jum.15188 https://onlinelibrary.wiley.com/doi/10.1002/jum.15188

Malone FD, Canick JA, Ball RH, Nyberg DA, Comstock CH, Bukowski R, et al. First-trimester or second-trimester screening, or both, for Down's syndrome. First- and Second-Trimester Evaluation of Risk (FASTER) Research Consortium. N Engl J Med 2005;353:2001–11. doi: 10.1056/NEJMoa043693 https://www.nejm.org/doi/10.1056/NEJMoa043693

Screening for fetal chromosomal abnormalities: ACOG Practice Bulletin No. 226. American College of Obstetricians and Gynecologists. Obstet Gynecol 2020;136:e48–69. doi: 10.1097/AOG.0000000000004084 https://journals.lww.com/greenjournal/Fulltext/2020/10000/Screening_for_Fetal_Chromosomal_Abnormalities_.44.aspx

Sotiriadis A, Papatheodorou S, Eleftheriades M, Makrydimas G. Nuchal translucency and major congenital heart defects in fetuses with normal karyotype: a meta-analysis. Ultrasound Obstet Gynecol 2013;42:383–9. doi: 10.1002/uog.12488 https://obgyn.onlinelibrary.wiley.com/doi/10.1002/uog.12488

21 Substance use disorder

A 32-year-old multigravida presents to establish prenatal care at 7 weeks of gestation. She reports recent heroin use and continued craving for heroin, although she wants to stop using and is interested in medication-assisted treatment. The most appropriate approach to decrease the severity of neonatal opioid withdrawal syndrome in her neonate is

* (A) buprenorphine
(B) disulfiram
(C) methadone
(D) naloxone
(E) supervised withdrawal

As the nationwide opioid epidemic has escalated, so too has opioid use in pregnancy. Opioids exert their effect by binding to the mu and kappa receptors; inducing euphoria, analgesia, and sedation; and sending a signal to dopamine terminals to release dopamine, which creates a positive emotional response. Pregnancy is a unique opportunity to identify and treat women with opioid use disorder, and screening for substance use should be performed universally as part of the first prenatal visit.

Opioid use disorder is a pattern of opioid use with tolerance, craving, inability to control use, and continued use despite adverse consequences. Untreated opioid use disorder is associated with adverse pregnancy outcomes, including fetal growth restriction, placental abruption, and stillbirth. Opioid use also is associated with neonatal opioid withdrawal syndrome, a syndrome characterized by respiratory distress, autonomic instability, central nervous system irritability, and gastrointestinal dysfunction. This syndrome was previously referred to as *neonatal abstinence syndrome*. Patients who screen positive for opioid use disorder should be referred for treatment with the goal of reducing maternal and fetal adverse effects.

Regular use of opioids leads to dependence and results in withdrawal with discontinuation of the drug. Treatment of opioid use disorder is aimed at preventing withdrawal and thereby reducing relapse risk and the associated consequences. Withdrawal is characterized by muscle pain, nausea, diarrhea, sweating, rhinorrhea, tearing, dilated pupils, tremor, restlessness, goose bumps, and anxiety. Withdrawal symptoms may develop 1–3 hours after use of short-acting opioids, peak at 1–3 days, and may last 5–7 days.

Treatment of opioid use disorder is associated with decreased risks of obstetric complications. There are several options for treatment of opioid use disorder. Ultimately, the best treatment choice may vary from patient to patient based on availability and patient preferences. Shared decision making should be used to determine which treatment option is best for the patient.

Buprenorphine acts as a partial mu receptor agonist with high affinity for the receptor. Buprenorphine has some advantages in that overdose is less likely, dosage adjustments are needed less frequently, and there are fewer drug interactions. Buprenorphine can be prescribed by select health care professionals and used on an outpatient basis without need for daily visits to an opioid treatment program. Because buprenorphine has a high affinity for the mu receptor, if one takes buprenorphine while the receptors are occupied with a full agonist, buprenorphine may displace the full receptor agonist as a partial receptor agonist and may precipitate withdrawal. For this reason, it is recommended that buprenorphine be initiated once patients have abstained from short-acting opiates, including heroin and oxycodone, for 12–24 hours; long-acting opiates, including oxycontin, for at least 24 hours; and methadone, for at least 36 hours. It is not recommended that a pregnant woman transition from methadone to buprenorphine because of the risk of precipitated withdrawal and relapse. Buprenorphine does have the potential for misuse with intravenous injection and diversion because it has a high value when sold illegally.

Disulfiram is a drug used to prevent alcohol use disorder by increasing sensitivity to ethanol. It works by inhibiting the enzyme acetaldehyde dehydrogenase and causing hangover-like symptoms to develop quickly. It causes a throbbing headache, nausea, and vomiting, and may cause palpitations or even cardiac arrythmias. It is no longer considered first line in alcohol use disorder, as naltrexone and acamprosate are now more commonly used. Disulfiram also is generally avoided in pregnancy unless benefits clearly outweigh risks because it is known to cross the placenta.

Methadone is a full mu receptor agonist and weak NMDA (N-methyl-d-aspartate) receptor antagonist and is the classic drug used for medication-assisted treatment. Methadone is dispensed daily and is available only in registered opioid treatment programs. Methadone dosage may be adjusted throughout pregnancy to avoid withdrawal symptoms; even if a patient was on a stable dosage before pregnancy, they may need methadone to be titrated up to avoid withdrawal symptoms. Patients may need more than a single daily dose in pregnancy secondary to more rapid metabolism during pregnancy. An inadequate maternal methadone dose may result in withdrawal symptoms, fetal stress, maternal cravings, and increased risk of relapse.

Naloxone is an opioid receptor antagonist that is used to reverse opioid overdose. To decrease the risk of misuse of buprenorphine, a combination drug containing naloxone also is available. This product does not cause withdrawal symptoms when taken sublingually as prescribed and decreases diversion for abuse because it precipitates withdrawal symptoms when injected. The buprenorphine mono product has been recommended during pregnancy to attempt to avoid fetal exposure to naloxone out of historical concerns for fetal naloxone exposure. More recent studies have illustrated no adverse effects of buprenorphine in combination with naloxone and have shown similar outcomes when compared to buprenorphine used alone, and use of the combination buprenorphine–naloxone product is becoming more common during pregnancy.

Pregnant patients are advised to pursue medication-assisted treatment rather than supervised or unsupervised withdrawal because of the high rates of relapse and adverse outcomes associated with withdrawal, including accidental overdose. Early case reports suggested that withdrawal from opioids during pregnancy could lead to fetal distress and stillbirth. More recent studies have not clearly demonstrated this association, and more research is needed to evaluate the long-term success rates and neonatal outcomes with medically supervised withdrawal in pregnancy.

Shared decision making should be used to determine the best treatment option for the patient. Several studies have evaluated the effects of different types of medication-assisted treatment on neonatal opioid withdrawal syndrome. A double-blind, randomized controlled trial, known as the MOTHER (Maternal Opioid Treatment: Human Experimental Research) study, compared the occurrence of neonatal opioid withdrawal syndrome among neonates born to women treated with methadone with those treated with buprenorphine. This study illustrated that buprenorphine use was associated with decreased severity of neonatal opioid withdrawal syndrome when compared with methadone. These results have been replicated in several clinical trials.

In the described patient, buprenorphine is the best choice to decrease the severity of neonatal opioid withdrawal syndrome and would be superior to methadone in terms of neonatal opioid withdrawal syndrome, based on previous studies. Methadone also is an acceptable choice for a medication-assisted treatment option, and it is not recommended that patients transition from methadone to buprenorphine because of the risk of precipitated withdrawal. Whereas there are increasing data regarding safety, naloxone and supervised withdrawal are not the best answers as they are less likely to yield sustainable results for the patient. Finally, disulfiram, used for the treatment of alcohol use disorder, would not have an effect on neonatal opioid withdrawal syndrome and would be inappropriate for the patient. Buprenorphine is the best answer for medication-assisted treatment that would decrease the risk of neonatal opioid withdrawal syndrome the most in this patient.

Bell J, Towers CV, Hennessy MD, Heitzman C, Smith B, Chattin K. Detoxification from opiate drugs during pregnancy. Am J Obstet Gynecol 2016;215:374.e1–6. doi: 10.1016/j.ajog.2016.03.015 https://www.ajog.org/article/S0002-9378(16)00477-4/fulltext

Centers for Disease Control and Prevention. About opioid use during pregnancy. 2021. https://www.cdc.gov/pregnancy/opioids/basics.html

McCarthy JJ, Leamon MH, Willits NH, Salo R. The effect of methadone dose regimen on neonatal abstinence syndrome. J Addict Med 2015;9:105–10. doi: 10.1097/ADM.0000000000000099 https://journals.lww.com/journaladdictionmedicine/Abstract/2015/03000/The_Effect_of_Methadone_Dose_Regimen_on_Neonatal.5.aspx

Opioid use and opioid use disorder in pregnancy. Committee Opinion No. 711. American College of Obstetricians and Gynecologists. Obstet Gynecol 2017;130:e81–94. doi: 10.1097/AOG.0000000000002235 https://journals.lww.com/greenjournal/Fulltext/2017/08000/Committee_Opinion_No__711__Opioid_Use_and_Opioid.57.aspx

22 High risk of open neural tube defects and recommendation of dosing†

A 32-year-old gravida 1, para 1, presents for a prepregnancy visit. Her previous pregnancy was significant for gestational diabetes mellitus treated with insulin. She is on levetiracetam for seizures. Her husband has no significant medical conditions and his sister's child has an open neural tube defect (ONTD). The patient's body mass index (BMI) is 31, and a recent hemoglobin A_{1C} was 5.9%. The most appropriate prepregnancy dose of folic acid to reduce the risk of an ONTD with her next pregnancy is

(A) 400 micrograms
(B) 800 micrograms
(C) 1,000 micrograms
* (D) 4,000 micrograms

Congenital anomalies affect 2–3% of all pregnancies. Open neural tube defects are the most common malformation of the central nervous system, occurring in approximately 0.1% of the general population with 3,000 cases in the United States and 300,000 cases worldwide each year. The neural plate transitions to the neural tube, closing bidirectionally in a cranial–caudal fashion. A defect can occur anywhere along the axis. The severity of an ONTD ranges from anencephaly or craniorachischisis, to spinal lipoma or spina bifida occulta. A caudal defect in the neural groove results in anencephaly, exencephaly, encephalocele, or iniencephaly. The spinal defects include spina bifida, meningocele, myelomeningocele, myeloschisis, holorachischisis, and craniorachischisis. Incomplete closure of spinal defects in the lumbosacral region is most common.

Every pregnancy is at risk of an ONTD. Moderate to high risk factors for having an ONTD include a previous child with ONTD, family history of an ONTD, use of anticonvulsant medications, pregestational diabetes, and prepregnancy obesity with BMI of greater than 30. Neural tube defects are a genetically complex group of lesions with as many as 100 genes involved. Large-scale genome-wide association studies on neural tube defects have not been conducted. Support for a genetic association includes a higher concordance of ONTD, regardless of zygosity, in twin studies of the same sex compared with the opposite sex (1.93 versus 1.00 per 1,000), although a clear Mendelian inheritance has not been identified. There are over 20 genes affecting closure of the neural tube in mouse models, and it is reasonable to assume there are at least as many in humans. Chromosomal trisomy (18 and 13) or triploidy, microdeletions, microduplications, and individuals with Waardenburg syndrome are linked with an increased risk of ONTD.

Factors that increase the risk of an ONTD, especially if exposure occurs within the first 28 days after fertilization, include maternal hyperglycemia, pregestational diabetes, obesity, antiepileptic medication, opioid use, and elevated body temperature. Disadvantaged socioeconomic status also is a risk factor. Among the medications linked with an increased risk of ONTD, carbamazepine and valproic acid carry the highest risk with a 10- to 20-fold increase. A maternal fever in the first 28 days of pregnancy increases the risk up to 3-fold, and using a hot tub or sauna increases the risk 1.7-fold. Finally, having a partner with a previous child with an ONTD or a previous pregnancy with an ONTD increases the risk to the current pregnancy. With one affected sibling, the risk of another ONTD is 3.2%, increasing to 10% with two affected siblings. Having a second-degree relative with ONTD confers a 0.5% risk, and a third-degree relative, a 0.17% risk of ONTD in the current pregnancy.

The described patient has a BMI of 31, a history of gestational diabetes, and a hemoglobin A_{1C} value in the prediabetic range (5.7–6.4%). All three factors increase her likelihood of maternal hyperglycemia. A twofold increased risk of ONTD was identified in women with extreme obesity compared with women who had a normal BMI in a case-controlled study, a result supported in subsequent meta-analyses. A dose relationship also has been described. For every BMI increase of 1 kg/m^2 over normal weight, the odds of an ONTD in the offspring increases 1.027 times. Maternal obesity in pregnancy is associated with increased risk of an ONTD, but the mechanism of this association has yet to be determined.

Folic acid (vitamin B_9) is a water-soluble micronutrient excreted in the urine and is 30% more bioavailable than naturally occurring folate. Folic acid is found in fortified grains, natural foods, and supplements. Many countries, including the United States, have mandatory food fortification with folic acid, and supplementation worldwide has reduced the incidence of ONTD by 15–70%. Supplementation has eliminated the tendency of ONTD to affect female fetuses and decreased the rate of anencephaly. Folic acid supplementation of 400 micrograms orally per day for 1 month before pregnancy and continuing through the first 12 weeks of gestation has been shown to prevent ONTD in low-risk individuals. For moderate- or high-risk individuals, 4,000 micrograms orally per day beginning 3 months before pregnancy and continuing until 12 weeks of gestation is recommended. Folic acid has not been shown to reduce the incidence of cleft lip or palate, congenital cardiovascular defects, or other birth defects. A Cochrane review reports that additional supplementation with folic acid has not been shown to prevent a pregnancy loss (relative risk, 1.1; 95% CI, 0.94–1.28; five studies; 7,391 pregnancies, moderate-quality evidence). The Centers for Disease Control and Prevention estimates that adequate folic acid (400 micrograms daily) for at least 1 month before pregnancy and continued through the first 12 weeks of gestation may prevent as many as 50% of ONTDs in resource-challenged countries. For the high-risk person, an estimated 70% of ONTDs may be prevented with at least 3 months of 4,000 micrograms of folic acid daily.

A 2019 study used the Slone Epidemiology Center Birth Defects study data and examined the association between neural tube defects and prepregnancy folic acid supplementation through standard interviews with women within 6 months of delivery in 1,201 cases of ONTD (anencephaly, spina bifida, and encephalocele) and 11,137 controls. The four high-risk groups were those with family history, antiepileptic medication use, pregestational diabetes, and prepregnancy obesity. This study found that daily folic acid above 400 micrograms was associated with a 67% reduced risk of ONTD, and that a further reduction of ONTD occurred using a dose greater than 1,000 micrograms when obesity, pregestational diabetes, and antiepileptic medication use were present. For individuals at high risk of an ONTD, such as the patient described above, 4,000 micrograms of folic acid beginning 3 months before pregnancy and continuing until 12 weeks of gestational age is recommended.

[†]The dosages in the text were published by ACOG in 2017. For the most up-to-date dosing information, please review ACOG's guidance at acog.org.

De-Regil LM, Peña-Rosas JP, Fernández-Gaxiola AC, Rayco-Solon P. Effects and safety of periconceptional oral folate supplementation for preventing birth defects. Cochrane Database of Systematic Reviews 2015, Issue 12. Art. No.: CD007950. doi: 10.1002/14651858.CD007950.pub3 https://www.cochranelibrary.com/cdsr/doi/10.1002/14651858.CD007950.pub3/full

Manandhar M, Beydoun H, Kancherla V. Association between body mass index and folate insufficiency indicative of neural tube defects risk among nonpregnant women of childbearing age in the United States, NHANES, 2007–2010. Birth Defects Res 2020;112:490–502. doi: 10.1002/bdr2.1658 https://onlinelibrary.wiley.com/doi/10.1002/bdr2.1658

Neural tube defects. Practice Bulletin No. 187. American College of Obstetricians and Gynecologists. Obstet Gynecol 2017;130:e279–90. doi: 10.1097/AOG.0000000000002412 https://journals.lww.com/green-journal/Fulltext/2017/12000/Practice_Bulletin_No__187__Neural_Tube_Defects.41.aspx

Petersen JM, Parker SE, Benedum CM, Mitchell AA, Tinker SC, Werler MM. Periconceptional folic acid and risk of neural tube defects among higher risk pregnancies. Birth Defects Res 2019;111:1501–12. doi: 10.1002/bdr2.1579 https://onlinelibrary.wiley.com/doi/10.1002/bdr2.1579

Ramya S, Shyamasundar S, Bay BH, Dheen ST. Maternal diabetes alters expression of microRNAs that regulate genes critical for neural tube development. Front Mol Neurosci 2017;10:237. doi: 10.3389/fnmol.2017.00237 https://www.frontiersin.org/articles/10.3389/fnmol.2017.00237/full

Wilson RD, Audibert F, Brock JA, Carroll J, Cartier L, Gagnon A, et al. Pre-conception folic acid and multivitamin supplementation for the primary and secondary prevention of neural tube defects and other folic acid-sensitive congenital anomalies. J Obstet Gynaecol Can 2015;37:534–52. doi: 10.1016/s1701-2163(15)30230-9 https://www.jogc.com/article/S1701-2163(15)30230-9/fulltext

23 Diagnosis of peripartum cardiomyopathy

A 40-year-old gravida 3, para 2, at 39 weeks of gestation presents for a visit with 2 weeks of fatigue, edema, and increasing shortness of breath with her normal activities. She reports feeling short of breath when lying flat. On physical examination, her blood pressure is 135/80 mm Hg, respiratory rate is 22 breaths per minute, temperature is 37 °C (98.6 °F), and heart rate is 110 beats per minute. She has jugular venous distension to the angle of her right jaw, pulmonary rales bilaterally, and peripheral edema. She reports two previous uncomplicated pregnancies and no medications or medical conditions. The best next diagnostic test to order to confirm a diagnosis is

(A) computed tomography angiography
(B) duplex Doppler ultrasonography
* (C) echocardiogram
(D) electrocardiogram
(E) magnetic resonance imaging

The physiologic changes in the cardiovascular system comprise adaptive mechanisms to maximize oxygenation to maternal and fetal tissues and begin as early as 5 weeks of gestational age. The heart is displaced to the left and the apex is rotated laterally, which increases the cardiac silhouette on radiographic examination. Cardiac output (stroke volume times heart rate) increases 30–50% above nonpregnant states through changes in heart rate and stroke volume. After 32 weeks, heart rate maintains cardiac output since stroke volume starts to drop (Table 23-1). Dyspnea, decreased exercise tolerance, fatigue, syncope, orthopnea, and chest discomfort all potentially are normal symptoms of pregnancy that mimic heart disease.

In 2015–2016, the Centers for Disease Control and Prevention reported rates of obstetric cardiomyopathy in the peripartum period of 0.8 per 100,000 live births (2015) and 0.9 per 100,000 live births (2016). Heart disease accounted for 22.3% of all maternal deaths in the same time frame. The incidence of peripartum cardiomyopathy ranges from 1 in 1,000 to 1 in 4,000, with an estimated background rate of 5% worldwide and 3% in twin gestations. Risk factors include age over 30 years (10-fold risk above the age of 40 years), hypertension (37% of cases of peripartum cardiomyopathy), preeclampsia (22% of cases), and multigestational pregnancies (7–14.5% of cases). Personal, family, or genetic history can be elicited in familial cardiomyopathy, recurrent cardiomyopathy, or prepregnancy cardiomyopathy. Additional important factors include a history of cardiotoxic chemotherapy, valvular disease, systemic lupus, antiphospholipid syndrome, hemochromatosis, sepsis, need for intensive care, or post-respiratory arrest.

Peripartum cardiomyopathy is defined as nonischemic systolic dysfunction, with a reduced left ventricular ejection fraction below 45% at the end of pregnancy or in the months after delivery in patients who previously did not have heart disease. The signs and symptoms of heart failure at the end of pregnancy may be similar to normal symptoms and include shortness of breath with exertion, fatigue, and edema. Additional symptoms more likely in heart failure than in normal pregnancy include orthopnea, paroxysmal nocturnal dyspnea, and chest tightness. Elevated jugular venous pressure, pulmonary rales, tachypnea, tachycardia, and edema are the physical examination findings that together are concerning for heart failure. Each one independently has a broad differential diagnosis. Since the peak increase in cardiac output is between 30 and 34 weeks of gestation, it is reasonable that cardiomyopathy develops in the late third trimester or postpartum.

Peripartum cardiomyopathy is a diagnosis of exclusion. At the end of the third trimester and the first few months postpartum, the signs and symptoms of peripartum cardiomyopathy overlap with normal pregnancy and postpartum symptoms. Etiologies for peripartum cardiomyopathy include autoimmune processes, nutritional deficiencies, prolactin, genetic mutations of cardiac genes, microchimeric mutations, viral myocarditis (coxsackie virus, echovirus, parvovirus B19), and hemodynamic factors. Outcomes range from complete recovery to

TABLE 23-1. Cardiovascular Changes in a Normal Pregnancy*

	FIRST TRIMESTER	SECOND TRIMESTER	THIRD TRIMESTER	STAGE 1 LABOR	STAGE 2 LABOR	EARLY POSTPARTUM	3-6 MONTHS POSTPARTUM
Cardiac output	↑5–10%	↑↑35–45%		↑30%	↑↑50%	↑↑↑60–80% immediately, then rapidly decreases within the first hour	Return to prepregnancy values
Heart rate	↑3–5%	↑10–15%	↑15–20%	During uterine contractions: ↑40–50%		↓5–10% within 24 h; continues to decrease throughout the first 6 wk	Return to prepregnancy values
Blood pressure	↓10%	↓5%	↑5%	During uterine contractions: ↑SBP 15–25% ↑DBP 10–15%		↓SBP 5–10% within 48 h; may increase again between days 3–6 due to fluid shifts	Return to prepregnancy values
Plasma volume	↑	↑↑40–50%		↑	↑↑	↑↑↑500 mL due to autotransfusion	Return to prepregnancy values

Abbreviations: DBP, diastolic blood pressure; SBP, systolic blood pressure.

*Hemodynamic changes that occur during pregnancy, labor, and postpartum (compared with prepregnancy) should be understood to identify early interventions (such as blood pressure control and diuresis) that may be needed to prevent clinical deterioration in a woman with cardiovascular disease.

Data from Kuhn JC, Falk RS, Langesaeter E. Haemodynamic changes during labour: continuous minimally invasive monitoring in 20 healthy parturients. Int J Obstet Anesth 2017;31:74–83; Ouzounian JG, Elkayam U. Physiologic changes during normal pregnancy and delivery. Cardiol Clin 2012;30:317–29; Sanghavi M, Rutherford JD. Cardiovascular physiology of pregnancy. Circulation 2014;130:1003–8; Shen M, Tan H, Zhou S, Smith GN, Walker MC, Wen SW. Trajectory of blood pressure change during pregnancy and the role of pre-gravid blood pressure: a functional data analysis approach. Sci Rep 2017;7:6227; Sohnchen N, Melzer K, Tejada BM, Jastrow-Meyer N, Othenin-Girard V, Irion O, et al. Maternal heart rate changes during labour. Eur J Obstet Gynecol Reprod Biol 2011;158:173–8; *and* Walters BN, Walters T. Hypertension in the puerperium [letter]. Lancet 1987;2:330.

Reprinted from Pregnancy and heart disease. ACOG Practice Bulletin No. 212. American College of Obstetricians and Gynecologists. Obstet Gynecol 2019;133:e320–56. doi: 10.1097/AOG.0000000000003243 https://journals.lww.com/greenjournal/Fulltext/2019/05000/ACOG_Practice_Bulletin_No__212__Pregnancy_and.40.aspx

death and may include long-term heart failure, arrhythmia, and thromboembolism. The left ventricular ejection fraction dictates the prognosis with a low fraction at the time of diagnosis, suggesting a worse prognosis or decreased likelihood of complete resolution. Other factors affecting outcome are dilation of the left ventricle and delayed diagnosis. The IPAC (Investigations of Pregnancy-Associated Cardiomyopathy) study reported that recovery occurs in most cases by 6 months. If the initial left ventricular ejection fraction was 0.30 or greater, 85% of patients had an ejection fraction above 0.50. There was little improvement in the ejection fraction after 6 months. If there is incomplete recovery of the heart function, there is an increased chance of recurrence with a subsequent pregnancy.

Diagnostic studies are used to distinguish causes of heart failure. In the described patient, the best next test to confirm the diagnosis is echocardiography. Typical findings include left ventricular systolic dysfunction, left ventricular dilation, ventricular and atrial enlargement, valvular regurgitation, and pulmonary hypertension. Echocardiography measures the function of the heart and, therefore, is the confirmatory test. The other tests—electrocardiogram, duplex Doppler ultrasonography, computed tomography angiography, and magnetic resonance imaging—may eliminate other possible etiologies; however, none will confirm the diagnosis of peripartum cardiomyopathy.

If left ventricular function is preserved, preeclampsia or a pulmonary embolism may be the underlying condition. Preeclampsia with resultant heart failure more often presents before delivery and is associated with preserved ejection fraction, cardiac hypertrophy, and better overall prognosis compared with peripartum cardiomyopathy. More than 50% of peripartum cardiomyopathy is not related to preeclampsia, and an estimated 90% of preeclampsia with severe features does not result in cardiomyopathy. Left ventricular hypertrophy may be seen with hypertensive disease or with hypertrophic cardiomyopathy. Congenital heart disease and noncompliant left ventricular function first can be seen in pregnancy with an echocardiogram.

The echocardiogram is the first-line test, and it should be completed as soon as possible. The criteria for diagnosis are as follows: heart failure within 1 month of delivery and up to 5 months postpartum in the absence of other causes; left ventricular dysfunction on echocardiography with an ejection fraction less than 45% or motion-mode fractional shortening less than 30%, or both; and a left ventricular end diastolic dimension of greater than 2.7 cm/m^2. Other diagnostic tests may reveal noncardiac causes or eliminate options in the differential diagnosis but are not specific enough to diagnose cardiomyopathy. For example, a chest X-ray may reveal an enlarged cardiac silhouette and pulmonary venous congestion. A spiral computed tomography can evaluate for a pulmonary embolism in patients with dyspnea, tachycardia, and preserved left ventricular ejection fraction and can provide limited information to narrow the diagnosis. An electrocardiogram often reveals sinus tachycardia and nonspecific changes in pregnancy alone, or in heart failure, or both. Magnetic resonance imaging assesses cardiac volumes, left ventricular ejection fraction, and evaluation of the cardiac muscle. Magnetic resonance imaging currently remains an adjunct imaging method for peripartum cardiomyopathy.

Treatment of peripartum cardiomyopathy focuses on controlling volume status (diuretics or nitrites), neutralizing hormonal responses (nitrites and hydralazine before birth followed by an angiotensin-converting enzyme inhibitor or angiotensin receptor blockers after delivery), and reducing arrhythmic and thromboembolic events (Fig. 23-1). A multidisciplinary planning with a cardio-obstetrics team or cardiology and maternal–fetal medicine subspecialists is ideal to optimize maternal status before delivery and limit fluid overload after delivery.

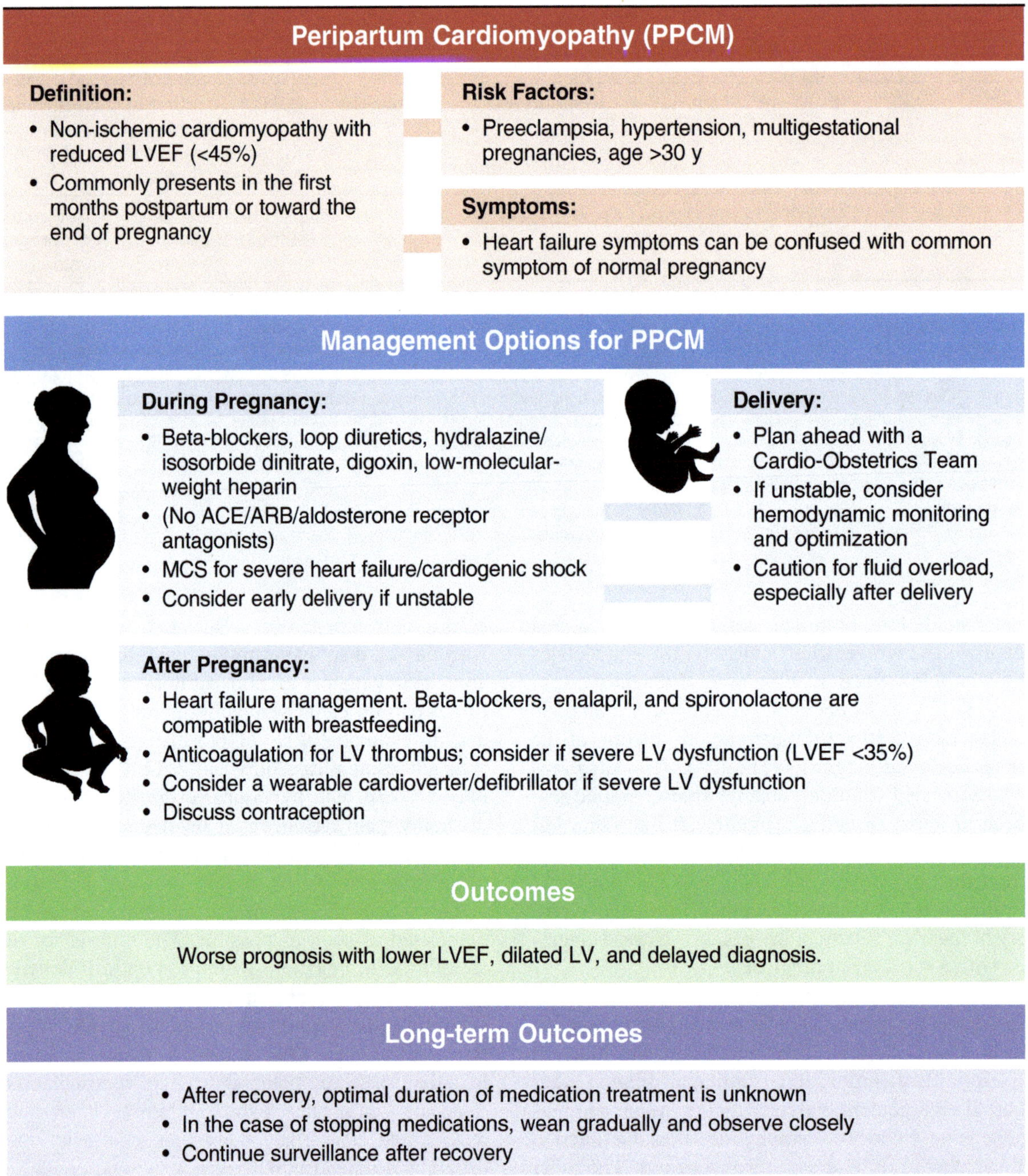

FIGURE 23-1. Diagnosis, management, and outcomes for peripartum cardiomyopathy. Diagnostic criteria, symptoms, and risk factors can aid in the diagnosis. Medications need to be tailored to pregnancy and breast-feeding status. Short- and long-term outcomes are variable and serial follow-up is important. Abbreviations: ACE, angiotensin converting enzyme inhibitor; ARB, angiotensin receptor blocker; LV, left ventricle; LVEF, left ventricular ejection fraction; MCS, mechanical circulatory support; PPCM, peripartum cardiomyopathy. Modified from Davis MB, Arany Z, McNamara DM, Goland S, Elkayam U. Peripartum cardiomyopathy: JACC state-of-the-art review. J Am Coll Cardiol 2020;75:207–21. doi: 10.1016/j.jacc.2019.11.014 https://www.sciencedirect.com/science/article/pii/S0735109719384578

Patients who have peripartum cardiomyopathy should receive counseling regarding contraception at the time of diagnosis and before hospital discharge with a goal of preventing a subsequent pregnancy for at least 6 months. During this time, cardiac function should be monitored for a return to normal function. Estrogen-containing contraceptives should be avoided because of the increased thromboembolic risk. Progesterone-only or long-acting reversible contraceptive methods are recommended with permanent sterilization only considered if the patient has completed her childbearing.

Arany Z, Elkayam U. Peripartum cardiomyopathy. Circulation 2016;133:1397–409. doi: 10.1161/CIRCULATIONAHA.115.020491 https://www.ahajournals.org/doi/10.1161/CIRCULATIONAHA.115.020491

Cunningham FG, Byrne JJ, Nelson DB. Peripartum cardiomyopathy. Obstet Gynecol 2019;133:167–79. doi: 10.1097/AOG.0000000000003011 https://journals.lww.com/greenjournal/Fulltext/2019/01000/Peripartum_Cardiomyopathy.23.aspx

Davis MB, Arany Z, McNamara DM, Goland S, Elkayam U. Peripartum cardiomyopathy: JACC state-of-the-art review. J Am Coll Cardiol 2020;75:207–21. doi: 10.1016/j.jacc.2019.11.014 https://www.sciencedirect.com/science/article/pii/S0735109719384578

Honigberg MC, Givertz MM. Peripartum cardiomyopathy. BMJ 2019;364:k5287. doi: 10.1136/bmj.k5287 https://www.bmj.com/content/364/bmj.k5287.long

Hoyert DL, Uddin SF, Miniño AM. Evaluation of the pregnancy status checkbox on the identification of maternal deaths. Natl Vital Stat Rep 2020;69:1–25. https://www.cdc.gov/nchs/data/nvsr/nvsr69/nvsr69_01-508.pdf

Pregnancy and heart disease. ACOG Practice Bulletin No. 212. American College of Obstetricians and Gynecologists. Obstet Gynecol 2019;133:e320–56. doi: 10.1097/AOG.0000000000003243 https://journals.lww.com/greenjournal/Fulltext/2019/05000/ACOG_Practice_Bulletin_No__212__Pregnancy_and.40.aspx

Schaufelberger M. Cardiomyopathy and pregnancy. Heart 2019;105:1543–51. doi: 10.1136/heartjnl-2018-313476 https://heart.bmj.com/content/105/20/1543.long

Schiau C, Schiau Ş, Dudea SM, Manole S. Cardiovascular magnetic resonance: contribution to the exploration of cardiomyopathies. Med Pharm Rep 2019;92:326–36. doi: 10.15386/mpr-1343 https://www.ncbi.nlm.nih.gov/pmc/articles/PMC6853046/

24 Anticoagulation for use postpartum and during breastfeeding

A 40-year-old multiparous patient had a spontaneous vaginal birth yesterday. Her pregnancy was notable for diagnosis of a deep vein thrombosis (DVT) at 34 weeks of gestation. She received a labor epidural that was removed yesterday morning after delivery. The patient plans to breastfeed. The best next step in management of her postpartum anticoagulation is initiation of

(A) antiplatelet agent
(B) direct thrombin inhibitor
(C) factor Xa inhibitor
* (D) heparin
(E) vitamin K antagonist

This patient experienced a venous thrombotic event (VTE) in the middle of the third trimester, and she must continue treatment for this VTE after giving birth. Multiple clinical issues influence when and how anticoagulation is administered. Recent regional anesthetic and delivery have increased her risk of bleeding if anticoagulation is started too soon. Furthermore, her intention to breastfeed also modifies agent selection during the postpartum, lactating period.

Pregnant women have a fourfold to fivefold increased risk of VTE when compared with nonpregnant women. Specific clotting events are spread evenly between the antenatal and postpartum periods, with approximately 75% occurring as DVT compared with around 25% as pulmonary embolism. The risk of VTE begins early in the first trimester with initial physiologic changes, although the actual incidence of clotting appears to be highest in the third trimester. The additional risks in later pregnancy appear to be caused by stasis from anatomic changes during the third trimester. After giving birth, the risk of a clotting event is higher than during pregnancy. Risk factors for VTE include a previous clot; presence of thrombophilia; pelvic surgery (such as with a cesarean birth); complications during delivery, such as infection or hemorrhage; and comorbidities, such as morbid obesity, sickle cell disease, autoimmune diseases, and preeclampsia.

Signs and symptoms that suggest the development of DVT, such as pain and swelling in the extremities, are nonspecific and can be confused with typical pregnancy symptoms. Larger venous clots may present with back pain, flank pain, or significant swelling of the entire leg. An evaluation for DVT includes initial compression ultrasonography of the proximal veins. When results are negative or equivocal and more extensive clot is suspected, as in iliac vein thrombosis, additional imaging with Doppler ultrasonography of the iliac vein, venography, or magnetic resonance imaging may be required. Although measurement of D-dimer levels is sometimes used in the nonpregnant population, false-negative D-dimer levels have been reported in pregnant women, and this modality currently is not recommended as part of the evaluation for VTE during pregnancy or in the postpartum period.

Once a DVT has been diagnosed during pregnancy, duration of therapy depends on gestational age at diagnosis and contributing factors, such as a woman's inherited thrombophilia status, her personal VTE history, route of delivery, and body mass index. Most often, given the hypercoagulable state of pregnancy, adjusted dose anticoagulation would be recommended for women with acute VTE occurring during pregnancy. Given this patient's VTE at 34 weeks of gestation, international consensus guidelines suggest that after initial treatment (3–6 months of anticoagulation), intensity can be decreased to intermediate or prophylactic anticoagulation. Coordination of care with a hematologist for specific case management is recommended. Table 24-1 shows recommended prophylaxis in several scenarios.

The Society for Obstetric Anesthesia and Perinatology has published consensus guidelines addressing specific considerations for regional anesthesia and thromboprophylaxis among pregnant and postpartum women. Practice-specific protocols may exist, and initiation of anticoagulation should be coordinated among practitioners. Specific recommendations are outlined in Table 24-2. When pharmacologic anticoagulation has been held or discontinued, such as intrapartum or before a procedure (cerclage or amniocentesis, for example), pneumatic compression devices are recommended when applicable (as in postpartum).

Although injectable therapies are strongly preferred during pregnancy given their inability to cross the placenta, a variety of options are available for postpartum therapy. Anticoagulation therapy should be selected based on the duration of therapy, lactation status, and patient preference. Heparin or low-molecular-weight heparin are the most frequently used agents during the initial postpartum and breastfeeding period for several reasons. In the scenario described, the patient has a relatively recent VTE (within 3 months) and needs therapeutic dosing of her anticoagulation. Postpartum, it often is simpler to resume the same medication that was used antepartum. Although some women may prefer a vitamin K antagonist, such as warfarin, they need to be bridged with dose-adjusted, low-molecular-weight heparin or unfractionated heparin to avoid paradoxical thrombosis until reaching the target international normalized ratio (INR), usually 2–3.

TABLE 24-1. Recommended Pharmacologic Thromboprophylaxis and the Postpartum Period

CLINICAL SCENARIO	POSTPARTUM MANAGEMENT
VTE diagnosed during pregnancy	Adjusted-dose LMWH/UFH for a minimum of 6 weeks postpartum. Longer duration of therapy may be indicated depending on the timing of VTE during pregnancy, prior VTE history, or presence of a thrombophilia. Oral anticoagulants may be considered postpartum based on planned duration of therapy, lactation, and patient preference.
Single provoked VTE, no known thrombophilia	Surveillance without anticoagulation therapy or postpartum prophylactic anticoagulation therapy if the patient has additional risk factors
History of single unprovoked VTE, not on long-term anticoagulation	Prophylactic, intermediate-dose, or adjusted-dose LMWH/UFH regimen for 6 weeks postpartum
Low-risk thrombophilia without previous VTE	Surveillance without anticoagulation therapy or postpartum prophylactic anticoagulation therapy if patient has additional risk factors
Low-risk thrombophilia with a family history of VTE	Postpartum prophylactic anticoagulation therapy or intermediate-dose LMWH/UFH
Low-risk thrombophilia with single previous VTE not on lifelong anticoagulation	Postpartum prophylactic anticoagulation therapy or intermediate-dose LMWH/UFH
High-risk thrombophilia without previous VTE	Postpartum prophylactic anticoagulation therapy or intermediate-dose LMWH/UFH
High-risk thrombophilia with single prior VTE not on lifelong anticoagulation	Postpartum prophylactic anticoagulation therapy or intermediate- or adjusted-dose LMWH/UFH for 6 weeks (therapy level should be equal to the selected antepartum treatment)
Two or more episodes of VTE not on lifelong anticoagulation regardless of thrombophilia status	Postpartum anticoagulation therapy with intermediate-dose or adjusted-dose LMWH/UFH for 6 weeks (therapy level should be equal to selected antepartum treatment)
Two or more episodes of VTE—receiving long-term anticoagulation therapy regardless of thrombophilia status	Resumption of long-term anticoagulation therapy. Oral anticoagulants may be considered postpartum based on planned duration of therapy, lactation, and patient preference.

Abbreviations: LMW, low molecular weight; H/UFH, heparin or unfractionated heparin.

Modified from Thromboembolism in pregnancy. ACOG Practice Bulletin No. 196. American College of Obstetricians and Gynecologists [published erratum appears in Obstet Gynecol 2018;132:1068]. Obstet Gynecol 2018;132:e1–17. doi: 10.1097/AOG.0000000000002706 https://journals.lww.com/greenjournal/Fulltext/2018/07000/ACOG_Practice_Bulletin_No__196__Thromboembolism_in.54.aspx

TABLE 24-2. Timing of Neuraxial Anesthesia in Relation to Pharmacologic Anticoagulation*

DOSAGE REGIMEN	POSTPARTUM
Unfractionated heparin prophylaxis twice daily	Wait at least 1 h after neuraxial blockade and catheter removal before restarting heparin.
Unfractionated heparin dose adjusted	Wait at least 1 h after neuraxial blockade or catheter removal before restarting heparin.
Low-dose LMWH prophylaxis	Wait at least 12 h after neuraxial blockade and at least 4 h after catheter removal to restart LMWH prophylaxis.
Intermediate-dose or adjusted-dose LMWH	Consider waiting at least 24 h after neuraxial blockade and at least 4 h after catheter removal to restart LMWH anticoagulation.

Abbreviation: LMWH, low-molecular-weight heparin.

*The dosages in the table were published by ACOG in 2018. For the most up-to-date dosing information, please review ACOG's guidance at acog.org.

Data from Thromboembolism in pregnancy. ACOG Practice Bulletin No. 196. American College of Obstetricians and Gynecologists [published erratum appears in Obstet Gynecol 2018;132:1068]. Obstet Gynecol 2018;132:e1–17. doi: 10.1097/AOG.0000000000002706 https://journals.lww.com/greenjournal/Fulltext/2018/07000/ACOG_Practice_Bulletin_No__196__Thromboembolism_in.54.aspx

Heparin, low-molecular-weight heparin, and warfarin are generally accepted as safe during breastfeeding and have not been shown to accumulate in breast milk. Currently, alternative agents for VTE treatment in nonpregnant adults, such as oral direct thrombin inhibitors, including dabigatran, are not used in pregnancy and during lactation because of the lack of data on safety and efficacy. Similarly, anti-Xa inhibitors, such as rivaroxaban, apixaban, edoxaban, and betrixaban, also lack supportive data for use during lactation. These agents have been found in human breast milk at detectable levels.

Bates SM, Jaeschke R, Stevens SM, Goodacre S, Wells PS, Stevenson MD, et al. Diagnosis of DVT: antithrombotic therapy and prevention of thrombosis, 9th ed: American College of Chest Physicians Evidence-Based Clinical Practice Guidelines. Chest 2012;141:e351S–418S. doi: 10.1378/chest.11-2299. https://journal.chestnet.org/article/S0012-3692(12)60128-7/fulltext

Chan WS, Rey E, Kent NE, Chan WS, Kent NE, Rey E, et al. Venous thromboembolism and antithrombotic therapy in pregnancy. VTE in Pregnancy Guideline Working Group, Society of Obstetricians and Gynecologists of Canada. J Obstet Gynaecol Can 2014;36:527–53. doi: 10.1016/s1701-2163(15)30569-7. https://www.jogc.com/article/S1701-2163(15)30569-7/fulltext

Middleton P, Shepherd E, Gomersall JC. Venous thromboembolism prophylaxis for women at risk during pregnancy and the early postnatal period. Cochrane Database of Systematic Reviews 2021, Issue 3. Art. No.: CD001689. DOI: 10.1002/14651858.CD001689.pub4

Thromboembolism in pregnancy. ACOG Practice Bulletin No. 196. American College of Obstetricians and Gynecologists [published erratum appears in Obstet Gynecol 2018;132:1068]. Obstet Gynecol 2018;132:e1–17. doi: 10.1097/AOG.0000000000002706. https://journals.lww.com/greenjournal/Fulltext/2018/07000/ACOG_Practice_Bulletin_No__196__Thromboembolism_in.54.aspx

25 Thrombocytopenia

A 39-year-old primiparous patient at 28 weeks of gestation presents for evaluation of hypertension, and vital signs include a blood pressure of 155/100 mm Hg, a pulse of 110 beats per minute, and brisk reflexes. Magnesium sulfate and betamethasone are initiated. Laboratory test results include creatinine of 1.2 mg/dL, aspartate aminotransferase (AST) and alanine aminotransferase (ALT) of 736 and 502 IU/L, respectively, and a platelet count of 30,000/mm^3. Ultrasonography reveals the fetus in breech presentation. The best next step in the treatment of this patient is

(A) cesarean birth
(B) intravenous dexamethasone
(C) intravenous immunoglobulin
(D) rebolus magnesium sulfate
* (E) transfuse platelets

The patient's most immediate need is to receive a transfusion of platelets given the severity of her thrombocytopenia, the diagnosis of HELLP (hemolysis, elevated liver enzymes, and low platelet count) syndrome, and the need for cesarean birth (because of malpresentation). Her diagnosis precludes expectant management, and treatment by delivery is indicated. Before surgery can be performed, platelet transfusion is indicated.

Hemolysis, elevated liver enzymes, and low platelet count syndrome is a more severe form of preeclampsia. Preeclampsia occurs in approximately 5% of pregnancies in the United States. The risk factors for preeclampsia can be found in Box 25-1. Preeclampsia is diagnosed with new-onset hypertension (blood pressure greater than 140/90 mm Hg) identified two times at least 4 hours apart, along with new-onset proteinuria in pregnancy at more than 20 weeks of gestation. Diagnostic criteria for preeclampsia also may include new-onset hypertension with thrombocytopenia (platelet count of less than 100,000/mm^3), serum creatinine concentration greater than 1.1 mg/dL or a doubling of serum creatinine in the absence of other renal disease, liver transaminases above twice the upper limit of normal, pulmonary edema, or new-onset headache unresponsive to usual treatments. To determine disease management, preeclampsia is divided into severe (including HELLP syndrome) and not severe features. Of women with preeclampsia, approximately 10% will have HELLP syndrome.

BOX 25-1

Risk Factors for Preeclampsia

Multifetal gestation	Prepregnancy body mass index greater than 30
Preeclampsia in a prior pregnancy	Antiphospholipid antibody syndrome
Chronic hypertension	Maternal age older than 35 years
Pregestational diabetes	Kidney disease
Gestational diabetes	Assisted reproductive technology
Thrombophilia	Obstructive sleep apnea
Nulliparity	Systemic lupus erythematosus

Reprinted from Gestational hypertension and preeclampsia. ACOG Practice Bulletin No. 222. American College of Obstetricians and Gynecologists. Obstet Gynecol 2020;135:e237–60. doi: 10.1097/AOG.0000000000003891 https://journals.lww.com/greenjournal/Fulltext/2020/06000/Gestational_Hypertension_and_Preeclampsia__ACOG.46.aspx

A diagnosis of HELLP syndrome is based on laboratory study findings including lactate dehydrogenase increased to 600 IU/L, AST and ALT concentrations greater than twice the upper limit of normal, and a platelet count of less than 100,000/mm^3. It often is diagnosed in the third trimester of pregnancy but may present after delivery. Symptoms include epigastric pain and generalized malaise, usually in combination with signs of preeclampsia. A minority of women (15%) with HELLP syndrome do not have hypertension or proteinuria at diagnosis. The etiology for declining platelet counts is uncertain but appears to be associated with platelet consumption and platelet activation and aggregation. In this case, platelet function can be impaired. The elevation in liver enzymes usually follows a pattern with AST concentrations increasing higher than ALT concentrations. Aspartate aminotransferase is the dominant transaminase released into maternal circulation in liver dysfunction from preeclampsia and is related to periportal necrosis. The pattern of transaminase elevation can help separate HELLP syndrome from other causes of liver disease. As hepatic function declines, increases in bilirubin and decreases in hepatic synthetic function can lead to abnormalities of prothrombin time, fibrinogen, and sometimes coagulation (either with significant liver dysfunction or when concurrent placental abruption is noted).

Regarding obstetric outcomes, HELLP syndrome is associated with prematurity and fetal growth restriction, which are thought to be independent of the low platelets but associated with preeclampsia. A diagnosis of HELLP syndrome generally precludes the option for inpatient expectant management. The treatment for HELLP syndrome is delivery, usually in conjunction with magnesium sulfate to prevent seizures. Delaying delivery for administration of antenatal corticosteroids is based on strict selection criteria and is best accomplished in a tertiary care center with resources for maternal and neonatal care. The route of delivery should be determined by routine obstetric indications. However, induction of labor in the setting of preeclampsia with severe features at less than 28 weeks of gestation often results in cesarean birth (as often as 97%).

After delivery, close monitoring of maternal clinical status and laboratory values is recommended with assessment of liver function testing at least at 12-hour intervals. On average, platelet nadir occurs at around 24 hours after delivery, whereas disease severity may peak up to 2 days after delivery. If platelet counts continue to drop and AST and ALT concentrations continue to increase at 4 days after delivery, alternate diagnoses should be considered. Additionally, for women with pregnancies notable for early-onset preeclampsia, alternate diagnoses should be entertained. Platelet transfusions should be considered if a platelet count is less than 50,000/mm^3, and cesarean birth is indicated or if disseminated intravascular coagulation is suspected.

The decision to transfuse platelets is either therapeutic, when bleeding poses an active clinical concern, or prophylactic, when platelets are low enough to give concern for spontaneous bleeding. A patient at risk of active bleeding with thrombocytopenia should be transfused to keep platelet counts above 50,000/mm^3. The need for ongoing platelet transfusion depends on the etiology of the thrombocytopenia and the presence or absence of active bleeding. For most major surgical procedures, the platelet count should be above 50,000/mm^3. The platelet count must be above 80,000–100,000/mm^3 to receive regional anesthesia. Administration of platelets to prevent spontaneous bleeding is initiated at a much lower platelet count—approximately 15,000–30,000/mm^3, depending on the etiology of the disease. Platelets are ordered as 4–6 units of pooled platelets or 1 pooled apheresis unit and are expected to increase platelets by 30,000/mm^3. One pooled apheresis unit of platelets or 6 units of pooled platelets are typically transfused over 20 to 30 minutes. In the case of massive blood product replacement, with risk of transfusion-associated circulatory overload, the transfusion rate may be much slower, at approximately 4 hours.

Thrombocytopenia, defined as a platelet count of less than 150,000/mm^3, is managed based on the clinical status, degree, and etiology of the thrombocytopenia. Some variation in platelet counts exists during pregnancy, with a trend toward lower averages observed during the third trimester. Hypertensive disorders in pregnancy are the cause of up to 20% of cases of maternal thrombocytopenia. The two mechanisms for thrombocytopenia are broadly grouped as either increased platelet destruction or decreased platelet production. Increased destruction is more commonly noted in pregnancy in immunologic activation, platelet consumption from bleeding, or abnormal platelet activation. Decreased production of platelets would be associated with bone marrow disorders or nutritional deficiencies.

In the scenario above, platelet transfusion is the best next step to increase this patient's platelet count from 30,000/mm^3 to a number safe for abdominal surgery. Although delivery by cesarean is indicated given the breech presentation and diagnosis of HELLP syndrome, it cannot be safely accomplished until the platelets are at or above 50,0000/mm^3. Repeating the magnesium bolus will not treat or alter her current course and would be used when a patient with eclampsia is seizing despite being on magnesium sulfate.

Intravenous dexamethasone has been evaluated for its effect on maternal outcomes in HELLP syndrome and has not been shown to be beneficial. Administration of intravenous immunoglobulin, often given in conjunction with corticosteroids, is used for the treatment of other causes of thrombocytopenia, such as immune thrombocytopenia and thrombotic thrombocytopenia purpura. There is no role for intravenous immunoglobulin in the treatment of HELLP syndrome unless platelet counts continue to decline through the fourth postpartum day, and then other etiologies should be considered.

Gestational hypertension and preeclampsia. ACOG Practice Bulletin No. 222. American College of Obstetricians and Gynecologists. Obstet Gynecol 2020;135:e237–60. doi: 10.1097/AOG.0000000000003891 https://journals.lww.com/greenjournal/Fulltext/2020/06000/Gestational_Hypertension_and_Preeclampsia__ACOG.46.aspx

Kaufman RM, Djulbegovic B, Gernsheimer T, Kleinman S, Tinmouth AT, Capocelli KE, et al. Platelet transfusion: a clinical practice guideline from the AABB. Ann Intern Med 2015;162:205–13. doi: 10.7326/M14-1589 https://www.acpjournals.org/doi/full/10.7326/M14-1589

Neiger R, Contag SA, Coustan DR. The resolution of preeclampsia-related thrombocytopenia. Obstet Gynecol 1991;77:692–5. https://journals.lww.com/greenjournal/Abstract/1991/05000/The_Resolution_of_Preeclampsia_Related.10.aspx

Schiffer CA, Bohlke K, Delaney M, Hume H, Magdalinski AJ, McCullough JJ, et al. Platelet transfusion for patients with cancer: American Society of Clinical Oncology Clinical Practice Guideline update. J Clin Oncol 2018;36:283–99. doi: 10.1200/JCO.2017.76.1734 https://ascopubs.org/doi/10.1200/JCO.2017.76.1734

Sibai BM. Evaluation and management of severe preeclampsia before 34 weeks' gestation. Publications Committee, Society for Maternal–Fetal Medicine. Am J Obstet Gynecol 2011;205:191–8. doi: 10.1016/j.ajog.2011.07.017 https://www.ajog.org/article/S0002-9378(11)00918-5/fulltext

Thrombocytopenia in pregnancy. ACOG Practice Bulletin No. 207. American College of Obstetricians and Gynecologists. Obstet Gynecol 2019;133:e181–93. doi: 10.1097/AOG.0000000000003100 https://journals.lww.com/greenjournal/Fulltext/2019/03000/ACOG_Practice_Bulletin_No__207__Thrombocytopenia.43.aspx

26 Hepatitis B treatment

A 31-year-old primiparous patient presents for initial prenatal care at 28 weeks of gestation. Her laboratory studies are notable for positive hepatitis B surface antigen, positive hepatitis B core antibodies, and negative immunoglobulin M antibody to hepatitis B core antigen, and her hepatitis B DNA viral load is greater than 10^8 copies/mL. Given her test results, the best next step in reducing the risk of neonatal infection is

(A) avoidance of breastfeeding
(B) avoidance of fetal scalp electrode
(C) cesarean birth at term
* (D) prenatal antiretroviral medication

The described patient's laboratory studies indicate chronic hepatitis B virus (HBV) infection. The best next step to reduce the risk of neonatal infection in a woman with high viral load is the initiation of antiretroviral medication during the third trimester and planned administration of hepatitis B immunoglobulin and the HBV vaccine to the neonate.

Hepatitis B is a DNA virus in the Hepadnaviridae family. Infection from hepatitis B may be acute or may result in a chronic carrier state. Hepatitis B virus can be passed by sexual or parenteral contact and by vertical transmission. The American College of Obstetricians and Gynecologists and the U.S. Preventive Services Task Force recognize the limitations of screening-based testing because most screening protocols have been shown to detect around 60% of HBV carriers. Instead, universal testing for HBV infection is recommended during pregnancy at the first prenatal visit. When either acute or chronic HBV infection is diagnosed, screening for hepatitis C and D also should be performed, and vaccination should be offered to household and sexual contacts who are not immune.

Acute infection with HBV usually is mild for the woman and often leads to an acute resolved infection and immunity. Hepatitis B infection is the most common etiology for jaundice in pregnancy. Treatment usually is supportive. Approximately 1% of individuals with acute infection will have liver failure.

The diagnosis of acute HBV infection is based on positive hepatitis B surface antigen (HBsAg) and immunoglobulin M (IgM) antibody to hepatitis B core antigen. Acute HBV infection has a high risk of mother-to-child transmission, and vertically acquired HBV is likely to lead to chronic infection in up to 90% of infants. During the first trimester, the risk of vertical infection is estimated at nearly 10%, increasing to as high as 60% at or near delivery with acute infections in the absence of neonatal prophylaxis.

As hepatitis infection progresses, immune response (through production of antibody) changes over time. Chronic HBV infection is based on the presence of HBsAg for more than 6 months, along with the presence of antibody to hepatitis B core antigen. Pregnancy in individuals with chronic HBV generally is well tolerated in the absence of severe liver disease. The immune tolerant state of pregnancy (shift toward humoral immune response) may result in hepatic flares. *Hepatic flares* are defined as a twofold to threefold rise in alanine aminotransferase (ALT) that is above the upper limits of normal. Predictors of hepatic flares are not known and remain relatively uncommon. Among women with chronic HBV infection, the hormonal milieu and the hemodynamic and immunologic changes of pregnancy can worsen or unmask underlying liver disease. Pregnancy outcomes among women with chronic HBV often are similar to those in women without HBV. Some studies have found possible associations with chronic HBV in pregnancy and increased risk of gestational diabetes, prematurity, and low-birth-weight infants. Women with liver cirrhosis have a significant risk of perinatal complications and adverse fetal outcomes, such as fetal growth restriction, preterm birth, and fetal death. Pregnant women with varices have an increased risk of esophageal bleeding given their increased plasma volume and increases in intra-abdominal pressure.

Positive surface antibody titers demonstrate clearance or immunity to the infection, either due to natural infection or immunization. Antibody to hepatitis B core is only demonstrated with actual infection (acute, chronic, or immune due to natural infection). Table 26-1 shows varying combinations of antigen and antibody test results and aids in interpretation of hepatitis B infection status.

Women with chronic HBV infection should have baseline liver function tests and hepatitis B viral load (DNA) drawn every trimester during pregnancy and be counseled on potential treatments and risks including transmission to the fetus. If a woman is being treated for chronic HBV infection with antiviral therapy and becomes pregnant, the risks and benefits of continuing therapy should be reviewed. If a therapeutic result (virologic remission) has been reached, then treatment can be ended. If the patient was on interferon or other antiviral agents, and ongoing therapy is warranted, tenofovir disoproxil fumarate, which has low incidence of HBV resistance and more favorable safety profile during pregnancy, can be substituted. Indications to start antiviral therapy in pregnant patients are similar to those in nonpregnant individuals, with elevated ALT greater than twice the upper limit of normal and HBV DNA greater than 200,000 IU/mL in the presence of positive HBsAg. In contrast, if a patient is in the second or third trimester and has a viral load over 2×10^5 IU/mL or over 10^6 copies/mL, even in the setting of normal ALT levels, they should be started on tenofovir disoproxil fumarate to further reduce the risk of transmission to the fetus. Tenofovir disoproxil fumarate and telbivudine have no increased risk of teratogenicity based on The Antiretroviral Pregnancy Registry, which began in 1989. When indicated, treatment with tenofovir disoproxil

TABLE 26-1. Interpretation of Hepatitis B Virus Testing

TEST	RESULTS	INTERPRETATION
HBsAg	Negative	Susceptible
Anti-HBc	Negative	
Anti-HBs	Negative	
HBsAg	Negative	Immune due to natural infection
Anti-HBc	Positive	
Anti-HBs	Positive	
HBsAg	Negative	Immune due to hepatitis B vaccination*
Anti-HBc	Negative	
Anti-HBs	Positive	
HBsAg	Positive	Acutely infected
Anti-HBc	Positive	
IgM anti-HBc	Positive	
Anti-HBs	Negative	
HBsAg	Positive	Chronically infected
Anti-HBc	Positive	
IgM anti-HBc	Negative	
Anti-HBs	Negative	
HBsAg	Negative	Four interpretations possible†
Anti-HBc	Positive	
Anti-HBs	Negative	

*Antibody response (anti-HGs) can be measured quantitatively or qualitatively. A protective antibody response is reported quantitatively as 10 or more milli-international units (10 mIU/mL) or qualitatively as positive. Postvaccination testing should be completed 1–2 months after the third vaccine dose for results to be meaningful.

†Four interpretations: might be recovering from acute HBV infections; might be distantly immune and test not sensitive enough to detect very low level of anti-HBs in serum; might be susceptible with a false-positive anti-HBc; might be undetectable level of HBsAg present in the serum and the person is actually chronically infected.

Modified from Centers for Disease Control and Prevention. Interpretation of hepatitis B serologic test results. CDC; 2008. Accessed February 11, 2022. https://www.cdc.gov/hepatitis/hbv/pdfs/serologicchartv8.pdf

fumarate usually is started at around 28 weeks of gestation to allow time for a decline in maternal viral level. After approximately 4 weeks on tenofovir therapy, a maternal HBV DNA level should be assessed, and is expected to decline by approximately 2–3 log copies.

The highest risk of perinatal infection likely occurs when the neonate is in contact with infected vaginal blood and bodily fluids. However, there are no conclusive data to support a cesarean birth exclusively for reduction in transmission to the neonate. Risks associated with operative vaginal delivery, episiotomy, and the use of fetal scalp electrodes remain theoretical. These procedures are not known to increase neonatal infection. Similarly, no differences in rate of infection have been noted among breast-fed versus formula-fed infants; thus, breastfeeding should be supported.

Higher viral loads in the patient and absence of active and passive neonatal immunization correlate with a higher risk of neonatal infection. Hepatitis B virus immunoglobulin and the first vaccine in the HBV series, given together within 12 hours after delivery, have been the mainstay of risk reduction and are approximately 90% successful in preventing infection in the neonate. Single use of either active or passive immunization is less successful. Furthermore, the current failure rate of approximately 10% of dual immunoprophylaxis among women with high viral levels is not ideal and, therefore, not recommended as the sole best prevention strategy. Instead, administration of oral antiviral therapy, such as tenofovir, started in the second or third trimester, lowers HBV DNA levels, and when combined with dual immunoprophylaxis, appears to offer ideal reduction in the rates of HBV mother-to-child transmission. Currently, the Society for Maternal-Fetal Medicine recommends tenofovir as the first-line agent in pregnant women with HBV infection who are candidates for antiviral therapy rather than other agents such as lamivudine and telbivudine. These medications have acceptable safety profiles when used in pregnancy but appear to have increased rates of antiviral resistance.

Antiretroviral Pregnancy Registry Steering Committee. Antiretroviral Pregnancy Registry interim report for 1 January 1989 through 31 July 2021. Registry Coordinating Center; 2021. Accessed February 11, 2022. http://www.apregistry.com/forms/interim_report.pdf

Brown RS Jr, McMahon BJ, Lok AS, Wong JB, Ahmed AT, Mouchli MA, et al. Antiviral therapy in chronic hepatitis B viral infection during pregnancy: a systematic review and meta-analysis. Hepatology 2016;63:319–33. doi: 10.1002/hep.28302 https://aasldpubs.onlinelibrary.wiley.com/doi/10.1002/hep.28302

Dionne-Odom J, Tita AT, Silverman NS. #38: Hepatitis B in pregnancy screening, treatment, and prevention of vertical transmission. Society for Maternal–Fetal Medicine (SMFM). Am J Obstet Gynecol 2016;214:6–14. doi: 10.1016/j.ajog.2015.09.100 https://www.ajog.org/article/S0002-9378(15)01214-4/fulltext

Sarkar M, Terrault NA. Ending vertical transmission of hepatitis B: the third trimester intervention. Hepatology 2014;60:448–51. doi: 10.1002/hep.27145 https://aasldpubs.onlinelibrary.wiley.com/doi/10.1002/hep.27145

Viral hepatitis in pregnancy. ACOG Practice Bulletin No. 86. American College of Obstetricians and Gynecologists. Obstet Gynecol 2007;110:941–56. doi: 10.1097/01.AOG.0000263930.28382.2a https://journals.lww.com/greenjournal/Citation/2007/10000/ACOG_Practice_Bulletin_No__86__Viral_Hepatitis_in.50.aspx

27 Asthma medications

A 30-year-old gravida 3, para 1, at 12 weeks of gestation presents for a routine prenatal visit. Her pregnancy is complicated by asthma and obesity. She uses albuterol approximately 4 days per week for wheezing. Her peak expiratory flow rate in the office is 85% of predicted, and she has no wheezing on examination. The best next step in management of her asthma is to initiate a(n)

(A) antihistamine
(B) leukotriene receptor agonist
(C) long-acting β_2-agonist
* (D) low-dose inhaled corticosteroid
(E) oral corticosteroid

Asthma is one of the most common medical complications in pregnancy, occurring in approximately 4–8% of pregnancies. During pregnancy, asthma may worsen, improve, or be unchanged, each occurring in approximately one-third of women with the condition. Asthma can be challenging to diagnose during pregnancy because of overlapping symptomatology. Asthma symptoms include wheezing, cough, chest tightness, and shortness of breath. Pregnancy is associated with physiologic dyspnea. Minute ventilation and tidal volume increase by almost 50%, but the respiratory rate remains unchanged from the nonpregnant state. Progesterone is thought to be responsible for the perceived dyspnea and increased ventilation because it stimulates respiratory drive. In addition, increasing girth from the growing gravid uterus results in diaphragmatic elevation.

Differentiating between normal pregnancy adaptation and pathologic processes such as asthma is important. Wheezing on pulmonary auscultation certainly supports the diagnosis of asthma. However, asthma is best confirmed by demonstrating reversible airway obstruction with the use of bronchodilator therapy. Specifically, a more than 12% increase in FEV_1 after therapy is confirmatory.

It is important to assess asthma control during pregnancy because poor control can lead to serious adverse outcomes, such as preterm birth, fetal growth restriction, preeclampsia, cesarean birth, and maternal morbidity and mortality. Evaluation includes patient-reported symptom control and an objective assessment of pulmonary function. Symptom severity assessment should include day and night symptoms, activity limitation, and rescue therapy use. Pulmonary function can be assessed by spirometry or peak expiratory flow assessment and pulmonary auscultation. Spirometry norms are essentially unchanged in pregnancy. A peak flow measurement less than 60–80% of predicted or personal best suggests suboptimal control (Fig. 27-1) and warrants a step-up in the therapy plan (Fig. 27-2).

Asthma classifications are outlined in Table 27-1. The medical management of asthma during pregnancy is similar to that

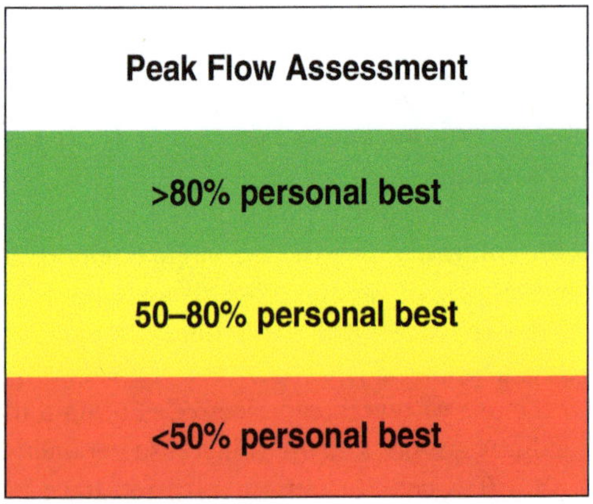

FIGURE 27-1. Peak flow assessment. In pregnant women, the peak expiratory flow rate is typically 380–550 L/min. When the patient is asymptomatic and feeling well, she should establish her "personal best."

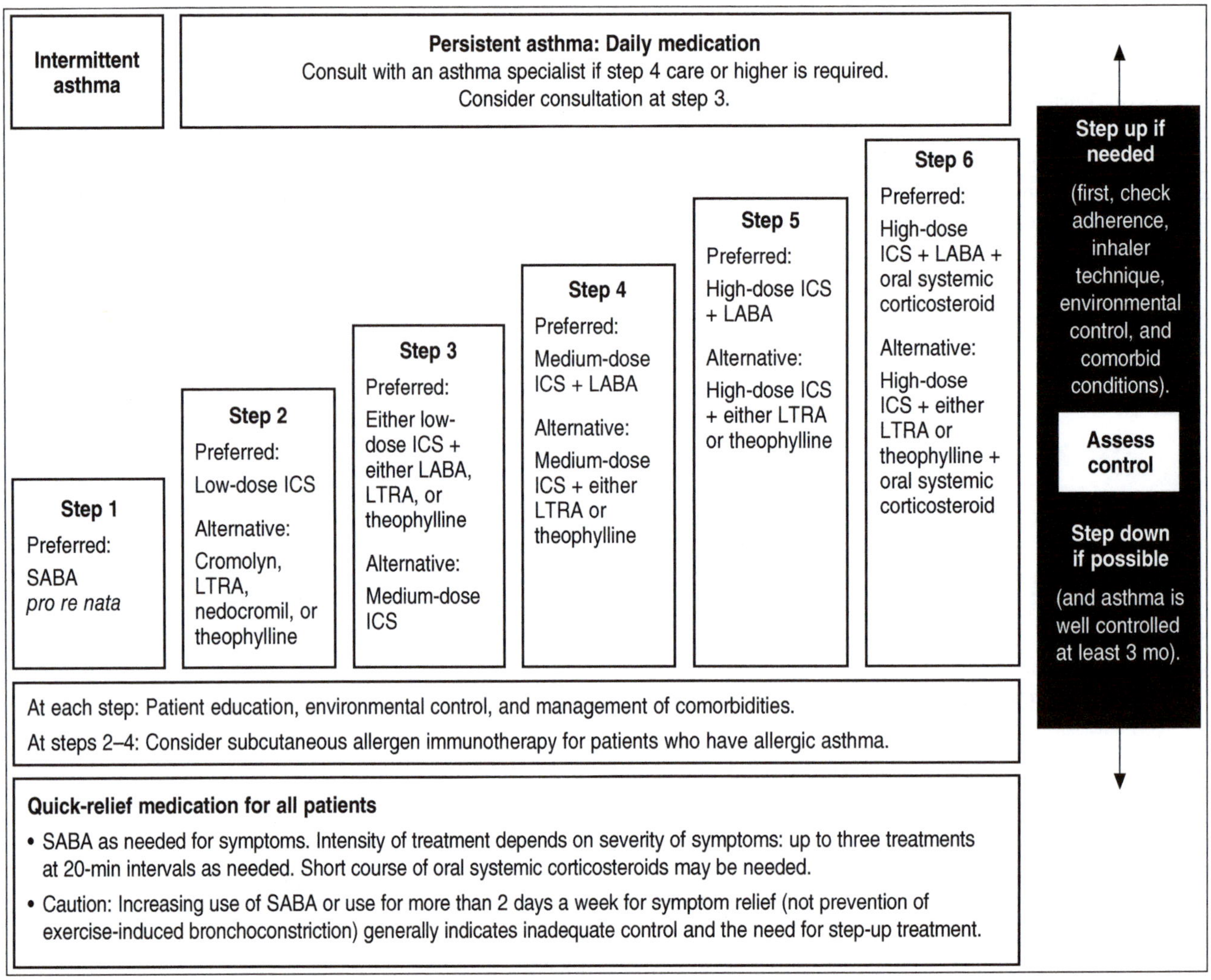

FIGURE 27-2. Stepwise approach for the management of asthma. Alphabetical order is used when more than one treatment option is listed within either preferred or alternative therapy. Abbreviations: ICS, inhaled corticosteroid; LABA, inhaled long-acting β2-agonist; LTRA, leukotriene receptor agonist; SABA, inhaled short-acting β2-agonist. (Modified from National Heart, Lung, and Blood Institute, National Asthma Education and Prevention Program. Expert Panel Report 3: guidelines for the diagnosis and management of asthma. NHLBI; 2007. Accessed February 28, 2022. https://www.nhlbi.nih.gov/health-topics/guidelines-for-diagnosis-management-of-asthma)

TABLE 27-1. Classification of Asthma Severity and Control in Pregnant Patients

ASTHMA SEVERITY* (CONTROL†)	SYMPTOM FREQUENCY	NIGHTTIME AWAKENING	INTERFERENCE WITH NORMAL ACTIVITY	FEV_1 OR PEAK FLOW (PREDICTED PERCENTAGE OF PERSONAL BEST)
Intermittent (well controlled)	2 days per week or less	Twice per month or less	None	More than 80%
Mild persistent (not well controlled)	More than 2 days per week, but not daily	More than twice per month	Minor limitation	More than 80%
Moderate persistent (not well controlled)	Daily symptoms	More than once per week	Some limitation	60–80%
Severe persistent (very poorly controlled)	Throughout the day	Four times per week or more	Extremely limited	Less than 60%

Abbreviation: FEV_1, forced expiratory volume in the first second of expiration.

*Assess severity for patients who are not taking long-term-control medications.

†Assess control in patients taking long-term-control medications to determine whether step-up therapy, step-down therapy, or no change in therapy is indicated.

in nonpregnant patients. The most commonly used medications to treat asthma appear to be safe during pregnancy and lactation. Inhaled corticosteroids are the preferred therapy for persistent asthma. The best next step for a patient who uses albuterol more than twice per week, even with a normal peak flow, such as the described patient, is the addition of a low-dose inhaled corticosteroid.

Allergic rhinitis is common in patients with asthma and may exacerbate asthma symptoms. Treatment of allergic rhinitis is an important component to maintaining asthma control. Commonly used antihistamines include loratadine or cetirizine. Intranasal corticosteroids also are an effective treatment. The described patient does not appear to have allergic rhinitis.

Although a leukotriene receptor agonist or a long-acting β_2-agonist could be considered as alternative therapy, neither of these would be the preferred therapy for the described patient (see Fig. 27-2). Inhaled corticosteroids are considered the mainstay of therapy for patients with persistent disease. Similarly, an oral corticosteroid is not the best next therapy for this patient. In the stepwise approach to asthma management, oral corticosteroids would be considered at step 6. Consultation with an asthma specialist is recommended with step 4 care or higher and can be considered at step 3.

Asthma in pregnancy. ACOG Practice Bulletin No. 90. American College of Obstetricians and Gynecologists. Obstet Gynecol 2008;111:457–64. doi: 10.1097/AOG.0b013e3181665ff4 https://journals.lww.com/greenjournal/Citation/2008/02000/ACOG_Practice_Bulletin_No__90__Asthma_in_Pregnancy.34.aspx

Namazy JA, Schatz M, Dombrowski M. Asthma. Clin Update Womens Health Care 2018;XVII(3):1–27. https://www.acog.org/clinical/journals-and-publications/clinical-updates/2018/05/asthma

National Heart, Lung, and Blood Institute, National Asthma Education and Prevention Program. Expert Panel Report 3: guidelines for the diagnosis and management of asthma. NHLBI; 2007. Accessed February 28, 2022. https://www.nhlbi.nih.gov/health-topics/guidelines-for-diagnosis-management-of-asthma

National Heart, Lung, and Blood Institute. 2020 focused updates to the asthma management guidelines: a report from the National Asthma Education and Prevention Program Coordinating Committee Expert Panel Working Group. NHLBI; 2020. Accessed February 28, 2022. https://www.nhlbi.nih.gov/health-topics/all-publications-and-resources/2020-focused-updates-asthma-management-guidelines

28 Postpartum mastitis

A 22-year-old gravida 1, para 1, presents 5 weeks postpartum with breast pain. The patient describes the pain as being in both nipples. The symptoms started 2 weeks ago and have progressively worsened. The pain is at its worst when her infant is nursing, with sharp pains occurring as the infant actively feeds. The pain does not improve when the breast is emptied. She has had minimal relief with use of over-the-counter analgesic medications. The patient's pregnancy was complicated by gestational diabetes mellitus. Her vital signs are normal. On physical examination, both nipples are erythematous. There is a scaly sheen overlying the areola. No fluctuance or mass is noted. A sample of breast milk is obtained by manual expression and examined under microscopy (Fig. 28-1). The most appropriate initial treatment is

(A) dicloxacillin
(B) fluconazole
(C) lanolin cream
* (D) miconazole gel
(E) nonsteroidal anti-inflammatory drugs

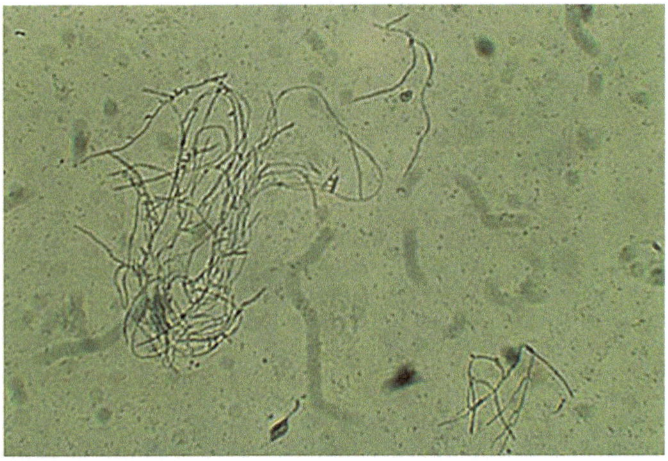

FIGURE 28-1. Breast milk cytology. (Reprinted from Sobel JD. Mucocutaneous candidiasis. In: Mandell GL, Diamond RD, editors. Atlas of infectious diseases: fungal infections. Current Medicine; 2000. p. 117–33.)

Nipple and breast pain are common challenges to breastfeeding patients and are a major contributor to breastfeeding cessation. Experts recommend exclusive breastfeeding for the first 6 months of life; however, only 25% of mother–infant pairs achieve this in the United States. In a study of 1,300 women who discontinued breastfeeding within 1 month of delivering, two-thirds reported pain and nipple trauma as major contributors. Obstetricians should promptly evaluate and treat women who report these symptoms in the postpartum period.

The most common cause of breast and nipple pain soon after birth is breast engorgement, which typically presents 3–5 days after delivery. Patients will describe bilateral breast fullness and a generalized dull ache. The pain improves with the onset of feeding and symptoms diminish as the breast is emptied. On examination the breast will be firm and tender. The first intervention for breast engorgement is to assess the neonate's latch and the breastfeeding technique; otherwise, for mild symptoms, expectant management is appropriate. Increasing the rate of milk expression to address engorgement can lead to overproduction, which increases the rate of plugged ducts and infection.

For persistent breast and nipple pain, the differential diagnoses include problems with latch and breastfeeding technique, trauma, dermatologic problems, infections, vasospasms, pain disorders, and other lactation problems. Improper latch can lead to nipple pain, nipple trauma, and incomplete emptying. All evaluations for breast and nipple pain in breastfeeding patients should include an observation of the patient's breastfeeding technique. Consultation with a lactation specialist often is beneficial. Infants can be evaluated for ankyloglossia and treated with frenotomy or frenectomy as indicated. Breast pumps can lead to mechanical trauma. Observing the patient's pump technique may be useful as the fit of the flange or the level of suction may need adjustment. For traumatic nipple injuries, address the cause of the trauma and treat symptomatically with topical emollient creams and over-the-counter pain medications. Superficial infections frequently accompany nipple trauma and are best treated with topical antibiotics, such as bacitracin or mupirocin ointments. Systemic antibiotics are reserved for severe cellulitis and mastitis.

Dermatologic conditions that can lead to breast and nipple pain during breastfeeding include eczema and psoriasis. Eczematous breast lesions can range from blisters and erosions to chronic findings such as scaly thickened tissue. In addition to pain, the patient will report burning and itching. Treatments include emollients, topical corticosteroids, and antihistamines. Oral corticosteroids are reserved for more severe or resistant cases. Psoriatic lesions usually are well-demarcated, erythematous plaques. Treatments again include emollients and topical corticosteroids, but immunomodulating agents should not be used because of the risk of infant exposure.

Infectious causes of breast and nipple pain during breastfeeding include bacterial mastitis, breast abscesses, *Candida* infection, and herpes simplex and herpes zoster outbreaks. Bacterial mastitis presents with localized breast tenderness, erythema, and induration. The breast symptoms commonly are accompanied by fevers, chills, nausea, and vomiting. Bacterial mastitis occurs in 2–10% of lactating postpartum patients, but in less than 1% of nonlactating postpartum women. The most common risk factor for bacterial mastitis is milk stasis, such as cases of maternal fatigue with abrupt reductions in breastfeeding frequency. Other risk factors include poor nursing technique and nipple trauma. The most common pathogens are *Staphylococcus aureus*, *Staphylococcus epidermidis*, streptococcal species, and occasionally Gram-negative rods. Treatment of bacterial mastitis includes mechanical breast support, fluids, continued feeding and emptying of both breasts, and antibiotic therapy. Dicloxacillin is the preferred antibiotic. In patients with a penicillin allergy, alternatives include cephalexin or clindamycin. Antibiotic therapy should be administered in 10- to 14-day courses. Ten percent of patients affected by breastfeeding mastitis will develop breast abscesses. The abscesses are most commonly located in the upper outer breast quadrants, with *S aureus* the most common bacteria isolated. Abscesses must be evacuated either by ultrasound-guided percutaneous needle aspiration or surgical incision and drainage.

Candida infection of the nipple during breastfeeding presents with erythema and scaly, shiny changes to the skin. The patients will describe severe pain and burning with nipple manipulation, such as during suckling. The pain will persist as long as the stimulation continues. Risk factors for *Candida* infection of the breast include recent maternal antibiotic use, maternal diabetes mellitus, and infant yeast infection such as thrush and diaper rash. Because of the nonspecific physical examination findings, the suspicion of *Candida* breast infection should be confirmed with a microscopic examination of the breast milk and a fungal culture of the milk. Characteristic findings of yeast, including spores and hyphae, will be visible within a high-powered field and are diagnostic. Otherwise, fungal culture with identification usually takes 10–14 days, and empiric therapy often is started. Topical antifungal therapy, such as miconazole, should be applied to the nipple after every feeding, and the infant's oral cavity should be treated with nystatin suspension or miconazole gel. This is the first-line regimen and generally is continued for 2 weeks. If symptoms do not resolve with miconazole gel or persist beyond 7 days, treatment with oral fluconazole is recommended.

Both herpes simplex and herpes zoster outbreaks can lead to breast pain during breastfeeding. Both are treated with oral antiviral therapy. Uniquely, women should neither directly breastfeed the infant on the affected breast nor provide them with expressed milk from the affected breast until the lesions have healed. It is safe to provide breast milk from the unaffected breast as long as it is obtained when the contralateral breast's lesions are covered.

Other conditions that can lead to breast and nipple pain in breastfeeding women include vasospasms, functional pain disorders, and plugged ducts. Vasospasms present as shooting or burning breast pain. The breast skin may appear discolored as the vessels constrict. Treatment includes applying warm compresses, avoiding cold temperatures, and using nifedipine for persistent symptoms. Functional pain disorders present in the breast characterized by pain with light touch, but no overlying skin changes or examination findings. Treatment can include nonsteroidal anti-inflammatory drugs, propranolol, antidepressants, and antihistamines. Plugged or blocked lactiferous ducts will present as discrete, tender cords in the breasts. Application of heat and expression techniques usually will allow passage of the plug and relief of symptoms.

This scenario represents a *Candida* mastitis based on the clinical presentation, physical examination, and laboratory findings. Bacterial mastitis is unlikely based on the bilateral findings and lack of accompanying constitutional symptoms. There is no mechanical trauma for which an emollient cream would be indicated. Nonsteroidal anti-inflammatory drugs are not therapeutic for a *Candida* mastitis. The first-line therapy for this infection is a topical antifungal.

Breastfeeding challenges. ACOG Committee Opinion No. 820. American College of Obstetricians and Gynecologists. Obstet Gynecol 2021;137:e42–53. doi: 10.1097/AOG.0000000000004253 https://journals.lww.com/greenjournal/Fulltext/2021/02000/Breastfeeding_Challenges__ACOG_Committee_Opinion,.46.aspx

Diagnosis and management of benign breast disorders. Practice Bulletin No. 164. American College of Obstetricians and Gynecologists [published erratum appears in Obstet Gynecol 2021;137:382]. Obstet Gynecol 2016;127:e141–56. doi: 10.1097/AOG.0000000000001482 https://journals.lww.com/greenjournal/Fulltext/2016/06000/Practice_Bulletin_No__164__Diagnosis_and.42.aspx

Newton ER, Stuebe AM. Lactation and breastfeeding. In: Landon MB, Galan HL, Jauniaux ER, Driscoll DA, Berghella V, Grobman WA, et al, editors. Gabbe's obstetrics: normal and problem pregnancies. 8th ed. Elsevier; 2021. p. 475–502.

Optimizing support for breastfeeding as part of obstetric practice. ACOG Committee Opinion No. 756. American College of Obstetricians and Gynecologists. Obstet Gynecol 2018;132:e187–96. doi: 10.1097/AOG.0000000000002890 https://journals.lww.com/greenjournal/Fulltext/2018/10000/ACOG_Committee_Opinion_No__756__Optimizing_Support.62.aspx

29 Severe rhesus disease in pregnancy

A 21-year-old gravida 3, para 2, presents at 27 weeks of gestation with a pregnancy complicated by Rh D alloimmunization. Her first pregnancy was uncomplicated, but her second pregnancy was affected by Rh D alloimmunization. This pregnancy has the same paternity, and the fetal antigenicity was confirmed Rh D positive with cell-free DNA testing in the second trimester. Doppler velocimetry measurements of the peak systolic velocity in the fetal middle cerebral artery have been conducted every 2 weeks for the last 2 months. The values of the Doppler measurements have ranged from 1.1 to 1.35 multiples of the mean for gestational age. Based on the current antenatal testing, delivery should be planned at a gestational age of

(A) 31 0/7 to 32 6/7 weeks
(B) 33 0/7 to 34 6/7 weeks
(C) 35 0/7 to 36 6/7 weeks
* (D) 37 0/7 to 38 6/7 weeks
(E) 39 0/7 to 40 6/7 weeks

Alloimmunization occurs with the development of maternal antibodies after a feto-maternal hemorrhage or an incompatible blood product transfusion. The Rh blood group system consists of five main erythrocyte antigens: C, c, D, E, and e, with the Rho D antigen causing most transfusion reactions and fetal hemolytic disease. There are more than 30 minor variants within the Rh blood group, including the weak D antigen. There are other blood group systems for which incompatibility can lead to alloimmunization. The degree of risk of fetal hemolytic disease varies among these other blood groups. The Lewis and I antigens are the most commonly encountered antigens outside of the Rh system, but they are cold agglutinins forming immunoglobulin M antibodies that carry no risk of erythroblastosis fetalis. For clinically relevant erythrocyte antigens, the degree of fetal hemolytic disease ranges from mild to severe anemia. With the introduction of Rho D immune globulin, the proportion of fetal hemolytic disease secondary to Rh alloimmunization has decreased dramatically with the other blood group systems now accounting for a greater proportion. Currently, Rh D alloimmunization affects 6.8 per 1,000 live births in countries where prophylaxis is routine.

Feto-maternal hemorrhage can occur as early as the first trimester and lead to alloimmunization. Approximately 3–11% of threatened abortions will have a feto-maternal hemorrhage with 1.5–2% leading to alloimmunization. The rate of alloimmunization is 4–5% in first-trimester abortions that require a dilation and curettage. Ectopic pregnancies have been associated with alloimmunization. Second-trimester invasive procedures, such as chorionic villus sampling and genetic amniocentesis, have feto-maternal hemorrhage rates of 14% and 2–6%, respectively. In the third trimester, 45% of deliveries will be complicated by feto-maternal hemorrhage. Risk factors for feto-maternal hemorrhage include cesarean birth, multiple gestations, abnormal placentation, and manual placental extraction.

Most pregnant patients undergo ABO blood group typing and have an antibody screen with the initiation of prenatal care. For Rh-negative patients who are not sensitized, alloimmunization prophylaxis is carried out with routine Rh D immune globulin administration. Patients who are weak D antigen positive also should receive prophylaxis. When first introduced, Rh D immune globulin was given postpartum to Rh-negative mothers who gave birth to Rh-positive neonates, successfully decreasing the rate of alloimmunization from 13–16% to 0.5–1.8%. With recognition that 1–2% of Rh D alloimmunization occurs in the antenatal period, routine administration also was instituted at 28 weeks of gestation after a third-trimester antibody screen, lowering the rate of alloimmunization to 0.14–0.2%.

Contemporary practice is to give susceptible patients Rh D immune globulin at 28 weeks of gestation and within 72 hours of delivering a Rh-positive neonate. Rh immune globulin administration is recommended in Rh-negative patients undergoing chorionic villus sampling and amniocentesis. It should be considered in women who have a spontaneous first-trimester miscarriage but is recommended for those who have instrumentation associated with a spontaneous miscarriage, for all patients who have a pregnancy termination by medical or surgical methods, and for those who have ectopic gestations. Rh immune globulin should be given to at-risk women who experience abdominal trauma or antenatal hemorrhage after 20 weeks of gestation and those who undergo external cephalic version. A standard 300-microgram vial of Rh immune globulin will provide adequate prophylaxis for a feto-maternal hemorrhage of 30 mL or less of fetal whole blood. When a larger feto-maternal hemorrhage is suspected, an erythrocyte rosette screen can be conducted on maternal blood samples. A positive screen indicates greater than 2 mL of whole fetal blood has been detected in the maternal circulation. This should be followed by a Kleihauer–Betke test or flow cytometry to further quantify the amount of hemorrhage, and the amount of Rh immune globulin that should be administered. Testing to quantify the feto-maternal hemorrhage is routine for postpartum Rh immune globulin administration.

For patients with a positive antibody screen of clinical significance, the first step is to assess the paternal erythrocyte antigen status. If the antigen status is positive, or if it is unknown or unavailable, fetal testing is required. Amniocentesis with polymerase chain reaction has a 98.7% sensitivity and 100% specificity for blood typing. Maternal cell-free DNA also can be obtained in the second trimester and has a 99% accuracy for fetal blood typing. However, this may not be widely available for this use.

For at-risk fetuses of alloimmunized mothers, the first step of surveillance is serial antibody titers. A critical titer is one at which there is a risk of severe erythroblastosis fetalis and hydrops. This critical threshold ranges from 1:8 to 1:32, depending on individual institutional experience. With a titer of 1:8 or less, repeat titers should be collected every 4 weeks until 24 weeks of gestation, then every 2 weeks. The titers should be conducted at the same laboratory each time. Different laboratories may use different enhancing media; thus, interlaboratory reliability is low. If a critical titer is reached, then fetal testing for anemia should be obtained. Titers are not followed in at-risk women who have had a previous pregnancy affected by hemolytic anemia because the titers are not predictive of the severity of the anemia in the subsequent pregnancy. Patients with Kell alloimmunization are not followed with serial titers for the same reason. Both of these situations should prompt testing for fetal anemia.

Fetal testing for anemia is accomplished with noninvasive ultrasonographic Doppler assessment of the peak systolic velocity in the middle cerebral artery. Spectral analysis of amniotic fluid is no longer contemporary practice. Doppler assessment of the peak systolic velocity in the middle cerebral artery requires proper technique and adequate experience and should be conducted at obstetric centers capable of treating high-risk pregnancies. A peak systolic velocity greater than 1.5 multiples of the mean for gestational age predicts moderate to severe fetal anemia with 100% sensitivity. The false-positive rate is 12% with the highest risk of false-positive results beyond 34–35 weeks of gestation. Doppler assessment of the middle cerebral artery should start by 24 weeks of gestation in alloimmunized women with critical titer levels. In patients who have had a previous pregnancy complicated by alloimmunization, Doppler assessment should begin by 18 weeks of gestation. Doppler assessments are conducted at 1- or 2-week intervals.

Percutaneous umbilical blood sampling is performed when middle cerebral artery peak systolic velocity exceeds 1.5 multiples of the mean. This procedure allows for direct fetal hematocrit assessment and intravascular, intrauterine fetal transfusion as indicated. Generally, transfusion is indicated when fetal hematocrit is less than 30% or more than 2 standard deviations below the mean for gestational age. Type O, Rh D negative, cytomegalovirus negative, leukocyte-reduced blood is transfused with a goal hematocrit of 40–50%.

In alloimmunized patients with mild disease or no evidence of hemolytic disease, delivery should be delayed until term (37 0/7 to 38 6/7 weeks of gestation). For patients requiring invasive transfusion procedures, recommendations vary on delivery timing. Some sources will plan the last transfusion for 30–32 weeks of gestation with delivery at 32–34 weeks of gestation after corticosteroid administration, whereas others advocate transfusing at up to 35 or 36 weeks of gestation with a goal of delivery at 37 weeks of gestation. The patient in this scenario has no evidence of moderate or severe fetal anemia based on middle cerebral artery Doppler assessment. Therefore, the most appropriate course would be continued surveillance with delivery in the early-term period. Maintaining the pregnancy beyond 39 weeks of gestation is not recommended because the risk of developing hemolytic disease outweighs any risk of iatrogenic delivery.

Management of alloimmunization during pregnancy. ACOG Practice Bulletin No. 192. American College of Obstetricians and Gynecologists. Obstet Gynecol 2018;131:e82–90. doi: 10.1097/AOG.0000000000002528 https://journals.lww.com/greenjournal/Fulltext/2018/03000/ACOG_Practice_Bulletin_No__192__Management_of.45.aspx

Medically indicated late-preterm and early-term deliveries. ACOG Committee Opinion No. 831. American College of Obstetricians and Gynecologists. Obstet Gynecol 2021;138:e35–9. doi: 10.1097/AOG.0000000000004447 https://journals.lww.com/greenjournal/Fulltext/2021/07000/Medically_Indicated_Late_Preterm_and_Early_Term.38.aspx

Moise KJ Jr. Management of rhesus alloimmunization in pregnancy. Obstet Gynecol 2008;112:164–76. doi: 10.1097/AOG.0b013e31817d453c https://journals.lww.com/greenjournal/Fulltext/2008/07000/Management_of_Rhesus_Alloimmunization_in_Pregnancy.26.aspx

Prevention of Rh D alloimmunization. Practice Bulletin No. 181. American College of Obstetricians and Gynecologists. Obstet Gynecol 2017;130:e57–70. doi: 10.1097/AOG.0000000000002232 https://journals.lww.com/greenjournal/Fulltext/2017/08000/Practice_Bulletin_No__181__Prevention_of_Rh_D.54.aspx

30 Recurrent spontaneous abortion

A 29-year-old gravida 4, para 0, presents a month after her fourth spontaneous first-trimester loss. Previously, she has had normal saline sonohysterography, maternal and paternal karyotype, and thyroid screening. She requests additional testing to evaluate the causes of her recurrent miscarriage. The most appropriate thrombophilia testing for this patient is

* (A) antiphospholipid syndrome
(B) antithrombin deficiency
(C) factor V Leiden mutation
(D) methylenetetrahydrofolate reductase mutation
(E) prothrombin mutation

The terms *miscarriage*, *spontaneous abortion*, and *early pregnancy loss* are used interchangeably and describe a nonviable, intrauterine pregnancy with an empty gestational sac or a gestational sac with an embryo without cardiac activity within the first 12 6/7 weeks of gestation. Pregnancy loss occurs in about 10–15% of all clinically recognized pregnancies with approximately 80% occurring in the first trimester. Many pregnancies are lost before the implantation of the embryo or before clinical recognition of pregnancy—this is estimated at 50–70% of fertilizations. A common cause of early pregnancy loss is chromosomal abnormality, occurring in approximately 60% of cases of early pregnancy loss, with the frequency increasing with maternal age. Most of these are autosomal trisomies, the most common being trisomy 16. Other causes of miscarriage include genetic abnormalities, such as single gene disorders, endocrine abnormalities, such as thyroid function abnormalities and diabetes mellitus, uterine müllerian defects, leiomyomas, infections, acquired thrombophilias, and exposure to known teratogens, such as irradiation and chemotherapeutic agents.

Recurrent pregnancy loss is defined as the loss of two or more clinical pregnancies after ultrasonographic evidence of a gestational sac or histopathology, and is estimated to affect 1–2% of couples. Evaluation of these couples is indicated and should start with a careful history, including all pregnancies and outcomes (Box 30-1). Screening for infections, thyroid disease, and diabetes mellitus is indicated in patients with risk factors or clinical signs of these diseases. An evaluation of the uterine cavity is recommended in women with recurrent pregnancy loss to screen for müllerian anomalies. This may be accomplished with sonohysterography, hysterosalpingography, hysteroscopy, or magnetic resonance imaging. Genetic testing of fetal tissue with karyotype and microarray may be helpful, and if an inherited genetic abnormality (such as chromosome translocation) is suspected, parental karyotyping is recommended.

A definitive causal link between hereditary thrombophilias and adverse pregnancy outcomes has not been clearly established. Retrospective studies have suggested a link between inherited thrombophilia and recurrent pregnancy loss, but no prospective studies support the association, and testing for thrombophilias is not recommended as part of routine assessment. The exception to this is antiphospholipid syndrome, which should be tested in the described patient by checking β_2-glycoprotein, anticardiolipin autoantibodies, and lupus anticoagulant. Antiphospholipid syndrome is diagnosed with clinical criteria and positive lupus anticoagulant, anti-cardiolipin antibody or β_2-glycoprotein antibodies above the 99th percentile or 40 IgG phospholipid/IgM phospholipid on two occasions with testing performed at least 12 weeks apart, or both. It is an acquired autoimmune disease that may present with venous, arterial, and microvascular thrombosis or obstetric complications, or both, including early pregnancy loss.

In women with antiphospholipid syndrome and recurrent pregnancy loss, treatment with anticoagulants and low-dose aspirin may decrease the risk of subsequent pregnancy loss by 50%. In women with unexplained recurrent pregnancy loss, supplementation with progestogen therapy may reduce the rate of loss in subsequent pregnancies. No other effective interventions have been demonstrated to reduce the risk of early pregnancy loss. Couples who have had as many as four losses have a good prognosis in a subsequent pregnancy, with a live birth rate of 60–70% without therapy or intervention, and support and encouragement can be given.

BOX 30-1

Evaluation for Couples With Recurrent Pregnancy Loss (After Two Consecutive Losses)

Recommended screening:

- Antiphospholipid antibodies
- Assessment of uterine anatomy
- Genetic testing of fetal tissue or parental karyotypes, or both
- Lifestyle factors (smoking, cocaine, excess alcohol or caffeine)
- Hormonal screening (thyroid, prolactin, diabetes)

Bender Atik R, Christiansen OB, Elson J, Kolte AM, Lewis S, Middeldorp S, et al. ESHRE guideline: recurrent pregnancy loss. ESHRE Guideline Group on RPL. Hum Reprod Open 2018;2018:hoy004. doi: 10.1093/hropen/hoy004 https://www.ncbi.nlm.nih.gov/pmc/articles/PMC6276652/

Early pregnancy loss. ACOG Practice Bulletin No. 200. American College of Obstetricians and Gynecologists. Obstet Gynecol 2018;132:e197–207. doi: 10.1097/AOG.0000000000002899 https://journals.lww.com/green-journal/Fulltext/2018/11000/ACOG_Practice_Bulletin_No__200__Early_Pregnancy.41.aspx

Evaluation and treatment of recurrent pregnancy loss: a committee opinion. Practice Committee of the American Society for Reproductive Medicine. Fertil Steril 2012;98:1103–11. doi: 10.1016/j.fertnstert.2012.06.048 https://www.fertstert.org/article/S0015-0282(12)00701-7/fulltext

Landon MB, Galan HL, Jauniaux ER, Driscoll DA, Berghella V, Grobman WA, et al, editors. Gabbe's obstetrics: normal and problem pregnancies. 8th ed. Elsevier; 2021.

31 Gestational diabetes

A 39-year-old gravida 3, para 0, presents for an initial prenatal visit at 13 weeks of gestation. She has a body mass index (BMI) of 26, and her medical history is significant for hypothyroidism and hypertension treated with nifedipine. She has had two first-trimester miscarriages and reports a family history of type 2 diabetes mellitus in her maternal grandmother. You recommend early diabetes screening with a 50-g, 1-hour glucose tolerance test based on her BMI and

(A) advanced maternal age
* (B) chronic hypertension
(C) family history
(D) hypothyroidism
(E) recurrent pregnancy loss

Gestational diabetes mellitus (GDM) is a condition of carbohydrate intolerance during pregnancy that affects up to 10% of pregnant women in the United States each year. In many cases, GDM can be controlled with diet and lifestyle changes, but some individuals will require treatment with medication. As obesity and sedentary lifestyles have become more common in the population, the prevalence of GDM also has increased. Universally screening for GDM between 24 and 28 weeks of gestation is recommended rather than screening only those with risk factors such as family history, previous pregnancy history, and obesity.

Because many women are not screened for diabetes mellitus before pregnancy, distinguishing GDM from preexisting diabetes may be challenging. Early pregnancy screening for undiagnosed type 2 diabetes is recommended in women with a BMI greater than 25 and with additional risk factors for diabetes, including a first-degree relative with diabetes, prior newborn weighing more than 4,000 g, prior diagnosis of GDM, hypertension, high cholesterol, A_{1c} of 5.7–6.4%, and polycystic ovary syndrome (Box 31-1). Early screening is recommended at the initiation of prenatal care; however, the best test

BOX 31-1

Screening Strategy for Detecting Pregestational Diabetes or Early Gestational Diabetes Mellitus

Consider testing in all women who are overweight or obese (ie, have a body mass index greater than 25 or greater than 23 in Asian Americans) and have one or more of the following additional risk factors:

- Physical inactivity
- First-degree relative with diabetes
- Have previously given birth to an infant weighing 4,000 g (approximately 9 lb) or more
- Previous gestational diabetes mellitus
- Hypertension (140/90 mm Hg or on therapy for hypertension)
- High-density lipoprotein cholesterol level less than 35 mg/dL (0.90 mmol/L), a triglyceride level greater than 250 mg/dL (2.82 mmol/L)
- Women with polycystic ovarian syndrome
- A_{1C} 5.7% or greater, impaired glucose tolerance, or impaired fasting glucose on previous testing
- Other clinical conditions associated with insulin resistance (eg, prepregnancy body mass index greater than 40 kg/m^2, acanthosis nigricans)
- History of cardiovascular disease

Reprinted from Gestational diabetes mellitus. ACOG Practice Bulletin No. 190. American College of Obstetricians and Gynecologists. Obstet Gynecol 2018;131:e49–64. doi: 10.1097/AOG.0000000000002501 https://journals.lww.com/greenjournal/Fulltext/2018/02000/ACOG_Practice_Bulletin_No__190__Gestational.37.aspx

Adapted from Classification and diagnosis of diabetes. American Diabetes Association. Diabetes Care 2017;40:S11–24. doi: 10.2337/dc17-S005 https://diabetesjournals.org/care/article/40/Supplement_1/S11/36898/2-Classification-and-Diagnosis-of-Diabetes.

for early screening is not clear. Options include the 2-hour, 75-g oral glucose tolerance test or the two-step screening test often used later in pregnancy (starting with a 1-hour, 50-g oral glucose tolerance test). In women who have negative early screening, routine GDM screening is recommended again at 24–28 weeks of gestation.

This patient is overweight with a BMI of 26, which does not alone qualify her for early pregnancy diabetes screening. The additional risk factor that qualifies her for early testing is her history of chronic hypertension. Women with hypothyroidism are not thought to be at increased risk of GDM. This patient has a second-degree relative with diabetes (her grandmother) but not a first-degree relative. Her history of two early pregnancy losses does not place her at increased risk of diabetes mellitus. Women at older ages are at higher risk of GDM; however, this risk is greatest in women older than 40 years. According to the American College of Obstetricians and Gynecologists and the American Diabetes Association, maternal age is not one of the risk factors that necessitates early screening.

Draznin B, Aroda VR, Bakris G, Benson G, Brown FM, Freeman R, et al. 15. Management of diabetes in pregnancy: Standards of Medical Care in Diabetes-2022. American Diabetes Association Professional Practice Committee. Diabetes Care 2022;45:S232–43. doi: 10.2337/dc22-S015 https://diabetesjournals.org/care/article/45/Supplement_1/S232/138916/15-Management-of-Diabetes-in-Pregnancy-Standards

Gestational diabetes mellitus. ACOG Practice Bulletin No. 190. American College of Obstetricians and Gynecologists. Obstet Gynecol 2018;131:e49–64. doi: 10.1097/AOG.0000000000002501 https://journals.lww.com/greenjournal/Fulltext/2018/02000/ACOG_Practice_Bulletin_No__190__Gestational.37.aspx

Landon MB, Galan HL, Jauniaux ER, Driscoll DA, Berghella V, Grobman WA, et al, editors. Gabbe's obstetrics: normal and problem pregnancies. 8th ed. Elsevier; 2021.

32 Postpartum contraception

A 27-year-old gravida 2, para 1, presents for a prenatal visit at 36 weeks of gestation. She plans to breastfeed, and she would like to discuss postpartum contraception. She previously had abnormal bleeding with the etonogestrel implant and prefers to avoid this method in the future. She wants to delay her next pregnancy for 2–3 years, and she is interested in highly effective contraception that she can start shortly after delivery. She will lose her health insurance 6 weeks after giving birth. For this patient, the contraceptive option you recommend is

(A) combined hormonal contraception
(B) depot medroxyprogesterone acetate
* (C) intrauterine device (IUD) placement
(D) progesterone-only oral contraceptives

Contraceptive planning is an important aspect of prenatal care. In the United States, 45% of pregnancies are unplanned, and approximately 40–67% of women report having intercourse before their 6-week postpartum visit. Short interval pregnancy of less than 18 months carries multiple increased risks, including low birth weight and preterm birth. Having an established plan before delivery will allow the patient to have access to all options for care.

Long-acting reversible contraceptive (LARC) methods have lower typical-use pregnancy rates compared with short-acting methods and are the most effective forms of contraception. Long-acting reversible contraceptive methods also have the highest rates of continuation compared with short-acting methods. Long-acting reversible contraceptive methods include IUDs and the etonogestrel contraceptive implant. Intrauterine devices and contraceptive implants can be placed immediately postpartum, reducing unintended pregnancy and a short interpregnancy interval. As many as 10–40% of women do not attend the postpartum visit, and many women who planned IUD insertion never receive one. Placement before hospital discharge prevents many barriers to access, and multiple studies have demonstrated the cost effectiveness of immediate postpartum insertion.

Immediate postpartum IUD insertion has few contraindications and is designated by the Centers for Disease Control and Prevention's U.S. Medical Eligibility for Contraception under categories 1 (no restriction) and 2 (benefits generally outweigh risks) (Fig. 32-1). Levonorgestrel and copper IUDs can be placed in the immediate postpartum period. Contraindications specific to immediate postpartum insertion include intra-amniotic infection and postpartum endometritis, as well as postpartum hemorrhage. Risks specific to the postpartum period include an increased risk of expulsion compared with interval placement (10–27% versus 2–10% in the first year). There is a theoretical risk of delayed lactogenesis in the setting of progesterone use in the postpartum period; however, the available evidence does not support this risk. Patients should be counseled about these risks to make an informed decision. In this case, because the patient desires highly effective contraception and will lose her insurance shortly after delivery, a LARC method is the most appropriate choice. A LARC method that is placed before discharge will allow years of contraception

Centers for Disease Control and Prevention
National Center for Chronic Disease Prevention and Health Promotion

Condition	Sub-Condition	Cu-IUD	LNG-IUD	Implant	DMPA	POP	CHC
		I C	I C	I C	I C	I C	I C
Age		Menarche to <20 yrs:**2** ≥20 yrs:**1**	Menarche to <20 yrs:**2** ≥20 yrs:**1**	Menarche to <18 yrs:**1** 18-45 yrs:**1** >45 yrs:**1**	Menarche to <18 yrs:**2** 18-45 yrs:**1** >45 yrs:**2**	Menarche to <18 yrs:**1** 18-45 yrs:**1** >45 yrs:**1**	Menarche to <40 yrs:**1** ≥40 yrs:**2**
Anatomical abnormalities	a) Distorted uterine cavity	4	4				
	b) Other abnormalities	2	2				
Anemias	a) Thalassemia	2	1	1	1	1	1
	b) Sickle cell disease‡	2	1	1	1	1	2
	c) Iron-deficiency anemia	2	1	1	1	1	1
Benign ovarian tumors	*(including cysts)*	1	1	1	1	1	1
Breast disease	a) Undiagnosed mass	1	2	2*	2*	2*	2*
	b) Benign breast disease	1	1	1	1	1	1
	c) Family history of cancer	1	1	1	1	1	1
	d) Breast cancer‡						
	i) Current	1	4	4	4	4	4
	ii) Past and no evidence of current disease for 5 years	1	3	3	3	3	3
Breastfeeding	a) <21 days postpartum			2*	2*	2*	4*
	b) 21 to <30 days postpartum						
	i) With other risk factors for VTE			2*	2*	2*	3*
	ii) Without other risk factors for VTE			2*	2*	2*	3*
	c) 30-42 days postpartum						
	i) With other risk factors for VTE			1*	1*	1*	3*
	ii) Without other risk factors for VTE			1*	1*	1*	2*
	d) >42 days postpartum			1*	1*	1*	2*
Cervical cancer	Awaiting treatment	I: 4 C: 2	I: 4 C: 2	2	2	1	2
Cervical ectropion		1	1	1	1	1	1
Cervical intraepithelial neoplasia		1	2	2	2	1	2
Cirrhosis	a) Mild *(compensated)*	1	1	1	1	1	1
	b) Severe‡ *(decompensated)*	1	3	3	3	3	4
Cystic fibrosis‡		1*	1*	1*	2*	1*	1*
Deep venous thrombosis (DVT)/Pulmonary embolism (PE)	a) History of DVT/PE, not receiving anticoagulant therapy						
	i) Higher risk for recurrent DVT/PE	1	2	2	2	2	4
	ii) Lower risk for recurrent DVT/PE	1	2	2	2	2	3
	b) Acute DVT/PE	2	2	2	2	2	4
	c) DVT/PE and established anticoagulant therapy for at least 3 months						
	i) Higher risk for recurrent DVT/PE	2	2	2	2	2	4*
	ii) Lower risk for recurrent DVT/PE	2	2	2	2	2	3*
	d) Family history *(first-degree relatives)*	1	1	1	1	1	2
	e) Major surgery						
	i) With prolonged immobilization	1	2	2	2	2	4
	ii) Without prolonged immobilization	1	1	1	1	1	2
	f) Minor surgery without immobilization	1	1	1	1	1	1
Depressive disorders		1*	1*	1*	1*	1*	1*

Key:	
1 No restriction (method can be used)	**3 Theoretical or proven risks usually outweigh the advantages**
2 Advantages generally outweigh theoretical or proven risks	**4 Unacceptable health risk (method not to be used)**

FIGURE 32-1. U.S. Medical Eligibility Criteria for Contraceptive Use, 2016. (Reprinted from Centers for Disease Control and Prevention. US Medical Eligibility Criteria [US MEC] for contraceptive use, 2016. CDC; 2021. Accessed April 21, 2022. https://www.cdc.gov/reproductivehealth/contraception/mmwr/mec/summary.html)

Condition	Sub-Condition	Cu-IUD		LNG-IUD		Implant		DMPA		POP		CHC	
		I	C	I	C	I	C	I	C	I	C	I	C
Diabetes	a) History of gestational disease	1		1		1		1		1		1	
	b) Nonvascular disease												
	i) Non-insulin dependent	1		2		2		2		2		2	
	ii) Insulin dependent	1		2		2		2		2		2	
	c) Nephropathy/retinopathy/neuropathy‡	1		2		2		3		2		3/4*	
	d) Other vascular disease or diabetes of >20 years' duration‡	1		2		2		3		2		3/4*	
Dysmenorrhea	Severe	2		1		1		1		1		1	
Endometrial cancer‡		4	2	4	2	1		1		1		1	
Endometrial hyperplasia		1		1		1		1		1		1	
Endometriosis		2		1		1		1		1		1	
Epilepsy‡	(*see also Drug Interactions*)	1		1		1*		1*		1*		1*	
Gallbladder disease	a) Symptomatic												
	i) Treated by cholecystectomy	1		2		2		2		2		2	
	ii) Medically treated	1		2		2		2		2		3	
	iii) Current	1		2		2		2		2		3	
	b) Asymptomatic	1		2		2		2		2		2	
Gestational trophoblastic disease‡	a) Suspected GTD (immediate postevacuation)												
	i) Uterine size first trimester	1*		1*		1*		1*		1*		1*	
	ii) Uterine size second trimester	2*		2*		1*		1*		1*		1*	
	b) Confirmed GTD												
	i) Undetectable/non-pregnant ß-hCG levels	1*	1*	1*	1*	1*		1*		1*		1*	
	ii) Decreasing ß-hCG levels	2*	1*	2*	1*	1*		1*		1*		1*	
	iii) Persistently elevated ß-hCG levels or malignant disease, with no evidence or suspicion of intrauterine disease	2*	1*	2*	1*	1*		1*		1*		1*	
	iv) Persistently elevated ß-hCG levels or malignant disease, with evidence or suspicion of intrauterine disease	4*	2*	4*	2*	1*		1*		1*		1*	
Headaches	a) Nonmigraine (mild or severe)	1		1		1		1		1		1*	
	b) Migraine												
	i) Without aura (includes menstrual migraine)	1		1		1		1		1		2*	
	ii) With aura	1		1		1		1		1		4*	
History of bariatric surgery‡	a) Restrictive procedures	1		1		1		1		1		1	
	b) Malabsorptive procedures	1		1		1		1		3		COCs: 3 P/R: 1	
History of cholestasis	a) Pregnancy related	1		1		1		1		1		2	
	b) Past COC related	1		2		2		2		2		3	
History of high blood pressure during pregnancy		1		1		1		1		1		2	
History of Pelvic surgery		1		1		1		1		1		1	
HIV	a) High risk for HIV	1*	1*	1*	1*	1		1		1		1	
	b) HIV infection					1*		1*		1*		1*	
	i) Clinically well receiving ARV therapy	1	1	1	1	If on treatment, see Drug Interactions							
	ii) Not clinically well or not receiving ARV therapy‡	2	1	2	1	If on treatment, see Drug Interactions							

Abbreviations: ARV = antiretroviral; C=continuation of contraceptive method; CHC=combined hormonal contraception (pill, patch, and, ring); COC=combined oral contraceptive; Cu-IUD=copper-containing intrauterine device; DMPA = depot medroxyprogesterone acetate; I=initiation of contraceptive method; LNG-IUD=levonorgestrel-releasing intrauterine device; NA=not applicable; POP=progestin-only pill; P/R=patch/ring; SSRI=selective serotonin reuptake inhibitor; ‡ Condition that exposes a woman to increased risk as a result of pregnancy. *Please see the complete guidance for a clarification to this classification: https://www.cdc.gov/reproductivehealth/contraception/contraception_guidance.htm.

FIGURE 32-1 *(continued).*

Condition	Sub-Condition	Cu-IUD	LNG-IUD	Implant	DMPA	POP	CHC
		I | C	I | C	I | C	I | C	I | C	I | C
Hypertension	a) Adequately controlled hypertension	1*	1*	1*	2*	1*	3*
	b) Elevated blood pressure levels (*properly taken measurements*)						
	i) Systolic 140-159 or diastolic 90-99	1*	1*	1*	2*	1*	3*
	ii) Systolic ≥160 or diastolic ≥100‡	1*	2*	2*	3*	2*	4*
	c) Vascular disease	1*	2*	2*	3*	2*	4*
Inflammatory bowel disease	(*Ulcerative colitis, Crohn's disease*)	1	1	1	2	2	2/3*
Ischemic heart disease‡	Current and history of	1	I: 2; C: 3	I: 2; C: 3	3	I: 2; C: 3	4
Known thrombogenic mutations‡		1*	2*	2*	2*	2*	4*
Liver tumors	a) Benign						
	i) Focal nodular hyperplasia	1	2	2	2	2	2
	ii) Hepatocellular adenoma‡	1	3	3	3	3	4
	b) Malignant‡ (hepatoma)	1	3	3	3	3	4
Malaria		1	1	1	1	1	1
Multiple risk factors for atherosclerotic cardiovascular disease	(e.g., older age, smoking, diabetes, hypertension, low HDL, high LDL, or high triglyceride levels)	1	2	2*	3*	2*	3/4*
Multiple sclerosis	a) With prolonged immobility	1	1	1	2	1	3
	b) Without prolonged immobility	1	1	1	2	1	1
Obesity	a) Body mass index (BMI) ≥30 kg/m²	1	1	1	1	1	2
	b) Menarche to <18 years and BMI ≥ 30 kg/m²	1	1	1	2	1	2
Ovarian cancer‡		1	1	1	1	1	1
Parity	a) Nulliparous	2	2	1	1	1	1
	b) Parous	1	1	1	1	1	1
Past ectopic pregnancy		1	1	1	1	2	1
Pelvic inflammatory disease	a) Past						
	i) With subsequent pregnancy	I: 1; C: 1	I: 1; C: 1	1	1	1	1
	ii) Without subsequent pregnancy	I: 2; C: 2	I: 2; C: 2	1	1	1	1
	b) Current	I: 4; C: 2*	I: 4; C: 2*	1	1	1	1
Peripartum cardiomyopathy‡	a) Normal or mildly impaired cardiac function						
	i) <6 months	2	2	1	1	1	4
	ii) ≥6 months	2	2	1	1	1	3
	b) Moderately or severely impaired cardiac function	2	2	2	2	2	4
Postabortion	a) First trimester	1*	1*	1*	1*	1*	1*
	b) Second trimester	2*	2*	1*	1*	1*	1*
	c) Immediate postseptic abortion	4	4	1*	1*	1*	1*
Postpartum (*nonbreastfeeding women*)	a) <21 days			1	1	1	4
	b) 21 days to 42 days						
	i) With other risk factors for VTE			1	1	1	3*
	ii) Without other risk factors for VTE			1	1	1	2
	c) >42 days			1	1	1	1
Postpartum (*in breastfeeding or non-breastfeeding women, including cesarean delivery*)	a) <10 minutes after delivery of the placenta						
	i) Breastfeeding	1*	2*				
	ii) Nonbreastfeeding	1*	1*				
	b) 10 minutes after delivery of the placenta to <4 weeks	2*	2*				
	c) ≥4 weeks	1*	1*				
	d) Postpartum sepsis	4	4				

FIGURE 32-1 *(continued).*

Condition	Sub-Condition	Cu-IUD I	Cu-IUD C	LNG-IUD I	LNG-IUD C	Implant I	Implant C	DMPA I	DMPA C	POP I	POP C	CHC I	CHC C
Pregnancy		4*		4*		NA*		NA*		NA*		NA*	
Rheumatoid arthritis	a) On immunosuppressive therapy	2	1	2	1	1		2/3*		1		2	
	b) Not on immunosuppressive therapy	1		1		1		2		1		2	
Schistosomiasis	a) Uncomplicated	1		1		1		1		1		1	
	b) Fibrosis of the liver‡	1		1		1		1		1		1	
Sexually transmitted diseases (STDs)	a) Current purulent cervicitis or chlamydial infection or gonococcal infection	4	2*	4	2*	1		1		1		1	
	b) Vaginitis (*including trichomonas vaginalis and bacterial vaginosis*)	2	2	2	2	1		1		1		1	
	c) Other factors relating to STDs	2*	2	2*	2	1		1		1		1	
Smoking	a) Age <35	1		1		1		1		1		2	
	b) Age ≥35, <15 cigarettes/day	1		1		1		1		1		3	
	c) Age ≥35, ≥15 cigarettes/day	1		1		1		1		1		4	
Solid organ transplantation‡	a) Complicated	3	2	3	2	2		2		2		4	
	b) Uncomplicated	2		2		2		2		2		2*	
Stroke‡	History of cerebrovascular accident	1		2		2	3	3		2	3	4	
Superficial venous disorders	a) Varicose veins	1		1		1		1		1		1	
	b) Superficial venous thrombosis (acute or history)	1		1		1		1		1		3*	
Systemic lupus erythematosus‡	a) Positive (or unknown) antiphospholipid antibodies	1*	1*	3*		3*		3*	3*	3*		4*	
	b) Severe thrombocytopenia	3*	2*	2*		2*		3*	2*	2*		2*	
	c) Immunosuppressive therapy	2*	1*	2*		2*		2*	2*	2*		2*	
	d) None of the above	1*	1*	2*		2*		2*	2*	2*		2*	
Thyroid disorders	Simple goiter/ hyperthyroid/hypothyroid	1		1		1		1		1		1	
Tuberculosis‡	a) Nonpelvic	1	1	1	1	1*		1*		1*		1*	
(see also Drug Interactions)	b) Pelvic	4	3	4	3	1*		1*		1*		1*	
Unexplained vaginal bleeding	(suspicious for serious condition) before evaluation	4*	2*	4*	2*	3*		3*		2*		2*	
Uterine fibroids		2		2		1		1		1		1	
Valvular heart disease	a) Uncomplicated	1		1		1		1		1		2	
	b) Complicated‡	1		1		1		1		1		4	
Vaginal bleeding patterns	a) Irregular pattern without heavy bleeding	1		1	1	2		2		2		1	
	b) Heavy or prolonged bleeding	2*		1*	2*	2*		2*		2*		1*	
Viral hepatitis	a) Acute or flare	1		1		1		1		1		3/4*	2
	b) Carrier/Chronic	1		1		1		1		1		1	1
Drug Interactions													
Antiretrovirals used for prevention (PrEP) or treatment of HIV	Fosamprenavir (FPV) All other ARVs are 1 or 2 for all methods.	1/2*	1*	1/2*	1*	2*		2*		2*		3*	
Anticonvulsant therapy	a) Certain anticonvulsants (phenytoin, carbamazepine, barbiturates, primidone, topiramate, oxcarbazepine)	1		1		2*		1*		3*		3*	
	b) Lamotrigine	1		1		1		1		1		3*	
Antimicrobial therapy	a) Broad spectrum antibiotics	1		1		1		1		1		1	
	b) Antifungals	1		1		1		1		1		1	
	c) Antiparasitics	1		1		1		1		1		1	
	d) Rifampin or rifabutin therapy	1		1		2*		1*		3*		3*	
SSRIs		1		1		1		1		1		1	
St John's wort		1		1		2		1		2		2	

Updated in 2020. This summary sheet only contains a subset of the recommendations from the U.S. MEC. For complete guidance, see: https://www.cdc.gov/reproductivehealth/contraception/contraception_guidance.htm. Most contraceptive methods do not protect against sexually transmitted diseases (STDs). Consistent and correct use of the male latex condom reduces the risk of STDs and HIV.

FIGURE 32-1 *(continued).*

Centers for Disease Control and Prevention. Summary chart of U.S. medical eligibility criteria for contraceptive use. Atlanta (GA): CDC 2017. Accessed March 31, 2021 https://www.cdc.gov/reproductivehealth/contraception/pdf/summary-chart-us-medical-eligibility-criteria_508tagged.pdf

Curtis KM, Tepper NK, Jatlaoui TC, Berry-Bibee E, Horton LG, Zapata LB, et al. U.S. medical eligibility criteria for contraceptive use, 2016. MMWR Recomm Rep 2016;65(RR-3):1–103. doi: 10.15585/mmwr.rr6503a1

Tepper NK, Krashin JW, Curtis KM, Cox S, Whiteman MK. Update to CDC's U.S. medical eligibility criteria for contraceptive use, 2016: revised recommendations for the use of hormonal contraception among women at high risk for HIV infection. MMWR Morb Mortal Wkly Rep 2017;66:990–4.

without a need for repeated visits. She should be counseled that there may be a cost associated with removal.

Depot medroxyprogesterone acetate is a highly effective contraception method; however, initiation in the immediate postpartum period or at her postpartum visit will allow her only 12–14 weeks of contraceptive benefit, after which she would not have coverage for repeated doses. Amenorrhea also can continue for 1 year after the last dose, making it difficult to plan the next pregnancy. Her stated desire for 2–3 years of contraception means this is not the best choice.

Similarly, although progesterone-only oral contraception is in U.S. Medical Eligibility for Contraception category 2 for breastfeeding women, after the loss of insurance coverage this patient may no longer have access. Additionally, progesterone-only oral contraception is less effective than LARC methods with typical use (91% effective versus 99% effective, respectively).

Immediate postpartum initiation of an IUD and or a contraceptive implant increases adherence to ongoing contraception, is cost effective, and improves access to care. All patients should be counseled about this option, and efforts should focus on making these contraceptive options available on labor and delivery units. For the described patient who has previously had bothersome side effects from the contraceptive implant, the most appropriate choice is a post-placental IUD.

Immediate postpartum long-acting reversible contraception. Committee Opinion No. 670. American College of Obstetricians and Gynecologists. Obstet Gynecol 2016;128:e32–7. doi: 10.1097/AOG.0000000000001587 https://journals.lww.com/greenjournal/Fulltext/2016/08000/Committee_Opinion_No__670__Immediate_Postpartum.56.aspx

Long-acting reversible contraception: implants and intrauterine devices Practice Bulletin No. 186. American College of Obstetricians and Gynecologists. Obstet Gynecol 2017;130:e251–69. doi: 10.1097/AOG.0000000000002400 https://journals.lww.com/greenjournal/pages/articleviewer.aspx?year=2017&issue=11000&article=00050&type=Fulltext

Optimizing support for breastfeeding as part of obstetric practice. ACOG Committee Opinion No. 756. American College of Obstetricians and Gynecologists. Obstet Gynecol 2018;132:e187–96. doi: 10.1097/AOG.0000000000002890 https://journals.lww.com/greenjournal/Fulltext/2018/10000/ACOG_Committee_Opinion_No__756__Optimizing_Support.62.aspx

33 Postexposure HIV prophylaxis

During an emergent cesarean birth, the surgical technologist, who is pregnant at 28 weeks of gestation, experiences an accidental needle stick. The patient had no prenatal care, and her rapid human immunodeficiency virus (HIV) test on admission to labor and delivery was positive. The best next step to decrease the risk of vertical transmission to the surgical technologist's fetus is

(A) administer zidovudine in labor
(B) await the surgical patient's fourth-generation HIV test results
* (C) begin postexposure prophylaxis (PEP) immediately
(D) perform HIV testing at 36 weeks of gestation

The risk of HIV seroconversion in occupational exposure from needlestick is approximately 0.3%. Postexposure prophylaxis for HIV should be started as soon as possible after high-risk exposure, including in pregnant women. High-risk exposures include percutaneous injury from a device visibly contaminated with the patient's blood, procedures in which the needle was directly in a vein or artery, and deep injury. High viral load at the time of exposure appears to increase the risk. Postexposure prophylaxis should be offered in all of these circumstances, even if the patient's viral load is undetectable. In situations in which the source patient's HIV status is unknown, PEP can be started while awaiting HIV testing results and discontinued if testing comes back negative.

The Centers for Disease Control and Prevention currently recommends 4 weeks of PEP. A multidrug regimen should be used, with at least three antiviral agents. The regimen selected should have a favorable adverse-effect profile with decreased toxicity to improve adherence. Older regimens often were poorly tolerated and patients often discontinued the treatment course early.

Postexposure prophylaxis should be offered to pregnant women with high-risk exposure to HIV, because HIV carries significant risk for the woman and acute HIV infection during pregnancy carries significantly higher risk of vertical transmission. Postexposure prophylaxis regimens in the first trimester should avoid efavirenz because of a possible increased risk of neural tube defects.

Those who are breastfeeding and have an HIV exposure should be counseled on the risks of transmission to the newborn if seroconversion occurs. Risks of PEP to the infant are low given the short duration of treatment, and breastfeeding is not a contraindication to PEP. Women should weigh the risks and benefits of breastfeeding in this setting.

In this scenario, the surgical technologist should be tested for HIV again in the third trimester, as should all those at high risk of HIV exposure. However, testing alone will not decrease the risk of transmission to the newborn. If seroconversion does occur, intravenous zidovudine should be administered in the setting of a high viral load, but again, this is not the best next step in management. Because the patient's rapid HIV is positive, PEP should not be delayed for a fourth-generation test result. Postexposure prophylaxis should be offered to the surgical technologist as soon as possible and could be discontinued if the patient's fourth-generation test is negative.

Kuhar DT, Henderson DK, Struble KA, Heneine W, Thomas V, Cheever LW, et al. Updated U.S. Public Health Service guidelines for the management of occupational exposures to HIV and recommendations for postexposure prophylaxis. USPHS Working Group on Occupational Postexposure Prophylaxis, National Center for Emerging and Zoonotic Infectious Diseases (U.S.), Division of Healthcare Quality Promotion. 2018. https://stacks.cdc.gov/view/cdc/20711

Prenatal and perinatal human immunodeficiency virus testing. ACOG Committee Opinion No. 752. American College of Obstetricians and Gynecologists. Obstet Gynecol 2018;132:e138–42. doi: 10.1097/AOG.0000000000002825 https://journals.lww.com/greenjournal/Fulltext/2018/09000/ACOG_Committee_Opinion_No__752__Prenatal_and.70.aspx

34 Induction in a patient undergoing a trial of labor after cesarean birth

A 34-year-old gravida 5, para 2, is at 39 weeks of gestation and has gestational hypertension without severe features. She delivered her first pregnancy vaginally at term, and her second was delivered at 38 weeks of gestation by cesarean birth for fetal intolerance of labor. She wants a trial of labor. Her cervix is 3-cm dilated and 50% effaced, in the anterior position, and soft, with the fetal vertex at −3 station and ballotable. The most appropriate management is

(A) dinoprostone
(B) expectant management
(C) misoprostol
* (D) oxytocin
(E) transcervical balloon

Successful vaginal birth after cesarean (VBAC) has several potential advantages for women and is associated with decreased maternal morbidity and fewer complications in future pregnancies. Most publications report a probability of successful VBAC in those undergoing trial of labor after cesarean (TOLAC) in the 60–80% range. There are several factors related to success in TOLAC, including demographic and obstetric characteristics. Several tools have been developed that calculate the likelihood of a VBAC for individual patients. Although no single prediction calculator has been shown to result in improved patient outcomes, use of these tools can provide helpful information for patients and obstetrician–gynecologists to consider in the shared decision making that occurs when considering TOLAC.

Induction of labor is an option for women considering TOLAC. Some studies have shown an increased risk of uterine rupture in patients with a previous cesarean birth who undergo labor induction, but the largest factor in these patients' outcomes was the use of prostaglandins. The risk of uterine rupture in patients undergoing TOLAC is not affected by cervical favorability. Oxytocin is not clearly associated with an increased risk of uterine rupture for either induction of labor or augmentation of labor in these patients, and it is the best next step for the patient in this scenario.

It is important to note that successful VBAC is associated with fewer complications than repeat cesarean birth; however, failed TOLAC requiring repeat cesarean delivery is associated with more complications than planned repeat cesarean delivery.

The Bishop pelvic scoring system (Appendix B) is a helpful guide in determining whether a patient is likely to benefit from cervical ripening before oxytocin augmentation or induction. The system assigns a score of 0–3 for each of the five components of the cervical examination: dilation, effacement, station, position, and consistency. Scores totaling less than 6 suggest that the cervix is unfavorable for oxytocin and should first be ripened. Scores greater than 8 suggest that the probability of vaginal birth with labor induction is similar to the probability of vaginal birth with spontaneous labor.

If cervical ripening is indicated to facilitate softening, thinning, and dilation of the cervix in anticipation of a successful vaginal birth, available cervical ripening agents include medical and mechanical options. Medical options include synthetic prostaglandin E1 (misoprostol) and E2 (dinoprostone) agents. Mechanical dilators typically consist of a double or single balloon catheter such as the Foley catheter. In the setting of a previous cesarean birth, misoprostol and dinoprostone typically are avoided because these prostaglandins have been associated with a higher risk of uterine rupture in some studies. After 28 weeks of gestation, the transcervical balloon has been associated with uterine rupture rates comparable to spontaneous labor and would be the best option in a patient requiring cervical ripening in the setting of a previous cesarean birth.

For the described patient who is selecting TOLAC, given the Bishop score of 8, she would not benefit from either medical or mechanical cervical ripening. Medical ripening agents (dinoprostone and misoprostol) typically are avoided in patients with a previous cesarean birth. Given the patient's desire for a vaginal birth, the best option is induction with oxytocin. Because she has gestational hypertension, delivery rather than expectant management is indicated.

Induction of labor. ACOG Practice Bulletin No. 107. American College of Obstetricians and Gynecologists. Obstet Gynecol 2009;114:386–97. doi: 10.1097/AOG.0b013e3181b48ef5 https://journals.lww.com/greenjournal/Citation/2009/08000/ACOG_Practice_Bulletin_No__107__Induction_of_Labor.30.aspx

Use of psychiatric medications during pregnancy and lactation. ACOG Practice Bulletin No. 92. American College of Obstetricians and Gynecologists. Obstet Gynecol 2008;111:1001–20. doi: 10.1097/AOG.0b013e31816fd910 https://journals.lww.com/greenjournal/Citation/2008/04000/ACOG_Practice_Bulletin_No__92__Use_of_Psychiatric.39.aspx

35 Aneuploidy screening

A 38-year-old gravida 4, para 2, at 12 weeks of gestation with a dichorionic twin pregnancy desires aneuploidy testing as early as possible. On ultrasonography, one twin has no fetal heart motion and measures about 4 weeks smaller than the co-twin with fetal heart motion. The appropriate aneuploidy test is

(A) amniocentesis
(B) cell-free DNA (cfDNA) screening
* (C) chorionic villus sampling
(D) first-trimester screening
(E) integrated screening

The incidence of all chromosomal abnormalities is approximately 1 in 150 live births. However, the prevalence is greater earlier in gestation because aneuploidy accounts for a significant percentage of pregnancy loss. All pregnant patients should be counseled regarding the risk of aneuploidy, regardless of age or risk of chromosomal abnormality. This counseling should include a discussion of the various screening and diagnostic tests. A wide variety of prenatal screening and tests is available, each with relative advantages and disadvantages, which are listed in Table 35-1.

The diagnostic tests include chorionic villus sampling, which can be performed between 10 and 14 weeks of gestation, and amniocentesis, typically not performed before 15 weeks of gestation. These diagnostic tests are invasive and carry a risk of complications. The complication rate of chorionic villus sampling is about 1%, and the complications include bleeding, infection, and pregnancy loss. The risk of complications from amniocentesis is less than 0.1%, with similar complications, including bleeding, infection, pregnancy loss, and rupture of membranes.

Cell-free DNA testing is the most sensitive and specific screening test for common aneuploidies. The sensitivity and specificity of cfDNA screening are similar across high-risk and low-risk populations. Cell-free DNA screening is more likely to be high risk of aneuploidy in the setting of a deceased co-twin, and is not advised. In this setting, nuchal translucency measurement or diagnostic testing is recommended.

First-trimester screening allows early and accurate detection of fetal chromosomal abnormalities, allowing for more choices in testing and diagnosis. First-trimester screening includes the measurement of the nuchal translucency and serial measurements of β-human chorionic gonadotropin (β-hCG) concentrations or total β-hCG and pregnancy-associated plasma protein A (PAPP-A) levels. These analytes are measured in multiples of the median, which standardizes values across gestational age. This test typically is performed when the crown–rump length is between 38–45 and 84 mm (generally between 10 0/7 and 13 6/7 weeks of gestation). The combination provides the detection rate of common aneuploidies of approximately 85%, with a false-positive test rate of 5%. Positive results for this test allow the patient the options of another screening with cfDNA or diagnostic tests, such as chorionic villus sampling or amniocentesis. Even without the analytes, an enlarged nuchal translucency measurement (ie, greater than the 99th percentile, or 3.0 mm) is an independent risk factor for a chromosomal abnormality. In these cases, patients often are offered additional testing without measuring the analytes.

The quadruple-marker screen ("quad" screen) can be performed during the second trimester (16–21 weeks of gestation). The serum test does not require specialized ultrasonography for measurement of the nuchal translucency, and it also provides information regarding the risk of open neural tube defects, in addition to risk assessment for trisomy 21 and 18. The quad screen involves measurement of four maternal serum analytes—β-hCG, α-fetoprotein, dimeric inhibin A, and unconjugated estriol—in combination with maternal factors such as age, weight, and the presence of pregestational diabetes to calculate risk estimate. Second-trimester quad screening has a detection rate for trisomy 21 of 80%, with a 5% false-positive rate.

With integrated screening, the patient undergoes a first-trimester nuchal translucency measurement and serum analyte screening followed by a second-trimester blood assessment obtained for the four analytes described previously in the quad

TABLE 35-1. Characteristics, Advantages, and Disadvantages of Common Screening Tests for Chromosomal Abnormalities

SCREENING APPROACH	APPROXIMATE GESTATIONAL AGE RANGE FOR SCREENING (WK)	DETECTION RATE (DR) FOR TRISOMY 21 (%)	SCREEN POSITIVE RATE* (%)	ADVANTAGES	DISADVANTAGES	METHOD
Cell-free DNA[†]	9–10 to term	99	2–4% Includes inability to obtain results, which is associated with increased risk[†]	1. Highest DR 2. Can be performed at any gestational age after 9–10 wk 3. Lowest false-positive rate	Results may reflect underlying maternal aneuploidy or maternal disease	Several molecular methods
First trimester[‡]	10–13 6/7[§]	82–87[‖]	5	1. Early screening 2. Single time point test	Lower DR than tests with first- and second-trimester component NT required	NT+PAPP-A, free β-hCG, +/– AFP[¶]
Quad screen[‡]	15–22	81	5	1. Single time point test 2. No specialized US required	Lower DR than first trimester and first and second trimester combined tests	hCG, AFP, uE3, DIA
Integrated[‡]	10–13 6/7[§], then 15–22	96	5	High DR	Two samples needed No first-trimester results NT required	NT+PAPP-A, then quad screen
Serum integrated[‡]	10–13 6/7[§], then 15–22	88	5	1. DR compares favorably with first-trimester screening 2. No specialized US required	Two samples needed No first-trimester results	PAPP-A + quad screen
Sequential**: stepwise	10–13 6/7[§], then 15–22	95	5	1. First-trimester results provided 2. Comparable performance to integrated, but FTS results provided	Two samples needed NT required	NT+ free β-hCG + PAPP-A, +/– AFP[¶], then quad screen
Contingent screening**		88–94	5	First-trimester test result: Positive: diagnostic test or cell-free DNA offered Negative: no further testing Intermediate: second-trimester test offered Final: risk assessment incorporates first- and second-trimester results	Possibly two samples needed NT required	NT+hCG+ PAPP-A, +/– AFP[¶], then quad screen
Nuchal translucency alone[#]	10–13 6/7[§]	70	5	Allows individual fetus assessment in multifetal gestations Provides additional screening for fetal anomalies	Poor sensitivity and specificity in isolation NT required	US only

TABLE 35-1 *(continued).*

Abbreviations: AFP, alpha-fetoprotein; DIA, dimeric inhibin-A; DR, detection rate; FTS, first-trimester screening; hCG, human chorionic gonadotropin; NPV, negative predictive value; NT, nuchal translucency; PAPP-A, pregnancy-associated plasma protein A; PPV, positive predictive value; uE3, unconjugated estriol; US, ultrasonography.

All patients should be offered second-trimester assessment for open fetal defects (by ultrasonography, with or without second-trimester serum AFP) and ultrasound screening for other fetal structural defects.

*A screen positive test result includes all positive test results: the true positives and false positives. For cell-free DNA, this includes the test failure rates given the association with increased risk of aneuploidy (see † below).

†Gil MM, Accurti V, Santacruz B, Plana MN, Nicolaides KH. Analysis of cell-free DNA in maternal blood in screening for aneuploidies: updated meta-analysis. Ultrasound Obstet Gynecol 2017;50:302–14.

‡First-trimester combined screening: 87%, 85%, and 82% for measurements performed at 11 weeks, 12 weeks, and 13 weeks, respectively (Malone FD, Canick JA, Ball RH, Nyberg DA, Comstock CH, Bukowski R, et al. First-trimester or second-trimester screening, or both, for Down's syndrome. First- and Second-Trimester Evaluation of Risk (FASTER) Research Consortium. N Engl J Med 2005;353:2001–11.)

§Because of variations in growth and pregnancy dating, some fetuses at the lower and upper gestational age limits may fall outside the required crown–rump length range. Also, different laboratories use slightly different gestational age windows for their testing protocol.

‖Use of free β-hCG in conjunction with nasal bone assessment increases the detection rate to 97% with a screen positive rate of 5% (Cicero S, Bindra R, Rembouskos G, Spencer K, Nicolaides KH. Integrated ultrasound and biochemical screening for trisomy 21 using fetal nuchal translucency, absent fetal nasal bone, free beta-hCG and PAPP-A at 11 to 14 weeks. Prenat Diagn 2003;23:306–10.)

¶Testing of first-trimester AFP depends on commercial lab used. First-trimester AFP should not be used in lieu of second-trimester AFP for open fetal defects screening.

#Alldred SK, Takwoingi Y, Guo B, Pennant M, Deeks JJ, Neilson JP, et al. First trimester ultrasound tests alone or in combination with first trimester serum tests for Down's syndrome screening. Cochrane Database of Systematic Reviews 2017, Issue 3. Art. No.: CD012600. doi: 10.1002/14651858.CD012600.

**Cuckle H, Benn P, Wright D. Down syndrome screening in the first and/or second trimester: model predicted performance using meta-analysis parameters. Semin Perinatol 2005;29:252–7.

Reprinted from Screening for fetal chromosomal abnormalities: ACOG Practice Bulletin No. 226. American College of Obstetricians and Gynecologists. Obstet Gynecol 2020;136:e48–69. doi: 10.1097/AOG.0000000000004084 https://journals.lww.com/greenjournal/Fulltext/2020/10000/Screening_for_Fetal_Chromosomal_Abnormalities_.44.aspx

screen. The patient receives a single test result in the second trimester. When specialized ultrasonography is not available, or an accurate nuchal translucency cannot be measured because of fetal position or maternal body habitus, serum integrated screening is an option. The detection rate with serum integrated screening is similar to first-trimester screening.

For the described patient, the appropriate test is a diagnostic one. In the setting of a death of one twin, screening by cfDNA testing or serum analyte measurement is less accurate, and, therefore, diagnostic testing should be offered. Because the patient requests testing as soon as possible, chorionic villus sampling is the best option.

Obesity in pregnancy. ACOG Practice Bulletin No. 230. American College of Obstetricians and Gynecologists. Obstet Gynecol 2021;137:e128–44. doi: 10.1097/AOG.0000000000004395 https://journals.lww.com/greenjournal/Fulltext/2021/06000/Obesity_in_Pregnancy__ACOG_Practice_Bulletin,.38.aspx

Screening for fetal chromosomal abnormalities: ACOG Practice Bulletin No. 226. American College of Obstetricians and Gynecologists. Obstet Gynecol 2020;136:e48–69. doi: 10.1097/AOG.0000000000004084 https://journals.lww.com/greenjournal/Fulltext/2020/10000/Screening_for_Fetal_Chromosomal_Abnormalities_.44.aspx

36 Smoking cessation

A 36-year-old multigravida presents at 22 weeks of gestation. She has been trying to quit smoking since early in pregnancy using cognitive behavioral techniques but has been unsuccessful. The patient is interested in additional therapy to help her quit. The best next step is to prescribe

* (A) bupropion
(B) nicotine replacement therapy
(C) sertraline
(D) venlafaxine

All pregnant women should be questioned regarding use of tobacco products and advised of the significant risks associated with tobacco use. Tobacco use in pregnancy is associated with preterm birth, fetal growth restriction, preterm prelabor rupture of membranes, placental abruption, and increased perinatal mortality. Children born to individuals who smoke are at increased risk of complications during childhood, such as asthma, obesity, and bone fractures, and sudden infant death syndrome. Tobacco cessation at any time during pregnancy provides benefit to the patient and fetus; therefore, tobacco use is an important modifiable risk factor that should be addressed by clinicians throughout their patients' pregnancies.

Many patients are motivated to quit smoking before or while pregnant. The U.S. Preventive Services Task Force recommends that practitioners ask patients about tobacco use, advise cessation, and offer behavioral interventions for those who use tobacco. Obstetricians should ask about all types of tobacco or nicotine use, including smoking, using e-cigarettes, vaping, and using hookahs. Both psychosocial interventions and pharmacologic therapy can be used. These interventions can be offered at initial prenatal visits and throughout pregnancy.

The five A's intervention has been shown to be effective in helping pregnant patients quit. This technique involves asking about tobacco or nicotine use, advising the patient to stop using tobacco or nicotine, assessing the patient's willingness to stop, assisting the patient with quitting with specific techniques, and arranging follow-up for the patient (Box 36-1). Patients can be given information on the national QUIT line network (1-800-QUIT-NOW). These effective psychosocial interventions can be used with pregnant patients.

In addition to psychosocial interventions, prescription medication and nicotine replacement often help with tobacco cessation. There are several categories of medication approved by the U.S. Food and Drug Administration. Bupropion, an atypical antidepressant that is a norepinephrine–dopamine reuptake inhibitor and nicotinic antagonist, has been shown to reduce the severity of craving for nicotine and reduce withdrawal symptoms. It helps with smoking cessation and is not associated with adverse effects in pregnancy. In doses of up to 300 mg, bupropion is associated with low levels of detection in breast milk, and no adverse effects have been shown in the infant. Bupropion is contraindicated in patients with a history of seizures or an eating disorder. Bupropion carries a warning regarding risk of increase in psychiatric symptoms associated with use, and clinicians must address psychiatric concerns before starting this medication. For the patient in this scenario, bupropion is the best answer as it is well studied in pregnancy and has been shown to be effective.

Nicotine replacement therapy may help with smoking cessation and is available in the form of a patch, gum, and nasal spray. However, nicotine replacement therapy may carry risks to pregnancy. The U.S. Preventive Services Task Force has concluded that there is insufficient evidence to assess the benefits and harms of nicotine replacement in pregnancy. Although nicotine replacement may increase rates of smoking cessation, recent studies have shown that nicotine replacement therapy is not the most effective approach during pregnancy. For these reasons, it is recommended that nicotine replacement therapy be used only after a detailed discussion with the patient regarding the risks and benefits and in patients who plan to use it for a defined time until smoking cessation is achieved. Nicotine replacement therapy is not the best answer choice in this patient as it is not the first-line therapy for smoking cessation in pregnancy.

In addition to bupropion, varenicline, although not listed in this question, is another medication available for smoking cessation in pregnancy. It is a partial agonist for nicotine receptors and is an effective pharmacologic assistant for smoking cessation. Several small studies have evaluated its use in pregnancy with no increase in teratogenicity or adverse pregnancy outcomes, although overall, data remain limited. In several studies varenicline has increased rates of smoking cessation without increasing adverse pregnancy outcomes.

Sertraline and venlafaxine are other antidepressants that are not helpful in smoking cessation and are not the best answer choices for this patient. Bupropion is well studied and effective and the best answer choice for the patient in this scenario.

BOX 36-1

Five A's of Tobacco and Nicotine Cessation

1. ASK the patient about smoking status* at the first prenatal visit and follow up with her at subsequent visits. The patient should choose the statement that best describes her tobacco or nicotine use status:
   A. I have never used tobacco or nicotine or have used minimal amounts of tobacco or nicotine in my lifetime (for example, less than 100 cigarettes in my lifetime).
   B. I stopped using tobacco or nicotine before I found out I was pregnant, and I am not using tobacco or nicotine now.
   C. I stopped using tobacco or nicotine after I found out I was pregnant, and I am not using tobacco or nicotine now.
   D. I use some tobacco or nicotine now, but I have cut down on the amount of tobacco or nicotine I use since I found out I was pregnant.
   E. I use tobacco or nicotine regularly now, about the same as before I found out I was pregnant.

   If the patient stopped using tobacco or nicotine before or after she found out she was pregnant (B or C), reinforce her decision to quit, congratulate her on success in quitting, and encourage her to stay tobacco and nicotine free throughout pregnancy and postpartum. If the patient is still using tobacco or nicotine (D or E), document tobacco and nicotine status in her medical record, and proceed to Advise, Assess, Assist, and Arrange.
2. ADVISE the patient who uses tobacco or nicotine to stop by providing advice about quitting with information about the risks of continued tobacco and nicotine use to the woman, fetus, and newborn.
3. ASSESS the patient's willingness to attempt to quit using tobacco or nicotine at the time. Quitting advice, assessment, and motivational assistance should be offered at subsequent prenatal care visits.
4. ASSIST the patient who is interested in quitting by providing pregnancy-specific, self-help tobacco and nicotine cessation materials. Support the importance of having tobacco- and nicotine-free space at home and seeking out a quitting buddy such as a former tobacco or nicotine user. Encourage the patient to talk about the process of quitting. Offer a direct referral to the national tobacco quit line (1-800-QUIT-NOW) to provide ongoing counseling and support.
5. ARRANGE follow-up visits to track the progress of the patient's attempt to quit using tobacco and nicotine. For current and former tobacco and nicotine users, use status should be monitored and recorded throughout pregnancy, providing opportunities to congratulate and support success, reinforce steps taken towards quitting, and encourage those still considering a cessation attempt.

*Includes smoking and use of e-cigarettes and vaping products, hookahs, snus, lozenges, patches, and gum.

Modified from Agency for Healthcare Research and Quality. Treating tobacco use and dependence: 2008 update. AHRQ; 2020. Accessed March 23, 2022. https://www.ahrq.gov/prevention/guidelines/tobacco/index.html.

Agency for Healthcare Research and Quality. Treating tobacco use and dependence: 2008 update. AHRQ; 2020. Accessed March 23, 2022. https://www.ahrq.gov/prevention/guidelines/tobacco/index.html

Agency for Healthcare Research and Quality. Five major steps to intervention (the "5 A's"). AHRQ; 2012. Accessed March 23, 2022. https://www.ahrq.gov/prevention/guidelines/tobacco/5steps.html

Hartmann-Boyce J, Chepkin SC, Ye W, Bullen C, Lancaster T. Nicotine replacement therapy versus control for smoking cessation. Cochrane Database of Systematic Reviews 2018, Issue 5. Art. No.: CD000146. doi: 10.1002/14651858.CD000146.pub5 https://www.cochranelibrary.com/cdsr/doi/10.1002/14651858.CD000146.pub5/full

National Library of Medicine. Bupropion. In: Drugs and Lactation Database (LactMed). NLM; 2021. https://www.ncbi.nlm.nih.gov/books/NBK501184

Siu AL. Behavioral and pharmacotherapy interventions for tobacco smoking cessation in adults, including pregnant women: U.S. Preventive Services Task Force Recommendation Statement. Ann Intern Med 2015;163:622–34. doi: 10.7326/M15-2023 https://pubmed.ncbi.nlm.nih.gov/26389730/

Tobacco and nicotine cessation during pregnancy: ACOG Committee Opinion No. 807. American College of Obstetricians and Gynecologists. Obstet Gynecol 2020;135:e221–9. doi: 10.1097/AOG.0000000000003822 https://journals.lww.com/greenjournal/pages/articleviewer.aspx?year=2020&issue=05000&article=00056&type=Fulltext

Turner E, Jones M, Vaz LR, Coleman T. Systematic review and meta-analysis to assess the safety of bupropion and varenicline in pregnancy. Nicotine Tob Res 2019;21:1001–10. doi: 10.1093/ntr/nty055 https://academic.oup.com/ntr/article/21/8/1001/4951455

37 Ultrasound screening

A patient presents for a fetal anatomy survey. She had low-risk cell-free DNA screening but declined other genetic testing. Her ultrasonographic findings are shown in Figure 37-1. The best next genetic carrier testing to recommend is

* (A) cystic fibrosis
(B) expanded carrier screening
(C) fragile X
(D) spinal muscular atrophy
(E) Tay-Sachs

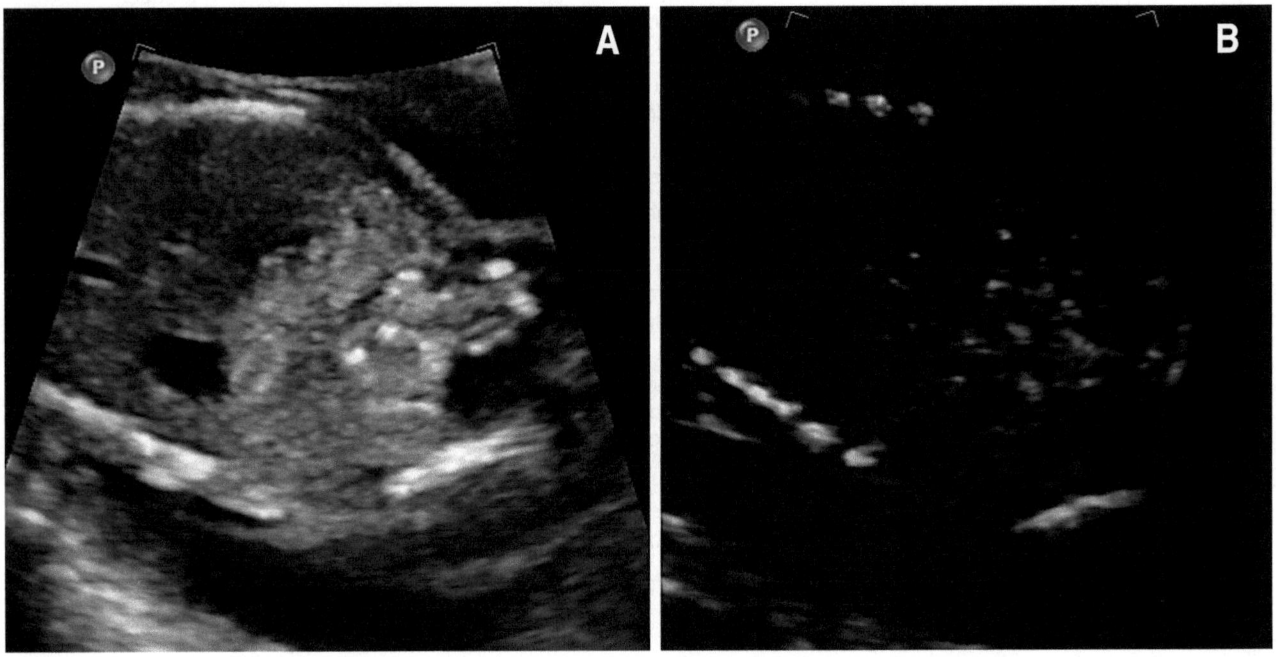

FIGURE 37-1. Ultrasonographic findings of the fetal abdomen for the described patient. Image B is the same as image A but with a modified transducer gain velocity curve.

Genetic carrier screening should be offered to all pregnant patients, ideally as a part of prepregnancy counseling, to detect the risk of autosomal recessive conditions and X-linked disorders. Certain carrier screening should be offered to all patients regardless of family history or ethnicity because of the high frequency of silent carriers in the general population. Screening for other conditions should be based on family history or ethnic background. Currently, the American College of Obstetricians and Gynecologists (ACOG) recommends universal screening for cystic fibrosis, hemoglobinopathies (with baseline blood count), and spinal muscular atrophy. If a patient is found to be a carrier for a condition, their partner should be offered testing to determine whether they are also a carrier, which would place the fetus at risk of an inheritable condition. Genetic counseling is advised for any at-risk pregnancy, with specific counseling regarding prenatal diagnosis if already pregnant, or the possibility of preimplantation diagnosis if the couple chooses in vitro fertilization as a method to achieve a future pregnancy.

Cystic fibrosis is the most common medically consequential genetic condition in the non-Hispanic White population with a carrier rate of 1:25. However, since race is difficult to assign and many patients self-ascribe to more than one race, ACOG recommends universal screening for cystic fibrosis. Cystic fibrosis carrier screening detects only the most common mutations, and the sensitivity of the test varies with different ethnic groups. This does mean that residual risk to the pregnancy is higher in Hispanic, Black, and Asian Americans because of the lower detection rates in these populations. In couples in which both individuals are carriers, prenatal diagnosis is possible with chorionic villus sampling or amniocentesis.

Fetuses affected with cystic fibrosis may have echogenic bowel found at the time of anatomical ultrasonography, and this should be considered a potential etiology of this marker in a patient with an unknown or positive carrier test. The pathophysiology of this is due to the meconium ileus that may be present in affected fetuses, and cystic fibrosis accounts for about 2% of echogenic bowel cases. The overall incidence of echogenic bowel is 0.4%, of which 72% are isolated. Echogenic bowel also may be associated with trisomy 21 (5%), intra-amniotic bleeding (9%), and fetal cytomegalovirus infection (2%). Approximately 13% of fetuses with echogenic bowel will develop fetal growth restriction. In this patient with low-risk cell-free DNA testing, the best genetic carrier test to perform is cystic fibrosis. If the patient is a cystic fibrosis carrier with echogenic fetal bowel, the risk to the fetus may be as high as 64%, and diagnostic testing should be offered.

Spinal muscular atrophy is a degenerative disease of the spinal cord motor neurons leading to muscle atrophy and weakness. Screening for this disease also is universally recommended to obstetric patients and has a carrier frequency of 1 in 40 to 1 in 60. Like cystic fibrosis, carrier frequencies vary by ethnicity, which will alter the residual risk of having an affected fetus in the setting of negative carrier testing. Carrier testing can detect how many copies of the survival of motor neuron 1 (*SMN1*) gene are present, with carriers identified as those with only one copy of the *SMN1* gene. However, carrier testing tests only the quantity of the *SMN1* gene and will not detect whether both genes are on one allele or whether there is a mutation in the gene itself. These factors are what contribute to the residual risk after negative screening. Spinal muscular atrophy has several types that are separated by age of onset. Type I (Werdnig Hoffmann) has symptom onset before age 6 months with death from respiratory failure in early childhood. Type 0 is proposed in cases with onset in the prenatal period. Although these cases may present with ultrasound findings of limited muscle movement, there is no association with echogenic bowel, and testing for spinal muscular atrophy would not be the recommended next step.

Fragile X syndrome, Tay–Sachs disease, and expanded carrier screening usually are performed only in selected populations. Genetic counseling should occur if a patient who does not meet clinical criteria desires more expansive genetic carrier screening. Fragile X premutation testing can be offered to patients who present with ovarian insufficiency before age 40 years or have a family history of fragile X–related disorders or intellectual disability that could be suggestive of fragile X syndrome, an X-linked condition. Tay–Sachs carrier testing is recommended for patients of Ashkenazi Jewish descent because of the high carrier frequency of 1 in 30. Patients with French Canadian and Cajun ancestry also have relatively high carrier frequency rate (1 in 50) and should be offered screening. The described patient's history does not state any specific ancestry consistent with a high carrier frequency for fragile X or Tay–Sachs disease, nor do these present with echogenic bowel on prenatal cases. Although expanded carrier screening may be the test of choice in the future, only directive carrier screening currently is recommended. Expanded carrier screening is an option for patients, but they should be fully counseled on the potential conditions being evaluated, and counseling should continue if screening results are positive. Expanded carrier screening through commercial laboratories may be more cost effective than testing for several individual carrier conditions, and this can be considered in these scenarios. However, directly testing for cystic fibrosis is most appropriate given the ultrasound findings.

Carrier screening for genetic conditions. Committee Opinion No. 691. American College of Obstetricians and Gynecologists. Obstet Gynecol 2017;129:e41–55. doi: 10.1097/AOG.0000000000001952 https://journals.lww.com/greenjournal/Fulltext/2017/03000/Committee_Opinion_No__691__Carrier_Screening_for.48.aspx

Goetzinger KR, Cahill AG, Macones GA, Odibo AO. Echogenic bowel on second-trimester ultrasonography: evaluating the risk of adverse pregnancy outcome. Obstet Gynecol 2011;117:1341–8. doi: 10.1097/AOG.0b013e31821aa739 https://journals.lww.com/greenjournal/Fulltext/2011/06000/Echogenic_Bowel_on_Second_Trimester.12.aspx

Ogino S, Wilson RB, Gold B, Hawley P, Grody WW. Bayesian analysis for cystic fibrosis risks in prenatal and carrier screening [published erratum appears in Genet Med 2005;7:460]. Genet Med 2004;6:439–49. doi: 10.1097/01.gim.0000139511.83336.8f https://www.nature.com/articles/gim200458

Screening for fetal chromosomal abnormalities: ACOG Practice Bulletin No. 226. American College of Obstetricians and Gynecologists. Obstet Gynecol 2020;136:e48–69. doi: 10.1097/AOG.0000000000004084 https://journals.lww.com/greenjournal/Fulltext/2020/10000/Screening_for_Fetal_Chromosomal_Abnormalities_.44.aspx

38 Hypertension in pregnancy

A previously healthy 38-year-old gravida 1 at 35 weeks of gestation presents to the labor and delivery unit with a severe headache and nausea. Her initial blood pressure is 182/108 mm Hg, and repeat blood pressure is 174/110 mm Hg. Hydralazine is administered intravenously. Ultrasonography on presentation showed the fetus in the cephalic presentation. The fetal heart tracing was reassuring upon arrival with a baseline of 120 beats per minute, moderate variability, and accelerations. Laboratory values are pending. You are called to the room after the patient experiences a tonic-clonic seizure. She is in the left lateral decubitus position, bedrails are padded, and oxygen is being administered through a nonrebreather face mask. The fetal heart tracing is shown in Figure 38-1. The most appropriate next step is to

(A) administer diazepam
* (B) administer magnesium sulfate
(C) initiate induction of labor
(D) perform imaging of the brain
(E) perform immediate cesarean delivery

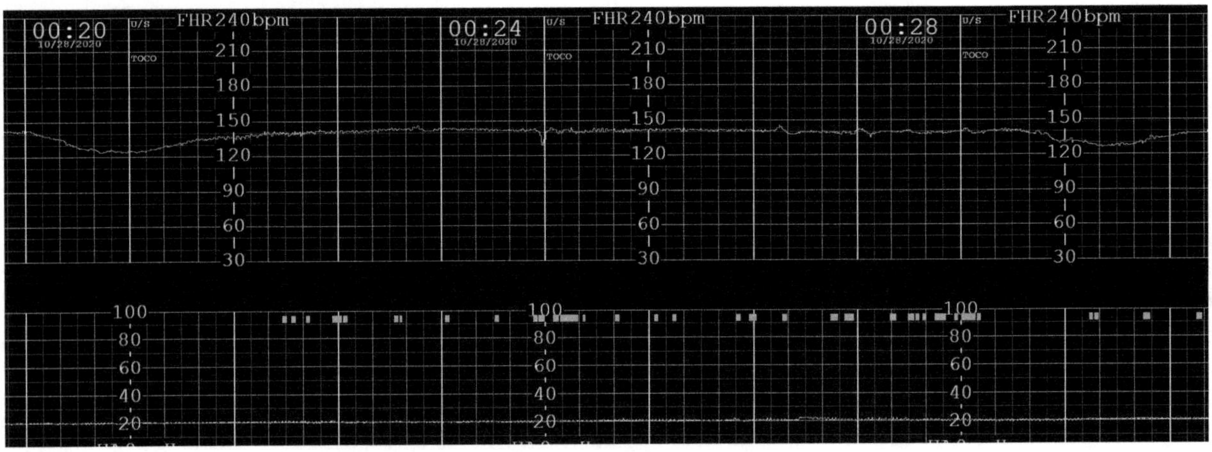

FIGURE 38-1. Fetal heart tracing after the patient experiences a tonic-clonic seizure.

Hypertensive disorders of pregnancy remain a major cause of maternal morbidity and mortality worldwide. The four major categories of hypertensive disorders during pregnancy include 1) chronic hypertension; 2) gestational hypertension; 3) preeclampsia, eclampsia, or HELLP (hemolysis, elevated liver enzymes, and low platelet count) syndrome; and 4) preeclampsia superimposed on chronic hypertension. Preeclampsia is new-onset hypertension occurring primarily after 20 weeks of gestation. In the United States, the incidence of preeclampsia has increased and currently affects approximately 4% of pregnancies. Approximately 1–2% of preeclampsia cases evolve into eclampsia, a severe manifestation of hypertension in pregnancy. The rate of eclampsia varies significantly and is increased in communities with limited resources. Most deaths attributed to hypertension in pregnancy could be prevented with timely and appropriate care.

In this scenario, the initial diagnosis is preeclampsia with severe features (Appendix C). The criteria for severe features are fulfilled based on blood pressures and neurologic symptoms. *Severe hypertension* is defined as a systolic blood pressure of 160 mm Hg or greater, a diastolic blood pressure of 110 mm Hg or greater, or both, on two occasions at least 4 hours apart. However, the 4-hour interval is not necessary if the elevations are persistent (two elevations in 15 minutes or more) to facilitate timely antihypertensive therapy. In this scenario, with two severe-range blood pressures, the goal is to administer antihypertensive medications as soon as possible, and within 30–60 minutes at most, to reduce the risk of maternal stroke. First-line antihypertensive agents for acute-onset severe hypertension include intravenous hydralazine or labetalol and oral nifedipine; any of these are appropriate to administer (Table 38-1). Maintenance antihypertensive therapy may

TABLE 38-1. Antihypertensive Agents Used for Urgent Blood Pressure Control in Pregnancy*

DRUG	DOSE	COMMENTS	ONSET OF ACTION
Labetalol	10–20 mg IV, then 20–80 mg every 10–30 min to a maximum cumulative dosage of 300 mg; or constant infusion 1–2 mg/min IV	Tachycardia is less common with fewer adverse effects. Avoid in women with asthma, preexisting myocardial disease, decompensated cardiac function, and heart block and bradycardia.	1–2 min
Hydralazine	5 mg IV or IM, then 5–10 mg IV every 20–40 min to a maximum cumulative dosage of 20 mg; or constant infusion of 0.5–10 mg/h	Higher or frequent dosage associated with maternal hypotension, headaches, and abnormal fetal heart rate tracings; may be more common than other agents.	10–20 min
Nifedipine (immediate release)	10–20 mg orally, repeat in 20 min if needed; then 10–20 mg every 2–6 h; maximum daily dose is 180 mg	May observe reflex tachycardia and headaches.	5–10 min

*The dosages in the table were published by ACOG in 2020. For the most up-to-date dosing information, please review ACOG's guidance at acog.org.

Modified from Gestational hypertension and preeclampsia. ACOG Practice Bulletin No. 222. American College of Obstetricians and Gynecologists. Obstet Gynecol 2020;135:e237–60. doi: 10.1097/AOG.0000000000003891 https://journals.lww.com/greenjournal/Fulltext/2020/06000/Gestational_Hypertension_and_Preeclampsia__ACOG.46.aspx

subsequently be required using oral medications—labetalol or nifedipine is frequently used. Women with preeclampsia with severe features should remain inpatient following diagnosis with expectant management until 34 weeks of gestation unless clinical status changes.

In this scenario, the patient subsequently develops *eclampsia*, defined as one or more new-onset seizures in a woman with preeclampsia or gestational hypertension in the absence of other causes. The seizures often are generalized, tonic-clonic seizures. Less commonly they are focal or multifocal. Eclampsia often is, but not always, preceded by premonitory signs and symptoms including hypertension; severe, persistent frontal, occipital, or thunderclap headaches; vision changes (scotomata, blurred vision, loss of vision, visual field defects); or right upper quadrant or epigastric pain. However, 20–38% of women do not exhibit these signs or symptoms before experiencing a seizure.

The initial management of eclampsia includes calling for help, maintaining the airway and preventing aspiration, taking steps to avoid maternal injury, positioning the patient on their left side, and administering oxygen. These supportive measures were performed in this scenario. The next step is to administer magnesium sulfate, primarily to prevent recurrent seizures, because the initial seizure is usually self-limited. Magnesium sulfate is administered intravenously as a bolus infusion followed by a maintenance dose. If intravenous access is not established, magnesium sulfate can be administered intramuscularly. Evidence suggests that magnesium sulfate is more efficacious in reducing recurrent seizures than diazepam, phenytoin, or other antiseizure medications. Magnesium sulfate also has been shown to provide fetal and neonatal benefits, including neuroprotection in gestations less than 32 weeks. The general recommendation is to continue magnesium sulfate for at least 24 hours after delivery. A small percentage of women will experience recurrent seizures after receiving magnesium sulfate, and an additional bolus can be administered in these cases. Further recurrences may require other medications, such as sodium amobarbital, thiopental, or phenytoin.

It is important to recognize that eclamptic seizures may be associated with prolonged fetal heart rate decelerations or bradycardia. After a seizure, the fetal heart rate may exhibit tachycardia, reduced variability, and recurrent decelerations. Urgent delivery is not recommended in this scenario. In most cases, stabilizing maternal status, including administering magnesium sulfate, and treating hypertension facilitates in utero resuscitation of the fetus with subsequent normalization of the fetal heart tracing. If the nonreassuring fetal heart rate changes persist for more than 10–15 minutes after maternal stabilization, urgent delivery may be required. Placental abruption may be the cause of a prolonged concerning fetal heart tracing and may necessitate immediate delivery.

Eclampsia should not be managed expectantly, and timely delivery is indicated. The most appropriate mode of delivery must be considered. Eclampsia is not necessarily an indication for cesarean birth; induction of labor may be attempted in certain situations. The decision to consider induction of labor versus cesarean birth will depend upon many factors, including gestational age, fetal presentation, Bishop score, and maternal–fetal status. Evidence suggests that the success of a vaginal birth increases with advancing gestational age (particularly when greater than 30 weeks of gestation). In those who undergo labor induction, the chances of ultimately requiring a cesarean birth may be as high as 93–97% when gestational age is less than 28 weeks of gestation and 53–65% from 28 to 32 weeks of gestation. Although induction of labor is an option with eclampsia, it would not be the most appropriate next step in this scenario.

Neurologic findings are common in women with eclampsia, although they typically are transient. Posterior reversible encephalopathy syndrome is a common finding on imaging and is a clinical syndrome characterized by headaches, seizures, altered mental status, and vision loss. Imaging findings include vasogenic edema, often in the parietal-occipital regions of the brain likely secondary to a failure of the normal autoregulation in cerebral blood flow. Cranial imaging is indicated if the patient continues to have neurologic deficits, seizures refractory to magnesium, prolonged coma, or an atypical seizure pattern.

Altman D, Carroli G, Duley L, Farrell B, Moodley J, Neilson J, et al. Do women with pre-eclampsia, and their babies, benefit from magnesium sulphate? The Magpie Trial: a randomised placebo-controlled trial. Magpie Trial Collaboration Group. Lancet 2002;359:1877–90. doi: 10.1016/s0140-6736(02)08778-0 https://www.thelancet.com/journals/lancet/article/PIIS0140-6736(02)08778-0/fulltext

Gestational hypertension and preeclampsia. ACOG Practice Bulletin No. 222. American College of Obstetricians and Gynecologists. Obstet Gynecol 2020;135:e237–60. doi: 10.1097/AOG.0000000000003891 https://journals.lww.com/greenjournal/Fulltext/2020/06000/Gestational_Hypertension_and_Preeclampsia__ACOG.46.aspx

Petersen EE, Davis NL, Goodman D, Cox S, Mayes N, Johnston E, et al. Vital signs: pregnancy-related deaths, United States, 2011-2015, and strategies for prevention, 13 States, 2013-2017. MMWR Morb Mortal Wkly Rep 2019;68:423–9. doi: 10.15585/mmwr.mm6818e1 https://www.cdc.gov/mmwr/volumes/68/wr/mm6818e1.htm?s_cid=mm6818e1_w

Sibai BM. Diagnosis, prevention, and management of eclampsia. Obstet Gynecol 2005;105:402–10. doi: 10.1097/01.AOG.0000152351.13671.99 https://journals.lww.com/greenjournal/Fulltext/2005/02000/Diagnosis,_Prevention,_and_Management_of_Eclampsia.31.aspx

Sibai BM. Evaluation and management of severe preeclampsia before 34 weeks' gestation. Publications Committee, Society for Maternal–Fetal Medicine. Am J Obstet Gynecol 2011;205:191–8. doi: 10.1016/j.ajog.2011.07.017 [doi] https://www.ajog.org/article/S0002-9378(11)00918-5/fulltext

Sibai BM. Magnesium sulfate prophylaxis in preeclampsia: lessons learned from recent trials. Am J Obstet Gynecol 2004;190:1520–6. doi: 10.1016/j.ajog.2003.12.057 https://www.ajog.org/article/S0002-9378(03)02177-X/fulltext

39 Gastric bypass surgery

A 34-year-old gravida 3, para 2, at 18 weeks of gestation with a history of laparoscopic cholecystectomy and Roux-en-Y gastric bypass procedure presents to the emergency department reporting nausea, vomiting, and upper abdominal pain for 3 days. You suspect internal herniation. The best imaging technique to evaluate this patient is

(A) computed tomography (CT)
* (B) magnetic resonance imaging (MRI)
(C) ultrasonography
(D) X-ray

The two primary approaches to bariatric surgery are restrictive and malabsorptive procedures. Restrictive procedures include vertical banded gastroplasty, adjustable gastric banding, and sleeve gastrectomy. Malabsorptive procedures include biliopancreatic diversion, jejunoileal bypass, and, most commonly, Roux-en-Y bypass, which is a combination of restrictive and malabsorptive procedures. The Roux-en-Y bypass creates a straight limb, or "Roux," connected to the gastric pouch with the Y portion downstream as the enteroenterostomy. The proximal stomach is separated from the remaining part of the stomach with staples.

Several small studies and case reports have identified significant complications during pregnancy after previous bariatric surgeries. These complications include anastomotic leaks, bowel obstructions, internal hernias, ventral hernias, band erosion, and band migration. Internal hernia causing small-bowel obstruction is the most common postbariatric surgery complication occurring in pregnancy and is more common after laparoscopic than open procedures. Postsurgical complications most often occur in the first pregnancy after gastric bypass surgery. Because of the increase in these complications in pregnancy, when a pregnant patient who has had bariatric surgery presents with abdominal complaints, the clinician must have a high index of suspicion for these complaints and involve a bariatric surgeon in the evaluation of abdominal pain.

The choice of diagnostic imaging for evaluation of a patient with abdominal pain and a history of bariatric surgery may be challenging. Evaluation should be performed by a bariatric surgeon or a radiologist experienced with bariatric patients. In considering the appropriate imaging for abdominal pain in a pregnant patient, one must consider the clinical scenario, availability of imaging modalities, and potential radiation from imaging. Patients should be counseled about risks of imaging modalities and how these risks relate to the risks of untreated or undiagnosed illness. In general, radiation exposure can be modified by imaging techniques, and the benefit of imaging often will outweigh the risks.

The risk to a fetus from ionizing radiation depends on the dose of radiation and the gestational age at exposure. Large doses very early in pregnancy may result in either death of the embryo or no consequences. As pregnancy advances, growth restriction and intellectual disability are the most likely consequences with high-dose radiation exposure. Complications of fetal anomalies, growth restriction, or miscarriage have not been reported with radiation exposure less than 50 milligray (mGy). The lowest clinically documented case of severe intellectual disability occurred with exposure to 610 mGy. Fetal radiation exposure doses associated with common radiological examinations are shown in Table 39-1. Although the higher exposure studies may reach 50 mGy, none of them exceeds that dose.

Abdominal ultrasonography uses sound waves, not ionizing radiation, and poses no known risk to a fetus. Although ultrasonography is low risk and may be useful in evaluating pregnant patients with abdominal pain, its diagnostic utility is limited in evaluating for internal hernia in patients who have undergone bariatric surgery. A recent systematic review demonstrated that abdominal ultrasonography was normal in all cases of internal herniation complicating pregnancy after Roux-en-Y gastric bypass. Because of its low utility in detecting complications following bariatric surgery, abdominal ultrasonography is not the best imaging choice in this patient.

Computed tomography also often is used for workup for abdominal pain in pregnancy. Although pelvic CT can result in exposure as high as 50 mGy, the dose that may cause harm, this can be reduced by radiologists using a low-exposure technique. Oral contrast agents may increase diagnostic capability of CT by increasing enhancement of soft tissues and vascular structures. These agents, which are often iodinated, are not absorbed by the patient and, although they may cross the placenta, have not been shown to cause adverse effects. Nevertheless, because of the theoretical concerns about negative effects of free iodide on the fetal thyroid gland, contrast generally is used only if required.

Magnetic resonance imaging offers some key advantages in that it can image deep soft tissue structures without ionizing radiation. There is no evidence of fetal harm caused by MRI. Unlike with CT, MRI can adequately image most soft tissue structure without the use of contrast. Despite this, contrast enhancement may be used to improve the specificity of MRI. Because of the risk of neonatal autoimmune disorders with

TABLE 39-1. Fetal Radiation Doses Associated With Common Radiologic Examinations

TYPE OF EXAMINATION	FETAL DOSE* (mGy)
Very low-dose examinations (less than 0.1 mGy)	
Cervical spine radiography (anteroposterior and lateral views)	Less than 0.001
Head or neck CT	0.001–0.01
Radiography of any extremity	Less than 0.001
Mammography (two views)	0.001–0.01
Chest radiography (two views)	0.0005–0.01
Low- to moderate-dose examinations (0.1–10 mGy)	
Radiography	
Abdominal radiography	0.1–3.0
Lumbar spine radiography	1.0–10
Intravenous pyelography	5–10
Double-contrast barium enema	1.0–20
CT	
Chest CT or CT pulmonary angiography	0.01–0.66
Limited CT pelvimetry (single axial section through the femoral heads)	Less than 1
Nuclear medicine	
Low-dose perfusion scintigraphy	0.1–0.5
Technetium-99m bone scintigraphy	4–5
Pulmonary digital subtraction angiography	0.5
Higher-dose examinations (10–50 mGy)	
Abdominal CT	1.3–35
Pelvic CT	10–50
^{18}F PET/CT whole-body scintigraphy	10–50

Abbreviations: CT, computed tomography; PET, positron emission tomography.

*Fetal exposure varies with gestational age, maternal body habitus, and exact acquisition parameters.

Note: Annual average background radiation = 1.1–2.5 mGy, ^{18}F = 2-[fluorine-18]fluoro-2-deoxy-d-glucose.

Modified from Tremblay E, Therasse E, Thomassin-Naggara I, Trop I. Quality initiatives: guidelines for use of medical imaging during pregnancy and lactation. Radiographics 2012;32:897–911.

Reprinted from Guidelines for diagnostic imaging during pregnancy and lactation. Committee Opinion No. 723. American College of Obstetricians and Gynecologists [published erratum appears in Obstet Gynecol 2018;132:786]. Obstet Gynecol 2017;130:e210–6. doi: 10.1097/AOG.0000000000002355 https://journals.lww.com/greenjournal/Fulltext/2017/10000/Committee_Opinion_No__723__Guidelines_for.60.aspx gadolinium exposure, it is recommended in pregnancy only when it would alter maternal treatment and is balanced with fetal risks. Gadolinium, which is the most commonly used contrast agent, is water soluble and can cross the placenta, which could theoretically cause harm. Therefore, MRI contrast use should be limited to situations in which the benefits clearly outweigh the risks. Because MRI often is comparable to CT, when MRI is readily available it is the preferred approach if it is expected to provide the information that is clinically needed. In the case of complications during pregnancy after bariatric surgery, MRI is very useful. The specificity and sensitivity of MRI for diagnosis of internal hernia are similar to those of CT. In a recent systematic review, MRI confirmed the diagnosis of internal hernia in 75% of cases. For the patient in question, MRI is the most acceptable choice because it can reasonably provide a diagnosis with no radiation. If MRI were not readily available, the benefits of CT scan for diagnosis would make it the best next choice.

X-ray procedures involve a relatively low amount of ionizing radiation and are often used for the evaluation of medical problems or trauma. Abdominal X-ray is a very low-dose examination but may not be helpful in diagnosing complications related to previous surgeries. A recent systematic review showed that abdominal X-ray was normal in two-thirds of women with internal herniation in pregnancy after bariatric surgery. An X-ray of the abdomen would not be useful as it would not rule out postoperative complications in this patient.

Bariatric surgery and pregnancy. ACOG Practice Bulletin No. 105. American College of Obstetricians and Gynecologists. Obstet Gynecol 2009;113:1405–13. doi: 10.1097/AOG.0b013e3181ac0544 https://journals.lww.com/greenjournal/Citation/2009/06000/ACOG_Practice_Bulletin_No__105__Bariatric_Surgery.48.aspx

Guidelines for diagnostic imaging during pregnancy and lactation. Committee Opinion No. 723. American College of Obstetricians and Gynecologists [published erratum appears in Obstet Gynecol 2018;132:786]. Obstet Gynecol 2017;130:e210–6. doi: 10.1097/AOG.0000000000002355 https://journals.lww.com/greenjournal/Fulltext/2017/10000/Committee_Opinion_No__723__Guidelines_for.60.aspx

Krishna S, McInnes MD, Schieda N, Narayanasamy S, Sheikh A, Kielar A. Diagnostic accuracy of MRI for diagnosis of internal hernia in pregnant women with prior Roux-en-Y gastric bypass. AJR Am J Roentgenol 2018;211:755–9. doi: 10.2214/AJR.17.19252 https://www.ajronline.org/doi/10.2214/AJR.17.19252

Torres-Villalobos GM, Kellogg TA, Leslie DB, Antanavicius G, Andrade RS, Slusarek B, et al. Small bowel obstruction and internal hernias during pregnancy after gastric bypass surgery. Obes Surg 2009;19:944–50. doi: 10.1007/s11695-008-9681-x https://link.springer.com/article/10.1007/s11695-008-9681-x

Vannevel V, Jans G, Bialecka M, Lannoo M, Devlieger R, Van Mieghem T. Internal herniation in pregnancy after gastric bypass: a systematic review. Obstet Gynecol 2016;127:1013–20. doi: 10.1097/AOG.0000000000001429 https://journals.lww.com/greenjournal/Fulltext/2016/06000/Internal_Herniation_in_Pregnancy_After_Gastric.5.aspx

40 Vaginal birth after multiple cesarean births

A 30-year-old and her husband present to the office at 24 weeks of gestation to discuss her mode of delivery. She was in your care for her two prior uncomplicated low transverse cesarean births. Her partner initially is supportive but appears less so as you review the risks and benefits of a trial of labor and another cesarean birth. She verbalizes understanding of her choices and would like a repeat cesarean birth. Her husband interrupts to say that she does not want another surgery and that he will not support her if she chooses to have a repeat cesarean birth. She turns to you and says she has changed her mind and would like a trial of labor. The best next step is to

(A) proceed with signing the consent for a trial of labor
(B) request a court order for a cesarean birth
(C) request a psychiatric consult evaluating capacity
* (D) speak with the patient alone
(E) terminate the patient-physician relationship

The four pillars of medical ethics are respect for autonomy, beneficence, nonmaleficence, and justice. Whereas no one principle is more important than another, autonomy is considered "the first among equals." A person's autonomy and self-determination form the basis of informed consent, which is composed of three elements: capacity, information, and freedom to choose. Shared decision making is the concept that an individual's self-determined goal is an acceptable outcome and should be supported by the health care professional. Informed consent and shared decision making complement each other and are distinct. The development of a relationship between an obstetrician–gynecologist and a patient is essential to both concepts and ideally occurs over time during antenatal care.

When engaging in informed consent, the obstetrician–gynecologist must determine whether the patient has the capacity to make a medical decision when clinical information is provided. *Capacity* is defined by three tenets:

- The ability, capability, or fitness to do something
- A legal right, power, or competency to perform some act
- An ability to comprehend both the nature and consequences of one's acts

Communication, understanding, and appreciation of a choice, as well as rationalization and reasoning, are necessary to assess an individual's capacity. The obstetrician–gynecologist presents the information and options, and then discusses the risks and benefits of each while listening to the patient express their goals and expectations. The patient verbalizes their understanding of what has been presented, including consequences of the options, and then determines their choice.

In addition to capacity and information, the final element of informed consent is the freedom to choose among the presented options. When combining the principles of autonomy, informed consent, and decision-making capacity, it is a person's free will that is the prerequisite necessary for any person to make a choice. A person can lack free will either by circumstance (riding in car when they prefer to ride a horse) or by medical condition (being in a coma). Once capacity and free will are established, the patient makes their own decision. There are situations when a previously made decision may be reversed, specifically when there is an unanticipated change in circumstance; for example, an individual who would like every life-sustaining intervention, and then tragically burns 80% of their body in a house fire. This person retains capacity to reevaluate the previous decision based on the new set of circumstances and may make a different decision. The assessment of decision-making capacity is more nuanced in life-and-death circumstances. For example, an individual requests all life-sustaining care and 10 years later has end-stage dementia, is nonverbal, and no longer recognizes their life partner or children. This individual no longer has the capability to understand presented information or the ability to communicate a new decision. Ethics boards at hospitals provide support in making these challenging decisions.

The described patient has the capacity to make her own decision; however, it is not clear that she has the free will to execute her choice. She makes one decision after reviewing the information. Her husband expresses displeasure at and disagreement with her decision using hurtful words. The partner is demonstrating behavior designed to assert power and control. Under this pressure, the patient changes her mind and conforms to his choice. The best next step is to speak with the patient alone to clarify her wishes independent of her partner. Additionally, this can be addressed over several visits. She is at 24 weeks of gestation with two previous full-term births, and another term birth is likely. This gives you future visits during which to discuss her goals and her decision independent of her partner. Finally, even though the patient and her partner are well known to you, in addition to asking the partner to step out of the room to speak to the patient alone, screening for intimate partner violence also is indicated.

Formal coercion occurs when a woman lacks the capacity to make a choice. The issue of coercion when making the decision for a cesarean birth has been part of the medical, legal, and ethics literature for decades. There is a continuum beginning with self-determination and moving to informal coercion and finally formal coercion. Patients are coerced by inducement, persuasion, manipulation, pressure, and threats. Informal coercion occurs more often than formal coercion. When deciding on an obstetric intervention, an individual may confront coercion if they do not have the information required and the time needed for agreement, informed consent, and the opportunity for opposition. The woman can feel intimidated or manipulated into a cesarean birth or other obstetric intervention. The laboring woman must have freedom of choice and the ability to accept or decline the offered intervention.

Intimidation as a form of coercion has been studied. In a Swiss study published in 2021, among women surveyed the previous year about their experiences during labor and delivery, 37% of those who underwent an emergency cesarean birth felt intimidated. Furthermore, women who had an induction of labor or unplanned cesarean birth reported insufficient time and information to make the required decision, with high ratings of opposition and feeling manipulated. Only 30% of surveyed women felt appropriately informed before making the decision for an operative birth and episiotomy. In the Giving Voice to Mothers–U.S. study, of the 2,138 women who completed the survey, 28% reported feeling mistreated because of unsupported care, being scolded or shouted at, having their privacy violated, or being forced to have a treatment they did not want. Additionally, 15% of women reported feeling pressured to accept an induction of labor, an epidural, or a cesarean birth. Of White women of low socioeconomic status, 18.7% reported any mistreatment compared with 27.2% of women of color of the same socioeconomic status. Finally, the study reported a lower likelihood of mistreatment when the woman was White, multiparous, over 30 years of age, having a vaginal birth, having a community birth, or using a midwife. It is challenging and important for obstetrician–gynecologists to take the necessary steps to minimize informal coercion during labor and delivery and antenatal care.

The patient in this scenario experiences coercion from a partner during the shared decision-making process for informed consent. Family, friends, or community support groups also can intimidate and manipulate a person when they are trying to make a medical decision. This patient does not have free will to sign the consent for a trial of labor; therefore, signing the document at this time would not be an accurate reflection of her choice. A court order for a cesarean birth would be a last resort and not indicated at 24 weeks of gestation. All options to ascertain her true decision need to be exhausted, and it would need to be clear that she no longer has the capacity to make her own decisions before a court order would be requested. A psychiatric evaluation would be indicated for a concern of emotional abuse, but not for her medical decision-making capacity.

As described, this patient has demonstrated that she has the capacity to make this decision. In the scenario, she demonstrates the ability to understand, acknowledges the situation and consequences, makes a treatment choice, and communicates her choice. After communication of this decision, she changes her mind after hearing the view expressed by her partner. It is not clear that her original reasoning or decision has changed. Termination of the patient–physician relationship would imply that the clinician can no longer meet the needs of the patient. However, there is no evidence that her decision is one that cannot be respected and executed. Therefore, the appropriate response in this situation is to defer further discussion until she is alone. With the patient alone, it is appropriate to screen for intimate partner violence and to ascertain precisely what her wishes are for her pregnancy.

Begley K, Daly D, Panda S, Begley C. Shared decision-making in maternity care: acknowledging and overcoming epistemic defeaters. J Eval Clin Pract 2019;25:1113–20. doi: 10.1111/jep.13243 https://onlinelibrary.wiley.com/doi/10.1111/jep.13243

Informed consent and shared decision making in obstetrics and gynecology. ACOG Committee Opinion No. 819. American College of Obstetricians and Gynecologists. Obstet Gynecol 2021;137:e34–41. doi: 10.1097/AOG.0000000000004247 https://journals.lww.com/greenjournal/Fulltext/2021/02000/Informed_Consent_and_Shared_Decision_Making_in.45.aspx

Oelhafen S, Trachsel M, Monteverde S, Raio L, Cignacco E. Informal coercion during childbirth: risk factors and prevalence estimates from a nationwide survey of women in Switzerland [published erratum appears in BMC Pregnancy Childbirth 2021;21:437]. BMC Pregnancy Childbirth 2021;21:369-1. doi: 10.1186/s12884-021-03826-1 https://bmcpregnancychildbirth.biomedcentral.com/articles/10.1186/s12884-021-03826-1

Vedam S, Stoll K, Taiwo TK, Rubashkin N, Cheyney M, Strauss N, et al. The Giving Voice to Mothers study: inequity and mistreatment during pregnancy and childbirth in the United States. GVtM-US Steering Council. Reprod Health 2019;16:77-2. doi: 10.1186/s12978-019-0729-2 https://reproductive-health-journal.biomedcentral.com/articles/10.1186/s12978-019-0729-2

Zürcher T, Elger B, Trachsel M. The notion of free will and its ethical relevance for decision-making capacity. BMC Med Ethics 2019;20:31-0. doi: 10.1186/s12910-019-0371-0 https://bmcmedethics.biomedcentral.com/articles/10.1186/s12910-019-0371-0

41 Vulvovaginal hematoma management

A 25-year-old gravida 1 at term delivered after a prolonged second stage of labor. A second-degree laceration was repaired. A few hours later, she reports increasing vulvar pain and inability to void. An indwelling Foley catheter was placed. Her vital signs show a blood pressure of 110/70 mm Hg, a heart rate of 100 beats per minute, and a respiratory rate of 18 breaths per minute. Her fundus is firm, and she has minimal lochia. Her external examination is shown in Figure 41-1, and the area appears to be enlarging. On bimanual examination, there is no palpable lesion along the vaginal side wall. Her hemoglobin on admission was 11 g/dL and a repeat measurement was 9 g/dL with normal coagulation studies. The best next step in management is

(A) external ice pack
(B) hypogastric artery ligation
* (C) incision and drainage
(D) transfusion
(E) vascular embolization

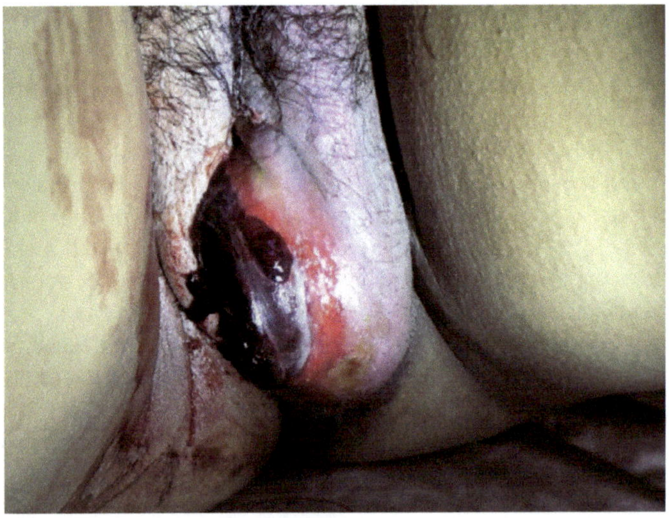

FIGURE 41-1. Left vulva hematoma with rupture and protruding blood clots. (Reprinted from Tseng JY, Lin IC, Lin JH, Chang CM, Chao WT, Wang PH. Optimal approach for management of postpartum vulva hematoma: Report of three cases. Taiwan J Obstet Gynecol 2020;59:780–3. doi: 10.1016/j.tjog.2020.07.030 https://www.sciencedirect.com/science/article/pii/S1028455920301844)

Common presenting symptoms of a vulvar hematoma include rapid onset of significant vulvar pain and swelling after vaginal delivery. Risk factors for vulvar or vaginal hematomas include prolonged second stage of labor, episiotomy, instrumental delivery, multifetal gestation, clotting disorders, vaginal laceration, vulvar or vaginal varicosities, macrosomia, and primigravid state. Altered mental status or hypotension can occur when vaginal lacerations and hematomas extend into the retroperitoneal space.

Vulvar hematomas can originate above or below the levator ani muscles and the urogenital diaphragm. The perineal branches of the internal pudendal artery supply blood to the vulva (Fig. 41-2). There are four nerves to the vulva: 1) pudendal, 2) ilioinguinal, 3) genital femoral, and 4) posterior femoral cutaneous. The round ligament also traverses the inguinal canal and terminates in the subcutaneous fat of the labia majora. An infralevator hematoma occurs in the anterior or posterior triangle with the Colles fascia (covering the space between the ischiocavernosus, bulbocavernosus, and superficial transverse perineal muscles) and the urogenital diaphragm to confine the bleeding. From this location a hematoma could extend inferiorly to the fascia lata of the thigh. A vulvar hematoma occurring in

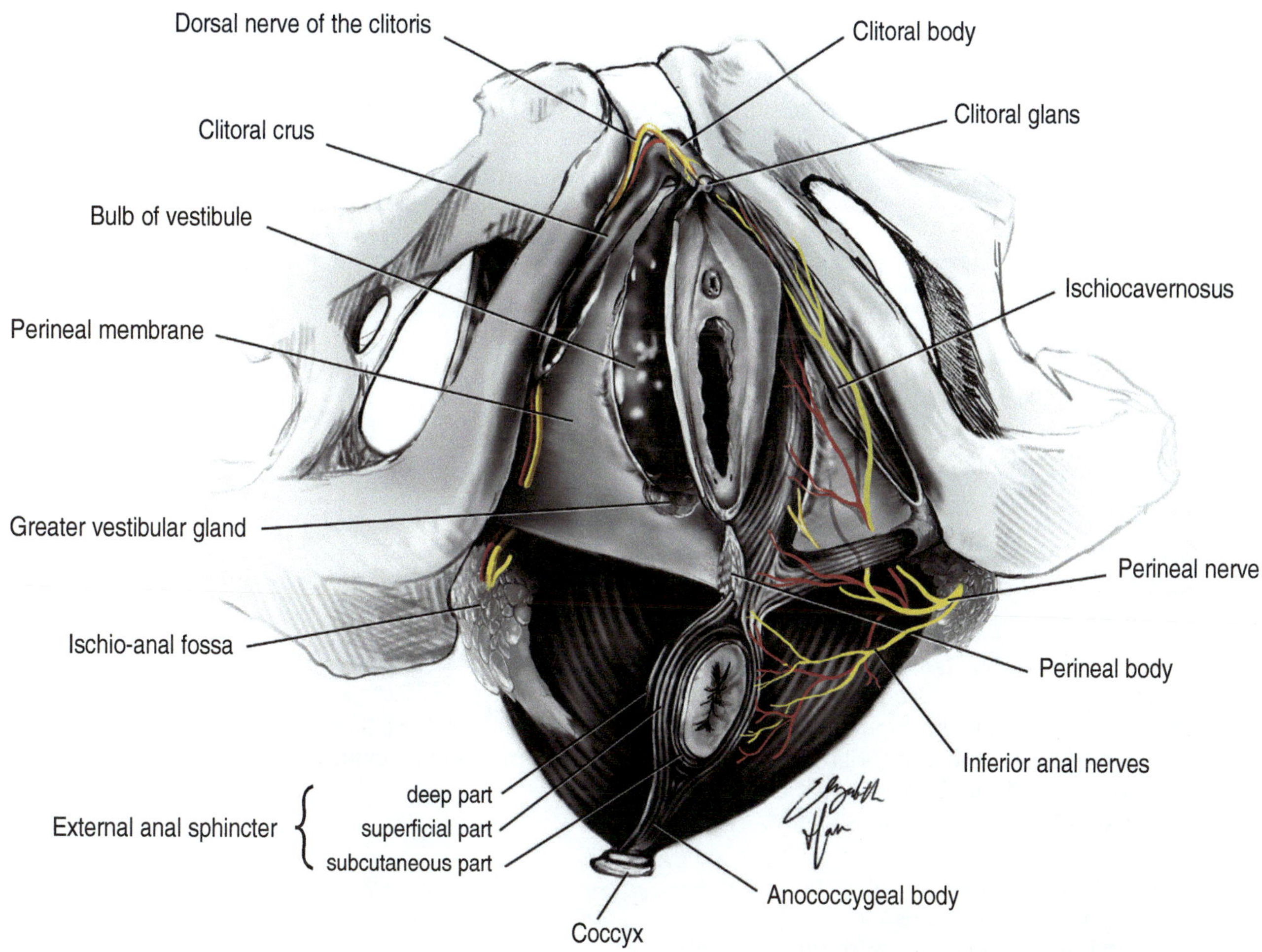

FIGURE 41-2. Inferior view of the female perineum and vulvar structures. (Reprinted from Hill AJ, Balgobin S, Mishra K, Jeppson PC, Wheeler T II, Mazloomdoost D, et al. Recommended standardized anatomic terminology of the posterior female pelvis and vulva based on a structured medical literature review. Society of Gynecologic Surgeons Pelvic Anatomy Group. Am J Obstet Gynecol 2021;225:169.e1–16. doi: 10.1016/j.ajog.2021.02.033 https://www.ajog.org/article/S0002-9378(21)00149-6/fulltext)

or above the levator ani muscles may extend cephalad along the vaginal wall medial to the obturator internus muscle and into the broad ligament. The vaginal artery is a branch of the internal iliac vessel or the uterine artery. The levator ani surrounds the middle third of the vagina. A hematoma originating lateral to the vagina and above Colles fascia has no barrier to limit expansion cephalad into the broad ligament and retroperitoneal space.

For the described patient, a speculum, bimanual vaginal examination, and a rectal examination will characterize the location and size of the hematoma. This patient is hemodynamically stable without concern for coagulopathy but has a large expanding hematoma resulting in significant pain and inability to void and, therefore, the best next step is an incision and drainage. Because the patient is hemodynamically stable, the bleeding is likely venous. Expectant management with serial examinations, ice packs, and pain control may be appropriate for a smaller, stable hematoma; however, the described patient has significant pain, an enlarging hematoma, and inability to void and requires active management. When the hematoma remains below the urogenital diaphragm, incision and drainage with figure-of-eight sutures placed to close the defect is the best next step with consideration for packing or drain placement if indicated.

In the setting of stable maternal blood pressure and heart rate, transfusion would not be immediately indicated. Should her clinical situation worsen, reevaluation for an evolving coagulopathy, factor replacement, and transfusion would be necessary. If there were concern for vaginal extension on bimanual examination and maternal vital signs remained stable, then interventional radiology and vascular embolization may be appropriate, as it would be a less invasive procedure to control the bleeding vessels and avoid abdominal hypogastric artery ligation. Also, the vagina is highly vascularized, and an incision and drainage in this setting may not reveal an identifiable vessel, making isolation of the bleeding vessel difficult. In such a situation, placement of vaginal packing or a Foley balloon may be considered to tamponade the area. Vascular embolization, if available, may be required to stop further bleeding.

Abedzadeh-Kalahroudi M, Talebian A, Sadat Z, Mesdaghinia E. Perineal trauma: incidence and its risk factors. J Obstet Gynaecol 2019;39:206–11. doi: 10.1080/01443615.2018.1476473 https://www.tandfonline.com/doi/abs/10.1080/01443615.2018.1476473

Denson LE, Terrell DR, Vesely SK, Peck JD, Quiroz LH, Shobeiri SA. The prevalence of pelvic floor hematoma after vaginal delivery. Female Pelvic Med Reconstr Surg 2021;27:393–7. doi: 10.1097/SPV.0000000000000895 https://journals.lww.com/fpmrs/Abstract/2021/06000/The_Prevalence_of_Pelvic_Floor_Hematoma_After.11.aspx

Hill AJ, Balgobin S, Mishra K, Jeppson PC, Wheeler T II, Mazloomdoost D, et al. Recommended standardized anatomic terminology of the posterior female pelvis and vulva based on a structured medical literature review. Society of Gynecologic Surgeons Pelvic Anatomy Group. Am J Obstet Gynecol 2021;225:169.e1–16. doi: 10.1016/j.ajog.2021.02.033 https://www.ajog.org/article/S0002-9378(21)00149-6/fulltext

Prevention and management of obstetric lacerations at vaginal delivery. ACOG Practice Bulletin No. 198. American College of Obstetricians and Gynecologists. Obstet Gynecol 2018;132:e87–102. doi: 10.1097/AOG.0000000000002841 https://journals.lww.com/greenjournal/Fulltext/2018/09000/ACOG_Practice_Bulletin_No__198__Prevention_and.66.aspx

Stobie W, Krishnan D. Large concealed paravaginal haematoma: a case report of an occult postpartum haemorrhage. Case Rep Womens Health 2021;30:e00311. doi: 10.1016/j.crwh.2021.e00311 https://www.sciencedirect.com/science/article/pii/S2214911221000291

Tseng JY, Lin IC, Lin JH, Chang CM, Chao WT, Wang PH. Optimal approach for management of postpartum vulva hematoma: report of three cases. Taiwan J Obstet Gynecol 2020;59:780–3. doi: 10.1016/j.tjog.2020.07.030 https://www.sciencedirect.com/science/article/pii/S1028455920301844

42 Gram-positive bacteria in pregnancy

A 28-year-old multiparous patient with term prelabor rupture of membranes undergoes an uncomplicated cesarean birth for arrest of the active phase of labor. On postoperative day 2, she reports severe abdominal pain, fever, and chills. Her vital signs include temperature of 39.8 °C (103.8 °F), a heart rate of 138 beats per minute, and blood pressure of 80/42 mm Hg. Laboratory studies reveal leukocytosis and lactic acidosis. Antibiotics are started, and several hours later a follow-up examination reveals the finding in Figure 42-1. The best next step in her treatment is

(A) administer intravenous immunoglobulin
(B) broaden antibiotic coverage
(C) expectant management with repeat cultures
* (D) surgical debridement

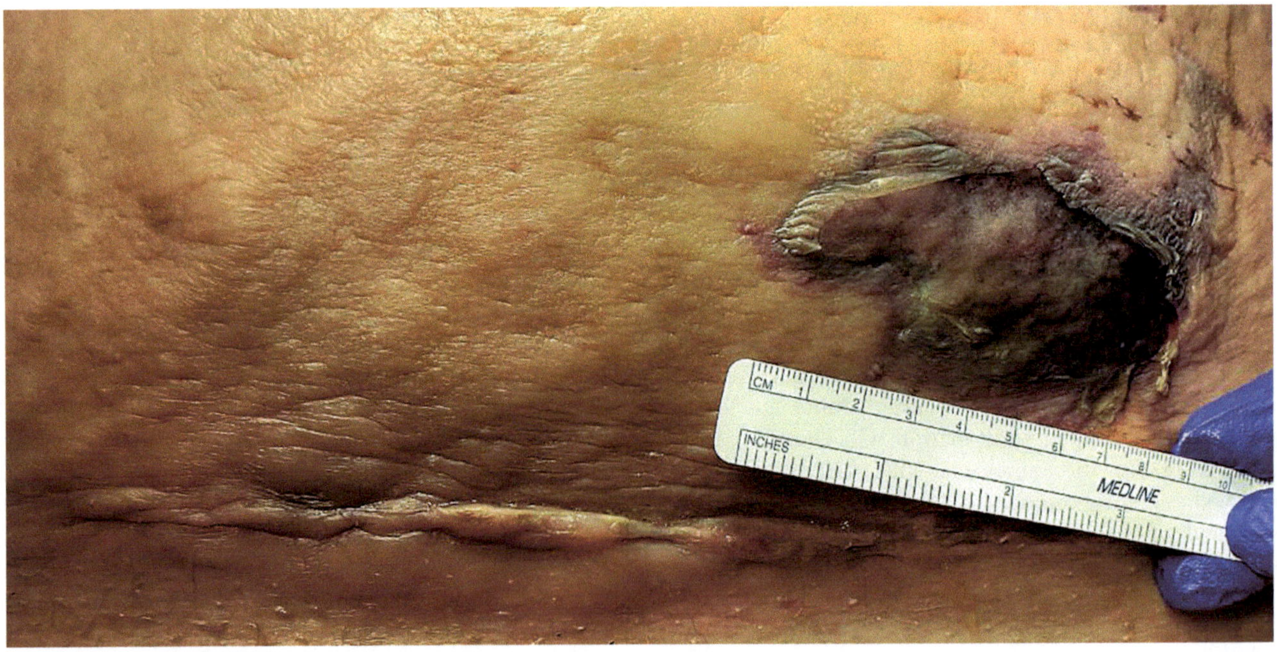

FIGURE 42-1. Maternal abdomen after cesarean birth. (Image courtesy of Rebecca Barbaresso, DO, Baystate Medical Center.)

Invasive infections caused by group A streptococcus carry an increased risk of morbidity and mortality, especially without prompt recognition and treatment. Mitigation of risks depends on a timely diagnosis, initiation of antibiotic therapy, and, when indicated, surgical intervention. Infections caused by group A streptococcus can be noninvasive or invasive. The noninvasive infections most often seen include streptococcal pharyngitis, otitis media, rheumatic fever, or acute glomerulonephritis. Invasive infections include pneumonia, sepsis, necrotizing fasciitis, streptococcal toxic shock syndrome, and focal infections, such as arthritis and skin and soft tissue infections. The estimated fatality rate for invasive infections depends on chronic illness and distribution, and location and type of disease and is estimated to be approximately 10%.

Among women of childbearing age, one-fifth of invasive infections with group A streptococcus are pregnancy related, including both infection specific to pregnancy (such as endometritis) or occurring during pregnancy. Of group A streptococcus infections in pregnancy, 85% of infections occur postpartum, and most are within the first 4 days of delivery. Most group A streptococcus infections appear to be community acquired with only about 15–25% tracked as nosocomial infections. Although precise biologic plausibility is unknown, contact with younger children and their carriage of group A streptococcus (pharyngeal) increases risk. Other factors increasing susceptibility to group A streptococcus include mucosal tears after delivery, more neutral vaginal pH, and pregnancy-related decline in cellular immunity.

Group A streptococcus infections usually present with fever, abdominal pain, leukocytosis, tachycardia, and hypotension (sepsis). The fever often is greater than 38.5 °C (101.3 °F) and usually occurs within the first 48 hours after delivery. Women may have rapid clinical deterioration, and those with toxic shock syndrome have higher mortality rates (up to 20%). Prompt diagnosis and initiation of antibiotics are critical but challenging given the relatively uncommon prevalence of disease and the ambiguity of early symptoms. Mother-to-child transmission also has been reported, and the newborn team should be advised of this maternal diagnosis.

The described patient is septic. Sepsis is not a specific diagnosis but is a life-threatening syndrome with organ dysfunction caused by immune responses to infection. Sepsis exists on a continuum, from bacteremia to septic shock to multiple organ dysfunction syndrome. Systemic inflammatory response syndrome is no longer included in this spectrum by several national professional societies because it is not always caused by infection. Septic shock is found in a subset of individuals with sepsis who have persistent hypotension requiring vasopressors to maintain mean arterial pressure of 65 mm Hg or greater and a serum lactate concentration greater than 2 mmol/L, despite volume resuscitation. Given the risks associated with sepsis in pregnancy and postpartum, early warning criteria are published to identify women at risk (Box 42-1). In maternal sepsis, the most frequently identified organisms are *Escherichia coli*, group A streptococcus, and group B streptococcus. During the antepartum period, the most common conditions that lead to maternal sepsis are septic abortion and chorioamnionitis, and in the postpartum period maternal sepsis often occurs with endometritis and wound infection.

BOX 42-1

Maternal Early Warning Criteria From the National Partnership for Maternal Safety

Maternal Early Warning Criteria

- Systolic BP (mm Hg) less than 90 or greater than 160
- Diastolic BP (mm Hg) greater than 100
- Heart rate (beats per min) less than 50 or greater than 120
- Respiratory rate (breaths per min) less than 10 or greater than 30
- Oxygen saturation on room air, at sea level, % less than 95
- Oliguria, mL/h, for 2 or more hours less than 35
- Maternal agitation, confusion, or unresponsiveness; patient with preeclampsia reporting a non-remitting headache or shortness of breath

Abbreviation: BP, blood pressure.

Adapted from Mhyre JM, D'Oria R, Hameed AB, Lappen JR, Holley SL, Hunter SK, et al. The maternal early warning criteria: a proposal from the National Partnership for Maternal Safety. Obstet Gynecol 2014;124:782–6. doi: 10.1097/AOG.0000000000000480.

When sepsis is suspected, cultures should be obtained based on examination (blood, sputum, urine, and wound cultures). Examination includes prompt evaluation of susceptible sites, such as the respiratory tract, uterus, external genitalia, episiotomy site, and cesarean incision. Serologic evaluation includes screening for elevated lactate levels, leukocytosis, or leukocytopenia with or without bandemia. Endometrial aspiration should be considered for Gram stain and culture in postpartum women. Broad-spectrum antibiotics should be initiated within 1 hour of diagnosis. Each hour of delay in treatment has been associated with an increase in mortality. Some hospitals have protocols for the treatment of sepsis, and guidance may be obtained from society guidelines, such as in the American College of Obstetricians and Gynecologists' Practice Bulletin No. 211, "Critical Care in Pregnancy." After taking these initial steps, the source of the infection should be evaluated, including a thorough history, clinical examination, and imaging as indicated. Imaging results, from modalities such as computed tomography or ultrasonography, can appear healthy in cases of group A streptococcus, and aggressive management should not be delayed, especially when gangrene or necrosis is noted, as in this patient. Fluid resuscitation is a key component when hypotension is present. Multidisciplinary care teams often are necessary, and patients may require admission to the intensive care unit.

The described scenario may have initially been suspicious for endometritis, which is treated with ampicillin, gentamicin, and metronidazole or clindamycin. However, with further fever and additional clinical findings, as seen in Figure 42-1, invasive infection should be suspected. When group A streptococcus or *Clostridium perfringens* is suspected, penicillin G plus clindamycin should be started and continued even after source control. Surgical debridement, resection, and often hysterectomy are the preferred procedures to obtain control of the source of the infection, with debridement occurring early and aggressively. Superficial infections are likely to require resection and debridement, whereas deep-tissue infections require hysterectomy and additional procedures as necessary. Surgery is coupled with continued antibiotic therapy and potential further debridement. Intravenous immunoglobulin has been attempted with severe cases of necrotizing fasciitis, but the efficacy has not been proved. Vancomycin plus piperacillin tazobactam are excellent additions when broader spectrum coverage is indicated with skin or soft tissue infection, excluding those associated with group A streptococcus or *C perfringens*.

Centers for Disease Control and Prevention. Group A streptococcal (GAS) disease: type II necrotizing fasciitis. CDC; 2018. Accessed February 11, 2022. https://www.cdc.gov/groupastrep/diseases-hcp/necrotizing-fasciitis.html

Nelson GE, Pondo T, Toews KA, Farley MM, Lindegren ML, Lynfield R, et al. Epidemiology of invasive group a streptococcal infections in the United States, 2005–2012. Clin Infect Dis 2016;63:478–86. doi: 10.1093/cid/ciw248 https://academic.oup.com/cid/article/63/4/478/2566560

Plante LA, Pacheco LD, Louis JM. SMFM Consult Series #47: sepsis during pregnancy and the puerperium. Society for Maternal-Fetal Medicine (SMFM) [published erratum appears in Am J Obstet Gynecol 2021;224:224]. Am J Obstet Gynecol 2019;220:B2–10. doi: 10.1016/j.ajog.2019.01.216 https://www.ajog.org/article/S0002-9378(19)30246-7/fulltext

43 Peripartum cardiomyopathy

A 38-year-old gravida 4, para 2, at 8 weeks of gestation presents for initial prenatal care. Her medical history includes chronic hypertension and peripartum cardiomyopathy. She is currently taking labetalol and aspirin. She reports feeling short of breath with physical activity but is otherwise asymptomatic. Her vital signs are within normal limits. A recent echocardiogram demonstrates a left ventricular ejection fraction (EF) of 25%. The best next step is to

(A) administer furosemide
* (B) discuss termination of pregnancy
(C) perform exercise stress test
(D) place a left ventricular assist device
(E) refer to maternal–fetal medicine

The modified World Health Organization (mWHO) risk assessment model is the most widely accepted and validated risk classification system for pregnant women with cardiovascular disease (Table 43-1). The model classifies women into five risk categories and provides recommendations for antenatal care. Women with *severe systemic ventricular dysfunction*, defined as an EF of less than 30% or history of peripartum cardiomyopathy with residual left ventricular dysfunction, are considered mWHO risk class IV. Women in this class carry an extremely high risk of maternal mortality or severe morbidity, with a major cardiac event rate of greater than 27%. For women in this class, pregnancy is contraindicated and termination of pregnancy should be discussed. In women who opt to continue pregnancy, follow-up cardiology examinations should be performed every month at a minimum. Women in this class should receive prenatal, intrapartum, and postpartum care at a maternal care Level IV facility or higher with a multidisciplinary care team available. Levels of maternal care are shown in Appendix D. The health care professionals who should be in the care team of a Level IV center include a maternal–fetal medicine subspecialist, a nursing service line leader, a nurse experienced in obstetric and critical care, an obstetric anesthesiologist, and at least one neurosurgeon, cardiac surgeon, or transplant surgeon.

Peripartum cardiomyopathy accounts for an increasing number of maternal cardiac deaths. Mortality rates have been reported to be as high as 25–50%. Approximately 30–50% of women fully recover, and there is a 35% risk of recurrence in a subsequent pregnancy. Poor prognostic factors include large left ventricular end-diastolic dimension at the time of diagnosis, an EF of less than 30% on initial testing, or failure of left ventricular function to normalize by 6 months.

Furosemide is a loop diuretic that acts by inhibiting resorption of sodium and chloride in the ascending loop of Henle and proximal and distal renal tubules. It is considered acceptable for use during pregnancy with no expected adverse fetal effects. Furosemide commonly is used in the treatment of heart failure for peripheral edema. Although it may be indicated for the treatment of the described patient, it is not the most appropriate immediate next step.

In women with cardiac disease, an exercise stress test can be used to predict a woman's ability to tolerate pregnancy. This test is performed before pregnancy to aid in prepregnancy counseling. In women with suspected heart disease who are already pregnant, it can be performed at 80% of predicted maximum heart rate (submaximal testing). The described patient feels short of breath with physical activity and might not be

TABLE 43-1. Modified World Health Organization Pregnancy Risk Classification for Women With Preexisting Cardiovascular Disease, Pregnancy, and Heart Disease

MODIFIED WHO PREGNANCY RISK CLASSIFICATION (RISK OF PREGNANCY BY MEDICAL CONDITION) SUGGESTED FOLLOW-UP*	SPECIFIC CARDIAC LESIONS	PREGNANCY CARE DELIVERY LOCATION
mWHO Risk Class I No detectable increased risk of maternal mortality and no or mild increase in morbidity (2–5% risk of maternal cardiac event rate) Follow-up: Cardiology evaluation once or twice during pregnancy	• Uncomplicated, small, or mild — Pulmonary stenosis — Patient ductus arteriosus — Mitral valve prolapse • Successfully repaired simple lesions (atrial or ventricular septal defect, patent ductus arteriosus, anomalous pulmonary venous drainage) • Atrial or ventricular ectopic beats, isolated	• Prepregnancy/pregnancy counseling • Care at local hospital • Delivery at local hospital*
mWHO Risk Class II Small increased risk of maternal mortality or moderate increase in morbidity (6–10% maternal cardiac event rate) Follow-up: cardiology, every trimester	• Unoperated atrial or ventricular septal defect • Repaired tetralogy of Fallot or aortic coarctation • Most arrhythmias (supraventricular arrhythmias) • Turner syndrome without congenital cardiac disease	• Prepregnancy/pregnancy counseling • Pregnancy Heart Team* consultation/counseling • Care at local hospital • Delivery at local hospital*
mWHO Risk Classes II and III Intermediate increased risk of maternal mortality or moderate to severe increase in morbidity (11–19% maternal cardiac event rate) Follow-up: cardiology, every trimester	• Mild left ventricular impairment (EF greater than 45%) • Hypertrophic cardiomyopathy • Native or bioprosthetic valve disease not considered mWHO Risk Class I or IV (mild mitral stenosis, moderate aortic stenosis) • Marfan or other HTAD syndrome without aortic dilation • Aorta less than 45 mm in bicuspid aortic valve pathology • Repaired coarctation without residua (non-Turner) • Atrioventricular septal defect	• Prepregnancy/pregnancy counseling • Pregnancy Heart Team* consultation/counseling • Care at an appropriate level hospital (critical members of the Pregnancy Heart Team* available depending on cardiac disease) • Delivery at an appropriate level hospital*†
Pre-mWHO Risk Class III Significantly increased risk of maternal mortality or severe morbidity (20–27% maternal cardiac event rate) Follow-up: cardiology, every 1–2 mo	• Moderate left ventricular impairment (EF 30–45%) • Previous peripartum cardiomyopathy without any residual left ventricular impairment • Mechanical valve • Systemic right ventricle with good or mildly decreased ventricular function • Uncomplicated Fontan circulation • Unrepaired cyanotic heart disease • Other complex heart disease • Moderate mitral stenosis • Severe asymptomatic aortic stenosis • Moderate aortic dilation (40–45 mm in Marfan syndrome or other HTAD; 45–50 mm in bicuspid aortic valve; Turner syndrome ASI 20–25 mm/m^2; tetralogy of Fallot less than 50 mm) • Ventricular tachycardia	• Prepregnancy/pregnancy counseling • Pregnancy Heart Team* consultation/counseling • Care at an appropriate level hospital† • Delivery at an appropriate level hospital*†

(continued)

Table 43-1 (continued)

mWHO Risk Class IV Pregnancy contraindicated Discuss induced abortion Extremely high risk of maternal mortality or severe morbidity (Greater than 27% maternal cardiac event rate) Follow-up: cardiology follow-up every month (minimum)	· Pulmonary arterial hypertension · Severe systemic ventricular dysfunction (EF less than 30%, NYHA III-IV) · Previous peripartum cardiomyopathy with any residual left ventricular dysfunction · Severe mitral stenosis · Severe symptomatic aortic stenosis · Systemic right ventricle with moderate to severely decreased ventricular function · Severe aortic dilation (greater than 45 mm in Marfan syndrome or other HTAD; greater than 50 mm in bicuspid aortic valve; Turner syndrome ASI greater than 25 mm/m²; tetralogy of Fallot greater than 50 mm) · Vascular Ehlers-Danlos · Severe (re)coarctation · Fontan circulation with any complication	· Pregnancy Heart Team* consultation/counseling · Care at an appropriate level hospital‡ (critical members of the Pregnancy Heart Team* available depending on cardiac disease) · Delivery at an appropriate level hospital*‡

Abbreviations: ASI, aortic size index; EF, ejection fraction; HTAD, hereditary thoracic aortic disease; mWHO, modified World Health Organization; NYHA, New York Heart Association.

*Pregnant women with a positive cardiac history or findings, or both, should receive prenatal, intrapartum, and postpartum care in a hospital setting that represents an appropriate maternal level of care that is at Level II or higher depending upon the specific cardiac lesion(s) that are present. "The goal of regionalized maternal care is for pregnant women at high risk to receive care in facilities that are prepared to provide the required level of specialized care, thereby reducing maternal morbidity and mortality in the United States." (Levels of maternal care. Obstetric Care Consensus No. 2. American College of Obstetricians and Gynecologists. Obstet Gynecol 2015;125:502–15).

†**mWHO Risk Class III**. Critical members of the Pregnancy Heart Team available depending on cardiac disease. For example: A mechanical valve patient requires care at a center with cardiologist/maternal-fetal medicine team who monitor and adjust anticoagulation weekly, delivery at a center with obstetric anesthesia, and advance cardiac care options including access to emergency cardiac surgery should acute prosthetic valve thrombosis necessitate emergency intervention.

‡**mWHO Risk Class IV**. For example, a severe pulmonary hypertension patient requires care and delivery at a center with maternal-fetal medicine, obstetric and cardiac anesthesia, a pulmonary hypertension specialist, and advanced heart failure care options, such as ventricular assist device and extracorporeal membrane oxygenator management.

Adapted from Thorne S, MacGregor A, Nelson-Piercy C. Risks of contraception and pregnancy in heart disease. Heart 2006;92:1520–5.

Reprinted from Pregnancy and heart disease. ACOG Practice Bulletin No. 212. American College of Obstetricians and Gynecologists. Obstet Gynecol 2019;133:e320–56. doi: 10.1097/AOG.0000000000003243 https://journals.lww.com/greenjournal/Fulltext/2019/05000/ACOG_Practice_Bulletin_No__212__Pregnancy_and.40.aspx.

able to complete an exercise stress test, and it is not the best immediate next step.

A left ventricular assist device (LVAD) is an intervention that may be indicated in patients with refractory heart failure. It is considered an intermediate or long-term mechanical circulatory support system and is primarily used for patients who have failed optimal pharmacologic therapy while awaiting heart transplantation. An LVAD eventually may be indicated for the described patient, but it would not be considered the best next step.

All pregnant women with cardiac disease should receive care from a multidisciplinary team including a cardiologist and their obstetrician. For women with mWHO class II or higher, maternal–fetal medicine consultation or care is recommended. The described patient warrants a multidisciplinary care team including a maternal–fetal medicine subspecialist if pregnancy is continued; however, because of the substantial risk of maternal morbidity and mortality, termination of pregnancy should be discussed first.

Levels of maternal care. Obstetric Care Consensus No. 9. American College of Obstetricians and Gynecologists [published erratum appears in Obstet Gynecol 2019;134:883]. Obstet Gynecol 2019;134:e41–55. doi: 10.1097/AOG.0000000000003383 https://journals.lww.com/greenjournal/Fulltext/2019/08000/Levels_of_Maternal_Care__Obstetric_Care_Consensus.44.aspx

Pregnancy and heart disease. ACOG Practice Bulletin No. 212. American College of Obstetricians and Gynecologists. Obstet Gynecol 2019;133:e320–56. doi: 10.1097/AOG.0000000000003243 https://journals.lww.com/greenjournal/Fulltext/2019/05000/ACOG_Practice_Bulletin_No__212__Pregnancy_and.40.aspx

Simpson LL. Maternal cardiac disease: update for the clinician. Obstet Gynecol 2012;119:345–59. doi: 10.1097/AOG.0b013e318242e260 https://journals.lww.com/greenjournal/Fulltext/2012/02000/Maternal_Cardiac_Disease__Update_for_the_Clinician.21.aspx

44 Electronic fetal monitoring

A 23-year-old gravida 1, para 0, at 38 weeks of gestation presents to the labor and delivery unit in spontaneous labor. Her pregnancy has been uncomplicated. Her labor is progressing normally with a Category I fetal tracing on electronic fetal monitoring (EFM). The use of continuous EFM in this patient reduces the risk of

(A) cerebral palsy
(B) cesarean birth
* (C) neonatal seizures
(D) operative vaginal delivery
(E) perinatal death

The purpose of EFM is to assess fetal well-being during labor. The efficacy of this intervention is based on its ability to reduce adverse perinatal outcomes, such as neonatal seizures, cerebral palsy, or intrapartum fetal death, in addition to a reduction in obstetric intervention such as operative delivery. However, continuous EFM has not been shown to reduce most of these adverse outcomes—only neonatal seizures have been reduced by continuous EFM. The American College of Obstetricians and Gynecologists has acknowledged that there are no known long-term benefits of continuous EFM as currently used.

The ability of continuous EFM to predict cerebral palsy is quite poor. The positive predictive value in singletons weighing more than 2,500 g is only 0.14%. In other words, of 1,000 fetuses with a nonreassuring fetal heart rate pattern, only one to two will develop cerebral palsy. This is further supported by the fact that the occurrence of cerebral palsy has remained unchanged despite the introduction of continuous EFM. The primary reason that continuous EFM does not predict or prevent cerebral palsy is that 70% of cases occur before the onset of labor, and only 4% of cases can be attributed solely to intrapartum events.

The only trials evaluating EFM for fetal assessment during labor have compared continuous EFM to intermittent auscultation. There are no studies comparing fetal monitoring with no monitoring. A Cochrane Systematic Review evaluated these trials to assess the effectiveness and safety of continuous EFM versus intermittent auscultation. A summary of these findings is presented in Table 44-1. The authors found that continuous EFM was associated with a reduced rate of neonatal seizures, but there were no clear differences in cerebral palsy, infant mortality, or other standard measures of neonatal well-being. The incidence of neonatal seizures was reduced by 50% in the continuous EFM group (relative risk, 0.50; 95% CI, 0.31–0.80; n=32,386; nine trials). However, a follow-up study of children who had seizures at 4 years of age found that the risk of cerebral palsy was no different. Additionally, continuous EFM was associated with an increased risk of cesarean delivery and operative vaginal delivery. The authors acknowledged the fact that translating this evidence into clinical practice is challenging. The limitations of the included studies—such as outdated studies; heterogeneity in protocols, including quick recourse to continuous monitoring, if indicated; and differences in nursing care—cannot be ignored.

Studying the utility of continuous EFM is challenging because the outcome of severe neonatal neurologic morbidity is very rare. There is no evidence to suggest that continuous EFM

TABLE 44-1. Outcomes With Continuous Electronic Fetal Heart Rate Tracing Versus Intermittent Auscultation

	NUMBER OF TRIALS	N	RISK RATIO (95% CI)
Operative vaginal delivery	9	18,515	1.16 (1.01, 1.32)
Cesarean delivery for abnormal fetal heart rate tracing	11	33,379	2.37 (1.88, 3.00)
Neonatal seizures	9	32,386	0.50 (0.31, 0.80)
Cerebral palsy	2	13,252	1.74 (0.97, 3.11)
Perinatal death	11	33,513	0.85 (0.59, 1.23)

Abbreviation: CI, confidence interval.

Data from Alfirevic Z, Devane D, Gyte GM. Continuous cardiotocography (CTG) as a form of electronic fetal monitoring (EFM) for fetal assessment during labour. Cochrane Database Syst Rev 2006;3:CD006066

Reprinted from Management of intrapartum fetal heart rate tracings. Practice Bulletin No. 116. American College of Obstetricians and Gynecologists . Obstet Gynecol 2010;116:1232-40. doi: 10.1097/AOG.0b013e3182004fa9 https://journals.lww.com/greenjournal/Citation/2010/11000/Practice_Bulletin_No__116__Management_of.53.aspx.

can predict severe neonatal neurologic morbidity or stillbirth. However, it is currently the most commonly used method of intrapartum fetal monitoring. As with any test, patients and clinicians should understand the limitations.

Alfirevic Z, Gyte GM, Cuthbert A, Devane D. Continuous cardiotocography (CTG) as a form of electronic fetal monitoring (EFM) for fetal assessment during labour. Cochrane Database of Systematic Reviews 2017, Issue 2. Art. No.: CD006066. doi: 10.1002/14651858.CD006066.pub3 http://dx.doi.org/10.1002/14651858.CD006066.pub3

American College of Obstetricians and Gynecologists, American Academy of Pediatrics. Neonatal encephalopathy and neurologic outcome. 2nd ed. ACOG; AAP; 2014. https://www.acog.org/clinical/clinical-guidance/task-force-report/articles/2014/neonatal-encephalopathy-and-neurologic-outcome

Intrapartum fetal heart rate monitoring: nomenclature, interpretation, and general management principles. ACOG Practice Bulletin No. 106. American College of Obstetricians and Gynecologists. Obstet Gynecol 2009;114:192–202. doi: 10.1097/AOG.0b013e3181aef106 https://journals.lww.com/greenjournal/Citation/2009/07000/ACOG_Practice_Bulletin_No__106__Intrapartum_Fetal.51.aspx

Management of intrapartum fetal heart rate tracings. Practice Bulletin No. 116. American College of Obstetricians and Gynecologists. Obstet Gynecol 2010;116:1232–40. doi: 10.1097/AOG.0b013e3182004fa9 https://journals.lww.com/greenjournal/Citation/2010/11000/Practice_Bulletin_No__116__Management_of.53.aspx

45 Breast cancer screening

A 42-year-old gravida 4, para 3, presents for a routine postpartum visit. The patient is exclusively breastfeeding. Her breast examination is normal. She reports no family history of breast cancer. After counseling about breast cancer screening recommendations from various societies, the patient opts to begin screening. The most appropriate breast cancer screening option for this patient is

(A) deferment while breastfeeding
(B) magnetic resonance imaging (MRI)
* (C) mammography
(D) ultrasonography

Breast cancer is the most common malignancy among reproductive-aged women. With advancing maternal age due to delayed childbearing, more women are breastfeeding around the time of screening initiation. The American College of Obstetricians and Gynecologists recommends that average-risk women be offered screening at age 40 years and initiate screening no later than age 50 years, with an interval of every 1–2 years. The U.S. Preventive Service Task Force recommends biennial screening beginning at age 50, whereas the American Cancer Society recommends yearly screening from ages 45 to 54 and screening every 1–2 years thereafter (Table 45-1). When reviewing breast cancer screening with patients, it is prudent to discuss the differences in these societal recommendations as well as the risks and benefits for each approach. For example, the benefits of screening may include earlier detection and reduced need for advanced treatment and decreased mortality risk. However, the risks of screening may include false-positive test results, unnecessary biopsies and procedures, anxiety, discomfort with examinations, overtreatment, and radiation exposure.

Breastfeeding women should undergo routine breast cancer screening with the same frequency and timing as women who are not lactating. The timing of initiation should be determined using informed counseling and shared decision making. Reproductive-aged women are more likely to be diagnosed with advanced-stage and more biologically aggressive subtypes of breast cancer. Furthermore, delays in the diagnosis and treatment of breast cancer are associated with increased mortality. Current evidence suggests that screening initiation at the age of 40 results in the greatest mortality reduction. The described patient should be offered a routine screening mammogram. Lactation is not a contraindication to mammography. Deferment until completion of breastfeeding is not appropriate.

The physiologic changes in the breasts in lactating women can affect the radiographic appearance of the breasts, including increased parenchymal density on mammography and increased echogenicity on ultrasonography. Lactating women should express milk just before the examination to decrease breast density and maximize the sensitivity of the study. Breastfeeding women have higher rates of false-positive test results and may undergo more biopsies.

Magnetic resonance imaging is an imaging modality that may be used in breast cancer screening, but it would not be the best choice for the described patient. Magnetic resonance imaging is associated with a higher sensitivity and, thus, a higher false-positive rate. Magnetic resonance imaging typically is reserved for women with moderate to high lifetime risk of breast cancer. Gadolinium contrast is considered safe in lactation; less than 0.0004% of the dose is excreted into breast milk. However, if women elect to discard their milk, they should be counseled to do so for 12–24 hours after contrast administration.

Breast ultrasonography is another imaging modality that may be considered in the evaluation. It is particularly useful in the setting of a palpable lesion. It has not been studied as a

TABLE 45-1. Recommendations for Breast Cancer Screening in Average-Risk Women

	AMERICAN COLLEGE OF OBSTETRICIANS AND GYNECOLOGISTS	U.S. PREVENTIVE SERVICES TASK FORCE	AMERICAN CANCER SOCIETY	NATIONAL COMPREHENSIVE CANCER NETWORK
Clinical breast examination	May be offered* every 1–3 y for women aged 25–39 y and annually for women 40 y and older.	Insufficient evidence to recommend for or against.†	Does not recommend.‡	Recommend every 1–3 y for women aged 25–39 y. Recommend annually for women 40 y and older.
Mammography initiation age	Offer starting at age 40 y.§ Initiate at ages 40–49 y after counseling, if patient desires. Recommend by no later than age 50 y if patient has not already initiated.	Recommend at age 50 y.‖ Age 40–49 y: The decision to start screening mammography in women before age 50 y should be an individual one.¶	Offer at ages 40–45 y. Recommend at age 45 y.#	Recommend at age 40 y.
Mammography screening interval	Annual or biennial§	Biennial‖	Annual for women aged 40–54 y‡ Biennial with the option to continue annual screening for women 55 y or older‡	Annual
Mammography stop age	Continue until age 75 y. Beyond age 75 y, the decision to discontinue should be based on a shared decision-making process that includes a discussion of the woman's health status and longevity.	The current evidence is insufficient to assess the balance of benefits and harms of screening mammography in women 75 y and older.†	When life expectancy is less than 10 y‡	When severe comorbidities limit life expectancy to 10 y or less

*Offer in the context of a shared, informed decision-making approach that recognizes the uncertainty of additional benefits and harms of clinical breast examination beyond screening mammography.

†Category I recommendation.

‡Qualified recommendation.

§Decision between options to be made through shared decision making after appropriate counseling.

‖Category B recommendation.

¶Category C recommendation. The Task Force notes that "Women who place a higher value on the potential benefit than the potential harms may choose to begin screening between the ages of 40 and 49 years."

#Strong recommendation.

Data from National Comprehensive Cancer Network. Breast cancer screening and diagnosis. Version 1.2016; Oeffinger KC, Fontham ET, Etzioni R, Herzig A, Michaelson JS, Shih YC, et al. Breast cancer screening for women at average risk: 2015 guideline update from the American Cancer Society [published erratum appears in JAMA 2016;315:1406]. JAMA 2015;314:1599–614; ***and*** Siu AL. Screening for breast cancer: U.S. Preventive Services Task Force recommendation statement. U.S. Preventive Services Task Force [published erratum appears in Ann Intern Med 2016;164:448]. Ann Intern Med 2016;164:279–96.

Reprinted from Breast cancer risk assessment and screening in average-risk women. Practice Bulletin No. 179. American College of Obstetricians and Gynecologists. Obstet Gynecol 2017;130:e1–16. doi: 10.1097/AOG.0000000000002158 https://journals.lww.com/greenjournal/Fulltext/2017/07000/Practice_Bulletin_Number_179__Breast_Cancer_Risk.50.aspx

primary screening tool and is less sensitive than mammography in the detection of calcifications. Therefore, ultrasonography would not be appropriate for the described patient. However, it can be a very useful supplemental test in lactating women.

Breast cancer risk assessment and screening in average-risk women. Practice Bulletin No. 179. American College of Obstetricians and Gynecologists. Obstet Gynecol 2017;130:e1–16. doi: 10.1097/AOG.0000000000002158 https://journals.lww.com/greenjournal/Fulltext/2017/07000/Practice_Bulletin_Number_179__Breast_Cancer_Risk.50.aspx

Guidelines for diagnostic imaging during pregnancy and lactation. Committee Opinion No. 723. American College of Obstetricians and Gynecologists [published erratum appears in Obstet Gynecol 2018;132:786]. Obstet Gynecol 2017;130:e210–6. doi: 10.1097/AOG.0000000000002355 https://journals.lww.com/greenjournal/Fulltext/2017/10000/Committee_Opinion_No__723__Guidelines_for.60.aspx

Johnson HM, Lewis TC, Mitchell KB. Breast cancer screening during lactation: ensuring optimal surveillance for breastfeeding women. Obstet Gynecol 2020;135:194–8. doi: 10.1097/AOG.0000000000003600 https://journals.lww.com/greenjournal/Fulltext/2020/01000/Breast_Cancer_Screening_During_Lactation__Ensuring.25.aspx

Kuo K, Caughey AB. Management strategy for breast cancer in pregnancy. Obstet Gynecol 2018;132:122–5. doi: 10.1097/AOG.0000000000002647 https://journals.lww.com/greenjournal/Fulltext/2018/07000/Management_Strategy_for_Breast_Cancer_in_Pregnancy.19.aspx

46 Hyperthyroidism

A 21-year-old gravida 1, para 0, presents at 33 weeks of gestation with fever and intermittent abdominal pain. The patient appears agitated and has proptosis. On physical examination, she has bilateral pedal edema and bibasilar rales. Her blood pressure is 102/60 mm Hg, heart rate is 140 beats per minute, temperature is 39.4 °C (102.9 °F), respiratory rate is 24 breaths per minute, and pulse oximetry is 96% on room air. A complete blood count is obtained, which shows a white blood cell count of 13×10^9/L. The most appropriate laboratory test to confirm the most likely diagnosis is a (an)

(A) amniotic fluid culture
(B) antinuclear antibodies test
(C) rapid human immunodeficiency virus (HIV) test
* (D) thyroid-stimulating hormone (TSH) test
(E) urine drug screen

The described patient has signs and symptoms of hyperthyroidism and thyrotoxicosis. A TSH test would be most likely to aid in the diagnosis. Hyperthyroidism is characterized by a decreased TSH concentration and elevated free thyroxine (T_4) or triiodothyronine (T_3) concentrations (Table 46-1). An assessment of the total T_3 is preferred to a free T_3 because assays for free T_3 are less robust than those used to measure free T_4. Women with overt hyperthyroidism may have goiter, nervousness, tremor, tachycardia, frequent stools, sweating or heat intolerance, insomnia, weight loss, palpitations, or hypertension. Graves disease often is characterized by ophthalmic-related presentations, including lid lag or retraction and dermopathy (pretibial myxedema). The treatment of hyperthyroidism is imperative to prevent thyroid storm. Thyrotoxicosis also can lead to preeclampsia and maternal heart failure.

The treatment of hyperthyroidism includes antithyroid medications (thioamides). In pregnancy, propylthiouracil or methimazole can be used. Methimazole typically is avoided in the first trimester because of teratogenicity risks, including esophageal or choanal atresia and aplasia cutis (a rare skin condition). Propylthiouracil rarely can cause hepatotoxicity, leading some obstetrician–gynecologists to recommend switching to methimazole in the second trimester. However, propylthiouracil should be considered in patients with T_3 predominant hyperthyroidism because it decreases peripheral conversion of T_4 to T_3. Thioamides may cause a transient leukopenia in approximately 10% of patients. In fewer than 1% of patients, agranulocytosis may occur, requiring discontinuation of the offending thioamide. Patients with fever or sore throat taking a thioamide should be evaluated immediately with a complete blood count.

TABLE 46-1. Guide to Thyroid Function Testing

CONDITION	FREE THYROXINE	TRIIODOTHYRONINE	THYROID-STIMULATING HORMONE	COMMENT
Primary hypothyroidism	↓	↓	↑	Caused by primary thyroid failure
Subclinical hypothyroidism	→	→	↑	Usually caused by autoimmune thyroid failure
Central hypothyroidism	↓	↓	↓, →, or ↑	Note that thyroid-stimulating hormone levels may be normal or rarely elevated
Hyperthyroidism	↑	↑	↓	Graves disease is the main cause
Triiodothyronine thyrotoxicosis	→	↑	↓	Seen in approximately 10% of hyperthyroidism cases caused by Graves disease or toxic multinodular goiter
Subclinical hyperthyroidism	→	→	↓	Usually seen in patients with underlying multinodular goiter
Nonthyroidal illness	→ or ↑	↓		Thyroid-stimulating hormone levels may be increased in recovery phase

Reprinted from Cooper DS, Ladenson PW. Thyroid disorders. Clin Update Womens Health Care 2013;XII(5):1–88. https://www.acog.org/clinical/journals-and-publications/clinical-updates/2013/11/thyroid-disorders

Thyroid storm is a rare but serious complication of severe thyrotoxicosis caused by excessive thyroid hormone. It occurs in the setting of inadequate treatment of hyperthyroidism, infection, preeclampsia, or in peripartum patients. Clinical signs include heart failure, fever, tachycardia, and central nervous system dysfunction. The cardiomyopathy of thyroid storm is reversible with treatment of hyperthyroidism. A high index of suspicion is required for the diagnosis, and if suspected, treatment should not be delayed while awaiting laboratory results.

Box 46-1 outlines the medical management of thyroid storm. Supportive therapy is recommended, including intravenous fluids, oxygen, and intensive care. Tachycardia is treated with β-blockers. Propranolol is most commonly used for this purpose. Beta-blockers should be used with caution in the setting of acute heart failure, however, because of the negative inotropic effects. High-dose antithyroid medications are administered immediately. Typically, propylthiouracil is given because of its ability to block peripheral conversion of T_4 to T_3. Approximately 1 hour after antithyroid medications are given, oral potassium iodide should be added to block further release of thyroid hormone from the thyroid gland. During maternal treatment and stabilization, nonreassuring fetal monitoring may occur, but this typically improves with resolution of acute maternal disease. Delivery should be avoided during this time.

An amniotic fluid culture is an important consideration in the diagnosis of intra-amniotic infection (chorioamnionitis). Intra-amniotic infection should be included in the differential of the described patient who has fever and abdominal pain. However, the other signs and symptoms point to an alternative diagnosis. In addition, a culture will take days to return. If intra-amniotic infection is suspected, more appropriate testing of amniotic fluid (in addition to culture) would include a Gram stain, cell count, and glucose.

Antinuclear antibody is a nonspecific test of autoimmune or rheumatologic disorder. A positive test does not reveal information regarding the specific underlying disease and would not be helpful in this case.

An HIV test may be included in the complete laboratory workup, but the presentation of the described patient does not suggest HIV. Similarly, a urine toxicology screen also may be warranted, but it would not be the most appropriate test to aid in this diagnosis. Although substance use with intravenous administration may lead to acute infection or sepsis, the described patient has other signs that suggest thyrotoxicosis, such as proptosis, pedal edema, agitation, and signs of cardiomyopathy (bibasilar rales).

BOX 46-1

Medical Management of Thyroid Storm or Thyrotoxic Heart Failure in Pregnancy*

- Inhibit thyroid release of T_3 and T_4
  Propylthiouracil, 1,000 mg load by mouth, then 200 mg by mouth every 6 h
  Iodine administration 1–2 h after propylthiouracil by
  — sodium iodide, 500–1,000 mg IV every 8 h
  or
  — potassium iodide, five drops by mouth every 8 h
  or
  — Lugol solution, 10 drops by mouth every 8 h
  or
  — lithium carbonate (if patient has an iodine anaphylaxis history), 300 mg by mouth every 6 h
- Further block peripheral conversion of T_4 to T_3
  Dexamethasone, 2 mg IV every 6 h for four doses
  or
  Hydrocortisone, 100 mg IV every 8 h for three doses
- Propranolol, labetalol, and esmolol have all been used successfully to control tachycardia. However, caution must be exercised if using a β-blocking drug in the presence of heart failure.
- Supportive measures, such as temperature control, as needed

*The dosages in the table were published by ACOG in 2020. For the most up-to-date dosing information, please review ACOG's guidance at acog.org

Abbreviations: IV, intravenous; T_3, triiodothyronine; T_4, thyroxine.

Reprinted from Thyroid disease in pregnancy. ACOG Practice Bulletin No. 223. American College of Obstetricians and Gynecologists. Obstet Gynecol 2020;135:e261–74. doi: 10.1097/AOG.0000000000003893 https://journals.lww.com/greenjournal/Fulltext/2020/06000/Thyroid_Disease_in_Pregnancy__ACOG_Practice.47.aspx

Cooper DS, Ladenson PW. Thyroid disorders. Clin Update Womens Health Care 2013;XII(5):1–88. https://www.acog.org/clinical/journals-and-publications/clinical-updates/2013/11/thyroid-disorders

Cooper DS, Laurberg P. Hyperthyroidism in pregnancy. Lancet Diabetes Endocrinol 2013;1:238 49. doi: 10.1016/S2213-8587(13)70086-X https://www.thelancet.com/journals/landia/article/PIIS2213-8587(13)70086-X/fulltext

Thyroid disease in pregnancy. ACOG Practice Bulletin No. 223. American College of Obstetricians and Gynecologists. Obstet Gynecol 2020;135:e261–74. doi: 10.1097/AOG.0000000000003893 https://journals.lww.com/greenjournal/Fulltext/2020/06000/Thyroid_Disease_in_Pregnancy__ACOG_Practice.47.aspx

47 Brachial plexus injury

A 24-year-old gravida 1 is in labor at 37 weeks of gestation. Her pregnancy has been complicated by gestational diabetes mellitus, which has been managed with subcutaneous insulin therapy, and maternal obesity. Her body mass index is 44. The estimated fetal weight from an obstetric ultrasonographic examination 1 week ago was 3,600 g. Her hospital course has lasted 48 hours and included intravenous oxytocin after cervical ripening. She has effective neuraxial anesthesia in place. After 45 minutes of pushing, the head delivers and retracts against the perineum. Downward axial traction to deliver the anterior shoulder is unsuccessful. The obstetrician alerts the care team to a shoulder dystocia. Two assistants hyperflex the patient's hips and lay the patient flat while a third assistant provides suprapubic pressure, but the shoulder dystocia persists. The best next maneuver is to

(A) apply fundal pressure
* (B) deliver the posterior arm
(C) fracture the anterior fetal clavicle
(D) perform an episiotomy
(E) reposition the patient to hands and knees

A shoulder dystocia is an obstetric emergency with risk to the mother and fetus. A *shoulder dystocia* can be defined as an impaction of the anterior fetal shoulder against the symphysis pubis that is not relieved with downward axial traction, thus requiring additional maneuvers. Shoulder dystocia occurs in 0.2–3% of births. Risk factors for shoulder dystocia include increased birth weight, maternal diabetes, and a history of a previous shoulder dystocia. Of infants born weighing greater than 4,500 g, 9–14% experience a shoulder dystocia. Of infants born weighing greater than 4,500 g to women with diabetes, the rate of shoulder dystocia increases to 20–50%. Recurrence rates of shoulder dystocia in subsequent deliveries range from 1.0% to 16.7%. Despite these risks, most shoulder dystocia emergencies occur in women without diabetes who give birth to neonates weighing less than 4,500 g, making shoulder dystocia a largely unpredictable event.

Maternal morbidity related to shoulder dystocia includes increased rates of hemorrhage and obstetric anal sphincter injuries. Neonatal complications can be severe, including brachial plexus injuries, clavicular and humeral fractures, and neonatal encephalopathy. One large multicenter study of 2,018 cases of shoulder dystocia found a total injury rate of 5.2%. There were 60 cases of Erb paralysis, four cases of Klumpke paralysis, 41 fractures of either the clavicle or humerus, and six cases of neonatal encephalopathy.

Although more than 50% of brachial plexus injuries occur in uncomplicated vaginal deliveries, they are among the most common neonatal injuries associated with a shoulder dystocia. The overall prevalence of brachial plexus injuries is 1.5 per 1,000 live births. The rate of injury is significantly higher in neonates born with weights greater than 4,500 g, with 2.6–7% experiencing injuries. For neonates who experience a shoulder dystocia event at birth, 4–23% demonstrate a brachial plexus injury immediately after delivery. Data on the rate of persistent injury are widely variable because of differences in defining persistent symptoms and differing timelines. In general, injuries that involve more spinal levels (C5–T1) have lower rates of complete recovery compared with injuries in which only a few spinal nerve levels are affected. Brachial plexus injuries in infants with birth weights of greater than 4,500 g also have lower rates of functional recovery.

When a shoulder dystocia is encountered, the first step is to recognize the obstetric emergency and alert all care team members in attendance. When downward axial traction fails to deliver the anterior shoulder, additional intervention is needed. Additional nursing, obstetric, and anesthesia staff should be called to the room. The time should be marked, and an event recorder identified. Maternal expulsive efforts should cease because these will add to the traction being placed on the brachial plexus. Although all maneuvers will increase the stretch of the brachial plexus, there is no place for either lateral traction or fundal pressure because neither will relieve the impacted anterior shoulder. Fundal pressure also will risk uterine rupture. Because a shoulder dystocia is a bony obstruction, there is no general indication for an episiotomy, but occasionally it may be necessary to allow better access for obstetric maneuvers.

The generally accepted first maneuver once a shoulder dystocia is identified is the McRoberts maneuver with suprapubic pressure from an assistant (Fig. 47-1). With the labor bed completely flat, two assistants actively flex the hips to rotate the maternal pubic symphysis cephalad and flatten the lumbar lordosis, while another assistant simultaneously applies suprapubic pressure to abduct and rotate the fetal anterior shoulder. This combination is simple and effective. When a McRoberts maneuver with suprapubic pressure is unsuccessful, there is evidence that moving to delivery of the posterior arm has a higher rate of achieving birth versus other maneuvers (Fig. 47-2). In this situation, one study noted that delivery of the posterior arm successfully achieved delivery in 84% of cases versus 24–72% for other maneuvers, such as the Rubin or Wood screw. The same study noted comparable levels of injury for each maneuver but a reduction in neonatal injuries when the total number of maneuvers performed was lower. Other studies, including geometric studies and computer modeling, have found evidence to support proceeding with delivery of the posterior arm after an unsuccessful McRoberts, noting a decreased degree of anterior nerve stretch and a reduction in the delivery force needed versus rotational maneuvers.

During a Rubin maneuver the obstetrician exerts force on the posterior aspect of the posterior shoulder to rotate towards the face (Fig. 47-3). A Wood screw maneuver involves the obstetrician exerting force on the anterior aspect of the posterior shoulder to rotate the fetus the contralateral direction to free the impacted shoulder (Fig. 47-4). Patients with mobility

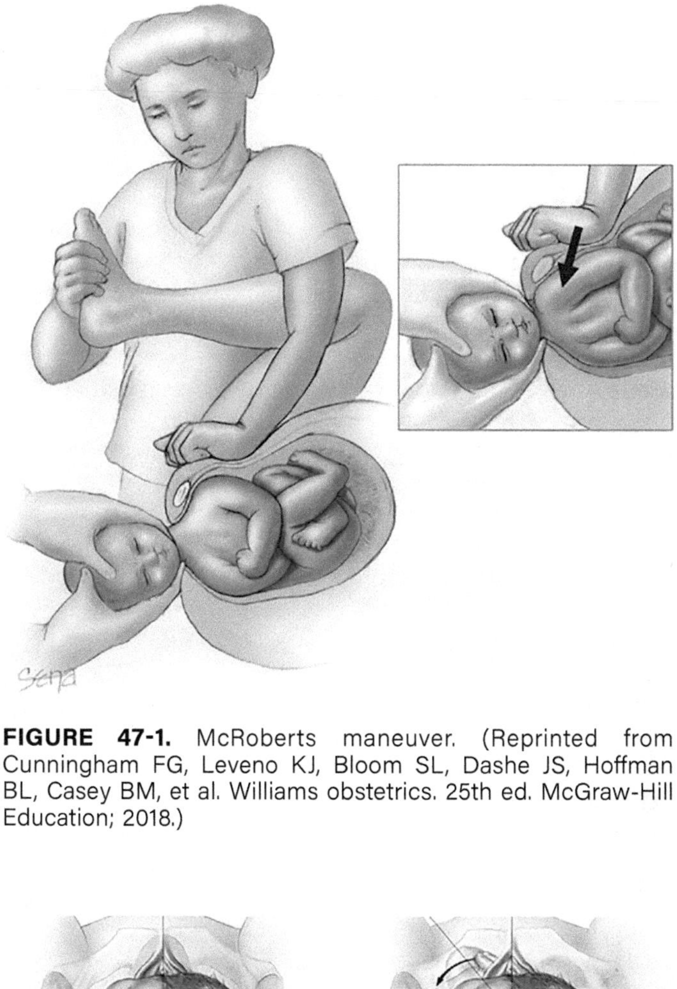

FIGURE 47-1. McRoberts maneuver. (Reprinted from Cunningham FG, Leveno KJ, Bloom SL, Dashe JS, Hoffman BL, Casey BM, et al. Williams obstetrics. 25th ed. McGraw-Hill Education; 2018.)

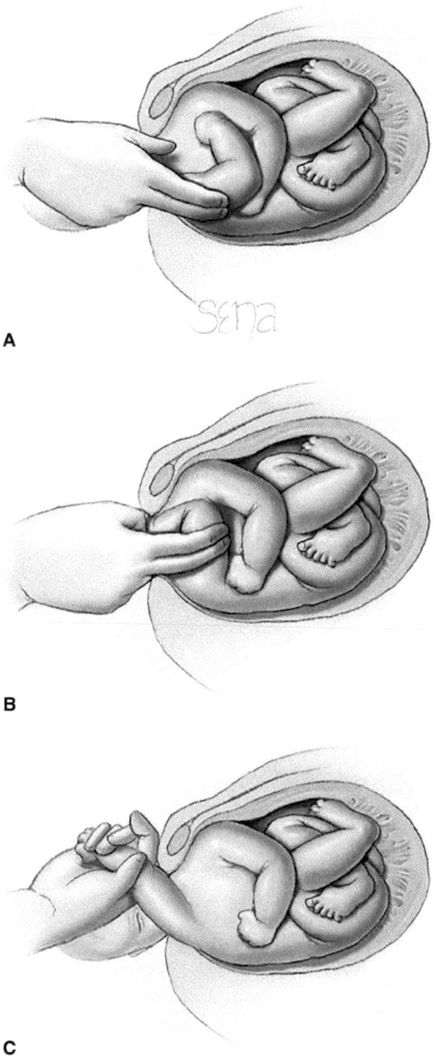

FIGURE 47-2. A, B, and C. Delivery of the posterior arm. (Reprinted from Cunningham FG, Leveno KJ, Bloom SL, Dashe JS, Hoffman BL, Casey BM, et al. Williams obstetrics. 25th ed. McGraw-Hill Education; 2018.)

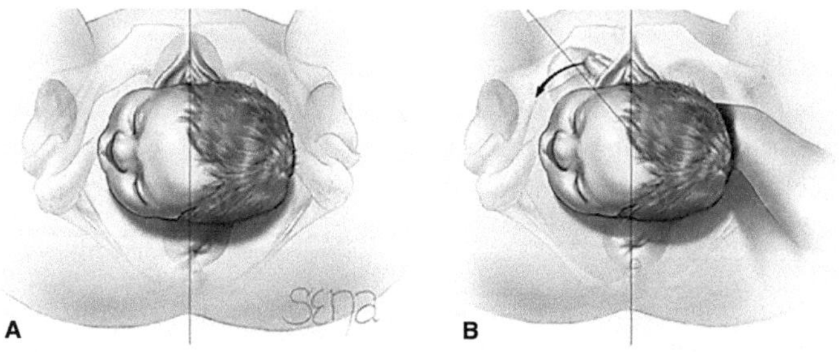

FIGURE 47-3. Rubin maneuver. (Reprinted from Cunningham FG, Leveno KJ, Bloom SL, Dashe JS, Hoffman BL, Casey BM, et al. Williams obstetrics. 25th ed. McGraw-Hill Education; 2018.)

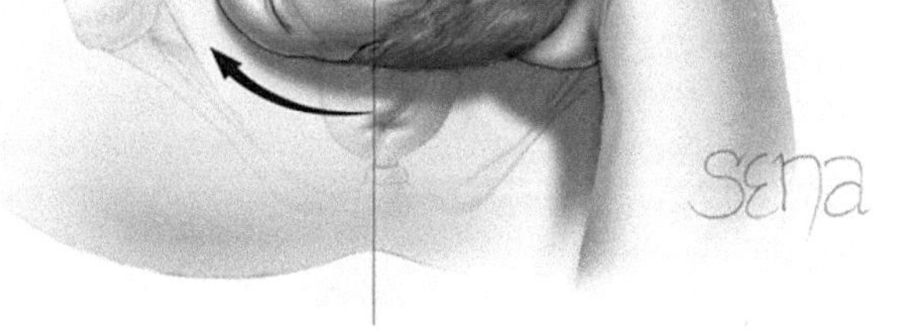

FIGURE 47-4. Woods maneuver. (Reprinted from Cunningham FG, Leveno KJ, Bloom SL, Dashe JS, Hoffman BL, Casey BM, et al. Williams obstetrics. 25th ed. McGraw-Hill Education; 2018.)

can be placed in a Gaskin position on hands and knees. Once repositioned, downward or upward axial traction can be applied to deliver the neonate. Neuraxial anesthesia can preclude a patient's ability to safely relocate to Gaskin position. When more conservative maneuvers fail, a fetal clavicle can be intentionally fractured, with manual traction directed away from the thoracic cavity. With a decrease in the bisacromial diameter, the previously attempted maneuvers can be repeated. The second clavicle can be intentionally fractured if the maneuvers again are unsuccessful, but these procedures are technically difficult to perform and risk major neonatal injury. Fetal clavicular fracture should never be performed with an instrument. Cephalic replacement with cesarean birth and laparotomy with manual reduction of the anterior shoulder are examples of extreme, life-saving interventions.

American College of Obstetricians and Gynecologists. Neonatal brachial plexus palsy. American College of Obstetricians and Gynecologists; 2014. Accessed March 2, 2022. https://www.acog.org/-/media/project/acog/acogorg/clinical/files/task-force-report/articles/2014/neonatal-brachial-plexus-palsy.pdf

Hoffman MK, Bailit JL, Branch DW, Burkman RT, Van Veldhusien P, Lu L, et al. A comparison of obstetric maneuvers for the acute management of shoulder dystocia. Consortium on Safe Labor. Obstet Gynecol 2011;117:1272–8. doi: 10.1097/AOG.0b013e31821a12c9 https://journals.lww.com/greenjournal/Fulltext/2011/06000/A_Comparison_of_Obstetric_Maneuvers_for_the_Acute.4.aspx

Macrosomia. ACOG Practice Bulletin No. 216. American College of Obstetricians and Gynecologists. Obstet Gynecol 2020;135:e18–35. doi: 10.1097/AOG.0000000000003606 https://journals.lww.com/greenjournal/Fulltext/2020/01000/Macrosomia__ACOG_Practice_Bulletin,_Number_216.50.aspx

Shoulder dystocia. Practice Bulletin No. 178. American College of Obstetricians and Gynecologists. Obstet Gynecol 2017;129:e123–33. doi: 10.1097/AOG.0000000000002043 https://journals.lww.com/greenjournal/Fulltext/2017/05000/Practice_Bulletin_No_178__Shoulder_Dystocia.47.aspx

48 Periviable birth

A 32-year-old gravida 4, para 3, at 23 4/7 weeks of gestation presented with preterm labor 3 days ago to a community hospital. Her cervix was 3-cm dilated, 50% effaced, and she was actively contracting. She received indomethacin tocolysis and was transferred to a hospital with a Level III neonatal intensive care unit. She received a two-dose betamethasone course and an intravenous magnesium sulfate infusion for the past 48 hours. She is now completely dilated, and delivery is imminent. After counseling with the neonatologists and considering neonatal resuscitation, the patient and her partner decline resuscitation and request palliative care for the neonate. The best next step in management is to

* (A) await delivery and provide neonatal comfort care
(B) consult psychiatry
(C) inform the hospital risk-management services
(D) report the patient's decision to the local government health agency
(E) review the case with the hospital ethics committee

Birth at a periviable gestational age is an evolving medical situation that can lead to difficult decisions for parents and physicians. The executive summary on *periviable birth* from the 2014 Joint Workshop by the *Eunice Kennedy Shriver* National Institute of Child Health and Human Development, the Society for Maternal–Fetal Medicine, the American Academy of Pediatrics, and the American College of Obstetricians and Gynecologists, defines this period as between 20 0/7 and 25 6/7 weeks of gestation. This period of rapid fetal development contributes significantly to neonatal survival. Data concerning survival at various gestational ages are often difficult to interpret, but in general survival progressively increases from 22 to 25 weeks of gestation with short- and long-term morbidity decreasing progressively. Birth earlier than 22 weeks of gestation is nearly universally fatal, and the American Academy of Pediatrics does not recommend resuscitation. According to data from the United States, England, and Australia, birth at 25 weeks of gestation has survival rates as high as 67–76%, and universal resuscitation is recommended. A large, multicenter study published in 2017 reviewed 4,000 births from 22–24 weeks of gestation from 2001 to 2011. The study authors noted improvements in overall survival and survival without neurodevelopmental impairment during the decade, reflecting improved techniques for the care of periviable neonates; however, overall mortality and morbidity remained high during this period.

Fetal survival and the chances of morbidity go beyond gestational age (Table 48-1). The limitations of gestational age as a predictor of mortality and morbidity include the inherent inaccuracy of dating pregnancies in general. Birth weight also is a significant factor in survival, with larger birth weight predicting better outcomes, but this can only be estimated with an obstetric ultrasonographic examination during the antenatal course with a significant margin of error.

Administration of maternal corticosteroids has a substantial effect on outcomes. Female gender and singleton status also are beneficial to survival and morbidity in the periviable birth setting. The location of delivery and neonatal resources available will dictate the resuscitation that is available.

TABLE 48-1. Factors That Affect the Reliability of Estimates of Survival or the Actual Outcomes Among Periviable Births

VARIABLE	EFFECT
Factors Affecting Reliability of Estimates of Probability of Clinical Outcomes	
Data source	International, national, regional, and single-institution data reflect variations in regional and local practices.
Cohort selection	Exclusion of newborns not surviving to NICU admission results in inclusion of those with higher potential for survival and higher reported rates of survival. Inclusion of nonresuscitated infants or stillbirths reduces overall reported rates of survival. Inclusion of anomalous infants may decrease reported survival estimates.
Gestational age assignment	In vitro fertilization and ovulation induction provide accurate gestational age assignment. Dating by last menstrual period assumes accurate recollection of this date as well as fertilization on day 14. Ultrasonography initially performed at less than 24 weeks of gestation estimates gestational age within 5–14 days.*
Factors Potentially Affecting Clinical Outcomes	
Nonmodifiable risk factors	Plurality (singleton versus multiple gestation), infant sex, birth weight, gestational age
Modifiable obstetric practices	Antenatal interventions (eg, corticosteroids, tocolysis, antibiotics for preterm PROM, or magnesium for neuroprotection), site and mode of delivery
Modifiable neonatal practices	Initial resuscitation and subsequent care (eg, approaches to ventilation and oxygenation, nutritional support, and treatment of newborn infections)
Approaches to comfort care	Influenced by institutional and physician philosophies, parental wishes, and religious convictions
Regional/hospital legal and practice guidelines	Policies concerning neonatal resuscitation

Modified from Raju TN, Mercer BM, Burchfield DJ, Joseph GF Jr. Periviable birth: executive summary of a joint workshop by the *Eunice Kennedy Shriver* National Institute of Child Health and Human Development, Society for Maternal–Fetal Medicine, American Academy of Pediatrics, and American College of Obstetricians and Gynecologists. Obstet Gynecol 2014;123:1083–96. doi: 10.1097/AOG.0000000000000243 https://journals.lww.com/greenjournal/Fulltext/2014/05000/Periviable_Birth__Executive_Summary_of_a_Joint.24.aspx

When counseling parents regarding the possible outcomes of a periviable birth, the physician should engage in a shared decision-making process. Some parents will want to know statistics, whereas others' decisions will be driven by cultural, religious, or other motivations. Some patients will focus on goals to maximize survival, whereas others will direct all care to minimize suffering. When appropriately counseled, parents of periviable neonates should be given the option of resuscitation or palliative care. As clinical circumstances change, the approach to resuscitation and ongoing intensive care can be reassessed.

The described scenario provides no suggestion that the patient lacks the capacity to understand the clinical scenario and make an informed decision; thus, a psychiatric evaluation is not warranted. There is no reason to contact risk management as the next step. Delivery is imminent, and the patient has the autonomy to make this decision. Likewise, there is no indication for an ethics committee consultation or reason to contact a government health agency because providing palliative care to a neonate in this situation is acceptable and appropriate medical care (Appendix E).

Cummings J. Antenatal counseling regarding resuscitation and intensive care before 25 weeks of gestation. Committee on Fetus and Newborn. Pediatrics 2015;136:588–95. doi: 10.1542/peds.2015-2336 https://publications.aap.org/pediatrics/article/136/3/588/61069/Antenatal-Counseling-Regarding-Resuscitation-and

Periviable birth. Obstetric Care Consensus No. 6. American College of Obstetricians and Gynecologists. Obstet Gynecol 2017;130:e187–99. doi: 10.1097/AOG.0000000000002352 https://journals.lww.com/greenjournal/Fulltext/2017/10000/Obstetric_Care_Consensus_No__6__Periviable_Birth.57.aspx

Raju TN, Mercer BM, Burchfield DJ, Joseph GF Jr. Periviable birth: executive summary of a joint workshop by the Eunice Kennedy Shriver National Institute of Child Health and Human Development, Society for Maternal–Fetal Medicine, American Academy of Pediatrics, and American College of Obstetricians and Gynecologists. Obstet Gynecol 2014;123:1083–96. doi: 10.1097/AOG.0000000000000243 https://journals.lww.com/greenjournal/Fulltext/2014/05000/Periviable_Birth__Executive_Summary_of_a_Joint.24.aspx

Younge N, Goldstein RF, Bann CM, Hintz SR, Patel RM, Smith PB, et al. Survival and neurodevelopmental outcomes among periviable infants. Eunice Kennedy Shriver National Institute of Child Health and Human Development Neonatal Research Network. N Engl J Med 2017;376:617–28. doi: 10.1056/NEJMoa1605566 https://www.nejm.org/doi/10.1056/NEJMoa1605566

49 Maternal cardiac arrest

A patient at 32 weeks of gestation arrives at the emergency department trauma bay. She suffered cardiac arrest while in the ambulance 7 minutes ago. Chest compressions were started along with bag mask ventilation. Intubation before arrival was unsuccessful because of poor visualization. The obstetric emergency response team and emergency department team are present on the patient's arrival. She is positioned supine with left lateral tilt. Chest compression and bag mask ventilation are continued. A defibrillator is placed, and the maternal rhythm is asystole. In addition to intravenous epinephrine, the best next step in management is

(A) biphasic defibrillation
(B) central venous access
* (C) cesarean birth
(D) endotracheal intubation
(E) transfer to the operating room

Maternal cardiac arrest during pregnancy is a rare but catastrophic event. Management of maternal cardiac arrest should include a multidisciplinary team, and because of its infrequent occurrence, maternal code teams should be formally organized and trained regularly through simulation drills. The differential diagnosis for maternal cardiac arrest is broad and has been organized alphabetically by the American Heart Institute (Table 49-1). For women who suffer cardiac arrest when admitted for delivery, the most common causes are hemorrhage (38.1% of cases) and amniotic fluid embolus (13.3% of cases). Pregnant patients with acute coronary syndrome have a 10% risk of cardiac arrest during the pregnancy or postpartum period. Pregnant patients who develop or have existing venous thrombotic emboli have a 4% chance of cardiac arrest during the pregnancy.

Maternal cardiac resuscitation during pregnancy is managed differently than it is in nonpregnant individuals. Simultaneous resuscitation versus a stepwise approach is the rule in pregnancy. Patients at more than 20 weeks of gestation will have aortocaval compression, and they should be positioned on a backboard with left-lateral tilt or manual displacement of the uterus to the left. The American Heart Institute recommends manual uterine displacement because left-lateral tilt can prohibit optimal chest compressions. The maternal airway should be secured early. Pharyngeal and laryngeal anatomy are altered in pregnancy, which raises the risk of aspiration during cardiac arrest and increases the difficulty of endotracheal tube placement, with an eightfold increase in the rate of failed intubation. A clinician possessing experience with maternal airways should be a part of every maternal code team.

Chest compressions are performed the same way in pregnant versus nonpregnant women with a rate of 100–120 compressions per minute over the mid-lower sternum while on a backboard. The compression-to-respiration ratio is 30:2 with 100% oxygen when bag masking the patient. Defibrillation should be performed for shockable rhythms, which include ventricular fibrillation and pulseless ventricular tachycardia. Fetal heart rate monitors should be removed during maternal rhythm analysis and defibrillation. For nonshockable rhythms, including asystole and pulseless electrical activity, epinephrine should be administered. If intravenous access is not obtainable, epinephrine can be given by the intraosseous route above the level of the diaphragm.

In pregnancies beyond 20 weeks of gestation or when the uterine fundus extends above the umbilicus, preparation for delivery should begin immediately in the case of maternal cardiac arrest and resuscitation. Decompression of the aorta and vena cava and evacuation of the uterus have beneficial effects for maternal resuscitation—mainly increased cardiac output. A review of published cases of perimortem cesarean births from 1980 to 2010 found that 31.7% of the procedures demonstrated maternal survival benefits, and no cases of perimortem cesarean birth were found to be harmful to maternal resuscitation. Both maternal and neonatal morbidity and mortality increase progressively as the cardiac arrest persists.

The goal of preparing for delivery with the onset of cardiac arrest is to achieve delivery by hysterotomy within 4–5 minutes if spontaneous circulation has not returned. Whereas earlier delivery improves maternal resuscitation and lessens neonatal harm, perimortem cesarean birth still can be beneficial more remote from cardiac arrest onset. Studies have found injury-free survival for the woman and the neonate to be as high as 33–50% even 25 minutes from the onset of cardiac arrest. Maternal code teams should have access to cesarean birth kits, but in these emergent situations personal protective equipment and a scalpel are sufficient supplies for the initial delivery.

The most appropriate next step in the management of this patient is to proceed with cesarean birth. She suffered cardiac arrest at least 7 minutes prior, and there is no reason to delay delivery another 4 minutes while continuing chest compressions. The maternal cardiac rhythm is asystole, which is nonshockable. Attempting to place a central venous catheter should not precede cesarean birth in this situation because of the time-critical nature of these events. A previous attempt at endotracheal intubation was unsuccessful, and delivery should not be delayed further to achieve this. Finally, it is not appropriate

TABLE 49-1. Most Common Etiologies of Maternal Arrest and Mortality

LETTER	CAUSE	ETIOLOGY
A	Anesthesia complications	High neuraxial block Hypotension Loss of airway Aspiration Respiratory depression Local anesthetic systemic toxicity
	Accidents/Trauma	Trauma Suicide
B	Bleeding	Coagulopathy Uterine atony Placenta accreta Placental abruption Placenta previa Retained products of pregnancy Uterine rupture Surgical Transfusion reaction
C	Cardiovascular causes	Myocardial infarction Aortic dissection Cardiomyopathy Arrhythmias Valve disease Congenital heart disease
D	Drugs	Oxytocin Magnesium Drug error Illicit drugs Opioids Insulin Anaphylaxis
E	Embolic causes	Amniotic fluid embolus Pulmonary embolus Cerebrovascular event Venous air embolus
F	Fever	Sepsis Infection
G	General	Metabolic abnormalities Electrolyte abnormalities
H	Hypertension	Preeclampsia Eclampsia HELLP syndrome Intracranial bleed

Abbreviation: HELLP, hemolysis, elevated liver enzymes, and low platelet count.

Modified from Jeejeebhoy FM, Zelop CM, Lipman S, Carvalho B, Joglar J, Mhyre JM, et al. Cardiac arrest in pregnancy: a scientific statement from the American Heart Association. American Heart Association Emergency Cardiovascular Care Committee, Council on Cardiopulmonary, Critical Care, Perioperative and Resuscitation, Council on Cardiovascular Diseases in the Young, and Council on Clinical Cardiology. Circulation 2015;132:1747–73. doi: 10.1161/CIR.0000000000000300 https://www.ahajournals.org/doi/10.1161/CIR.0000000000000300.

to transfer the patient from their current location during active resuscitation efforts. Even relocation to an operating room is not a priority over ongoing resuscitation efforts and could further delay the resuscitative hysterotomy.

Critical care in pregnancy. ACOG Practice Bulletin No. 211. American College of Obstetricians and Gynecologists. Obstet Gynecol 2019;133:e303–19. doi: 10.1097/AOG.0000000000003241 https://journals.lww.com/greenjournal/Fulltext/2019/05000/ACOG_Practice_Bulletin_No__211__Critical_Care_in.39.aspx

Cunningham FG, Leveno KJ, Bloom SL, Dashe JS, Hoffman BL, Casey BM, et al. Williams obstetrics. 25th ed. McGraw-Hill Education; 2018.

Einav S, Kaufman N, Sela HY. Maternal cardiac arrest and perimortem caesarean delivery: evidence or expert-based? Resuscitation 2012;83:1191–200. doi: 10.1016/j.resuscitation.2012.05.005 https://www.resuscitationjournal.com/article/S0300-9572(12)00254-7/fulltext

Jeejeebhoy FM, Zelop CM, Lipman S, Carvalho B, Joglar J, Mhyre JM, et al. Cardiac arrest in pregnancy: a scientific statement from the American Heart Association. American Heart Association Emergency Cardiovascular Care Committee, Council on Cardiopulmonary, Critical Care, Perioperative and Resuscitation, Council on Cardiovascular Diseases in the Young, and Council on Clinical Cardiology. Circulation 2015;132:1747–73. doi: 10.1161/CIR.0000000000000300 https://www.ahajournals.org/doi/10.1161/CIR.0000000000000300

Pregnancy and heart disease. ACOG Practice Bulletin No. 212. American College of Obstetricians and Gynecologists. Obstet Gynecol 2019;133:e320–56. doi: 10.1097/AOG.0000000000003243 https://journals.lww.com/greenjournal/Fulltext/2019/05000/ACOG_Practice_Bulletin_No__212__Pregnancy_and.40.aspx

50 Multifetal birth

A healthy 32-year-old gravida 3, para 2, at 34 weeks of gestation has a dichorionic–diamniotic twin pregnancy. She has had two previous low transverse cesarean births and desires a repeat cesarean birth. Her pregnancy is uncomplicated other than her experiencing significant pelvic pain with movement, standing, or walking, and she is undergoing physical therapy for pubic symphysis laxity. You recommend delivery at a gestational age of

(A) 36 0/7 to 36 6/7 weeks
(B) 37 0/7 to 37 6/7 weeks
* (C) 38 0/7 to 38 6/7 weeks
(D) 39 0/7 to 39 6/7 weeks
(E) 40 0/7 to 40 6/7 weeks

The risks to neonates from late-preterm (34 0/7 to 36 6/7 weeks of gestation) and early-term (37 0/7 to 38 6/7 weeks of gestation) delivery include respiratory complications, neonatal intensive care unit admission, hypoglycemia, low Apgar scores, and an increase in neonatal mortality. Unless there is a medical or obstetric indication, delivery before 39 weeks of gestation should be avoided, and policies to decrease these nonindicated deliveries have been found to improve neonatal outcomes. These recommendations are dependent on accurate determination of gestational age.

There are clinical situations in which delivery before 39 weeks of gestation is warranted for maternal or fetal indications, and often clinicians will need to weigh competing risks and benefits for the patient and the fetus. The timing of delivery in these cases always must balance the risks of continuing the pregnancy with the risks of late-preterm and early-term delivery. The American College of Obstetricians and Gynecologists has made recommendations for delivery timing based on the available research and expert opinion for a variety of indications (Table 50-1). Some common maternal indications for delivery before 39 weeks include preeclampsia, poorly controlled diabetes mellitus, and intrahepatic cholestasis of pregnancy. Some common fetal indications for medically indicated delivery include intrauterine growth restriction, oligohydramnios, and multiple gestations.

On average, women with twin pregnancies give birth around 35–36 weeks of gestation because of the increased risk of spontaneous preterm birth, which may be secondary to cervical insufficiency, preterm labor, and preterm prelabor rupture of membranes. These patients also have an increased risk of indicated preterm birth because of complications such as hypertensive disorders of pregnancy and fetal growth restriction. Patients with monochorionic multiple gestations have a higher risk of developing complications, including twin–twin transfusion syndrome, twin anemia–polycythemia syndrome, higher risks of fetal anomalies, and stillbirth. It is recommended that patients having monochorionic–monoamniotic twins undergo delivery between 32 0/7 and 34 0/7 weeks of gestation, and those having monochorionic–diamniotic twins undergo delivery between 34 0/7 and 37 6/7 weeks of gestation.

Patients with dichorionic–diamniotic twin pregnancies have fewer complications than patients with monochorionic twins, but more than those with singleton pregnancies. The risk of perinatal morbidity and mortality in dichorionic twin pregnancies increases starting around 38 weeks of gestation, and planned delivery is recommended at 38 0/7 to 38 6/7 weeks of gestation in women with uncomplicated dichorionic–diamniotic twin gestations. In the described patient, delivery is recommended for 38 0/7 to 38 6/7 weeks of gestation despite her pelvic pain.

Pelvic pain in pregnancy can be secondary to the ligamentous laxity and, consequently, hypermobility of the sacroiliac joint connecting the sacrum to the ilium (sacroiliac dysfunction) or the pubic symphysis connecting the two sides of the pelvis (pubic symphysis dysfunction). These conditions cause pain with movement, which may not resolve after delivery and can persist even decades later. This pain can be treated with conservative measures, such as avoiding more painful activities, using accessory muscles for support (like the gluteal muscles), and using a pelvic compression belt. Referral to physical therapy can be helpful for the use of manual therapy techniques and to learn stabilizing exercises and stretches as well as instruction in the proper body mechanics. Musculoskeletal pain, even severe pain requiring physical therapy, is not a medical indication for delivery before 39 weeks.

TABLE 50-1. Recommendations for the Timing of Delivery When Conditions Complicate Pregnancy*

CONDITION	GENERAL TIMING	SUGGESTED SPECIFIC TIMING
PLACENTAL/UTERINE CONDITIONS		
Placenta previa[†]	Late preterm/early term	36 0/7–37 6/7 wk of gestation
Suspected accreta, increta, or percreta[†]	Late preterm	34 0/7–35 6/7 wk of gestation
Vasa previa	Late preterm/early term	34 0/7–37 0/7 wk of gestation
Prior classical cesarean delivery	Late preterm/early term	36 0/7–37 0/7 wk of gestation
Prior myomectomy requiring cesarean delivery[‡]	Early term (individualize)	37 0/7–38 6/7 wk of gestation
Previous uterine rupture	Late preterm/early term	36 0/7–37 0/7 wk of gestation
FETAL CONDITIONS		
Oligohydramnios (isolated or otherwise uncomplicated [deepest vertical pocket less than 2 cm])	Late preterm/early term	36 0/7–37 6/7 wk of gestation or at diagnosis if diagnosed later
Polyhydramnios (mild, idiopathic)[†]	Full term (early term birth not routinely recommended)	39 0/7–40 6/7 wk of gestation
Growth restriction (singleton)		
Otherwise uncomplicated, no concurrent findings, EFW between 3rd and 10th percentile	Early term/full term	38 0/7–39 0/7 wk of gestation
Otherwise uncomplicated, no concurrent findings, EFW less than 3rd percentile	Early term	37 0/7 wk of gestation or at diagnosis if diagnosed later
Abnormal umbilical artery Doppler studies: elevated impedance to flow (eg, S/D ratio, pulsatility index, or resistance index greater than 95th percentile for gestational age) with end-diastolic flow still present	Early term	37 0/7 wk of gestation or at diagnosis if diagnosed later
Abnormal umbilical artery Doppler studies: absent end-diastolic flow	Preterm/late preterm	33 0/7–34 0/7 wk of gestation or at diagnosis if diagnosed later[§]
Abnormal umbilical artery Doppler studies: reversed end-diastolic flow	Preterm	30 0/7–32 0/7 wk of gestation or at diagnosis if diagnosed later[§]
Concurrent conditions (oligohydramnios, maternal comorbidity [eg, preeclampsia, chronic hypertension])	Late preterm/early term	34 0/7–37 6/7 wk of gestation
Multiple gestations—uncomplicated		
Dichorionic-diamniotic twins	Early term	38 0/7–38 6/7 wk of gestation
Monochorionic-diamniotic twins	Late preterm/early term	34 0/7–37 6/7 wk of gestation
Monochorionic-monoamniotic twins	Preterm/late preterm	32 0/7–34 0/7 wk of gestation
Triplet and higher order multiples	Preterm/late preterm	Individualized
Multiple gestations—complicated		
Dichorionic-diamniotic twins with isolated fetal growth restriction	Late preterm/early term	36 0/7–37 6/7 wk of gestation
Dichorionic-diamniotic twins with concurrent condition	Late preterm	Individualized
Monochorionic-diamniotic twins with isolated fetal growth restriction	Preterm/late preterm	32 0/7–34 6/7 wk of gestation

(continued)

Table 50-1 *(continued)*

CONDITION	GENERAL TIMING	SUGGESTED SPECIFIC TIMING
Alloimmunization		
At-risk pregnancy not requiring intrauterine transfusion	Early term	37 0/7–38 6/7 wk of gestation
Requiring intrauterine transfusion	Late preterm or early term	Individualized
MATERNAL CONDITIONS		
Hypertensive disorders of pregnancy		
Chronic hypertension: isolated, uncomplicated, controlled, not requiring medications	Early term/full term	38 0/7–39 6/7 wk of gestation[‖]
Chronic hypertension: isolated, uncomplicated, controlled on medications	Early term/full term	37 0/7–39 6/7 wk of gestation[‖]
Chronic hypertension: difficult to control (requiring frequent medication adjustments)	Late preterm/early term	36 0/7–37 6/7 wk of gestation
Gestational hypertension, without severe-range blood pressure	Early term	37 0/7 wk of gestation or at diagnosis if diagnosed later
Gestational hypertension with severe-range blood pressures	Late preterm	34 0/7 wk of gestation or at diagnosis if diagnosed later
Preeclampsia without severe features	Early term	37 0/7 wk of gestation or at diagnosis if diagnosed later
Preeclampsia with severe features, stable maternal and fetal conditions, after fetal viability (includes superimposed)	Late preterm	34 0/7 wk of gestation or at diagnosis if diagnosed later
Preeclampsia with severe features, unstable or complicated, after fetal viability (includes superimposed and HELLP)	Soon after maternal stabilization	Soon after maternal stabilization
Preeclampsia with severe features, before viability	Soon after maternal stabilization[¶]	Soon after maternal stabilization[¶]
Diabetes		
Pregestational diabetes well-controlled[†]	Full term	39 0/7–39 6/7 wk of gestation
Pregestational diabetes with vascular complications, poor glucose control, or prior stillbirth	Late preterm/early term	36 0/7–38 6/7 wk of gestation
Gestational: well controlled on diet and exercise	Full term	39 0/7–40 6/7 wk of gestation
Gestational: well controlled on medications	Full term	39 0/7–39 6/7 wk of gestation
Gestational: poorly controlled	Late preterm/early term	Individualized
HIV		
Intact membranes and viral load greater than 1,000 copies/mL	Early-term cesarean delivery	38 0/7 wk of gestation
Viral load less than or equal to 1,000 copies/mL with antiretroviral therapy	Full term (early term birth not indicated)	39 0/7 wk of gestation or later
Intrahepatic cholestasis of pregnancy: total bile acid levels less than 100 micromol/L	Late preterm/early term	36 0/7–39 0/7 wk of gestation or at diagnosis if diagnosed later[#]
Intrahepatic cholestasis of pregnancy: total bile acid levels greater than or equal to 100 micromol/L	Late preterm	36 0/7 wk of gestation or at diagnosis if diagnosed later[#]

(continued)

Table 50-1 *(continued)*

CONDITION	GENERAL TIMING	SUGGESTED SPECIFIC TIMING
OBSTETRIC CONDITIONS		
Preterm PROM	Late preterm	34 0/7–36 6/7 wk of gestation**
PROM (37 0/7 wk of gestation and beyond)	Generally, at diagnosis	Generally, at diagnosis
Previous stillbirth	Full term (early term birth not routinely recommended)	Individualized††

Abbreviations: EFW, estimated fetal weight; HELLP, hemolysis, elevated liver enzymes, and low platelet count; PROM, prelabor rupture of membranes (also referred to as premature rupture of membranes); S/D, systolic/diastolic.

*In situations in which there is a wide gestational age range for acceptable delivery thresholds, the lower range is not automatically preferable, and medical decision making for the upper or lower part of a range should depend on individual patient factors and risks and benefits.

†Uncomplicated, thus no fetal growth restriction, superimposed preeclampsia, or other complication. If these conditions are present, then the complicating conditions take precedence and earlier delivery may be indicated.

‡Prior myomectomy may require earlier delivery similar to prior classical cesarean (36 0/7 to 37 0/7 weeks of gestation) in situations with more extensive or complicated myomectomy. Data are conflicting regarding specific timing of delivery. Furthermore, timing of delivery may be influenced by the degree and location of the prior uterine surgery, with the possibility of delivering as late as 38 6/7 weeks of gestation for a patient with a less extensive prior surgery. Timing of delivery should be individualized based on prior surgical details available and the clinical situation.

§Consultation with maternal–fetal medicine subspecialist is recommended.

||Expectant management beyond 39 0/7 weeks of gestation should only be done after careful consideration of the risks and benefits and with appropriate surveillance.

¶Management individualized to particulars of maternal–fetal condition and gestational age.

#Measurement of serum bile acid levels and liver transaminase is recommended in patients with suspected intrahepatic cholestasis of pregnancy. Delivery before 36 weeks of gestation occasionally may be indicated depending on laboratory and clinical circumstances.

**The balance between benefit and risk, from both maternal and neonatal perspectives, should be carefully considered, and patients should be counseled clearly. Although a period of expectant management may be considered for women who request additional time for the onset of spontaneous labor, the potential maternal and neonatal risks associated with prolonged expectant management should be discussed. Care should be individualized through shared decision making, and expectant management should not extend beyond 37 0/7 weeks of gestation. Outside the scenario of unknown GBS status, latency antibiotics are not appropriate in this setting. If expectant management is being considered in a patient with unknown GBS status, an initial GBS culture should be obtained, and an antibiotic regimen active against GBS should be started until results of the GBS culture return. Women with PPROM who are colonized with GBS are at an increased risk of neonatal infection with expectant management. The potential additional neonatal risks associated with prolonged expectant management in the setting of maternal GBS colonization should be discussed and the reasons for discouraging such management reviewed and documented in the medical record.

††Deliveries before 39 weeks of gestation are associated with an increased risk of admission to neonatal special care units for respiratory complications and other neonatal morbidities; however, maternal anxiety with a history of stillbirth should be considered and may warrant an early-term delivery (37 0/7 to 38 6/7 weeks) in women who are educated regarding, and accept, the associated neonatal risks.

Reprinted from Medically indicated late-preterm and early-term deliveries. ACOG Committee Opinion No. 831. American College of Obstetricians and Gynecologists. Obstet Gynecol 2021;138:e35–9. doi: 10.1097/AOG.0000000000004447 https://journals.lww.com/greenjournal/Fulltext/2021/07000/Medically_Indicated_Late_Preterm_and_Early_Term.38.aspx.

Avoidance of nonmedically indicated early-term deliveries and associated neonatal morbidities. ACOG Committee Opinion No. 765. American College of Obstetricians and Gynecologists. Obstet Gynecol 2019;133:e156–63. doi: 10.1097/AOG.0000000000003076 https://journals.lww.com/greenjournal/Fulltext/2019/02000/ACOG_Committee_Opinion_No__765__Avoidance_of.43.aspx

Butler R. The role of physical therapy in obstetric–gynecologic practice. Clin Update Womens Health Care 2018;XVII(5):1–44. https://www.acog.org/clinical/journals-and-publications/clinical-updates/2018/09/the-role-of-physical-therapy-in-obstetricgynecologic-practice

Landon MB, Galan HL, Jauniaux ER, Driscoll DA, Berghella V, Grobman WA, et al, editors. Gabbe's obstetrics: normal and problem pregnancies. 8th ed. Elsevier; 2021.

Medically indicated late-preterm and early-term deliveries. ACOG Committee Opinion No. 831. American College of Obstetricians and Gynecologists. Obstet Gynecol 2021;138:e35–9. doi: 10.1097/AOG.0000000000004447 https://journals.lww.com/greenjournal/Fulltext/2021/07000/Medically_Indicated_Late_Preterm_and_Early_Term.38.aspx

Multifetal gestations: twin, triplet, and higher-order multifetal pregnancies. ACOG Practice Bulletin No. 231. American College of Obstetricians and Gynecologists. Obstet Gynecol 2021;137:e145–62. doi: 10.1097/AOG.0000000000004397 https://journals.lww.com/greenjournal/Fulltext/2021/06000/Multifetal_Gestations__Twin,_Triplet,_and.39.aspx

Resnik R, Lockwood CJ, Moore TR, Greene MF, Copel JA, Silver RM, editors. Creasy & Resnik's maternal–fetal medicine: principles and practice. 8th ed. Elsevier; 2019.

51 Obstetric anesthesia

A 30-year-old gravida 1, para 0, at 34 weeks of gestation is undergoing induction of labor. An urgent cesarean birth is planned because of fetal heart rate decelerations, and spinal anesthesia is placed with the patient in a seated position. Shortly after the abdominal incision, the patient exhibits upper extremity weakness and difficulty breathing. She attempts to speak but is unable to form words. The most likely diagnosis is

(A) amniotic fluid embolism
* (B) high neuraxial block
(C) myocardial infarction
(D) spinal hematoma
(E) stroke

There are several approaches to analgesia during labor and delivery. Neuraxial and regional anesthesia are the most commonly used forms of pain relief for women in labor and during operative delivery in the United States, and techniques include epidural and spinal injection. Solutions usually are composed of local anesthetic with or without opioids and may be administered through a catheter as a single bolus, with continuous infusion, or by patient-controlled pump.

Obstetric analgesia and anesthesia have low risks of complications, morbidity, and mortality. The most common complications include fever, hypotension, transient fetal heart rate decelerations, and pruritus. More serious complications occur in less than 0.001% of cases and include epidural hematoma, complete spinal blockade, abscess, meningitis, and neurotoxicity.

This patient likely has a high neuraxial block, or total spinal anesthesia, which is one of the more serious complications related to obstetric anesthesia, occurring between 1 in 2,971 and 1 in 16,200 procedures. This complication usually occurs within a few minutes of anesthesia administration, and symptoms include rapid ascending sympathetic, sensory, and motor block with bradycardia, hypotension, dyspnea, and difficulty with swallowing or speaking. It can progress to unconsciousness and respiratory depression and arrest. Risk factors include obesity, spinal technique used after failed epidural anesthesia, and short maternal stature. High neuraxial block likely results from injection of medication into the subdural or subarachnoid space rather than the intended epidural space or from an overdose of medication in the epidural space. Treatment usually requires general anesthesia and patient intubation until the medication wears off.

Amniotic fluid embolism is a rare and life-threatening emergency that occurs when amniotic fluid enters the maternal circulation, and it may cause sudden cardiovascular collapse, respiratory distress, hypoxia, and seizure, as well as disseminated intravascular coagulopathy. The diagnosis is clinical and is based on characteristic findings and exclusion of other potential causes. Amniotic fluid embolism occurs during labor or within 30 minutes after birth. Treatment generally is supportive and consists of stabilization, cardiopulmonary resuscitation, if indicated, control of hemorrhage, and reversal of coagulopathy.

Cardiac arrest and myocardial infarction are rare complications during pregnancy. These complications can be caused directly by local anesthetic toxicity or can be exacerbated by other risk factors, including hemorrhage, preexisting cardiac disease, anaphylaxis, amniotic fluid embolism, pulmonary embolism, hypoxia, and maternal drug use.

Spinal epidural hematoma can occur after spinal dural puncture and rarely occurs spontaneously. Patients present with pain and loss of sensory, motor, and bowel and bladder function. It occurs more often in patients with thrombocytopenia or a predisposition to bleeding, including anticoagulation. Spinal epidural hematoma may be diagnosed with magnetic resonance imaging and usually is treated with surgical intervention and blood evacuation.

Stroke, or cerebrovascular accident, may be caused by cerebral ischemia or intracerebral or subarachnoid hemorrhage. This is a rare complication in pregnancy, usually related to preeclampsia or coagulopathy. Stroke is the leading cause of death in women with preeclampsia, and the primary method of prevention is blood pressure control during pregnancy and the peripartum period. Symptoms include weakness or numbness, especially on one side of the body, confusion or trouble speaking, dizziness and loss of balance, and sudden severe headache. Stroke should be on the differential diagnosis for the described patient, but is less likely given the timing of anesthesia administration as well as her lack of risk factors.

Combs CA, Montgomery DM, Toner LE, Dildy GA. Society for Maternal–Fetal Medicine Special Statement: checklist for initial management of amniotic fluid embolism. Patient Safety and Quality Committee, Society for Maternal–Fetal Medicine. Am J Obstet Gynecol 2021;224:B29–32. doi: 10.1016/j.ajog.2021.01.001 https://www.ajog.org/article/S0002-9378(21)00001-6/fulltext

D'Angelo R, Smiley RM, Riley ET, Segal S. Serious complications related to obstetric anesthesia: the serious complication repository project of the Society for Obstetric Anesthesia and Perinatology. Anesthesiology 2014;120:1505–12. doi: 10.1097/ALN.0000000000000253 https://pubs.asahq.org/anesthesiology/article/120/6/1505/11867/Serious-Complications-Related-to-Obstetric

Dyer RA, Swanevelder JL, Bateman BT. Hypertensive disorders. In: Chestnut DH, Wong CA, Tsen LC, Ngan Kee WD, Beilin Y, Mhyre JM, et al, editors. Chestnut's obstetric anesthesia: principles and practice. 6th ed. Elsevier; 2020. p. 840–78.

Obstetric analgesia and anesthesia. ACOG Practice Bulletin No. 209. American College of Obstetricians and Gynecologists. Obstet Gynecol 2019;133:e208–25. doi: 10.1097/AOG.0000000000003132 https://journals.lww.com/greenjournal/Fulltext/2019/03000/ACOG_Practice_Bulletin_No__209__Obstetric.45.aspx

Wong CA. Epidural and spinal analgesia: anesthesia for labor and vaginal delivery. In: Chestnut DH, Wong CA, Tsen LC, Ngan Kee WD, Beilin Y, Mhyre JM, et al, editors. Chestnut's obstetric anesthesia: principles and practice. 6th ed. Elsevier; 2020. p. 474–539.

52 Treatment of gestational diabetes mellitus

A 24-year-old gravida 1 is diagnosed with gestational diabetes mellitus (GDM) at 26 weeks of gestation. She is following the diet recommended by her nutritionist and is exercising 30 minutes daily. She uses a continuous glucose monitor because of a needle phobia. Her blood glucose values have been consistently elevated for several weeks. She declines insulin treatment. The best next step in management of her GDM is

(A) a ketogenic diet
(B) exercise for 60 minutes daily
(C) glyburide
* (D) metformin
(E) needle exposure therapy

Gestational diabetes mellitus is a common medical complication of pregnancy in which women develop carbohydrate intolerance, usually in the late-second or third trimester. Gestational diabetes increases the risk of maternal complications, including preeclampsia, cesarean birth, and diabetes later in life. Fetal and neonatal complications also are increased, including macrosomia, shoulder dystocia, birth trauma, and hypoglycemia. Treating GDM is associated with a reduction in the risks of these complications. First-line treatment includes lifestyle interventions, such as improving nutrition and exercising moderately. The ideal diet to optimize perinatal outcomes is not determined, but a very low carbohydrate, or ketogenic, diet is not recommended in pregnancy. This patient already is participating in a moderate exercise program (30 minutes of moderate-intensity aerobic exercise at least 5 days a week or a minimum of 150 minutes of exercise a week). Increasing her exercise intensity or duration would not be expected to improve her glycemic control.

When glucose targets cannot be reached with appropriate diet and exercise, pharmacologic treatment is recommended. Insulin has been used for many years in pregnancy and is the recommended first-line medication for GDM. It does not cross the placenta and helps achieve tight glycemic control with focused, shorter-acting doses at certain times of day or longer-lasting doses throughout the day and night. Two large randomized controlled trials in the past several decades provided evidence that treatment of gestational diabetes with insulin, even for mild GDM, decreased the risks for complications such as fetal overgrowth, shoulder dystocia, cesarean birth, and hypertensive disorders of pregnancy.

Oral medications, such as metformin and glyburide, also are commonly used and have been studied in pregnant women. Both medications cross the placenta, and metformin has been shown to have fetal levels as high as the maternal concentration. Metformin's long-term neonatal outcomes and metabolic influence on offspring are not known, but pregnancy outcomes and immediate neonatal outcomes seem to be similar between metformin and insulin when compared in randomized trials and meta-analyses. Metformin is a reasonable alternative for GDM treatment in women who cannot or prefer not to use insulin in pregnancy, such as the described patient. Treatment with glyburide, when compared in studies with insulin, is associated with an increased risk of macrosomia and neonatal hypoglycemia despite demonstrating a similar degree of glycemic control during pregnancy. Glyburide is not recommended as a first-line treatment for GDM. If an oral agent is used, metformin is the preferred medication.

Exposure-based interventions have been described for patients with high levels of needle fear, which is seen in up to 38% of adults. This type of cognitive behavioral therapy may be effective for pregnant patients, but it is not currently recommended in women with GDM who decline insulin treatment.

Crowther CA, Hiller JE, Moss JR, McPhee AJ, Jeffries WS, Robinson JS. Effect of treatment of gestational diabetes mellitus on pregnancy outcomes. Australian Carbohydrate Intolerance Study in Pregnant Women (ACHOIS) Trial Group. N Engl J Med 2005;352:2477–86. doi: 10.1056/NEJMoa042973 https://www.nejm.org/doi/10.1056/NEJMoa042973

Draznin B, Aroda VR, Bakris G, Benson G, Brown FM, Freeman R, et al. 15. Management of diabetes in pregnancy: Standards of Medical Care in Diabetes-2022. American Diabetes Association Professional Practice Committee. Diabetes Care 2022;45:S232–43. doi: 10.2337/dc22-S015 https://diabetesjournals.org/care/article/45/Supplement_1/S232/138916/15-Management-of-Diabetes-in-Pregnancy-Standards

Gestational diabetes mellitus. ACOG Practice Bulletin No. 190. American College of Obstetricians and Gynecologists. Obstet Gynecol 2018;131:e49–64. doi: 10.1097/AOG.0000000000002501 https://journals.lww.com/greenjournal/Fulltext/2018/02000/ACOG_Practice_Bulletin_No__190__Gestational.37.aspx

Landon MB, Spong CY, Thom E, Carpenter MW, Ramin SM, Casey B, et al. A multicenter, randomized trial of treatment for mild gestational diabetes. *Eunice Kennedy Shriver* National Institute of Child Health and Human Development Maternal–Fetal Medicine Units Network. N Engl J Med 2009;361:1339–48. doi: 10.1056/NEJMoa0902430 https://www.nejm.org/doi/10.1056/NEJMoa0902430

McMurtry CM, Taddio A, Noel M, Antony MM, Chambers CT, Asmundson GJ, et al. Exposure-based interventions for the management of individuals with high levels of needle fear across the lifespan: a clinical practice guideline and call for further research. Cogn Behav Ther 2016;45:217–35. doi: 10.1080/16506073.2016.1157204 https://www.tandfonline.com/doi/full/10.1080/16506073.2016.1157204

SMFM Statement: pharmacological treatment of gestational diabetes. Society for Maternal–Fetal Medicine (SMFM) Publications Committee. Am J Obstet Gynecol 2018;218:B2–4. doi: 10.1016/j.ajog.2018.01.041 https://www.ajog.org/article/S0002-9378(18)30092-9/fulltext

53 Vulvar lesions

A 24-year-old primigravida at 24 weeks of gestation presents to your office reporting a painful vulvar rash. On examination you note clusters of vesicles on the labia that are tender to touch. She reports no prior history of sexually transmitted infection. She undergoes confirmatory testing and treatment, and the lesions resolve. The best next step to prevent neonatal transmission is

(A) cesarean birth
(B) herpes zoster immunization
(C) imiquimod therapy
* (D) valacyclovir prophylaxis

Genital herpes simplex virus (HSV) is a viral illness that poses significant risk to the neonate. Both HSV-1 and HSV-2 can cause genital disease, which carries a high risk of neonatal transmission. Neonatal HSV is classified into the categories of disseminated disease, central nervous system disease, and disease of the skin, eyes, or mouth. Mortality can reach as high as 30% with disseminated disease, and long-term neurologic disease occurs in 20% of newborns who survive. The risks to the neonate are significant, making the identification and management of HSV an important public health concern.

Herpes simplex virus should be suspected in the presence of vesicular eruption of the genitals, but new infections in pregnant women often are asymptomatic. Lesions usually are painful and should be swabbed to determine the diagnosis. To sample correctly, vesicles should be unroofed and vesicular fluid sampled. Culture sensitivity is low, with a false-negative rate of 60%. Polymerase chain reaction testing improves detection significantly and is preferred. In the setting of clinical history consistent with HSV but with a negative culture or polymerase chain reaction test, serologic testing can be helpful to determine the diagnosis. The presence of antibodies to HSV-2 can be considered diagnostic of genital infection, because it is an uncommon cause of oral infection. In the setting of a primary infection, serology may not be positive for 2 or more weeks after the presence of lesions.

Vaginal delivery should be avoided during an outbreak of HSV and when prodromal symptoms are present. Women with a history of HSV should be asked about symptoms on admission and examined again when admitted to labor and delivery. A thorough inspection of the vulva, vagina, and cervix is important. In the setting of HSV outbreak or prodrome, cesarean birth often is recommended unless the lesion is distant from the genital area and can be covered by an occlusive dressing.

In the setting of known HSV in pregnancy, patients should be treated for symptoms with an antiviral medication, usually acyclovir or valacyclovir, to decrease duration and severity of symptoms. Famciclovir also is acceptable, although it is less well studied in pregnancy. The best next step for this patient is to start prophylactic acyclovir or valacyclovir at 36 weeks of gestation, which will help prevent disease recurrence around the time of birth. This strategy has been shown to reduce the risk of outbreak at delivery, which in turn reduces the need for cesarean birth for active HSV. It also decreases asymptomatic shedding.

Cesarean birth is indicated for patients with active genital infection; however, prophylaxis at 36 weeks to avoid cesarean birth is a more appropriate next step. Herpes zoster immunization is contraindicated in pregnancy because it is a live attenuated vaccine. Additionally, this vaccine prevents herpes zoster, not herpes simplex. Imiquimod is an acceptable option for treatment of genital warts, but it is not an appropriate treatment for herpes.

Cunningham FG, Leveno KJ, Bloom SL, Dashe JS, Hoffman BL, Casey BM, et al. Williams obstetrics. 25th ed. McGraw-Hill Education; 2018.

Management of genital herpes in pregnancy. ACOG Practice Bulletin No. 220. American College of Obstetricians and Gynecologists. Obstet Gynecol 2020;136:850–1. doi: 10.1097/AOG.0000000000004115 https://journals.lww.com/greenjournal/Fulltext/2020/05000/Management_of_Genital_Herpes_in_Pregnancy__ACOG.53.aspx

54 Acute right-sided abdominal pain

A 37-year-old gravida 3, para 2, at 32 weeks of gestation presents to the emergency department reporting right lower quadrant abdominal pain that has worsened over the course of the day. She also has associated nausea and vomiting. The fetal heart rate is 155 beats per minute. Ultrasonography of the abdomen is remarkable for an inflamed appendix, and the general surgeon starts intravenous antibiotics and recommends appendectomy. The best approach to assess fetal well-being around the time of surgery is to

(A) obtain fetal heart tones before and after surgery
* (B) perform a nonstress test before and after surgery
(C) perform continuous fetal monitoring during surgery
(D) perform intermittent fetal monitoring during surgery

The management of appendicitis in a pregnant patient is similar to that in a nonpregnant one; however, immediate surgical management usually is first-line, except in the case of a periappendiceal abscess. Although medical management can be appropriate in the nonpregnant patient, surgical management is preferred in the pregnant woman because of the increased risk of peritonitis, fetal death, septic shock, and venous thromboembolism. Appendectomy is appropriate at any stage of pregnancy, although if appendicitis is diagnosed during active labor, it can be deferred to immediately postpartum. Surgery should not be delayed, because it places the patient at significant risk of morbidity due to sepsis.

When nonobstetric surgery is planned during pregnancy, the obstetrician should be involved in the planning of care when possible. Fetal monitoring may be used for a viable fetus, and surgery should be performed in a facility with obstetric and neonatal services available. Personnel able to interpret fetal monitoring also should be present. An obstetrician qualified to perform an urgent cesarean birth should be available, especially if hypotension or significant blood loss is anticipated. At a minimum, fetal monitoring with nonstress testing should be assessed preoperatively and postoperatively. Intraoperative continuous fetal monitoring can be considered when it is technically feasible and when the patient has given informed consent for urgent cesarean birth. In the case of abdominal surgery, such as in this patient, neither continuous nor intermittent fetal monitoring is technically possible. Simple auscultation of fetal heart tones would be insufficient at this gestational age. Therefore, the correct answer is nonstress testing before and after surgery.

Laparoscopy is feasible in any trimester of pregnancy, with care taken to avoid the uterine fundus with port placement. The patient should be placed in the left lateral recumbent position to avoid compression on the vena cava and aorta during surgery. There is a risk of preterm labor with some surgical procedures during pregnancy, so consideration should be given to administration of corticosteroids for fetal benefit at viable premature gestational age, and patients should be monitored postoperatively for signs of preterm labor. Tocolytics are not indicated prophylactically but may be indicated if there are signs of preterm labor.

Nonobstetric surgery during pregnancy. ACOG Committee Opinion No. 775. American College of Obstetricians and Gynecologists. Obstet Gynecol 2019;133:e285–6. doi: 10.1097/AOG.0000000000003174 https://journals.lww.com/greenjournal/pages/articleviewer.aspx?year=2019&issue=04000&article=00060&type=Fulltext

Pearl JP, Price RR, Tonkin AE, Richardson WS, Stefanidis D. SAGES guidelines for the use of laparoscopy during pregnancy. Surg Endosc 2017;31:3767–82. doi: 10.1007/s00464-017-5637-3 https://link.springer.com/article/10.1007/s00464-017-5637-3

Resnik R, Lockwood CJ, Moore TR, Greene ME, Copel JA, Silver RM, editors. Creasy and Resnik's maternal–fetal medicine: principles and practice. 8th ed. Elsevier; 2019.

55 Fetal tachycardia

A 21-year-old gravida 2, para 1, at 33 weeks of gestation calls with nausea and vomiting and decreased fetal movement. Her pregnancy is complicated by sickle cell trait. She denies any sick contacts at home. In triage, she has a temperature of 38.9 °C (102 °F). Her examination is unremarkable, with a closed cervix. There is no uterine activity. The fetal heart rate tracing shows fetal tachycardia at 185 beats per minute (bpm), with minimal variability. The patient is admitted for observation, and intravenous fluids are started. Respiratory pathogen testing, serum blood tests, and urine analysis are ordered. The best next step in management is

* (A) acetaminophen
(B) antibiotics
(C) betamethasone
(D) cesarean birth
(E) induction of labor

Fetal tachycardia is defined as a baseline fetal heart rate of greater than 160 bpm for at least 10 minutes. The estimated prevalence is 0.4–1% of pregnancies. When fetal tachycardia is observed, it is important to assess for an underlying cause. The most common causes are maternal infection and fever (eg, pyelonephritis, chorioamnionitis, viral infection, or other infections), medications (eg, terbutaline or stimulants), maternal medical conditions (eg, hyperthyroidism), and obstetric or fetal conditions (eg, abruption, fetal bleeding, and fetal tachyarrhythmia).

Once the underlying cause is identified, treatment should be targeted to the cause. Fetal tachycardia will resolve in most situations. In the scenario above, given maternal fever, the most likely etiology of the fetal tachycardia is maternal infection. The first step is the administration of antipyretics, such as acetaminophen, to reduce fever. Antibiotics or antiviral agents should be administered based on the identified source of infection and after a full assessment, including laboratory studies. In a patient with sickle cell trait, urinary tract infections are common, and a urinalysis or culture should be evaluated. In the present scenario, chorioamnionitis is unlikely given that the uterus is not tender and there is no uterine activity. Corticosteroids are not indicated because the risk of delivery is not imminent. Neither cesarean birth nor induction of labor is the best initial step in the setting of fetal tachycardia likely secondary to maternal infection.

Intrapartum fetal heart rate monitoring: nomenclature, interpretation, and general management principles. ACOG Practice Bulletin No. 106. American College of Obstetricians and Gynecologists. Obstet Gynecol 2009;114:192–202. doi: 10.1097/AOG.0b013e3181aef106 https://journals.lww.com/greenjournal/Citation/2009/07000/ACOG_Practice_Bulletin_No__106__Intrapartum_Fetal.51.aspx

Management of intrapartum fetal heart rate tracings. Practice Bulletin No. 116. American College of Obstetricians and Gynecologists . Obstet Gynecol 2010;116:1232–40. doi: 10.1097/AOG.0b013e3182004fa9 https://journals.lww.com/greenjournal/Citation/2010/11000/Practice_Bulletin_No__116__Management_of.53.aspx

56 Maternal hemorrhage protocol

A 31-year-old gravida 3, para 1, underwent repeat cesarean birth. Blood loss in the operating room was 850 mL. Three hours later, she develops vaginal bleeding. Fundal massage is started. Blood and clot measuring 450 mL are expressed. The patient is asymptomatic. Her blood pressure is 115/70 mm Hg, pulse is 100 beats per minute, and her respiratory rate is 16 breaths per minute. She has had 85 mL of urine output in the last hour. An oxytocin infusion has been continuous since her transfer to the postpartum unit. The best next step is to

* (A) administer additional uterotonic agent
(B) call for a critical care team
(C) initiate blood transfusion
(D) obtain coagulation studies
(E) transfer her to the operating room for further assessment

Maternal hemorrhage within the first 24 hours after delivery occurs in 4–6% of pregnancies, with 80% of cases resulting from uterine atony. Risk factors for postpartum hemorrhage include rapid or augmented labor, previous postpartum hemorrhage, chorioamnionitis, and an overdistended uterus. Often bleeding occurs in the absence of any identifiable risk factors.

In a review of patients with estimated blood loss of 1,500 mL or greater, many cases had significant opportunities for improvement, which, if recognized, may have led to reduction in morbidity. For this reason, The Joint Commission and the Society for Maternal-Fetal Medicine recommend adopting protocols to reduce maternal morbidity and mortality resulting from postpartum hemorrhage.

Protocols that involve the implementation of standard procedures and escalate care based on patient acuity have been successfully adopted in many hospital systems. The patient's bleeding status is assessed and assigned a clinical stage ranging from stage 0 through stage 3 hemorrhage. *Stage 0 hemorrhage* represents normal postpartum bleeding for a normal vaginal birth or cesarean birth (ie, less than 1,000 mL). Although the definition of Stage 0 hemorrhage is a blood loss of less than 1,000 mL, a loss of more than 500 mL at the time of vaginal birth should be considered increased. Quantitative methods of measuring obstetric blood loss are more accurate than visual estimation. Although quantitative methods of estimating blood loss have not been demonstrated to improve outcomes, many centers have incorporated quantitative blood loss measurement into obstetric hemorrhage bundles.

Stage 1 hemorrhage indicates greater bleeding than expected. Initial measures include calling for assistance, increasing intravenous fluid rate, continuing oxytocin, monitoring vital signs every 5 minutes (including pulse oximetry), performing uterine massage, emptying the bladder, and notifying the physician. *Stage 2* is defined as bleeding that does not respond to conservative treatment used in Stage 1, and *Stage 3 hemorrhage* involves continued bleeding with blood loss greater than 1,500 mL. Figures 56-1–4 outline detailed management of each stage of bleeding.

Using a standard protocol such as this one, obstetricians, nurses, and anesthesiologists can be prepared to quickly recognize and

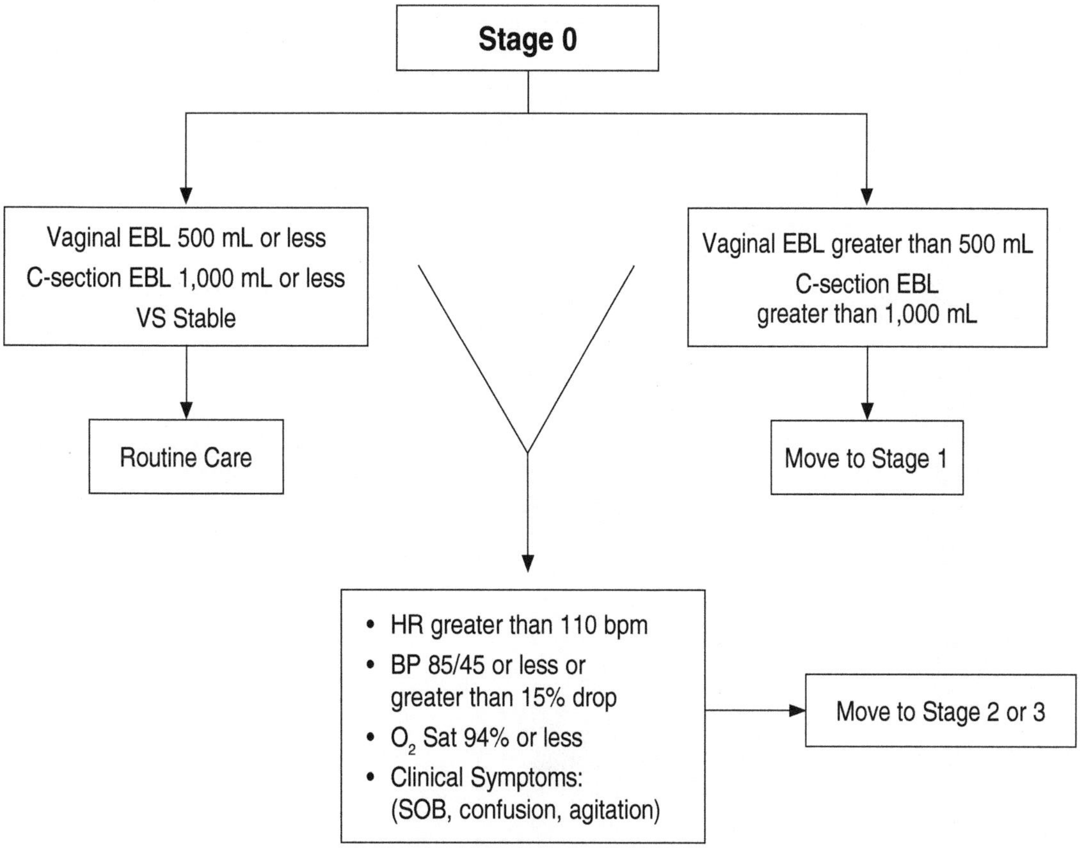

FIGURE 56-1. Protocol algorithm for stage 0 hemorrhage. Abbreviations: BP, blood pressure; C, cesarean; EBL, estimated blood loss; HR, heart rate; O_2, oxygen; SOB, shortness of breath; VS, vital signs. (Reprinted from Shields LE, Wiesner S, Fulton J, Pelletreau B. Comprehensive maternal hemorrhage protocols reduce the use of blood products and improve patient safety. Am J Obstet Gynecol 2015;212:272–80, with permission from Elsevier. doi: 10.1016/j.ajog.2014.07.012. https://www.ajog.org/article/S0002-9378(14)00694-2/fulltext)

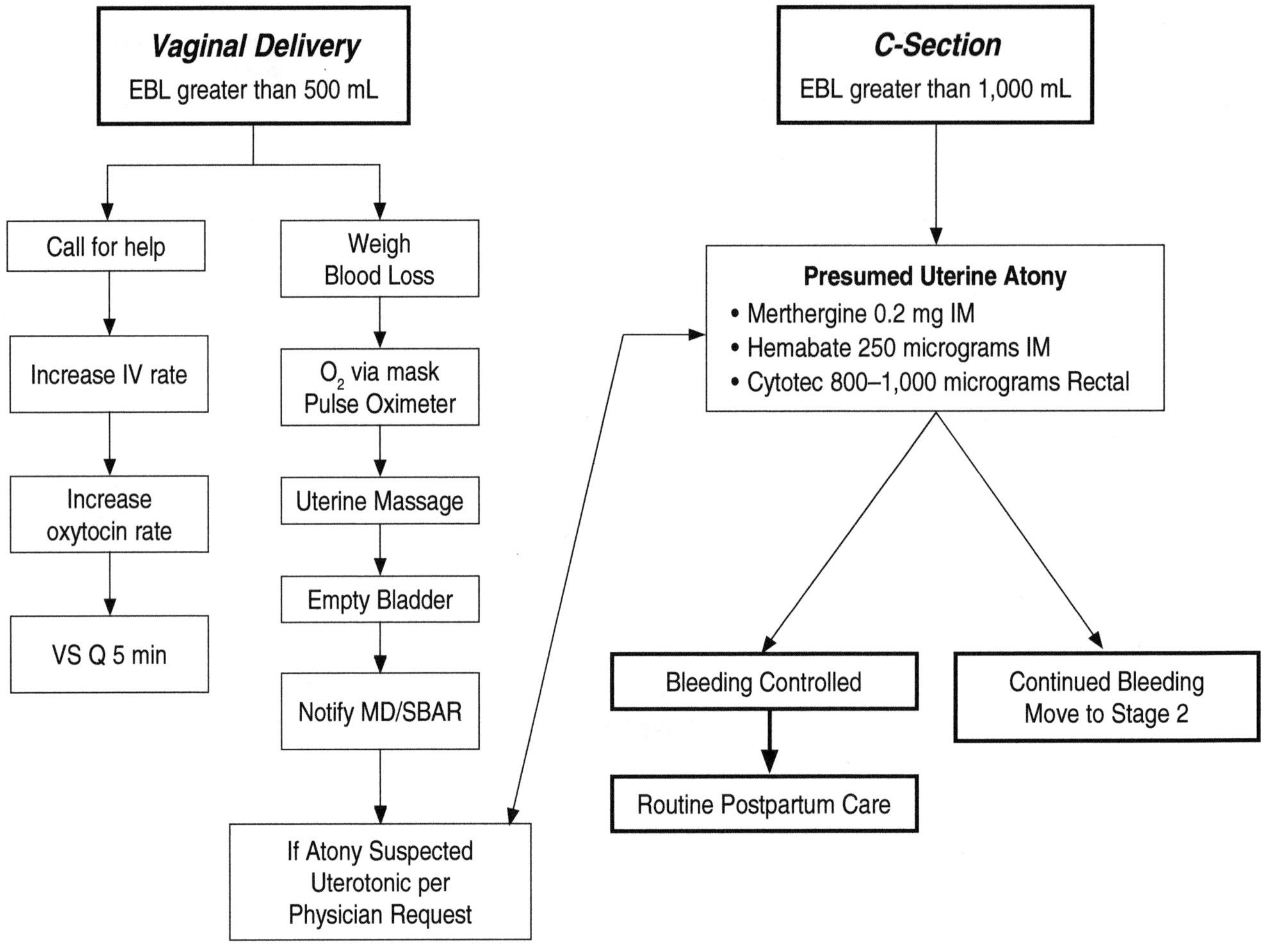

FIGURE 56-2. Protocol algorithm for stage 1 hemorrhage. Abbreviations: C, cesarean; EBL, estimated blood loss; IM, intramuscularly; IV, intravenously; O_2, oxygen; SBAR, situation, background, assessment, recommendation; VS, vital signs. (Reprinted from Shields LE, Wiesner S, Fulton J, Pelletreau B. Comprehensive maternal hemorrhage protocols reduce the use of blood products and improve patient safety. Am J Obstet Gynecol 2015;212:272–80, with permission from Elsevier. doi: 10.1016/j.ajog.2014.07.012. https://www.ajog.org/article/S0002-9378(14)00694-2/fulltext)

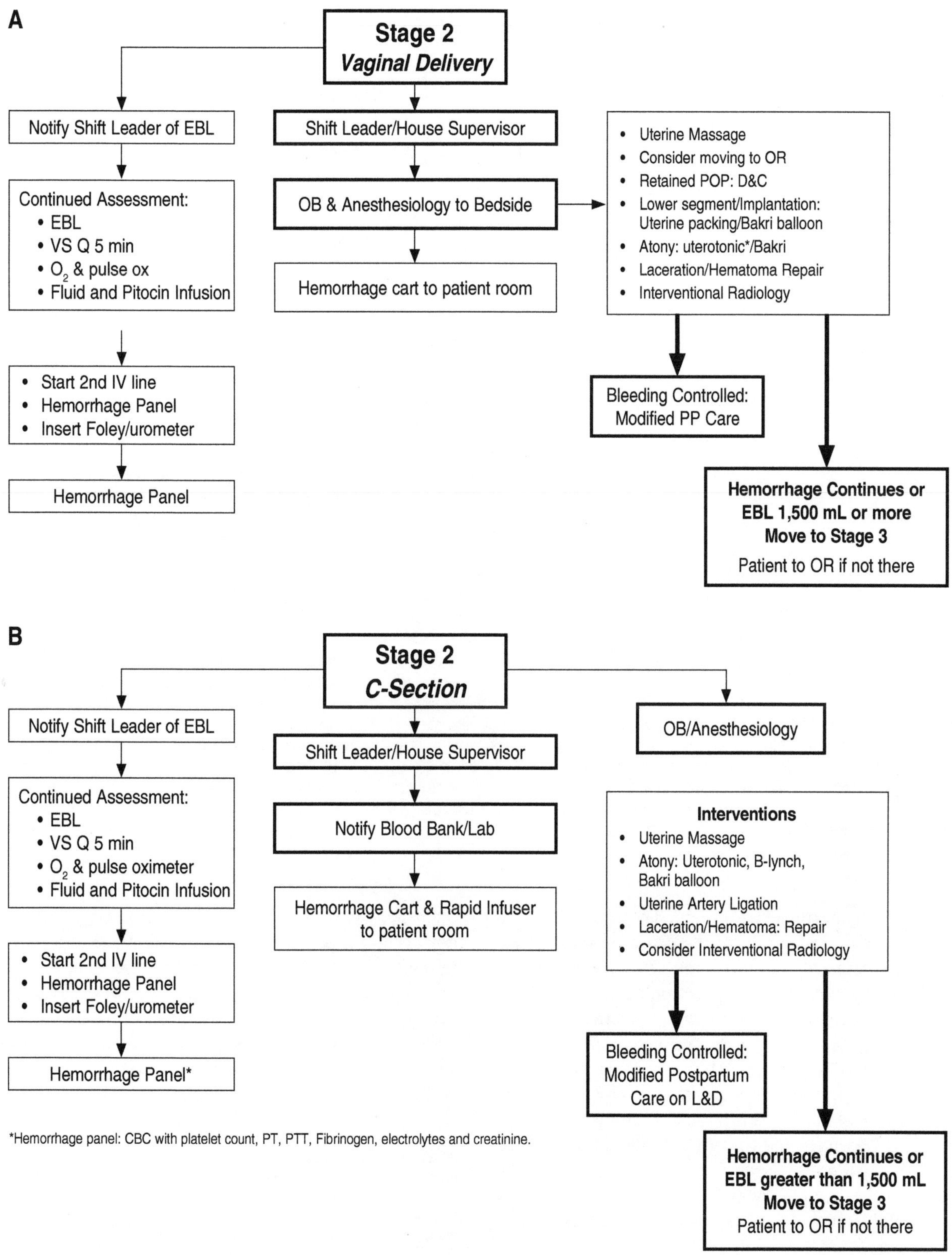

FIGURE 56-3. Protocol algorithms for stage 2 vaginal delivery (A) and stage 2 cesarean delivery (B). Abbreviations: C, cesarean; D&C, dilation; EBL, estimated blood loss; IV, intravenously; L&D, labor and delivery; O_2, oxygen; OB, obstetrics; OR, operating room; POC, products of conception; PP, postpartum; VS, vital signs. *Hemorrhage panel: CBC with platelet count, PT, PTT, fibrinogen, electrolytes, and creatinine. (Reprinted from Shields LE, Wiesner S, Fulton J, Pelletreau B. Comprehensive maternal hemorrhage protocols reduce the use of blood products and improve patient safety. Am J Obstet Gynecol 2015;212:272–80, with permission from Elsevier. doi: 10.1016/j.ajog.2014.07.012. https://www.ajog.org/article/S0002-9378(14)00694-2/fulltext)

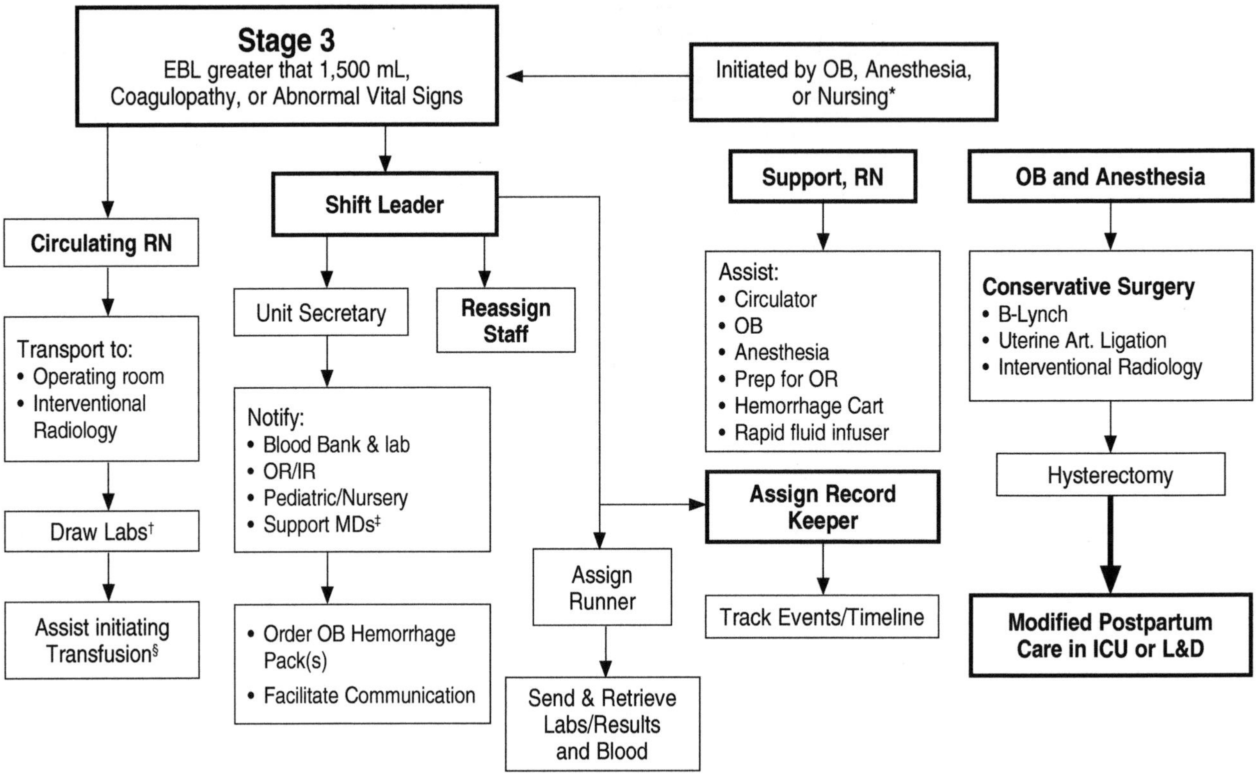

FIGURE 56-4. Protocol algorithm for stage 3 hemorrhage. Abbreviations: Art, artery; ICU, intensive care unit; IR, interventional radiology; L&D, labor and delivery; Labs, laboratory results; Prep, preparation; RN, registered nurse. *Stage 3 could be activated by the attending obstetrician, the anesthesiologist, or the treating nurse; †laboratory results include complete blood count with platelet count, partial thromboplastin time, plasma thromboplastin, fibrinogen, chemistry panel, ionized calcium, pH, and blood gases; ‡support doctors include general surgery, urology, and/or a second obstetrician or anesthesiologist, as deemed necessary; §the goal of transfusion was to maintain the hematocrit level at greater than 24%, international normalized ratio at greater than 1.4%, platelet count at greater than 50,000 per microliter, and fibrinogen level at greater than 100,000 mg/dL. (Reprinted from Shields LE, Wiesner S, Fulton J, Pelletreau B. Comprehensive maternal hemorrhage protocols reduce the use of blood products and improve patient safety. Am J Obstet Gynecol 2015;212:272–80, with permission from Elsevier. doi: 10.1016/j.ajog.2014.07.012. https://www.ajog.org/article/S0002-9378(14)00694-2/fulltext)

manage maternal hemorrhage as a team. The team approach allows for diagnostic evaluation for the cause of hemorrhage alongside simultaneous interventions for treatment.

Although uterine atony is the most common cause of hemorrhage, physical examination may identify laceration, hematoma, or retained placenta as other causes of hemorrhage. If no other causes are found, and uterine atony is suspected, medical treatment includes oxytocin, misoprostol, methylergonovine maleate, intramuscular 15-methyl prostaglandin F2α, and tranexamic acid. Methylergonovine maleate should be avoided in patients with hypertension, and 15-methyl prostaglandin F2α should be avoided in patients with asthma. Most patients with uterine atony will respond to uterotonic medication, as well as to fundal massage.

In the described patient, the stage of hemorrhage has progressed from Stage 0 to Stage 1, with estimated blood loss greater than 1,000 mL (850 mL in the operating room and 450 mL while on the postpartum unit). Administration of additional uterotonic agents is the best next step for this patient. A critical care team can be called when additional help is needed to care for a patient who is clinically deteriorating. In this scenario, however, the patient does not display abnormal vital signs. Initiating a rapid response team may become necessary if the patient does not respond to uterine massage and administration of uterotonic agents. Blood transfusion should be initiated based on evidence of continued bleeding and abnormal vital signs. Likewise, coagulation studies should be obtained if the patient does not respond to additional uterotonic agents.

Postpartum hemorrhage. Practice Bulletin No. 183. American College of Obstetricians and Gynecologists. Obstet Gynecol 2017;130:e168–86. doi: 10.1097/AOG.0000000000002351 https://journals.lww.com/greenjournal/Fulltext/2017/10000/Practice_Bulletin_No__183__Postpartum_Hemorrhage.56.aspx

Quantitative blood loss in obstetric hemorrhage. ACOG Committee Opinion No. 794. American College of Obstetricians and Gynecologists. Obstet Gynecol 2019;134:e150–6. doi: 10.1097/AOG.0000000000003564 https://journals.lww.com/greenjournal/Fulltext/2019/12000/Quantitative_Blood_Loss_in_Obstetric_Hemorrhage_.40.aspx

Shields LE, Wiesner S, Fulton J, Pelletreau B. Comprehensive maternal hemorrhage protocols reduce the use of blood products and improve patient safety. Am J Obstet Gynecol 2015;212:272–80. doi: 10.1016/j.ajog.2014.07.012 https://www.ajog.org/article/S0002-9378(14)00694-2/fulltext

57 Evaluation of first-trimester bleeding

A patient at 8 weeks of gestation (dated by last menstrual period) presents for evaluation of vaginal spotting. Her ultrasonographic findings are shown in Figures 57-1 and 57-2. Fetal cardiac activity was not seen with M-mode or the video images obtained. She is Rh-positive, and this is a desired pregnancy. The best next step in management is to

(A) administer mifepristone and misoprostol
(B) obtain serial β-human chorionic gonadotropin (β-hCG) concentrations
(C) perform dilation and curettage
* (D) repeat ultrasonography

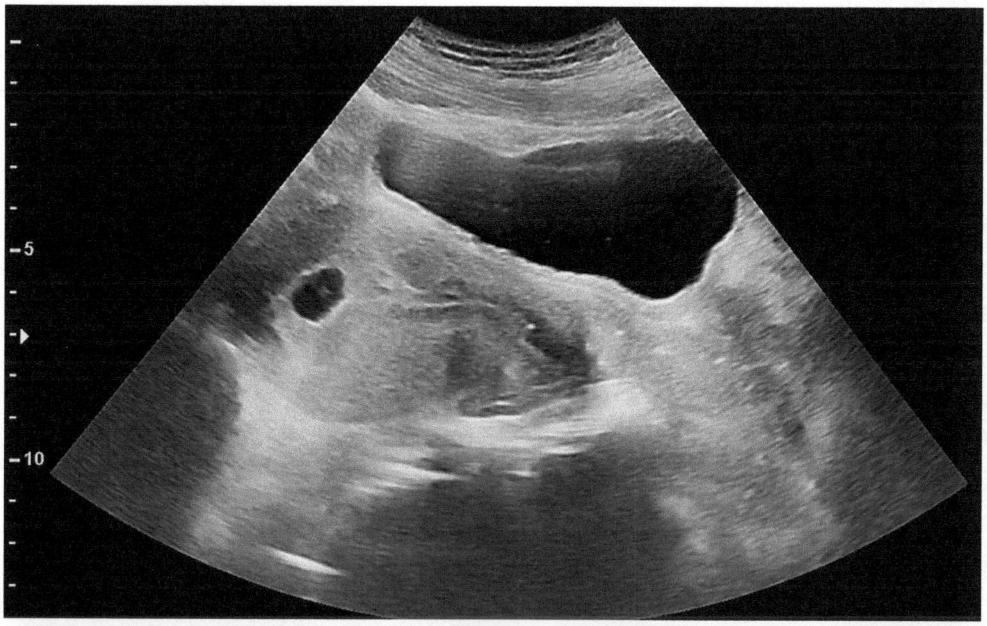

FIGURE 57-1. Described patient's abdominal ultrasonography.

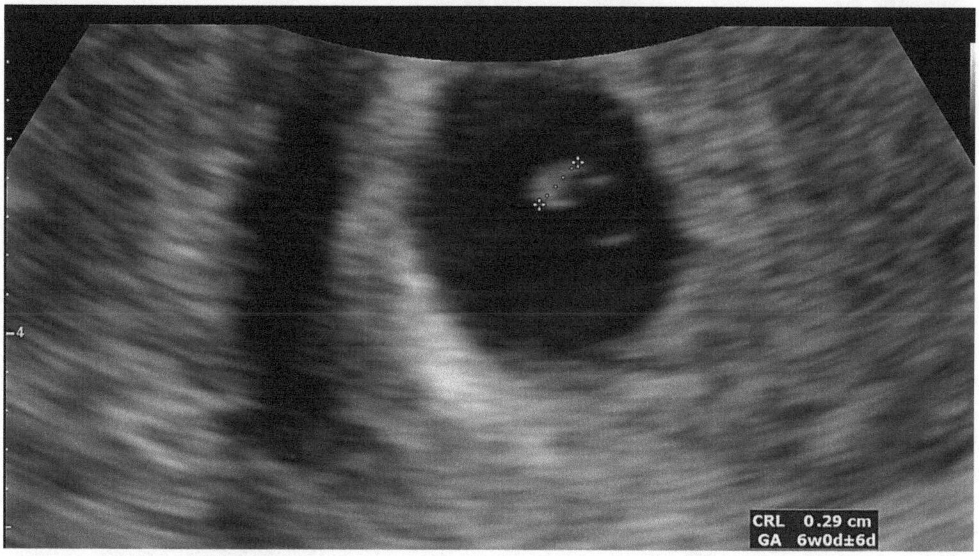

FIGURE 57-2. Described patient's transvaginal ultrasonography.

Early pregnancy loss occurs in 10% of clinically recognized pregnancies. Symptoms of pregnancy loss can include vaginal bleeding or uterine cramping, but these symptoms may be present in normal pregnancies or ectopic pregnancies. Diagnostic accuracy is of utmost importance, as a false-positive diagnosis of pregnancy loss can lead to the interruption of a desired pregnancy. Clinical presentation and physical examination are useful in aiding the clinician in an appropriate diagnosis, but ultrasonography and β-hCG concentrations can lead to a more accurate diagnosis. However, even this testing may not be useful in isolation or as a one-time clinical assessment.

Ultrasonography is an extremely useful tool to determine fetal viability when used in the appropriate clinical context. A collaboration of national U.S. societies has made recommendations for imaging criteria in the first trimester and has provided consensus recommendations as to what determines a first-trimester pregnancy loss (Table 57-1). First-trimester pregnancy imaging may be performed transabdominally or transvaginally, but transvaginal imaging is recommended if transabdominal imaging is not definitive. The uterus, cervix, and adnexa should be imaged, and the presence of a gestational sac should be documented. The presence or absence of the yolk sac or embryo should be determined, and the crown–rump length measured if an embryo is present. Cardiac activity in the embryo should be recorded in M-mode or in a video clip and is usually present on transvaginal ultrasonography if the crown–rump length is greater than 2 mm. The presence of multiple gestations and chorionicity should be recorded.

Prospective cohort studies have determined that the criteria used in the 1990s to determine pregnancy loss have a false-positive rate of 4.4% and 8.3% for a gestational sac size of 16 mm and a crown–rump length of 5 mm, respectively. There were no false-positive cases when the cutoffs were increased to 21 mm for gestational sac size and 5.3 mm for crown–rump length. The Society of Radiologists in Ultrasound Multispecialty Panel of Early First Trimester Diagnosis of Miscarriage Consensus Committee statement supports a more conservative approach to account for interobserver differences outside the strict setting of a research environment. The consensus committee agreed that a crown–rump length of 7 mm or a mean sac diameter of 25 mm without an embryo is diagnostic for pregnancy loss. Diagnostic criteria are listed in Table 57-1. If findings are suspicious for pregnancy loss, repeat ultrasonography in 7–10 days should be considered.

This patient has a documented intrauterine pregnancy, and serial β-hCG determinations would not be diagnostic for pregnancy loss, although they would be suggestive of a pregnancy failure or an abnormal pregnancy if an appropriate increase is not seen. The crown–rump length is 2.9 mm without cardiac activity, so repeat ultrasonography in 7–10 days is the best next step to determine fetal viability. Fetal viability is uncertain at the time of presentation; therefore, treatment for pregnancy loss with medical or surgical management is not appropriate because this treatment could lead to interruption of a desired pregnancy.

Once early pregnancy loss is confirmed, several treatment options are available to patients. Expectant management can be considered if the pregnancy loss is in the first trimester. This strategy is most successful for symptomatic patients or those with an incomplete abortion on diagnosis. Medical

TABLE 57-1. Guidelines for Transvaginal Ultrasonographic Diagnosis of Pregnancy Failure in a Woman With an Intrauterine Pregnancy of Uncertain Viability*

FINDINGS DIAGNOSTIC OF PREGNANCY FAILURE	FINDINGS SUSPICIOUS FOR, BUT NOT DIAGNOSTIC OF, PREGNANCY FAILURE†
Crown–rump length of 7 mm or greater and no heartbeat	Crown–rump length of less than 7 mm and no heartbeat
Mean sac diameter of 25 mm or greater and no embryo	Mean sac diameter of 16–24 mm and no embryo
Absence of embryo with heartbeat 2 wk or more after a scan that showed a gestational sac without a yolk sac	Absence of embryo with heartbeat 7–13 d after a scan that showed a gestational sac without a yolk sac
Absence of embryo with heartbeat 11 d or more after a scan that showed a gestational sac with a yolk sac	Absence of embryo with heartbeat 7–10 d after a scan that showed a gestational sac with a yolk sac Absence of embryo for 6 wk or longer after last menstrual period Empty amnion (amnion seen adjacent to yolk sac, with no visible embryo) Enlarged yolk sac (greater than 7 mm) Small gestational sac in relation to the size of the embryo (less than 5-mm difference between mean sac diameter and crown–rump length)

*Criteria are from the Society of Radiologists in Ultrasound Multispecialty Consensus Conference on Early First Trimester Diagnosis of Miscarriage and Exclusion of a Viable Intrauterine Pregnancy, October 2012.

†When there are findings suspicious for pregnancy failure, follow-up ultrasonography at 7–10 d to assess the pregnancy for viability is generally appropriate.

(Reprinted from Doubilet PM, Benson CB, Bourne T, Blaivas M, Barnhart KT, Benacerraf BR, et al. Diagnostic criteria for nonviable pregnancy early in the first trimester. Society of Radiologists in Ultrasound Multispecialty Panel on Early First Trimester Diagnosis of Miscarriage and Exclusion of a Viable Intrauterine Pregnancy. N Engl J Med 2013;369:1443–51. doi: 10.1056/NEJMra1302417 https://www.nejm.org/doi/10.1056/NEJMra1302417.)

management is an option for patients without infection, hemorrhage, severe anemia, or bleeding disorders. Vaginal misoprostol is recommended, with one repeat dose between 3 hours and 7 days if there is no response to the first dose. Mifepristone can increase the chance of successful medical treatment of first-trimester pregnancy loss; however, it is not available in all locations. If this is an option for the patient, mifepristone 24 hours before giving misoprostol should be considered.

Complete passage of tissue can be confirmed with ultrasonography 7–14 days after reported symptoms or by serial β-hCG assessment when ultrasonography is not available. Incomplete passage can be treated with suction dilation and curettage. Some patients may choose to be treated with suction dilation and curettage as first-line treatment. Surgical treatment is associated with higher patient satisfaction compared with medical management. Higher satisfaction rates may be due to the convenience for the patient of having a scheduled visit without risk of bleeding at an inopportune time and fewer follow-up requirements.

Suction dilation and curettage also may be preferable for patients who are at a higher risk of medical complications, including those with active hemorrhage, infection, severe anemia, bleeding disorders, or significant maternal cardiac disease. In patients for whom genetic testing is warranted, surgical treatment will facilitate collection of pregnancy tissue.

AIUM-ACR-ACOG-SMFM-SRU practice parameter for the performance of standard diagnostic obstetric ultrasound examinations. J Ultrasound Med 2018;37:E13–24. doi: 10.1002/jum.14831 https://onlinelibrary.wiley.com/doi/10.1002/jum.14831

Early pregnancy loss. ACOG Practice Bulletin No. 200. American College of Obstetricians and Gynecologists. Obstet Gynecol 2018;132:e197–207. doi: 10.1097/AOG.0000000000002899 https://journals.lww.com/greenjournal/Fulltext/2018/11000/ACOG_Practice_Bulletin_No__200__Early_Pregnancy.41.aspx

58 Medication management in sickle cell disease

A patient at 18 weeks of gestation with a history of sickle cell disease presents with fever. She has chest pain, cough, and shortness of breath that have been present for 1 day. Her temperature is 38.2 °C (100.8 °F), her pulse is 115 beats per minute, and pulse oximetry is 92% on room air. She appears ill on examination with an expiratory wheeze. Her COVID-19 polymerase chain reaction test is negative. Her chest X-ray is normal, and chest computed tomography angiogram is positive for a right segmental thrombus. Electrocardiogram shows sinus tachycardia, and cardiac troponin levels are normal. In addition to pulmonary embolism, the most likely concurrent diagnosis is

* (A) acute chest syndrome
(B) myocardial infarction
(C) myocarditis
(D) sickle cell pain crisis

Sickle cell disease is a hemoglobinopathy with almost all hemoglobin in the form of hemoglobin S. The abnormal protein structure leads red blood cells to be distorted. These cells become sickle shaped during periods of stress, infection, and reduced oxygen, leading to increased hemolysis and vaso-occlusive disease. This disease process then causes the chronic pain, acute pain, and acute-on-chronic pain patient experience. Treatment for sickle cell disease involves not only reducing acute pain episodes but also managing these episodes when they occur.

Hydroxyurea, L-glutamine, and crizanlizumab reduce the rate of acute pain episodes that require treatment in acute care settings. L-Glutamine is an amino acid and is not anticipated to increase the risk of congenital anomalies. Crizanlizumab was approved by the U.S. Food and Drug Association in 2019 for treatment of sickle cell disease, but there are no data on its use during pregnancy. Hydroxyurea has been shown to have teratogenic effects in animals, although there were no teratogenic effects seen in one small series that studied human pregnancies. Hydroxyurea is not routinely used during pregnancy, especially during the first trimester, because of the effects seen in animals and the limited evidence in pregnant women.

Current guidelines for treating adults with chronic pain due to sickle cell disease suggest the use of serotonin norepinephrine reuptake inhibitors, tricyclic antidepressants, or gabapentinoids. Although selective serotonin reuptake inhibitors and serotonin norepinephrine reuptake inhibitors have been used safely in pregnancy without risk of congenital birth defects, tricyclic antidepressants can interfere with embryonic development, as seen in some animals. Gabapentinoids are associated with fetal growth impairments and developmental delay in exposed fetuses.

Chronic transfusions are not recommended for the treatment of recurrent or chronic pain in patients with sickle cell disease in the nonpregnant or pregnant population. Nonsteroidal anti-inflammatory drugs are a mainstay of pain treatment but are not recommended during pregnancy. Opioids have been used as needed to control pain in pregnancy.

Patients with sickle cell disease have increased rates of obstetric complications, including preeclampsia, preterm birth, preterm rupture of membranes, fetal growth restriction, and postpartum infection. There is a higher level of red blood cell turnover during pregnancy, so additional folic acid is needed for pregnant patients with sickle cell disease and supplementation is recommended.

Acute chest syndrome is an acute illness in patients with sickle cell disease that presents with fever and usually respiratory symptoms. The etiology of acute chest syndrome is multifactorial but is frequently associated with an infectious cause or may present after or during a severe pain episode, pulmonary embolism or infarction, fat embolism, hypoventilation, or atelectasis. Pulmonary infiltrates usually are seen on chest X-ray but may not be present early in the illness, as is the case with the described patient. Repeat chest X-ray should be performed if there are ongoing signs and symptoms of acute chest syndrome. Adult patients may present with fever, cough, chest pain, and dyspnea. Over 80% of patients will have some degree of hypoxia.

Initial investigation for acute chest syndrome includes a chest X-ray, complete blood count, creatinine level, liver function tests, blood type and screen, and arterial blood gas (if Spo_2 is 94% or less on room air). Blood and urine cultures should be obtained in addition to sputum and nasopharyngeal aspiration cultures for patients with upper respiratory symptoms. Additional testing may be required depending on clinical presentation. Computed tomography angiogram of the chest is recommended for patients with suspicion of pulmonary embolism. D-dimer is less useful because of the baseline elevation in sickle cell disease patients as well as typical elevations seen in pregnancy. A ventilation perfusion scan is not recommended to diagnose pulmonary embolism if there is a possible coexisting diagnosis of acute chest syndrome, because this usually reveals widespread perfusion defect and normal ventilation during acute chest syndrome.

Although a cardiac etiology should always be considered for patients who present with chest pain, this patient's presentation most closely represents acute chest syndrome because she has respiratory symptoms, fever, and hypoxia. Myocardial infarction and myocarditis are not likely given an electrocardiogram with only sinus tachycardia and no ST segment changes. Pneumonia can precipitate acute chest syndrome, but this patient's chest X-ray and computed tomography angiogram showed no evidence of infiltrate. Sickle cell crises also can lead to acute chest syndrome, but this patient does not report any pain symptoms leading up to presentation or any other pain symptoms outside the chest, making a concurrent pain crisis unlikely.

Acute chest syndrome is a life-threatening condition, and early diagnosis and treatment are key to minimize lung damage and long-term morbidity. A multidisciplinary team is recommended, including an obstetrician, maternal–fetal medicine subspecialist, hematologist, and intensivist. Spo_2 should be maintained above 95% in pregnancy. Intravenous fluids are usually required during the acute illness to maintain fluid balance, with careful attention to avoid overhydration and pulmonary edema. Antibiotics with coverage for atypical organisms are recommended even if blood and sputum cultures are negative. Pain relief with acetaminophen or opioids is recommended during sickle cell crises or acute chest syndrome. Decision for exchange transfusion or transfusion of red blood cells should be made by physicians experienced in the treatment of this disease process.

Fever is not a sign of myocardial infarction, and there were no electrocardiogram changes to suggest ischemia such as ST segment elevations or depression. Additionally, cardiac troponin levels will increase in the setting of cardiac ischemia. Electrocardiogram changes and elevated troponin levels would also be expected in myocarditis. A recent respiratory illness or enteritis was reported in 36% of patients who went on to biopsy-proven myocarditis; however, the onset of myocarditis usually presented about 1–4 weeks after the initial viral illness. C-reactive proteins often are increased in acute myocarditis, but this is a nonspecific test. Lastly, the patient does not report pain other than in her chest, making this unlikely to be a typical sickle cell pain crisis. Infection can predispose patients to a pain crisis, but they do not present as acutely ill with respiratory symptoms or deoxygenation. Acute chest syndrome explains all of the patient's symptoms and clinical evaluation.

Brandow AM, Carroll CP, Creary S, Edwards-Elliott R, Glassberg J, Hurley RW, et al. American Society of Hematology 2020 guidelines for sickle cell disease: management of acute and chronic pain. Blood Adv 2020;4:2656–701. doi: 10.1182/bloodadvances.2020001851 https://ashpublications.org/bloodadvances/article/4/12/2656/460974/American-Society-of-Hematology-2020-guidelines-for

Caforio AL, Calabrese F, Angelini A, Tona F, Vinci A, Bottaro S, et al. A prospective study of biopsy-proven myocarditis: prognostic relevance of clinical and aetiopathogenetic features at diagnosis. Eur Heart J 2007;28:1326–33. doi: 10.1093/eurheartj/ehm076 https://academic.oup.com/eurheartj/article/28/11/1326/2887425

Carrier screening for genetic conditions. Committee Opinion No. 691. American College of Obstetricians and Gynecologists. Obstet Gynecol 2017;129:e41–55. doi: 10.1097/AOG.0000000000001952 https://journals.lww.com/greenjournal/Fulltext/2017/03000/Committee_Opinion_No__691__Carrier_Screening_for.48.aspx

Hemoglobinopathies in pregnancy. ACOG Practice Bulletin No. 78. American College of Obstetricians and Gynecologists. Obstet Gynecol 2007;109:229–37. doi: 10.1097/00006250-200701000-00055 https://journals.lww.com/greenjournal/Citation/2007/01000/ACOG_Practice_Bulletin_No__78__Hemoglobinopathies.55.aspx

Howard J, Hart N, Roberts-Harewood M, Cummins M, Awogbade M, Davis B. Guideline on the management of acute chest syndrome in sickle cell disease. BCSH Committee. Br J Haematol 2015;169:492–505. doi: 10.1111/bjh.13348 https://onlinelibrary.wiley.com/doi/10.1111/bjh.13348

Resnik R, Lockwood CJ, Moore TR, Greene ME, Copel JA, Silver RM, editors. Creasy and Resnik's maternal–fetal medicine: principles and practice. 8th ed. Elsevier; 2018.

59 Preterm labor

A 17-year-old gravida 1 presents at 27 weeks of gestation with increased pelvic pressure and back pain for 3 days. On cervical examination, she is 3-cm dilated and 50% effaced, with an unchanged examination over 2 hours. Fetal tracing shows a normal baseline with contractions every 4 minutes on tocodynamometer. She is given penicillin, betamethasone, magnesium sulfate, and indomethacin. Ultrasonography is performed 2 days later, and the maximum vertical pocket of amniotic fluid is 1.6 cm. The medication mostly likely responsible for the ultrasonographic finding is

(A) betamethasone
* (B) indomethacin
(C) magnesium
(D) penicillin

This patient is at risk of preterm delivery given her cervical examination and regular contractions, although it does not appear imminent given the stable examination over the course of her initial evaluation. If the patient progresses to active labor, consideration should be given to a planned neonatal transport to a Level III center to avoid extramural birth during transport. However, if the patient and fetus are stable, transport is the most ideal situation to ensure birth in the appropriate-level center.

Tocolysis may be considered for short-term periods to prolong pregnancy for up to 48 hours to allow for corticosteroid administration for fetal lung maturity and transfer to a tertiary center for delivery. Corticosteroids have been shown to reduce the risk of respiratory compromise, intraventricular hemorrhage, and necrotizing enterocolitis in the early preterm period. Penicillin reduces the risk of early-onset group B streptococcus sepsis in newborns. However, unlike corticosteroid and penicillin treatment, there is no evidence of direct neonatal benefits with tocolytic therapy. If tocolysis is initiated, use beyond 48 hours of therapy is not recommended because of the risk of drug-induced complications, and because the effectiveness of prolonged therapy to reduce preterm birth has not been proved. The patient has developed oligohydramnios, which is not a complication of penicillin or corticosteroid treatment.

Indomethacin is considered as a tocolytic agent for patients who present with preterm labor. It is a cyclooxygenase inhibitor, and its use after 32 weeks of gestation increases the risk of premature closure or narrowing of the ductus arteriosus and oligohydramnios. It should be avoided for gestational ages over 32 weeks and in certain maternal medical conditions, including hepatic disease, renal disease, platelet dysfunction, and bleeding disorders. Maternal adverse effects include gastritis and esophageal reflux.

Nifedipine is a calcium channel blocker that is considered one of the first-line agents for tocolytic therapy. It has been shown to prolong pregnancy longer than β-adrenergic agonists, and there are no known fetal or neonatal adverse effects associated with its use. However, placebo-controlled trials did not show a difference in delivery within 48 hours of treatment or in birth before 37 weeks of gestation. There are some contraindications to its use, including hypotension and preload-dependent cardiac lesions. Adverse effects can include headache, flushing, pulmonary edema, and increased heart rate. Another tocolytic is terbutaline, a β-adrenergic agonist, which may be used for tocolysis in the acute period. However, there is a significantly higher risk of maternal complications with use of this medication, and prolonged use is not advised. In 2011, the U.S. Food and Drug Administration (FDA) issued a warning against its use to treat preterm labor because of maternal adverse effects, including tachycardia, hypotension, pulmonary edema, and hyperglycemia.

Magnesium sulfate has been shown to reduce the incidence of cerebral palsy when given to fetuses at risk of preterm birth at less than 32 weeks of gestation. The intent is to provide neuroprotection, usually when delivery is anticipated within the next 12 hours. However, in a meta-analysis comparing magnesium sulfate to placebo, there was no difference in delaying birth for 48 hours or preventing preterm birth, making this a suboptimal choice for a tocolytic agent. Prolonged therapy with magnesium sulfate should be avoided. In 2013, the FDA issued a black box warning because of the increase in fetal and neonatal toxicity with magnesium use over 5–7 days. Magnesium can cause flushing, diaphoresis, and nausea, but is not associated with oligohydramnios. It should not be used for women who have a history of myasthenia gravis. At supratherapeutic levels, magnesium will lead to a loss of deep tendon reflexes, suppressed cardiac contractility, respiratory depression, cardiac arrhythmia, and eventually, cardiac arrest at toxic levels.

Patients who present in preterm labor should have care to optimize fetal outcomes depending on gestational age. Risks and benefits of these interventions, including tocolytic therapy, should be reviewed with patients. Oligohydramnios is a known potential complication of indomethacin because of the decreased fetal urine output associated with its use.

Crowther CA, Brown J, McKinlay CJ, Middleton P. Magnesium sulphate for preventing preterm birth in threatened preterm labour. Cochrane Database of Systematic Reviews 2014, Issue 8. Art. No.: CD001060. doi: 10.1002/14651858.CD001060.pub2. https://www.cochranelibrary.com/cdsr/doi/10.1002/14651858.CD001060.pub2/full

Flenady V, Wojcieszek AM, Papatsonis DN, Stock OM, Murray L, Jardine LA, et al. Calcium channel blockers for inhibiting preterm labour and birth. Cochrane Database of Systematic Reviews 2014, Issue 6. Art. No.: CD002255. doi: 10.1002/14651858.CD002255.pub2. https://www.cochranelibrary.com/cdsr/doi/10.1002/14651858.CD002255.pub2/full

Hawkins JS, Wells CE, Casey BM, McIntire DD, Leveno KJ. Nifedipine for acute tocolysis of preterm labor: a placebo-controlled randomized trial. Obstet Gynecol 2021;138:73–8. doi: 10.1097/AOG.0000000000004436 https://journals.lww.com/greenjournal/Fulltext/2021/07000/Nifedipine_for_Acute_Tocolysis_of_Preterm_Labor__A.11.aspx

Management of preterm labor. Practice Bulletin No. 171. American College of Obstetricians and Gynecologists. Obstet Gynecol 2016;128:e155–64. doi:10.1097/AOG.0000000000001711 https://journals.lww.com/greenjournal/pages/articleviewer.aspx?year=2016&issue=10000&article=00061&type=Fulltext

Reinebrant HE, Pileggi-Castro C, Romero CL, Dos Santos RA, Kumar S, Souza JP, et al. Cyclo-oxygenase (COX) inhibitors for treating preterm labour. Cochrane Database of Systematic Reviews 2015, Issue 6. Art. No.: CD001992. doi: 10.1002/14651858.CD001992.pub3 https://www.cochranelibrary.com/cdsr/doi/10.1002/14651858.CD001992.pub3/full

60 Intrahepatic cholestasis of pregnancy

A 35-year-old gravida 1 at 34 weeks of gestation presents with pruritus, concentrated on the palms of her hands and soles of her feet, that keeps her awake at night. She does not have a rash or other skin lesions. Her blood pressure is normal. Her total bile acid level is 102 micromoles/L. The proposed mechanism most likely associated with an increased risk of fetal death is

(A) bile salts in the fetal liver causing cirrhosis
(B) chronic placental insufficiency
* (C) fetal arrhythmia
(D) placental abruption
(E) thrombi in the placental vessels

Intrahepatic cholestasis of pregnancy is the most common liver disease affecting pregnancy. The incidence of intrahepatic cholestasis ranges from 0.3% to 15% and varies widely depending on ethnicity and geographic location. It is most commonly seen in patients originally from South America and Northern Europe.

The patient in this clinical scenario meets diagnostic criteria for intrahepatic cholestasis. Classic symptoms usually present in the late-second or third trimester and include pruritis localized to the palms of the hands and soles of the feet that often is worse at night. Intrahepatic cholestasis of pregnancy does not usually involve a rash, but excoriations can develop secondary to scratching. The primary laboratory finding with intrahepatic cholestasis is an elevated total serum bile acid level without an alternative cause. Although laboratory-specific values may be used for diagnosis, most laboratories do not have pregnancy-specific reference ranges; therefore, a level of greater than 10 micromoles/L often is used to diagnose intrahepatic cholestasis. Importantly, symptoms of pruritis often precede the rise in bile acids by approximately 3 weeks. Liver transaminase concentrations also may be increased but are not required for diagnosis. Alterations in transaminases also may precede the increase in bile acids by 1–2 weeks.

Intrahepatic cholestasis of pregnancy has been associated with increased risk of stillbirth as well as other adverse perinatal outcomes, including spontaneous preterm birth, meconium-stained amniotic fluid and aspiration, and neonatal respiratory distress syndrome. The pathophysiology explaining the increased risk of fetal death is not well understood. One of the leading hypotheses is that fetal death is secondary to an acute, unpredictable event, such as a fetal arrhythmia. Animal and in vitro studies have shown that bile acids impair fetal cardiomyocyte function, including abnormal cardiomyocyte contraction and rhythm, leading to arrhythmias. Therefore, fetal arrhythmia is the mechanism most associated with increased risk of stillbirth for the patient in this scenario.

Accumulation of bile acids in the fetus is considered harmful; however, fetal cirrhosis of the liver has not been proposed as a mechanism underlying stillbirth risk. Studies have shown that stillborn fetuses in women with intrahepatic cholestasis typically are not growth restricted, and oligohydramnios often is not present; thus, chronic placental insufficiency is not considered to be a cause. Although placental abruption is a known cause of stillbirth, intrahepatic cholestasis is not a risk factor for placental abruption. Moreover, there is no evidence to suggest that intrahepatic cholestasis results in thrombosis in the placenta.

The goal of antenatal fetal surveillance is to identify a fetus at risk of stillbirth so that delivery can be performed before the occurrence of an adverse event. Although fetal monitoring often is recommended in pregnancies complicated by intrahepatic cholestasis, it has not been shown to reduce the risk of stillbirth. This further supports the hypothesis that stillbirth in intrahepatic cholestasis is an acute, unpredictable event.

The level of total bile acids is important for stratifying risk. A level of 40 micromoles/L or greater is consistently associated with adverse perinatal outcomes, and it has been suggested that risk of stillbirth is increased only when bile acid levels are 100 micromoles/L or higher. Nevertheless, lower levels of bile acids still represent some level of risk and late-preterm or early-term delivery should be considered in all women diagnosed with intrahepatic cholestasis. The American College of Obstetricians and Gynecologists recommends that delivery be considered anytime between 36 0/7 and 39 0/7 weeks of gestation in women with intrahepatic cholestasis and total bile acid concentrations less than 100 micromoles/L. If bile acids are 100 micromoles/L or greater, delivery at 36 0/7 weeks of gestation is recommended.

Ursodeoxycholic acid therapy is considered first-line treatment for intrahepatic cholestasis. Its primary benefit is reducing maternal symptoms. It also may improve laboratory values; however, there is no definitive evidence that therapy decreases fetal risk. The symptoms of intrahepatic cholestasis begin to resolve several days after delivery. Intrahepatic cholestasis of pregnancy has a high rate of recurrence in a subsequent pregnancy, with reported rates ranging from 60–70% to as high as 90%.

Indications for outpatient antenatal fetal surveillance. ACOG Committee Opinion Number 828. American College of Obstetricians and Gynecologists. Obstet Gynecol 2021;137:e177–97. doi: 10.1097/AOG.0000000000004407 https://journals.lww.com/greenjournal/Fulltext/2021/06000/Indications_for_Outpatient_Antenatal_Fetal.42.aspx

Lee RH. Society for Maternal–Fetal Medicine Consult Series #53: intrahepatic cholestasis of pregnancy: replaces consult #13, April 2011. Am J Obstet Gynecol 2021;224:B2–9. doi: 10.1016/j.ajog.2020.11.002 https://www.ajog.org/article/S0002-9378(20)31284-9/fulltext

Ovadia C, Seed PT, Sklavounos A, Geenes V, Di Ilio C, Chambers J, et al. Association of adverse perinatal outcomes of intrahepatic cholestasis of pregnancy with biochemical markers: results of aggregate and individual patient data meta-analyses [published erratum appears in Lancet 2019;393:1100]. Lancet 2019;393:899–909. doi: 10.1016/S0140-6736(18)31877-4 https://www.thelancet.com/journals/lancet/article/PIIS0140-6736(18)31877-4/fulltext

Ovadia C, Williamson C. Intrahepatic cholestasis of pregnancy: recent advances. Clin Dermatol 2016;34:327–34. doi: 10.1016/j.clindermatol.2016.02.004 https://www.cidjournal.com/article/S0738-081X(16)30019-0/fulltext

Wood AM, Livingston EG, Hughes BL, Kuller JA. Intrahepatic cholestasis of pregnancy: a review of diagnosis and management. Obstet Gynecol Surv 2018;73:103–9. doi: 10.1097/OGX.0000000000000524 https://journals.lww.com/obgynsurvey/Abstract/2018/02000/Intrahepatic_Cholestasis_of_Pregnancy__A_Review_of.18.aspx

61 Monochorionic twins

A 26-year-old gravida 1 with a monochorionic–diamniotic twin pregnancy had normal nuchal translucency measurements at 13 weeks of gestation. At 20 weeks of gestation, ultrasonographic evaluation revealed normal fetal anatomical surveys for both twins, appropriate fetal growth, a transvaginal cervical length of 3.4 cm, and a fetal weight discordance of 5%. There was no evidence of twin-to-twin transfusion syndrome. She is scheduled for ultrasonographic evaluations every 2 weeks to assess amniotic fluid volume and bladder filling. At 22 weeks of gestation, the most appropriate additional evaluation is

(A) amniocentesis
(B) biophysical profiles
* (C) fetal echocardiography
(D) transvaginal cervical length
(E) umbilical artery Doppler velocimetry

Zygosity, chorionicity, and amnionicity are important concepts to understand in twin pregnancies. *Zygosity* refers to the genetic makeup of the twins. Monozygotic twins, often referred to as "identical," result from one zygote, and dizygotic, or "fraternal," twins result from two zygotes. *Chorionicity* refers to the number of placentas and is most accurately identified by ultrasonography before 14 weeks of gestation. *Amnionicity* refers to the number of amniotic membranes between the twins.

Dizygotic twins have two separate placentas and two amniotic sacs (dichorionic–diamniotic). Monozygotic twins can have one shared placenta or two separate placentas, and they may have their own or a shared amniotic sac depending on when the embryo divided. Accordingly, they can be either dichorionic–diamniotic (division on days 1–3), monochorionic–diamniotic (division on days 4–8), monochorionic–monoamniotic (division on days 8–13), or conjoined (division 13 days or later). Monochorionic–diamniotic twins are the most common type, accounting for approximately 60–70% of all monozygotic twins.

The risks of a multiple gestation include preterm delivery, hypertensive disorders of pregnancy, anemia, gestational diabetes mellitus, hyperemesis, cesarean birth, and postpartum hemorrhage. In addition, compared with dichorionic twins, monochorionic twins are at risk of a number of unique complications as a result of unequal sharing of the single placenta. These complications of monochorionicity include twin-to-twin transfusion syndrome, which occurs in 10–15% of twins; twin anemia–polycythemia sequence, which occurs in 5% of twins; selective intrauterine growth restriction, which occurs in 10–15% of twins; and twin reversed arterial perfusion sequence, which occurs in 2–3% of twins. Congenital anomalies also are more prevalent in monochorionic twins than in dichorionic twins.

Congenital heart defects are the most prevalent group of congenital anomalies, affecting approximately 1% of singleton births. The risk of congenital heart defects is significantly greater in monochorionic twins, with the prevalence varying depending upon the study population, but ranging from sixfold to ninefold that of singleton pregnancies. Some of these defects represent embryologic malformations, whereas others are acquired prenatally, usually as a result of changes in blood flow secondary to twin-to-twin transfusion syndrome. For instance, right ventricular outflow tract abnormalities affect approximately 9% of recipient twins in twin-to-twin transfusion syndrome, and these abnormalities often persist after successful twin-to-twin transfusion syndrome therapy.

The etiology explaining the increased risk of congenital heart defects in monochorionic twins is not completely understood. Although genetically identical, monochorionic twins can develop discordant anomalies. Possible etiologies include unequal allocation of progenitor cells during the twinning process, environmental influences affecting epigenetic processes resulting in variable gene expression, unequal sharing of the placental parenchyma leading to blood flow imbalance and hypoperfusion, and aberrant angiogenic factors, such as vascular endothelial growth factor.

Timely diagnosis of congenital heart defects and appropriate intervention have been shown to improve neonatal outcomes. Thus, antenatal diagnosis plays an important role in reducing morbidity and mortality related to congenital heart defects. When a cardiac anomaly is detected antenatally, patients are able to make more informed decisions, including choosing a delivery location that can provide appropriate postnatal care.

Because of the increased risks in a monochorionic twin pregnancy, there are additional management considerations compared with dichorionic twins. First-trimester ultrasonography should confirm dating and chorionicity. Subsequently, ultrasonographic evaluation every 2 weeks is recommended starting at 16 weeks of gestation to detect twin-to-twin transfusion syndrome. Even more frequent ultrasound evaluation may be required in complicated monochorionic twins.

With the specific increase in congenital heart defects risk, monochorionicity is considered an indication for fetal echocardiography, which is recommended in all monochorionic twin pregnancies. Fetal echocardiography involves a detailed evaluation of cardiac structure and function and commonly is performed between 18 and 22 weeks of gestation. Therefore, in the described patient, fetal echocardiography is the next most appropriate evaluation.

Amniocentesis is not necessarily indicated because the woman is not of advanced maternal age, had normal nuchal translucency measurements at 13 weeks of gestation, underwent normal fetal anatomical surveys, and does not have fetuses with growth restriction. Antenatal fetal surveillance is recommended for monochorionic twins, although there is no consensus on what gestational age to begin surveillance, how frequently to perform the surveillance, or which test to perform. Biophysical profiles are not performed as early as 22 weeks of gestation.

There also is no consensus on cervical length surveillance in monochorionic twins, particularly in uncomplicated monochorionic twins. The International Society of Ultrasound in Obstetrics and Gynecology recommends cervical length assessment at the same ultrasonographic visit as the anatomy survey in the second trimester to identify women at risk of extreme preterm birth; however, this society does not recommend serial evaluations. Because she had a normal cervical length at 20 weeks of gestation and this is her first pregnancy, the patient in this scenario does not require a repeat examination at 22 weeks of gestation.

The role of Doppler assessment in routine uncomplicated monochorionic twins has not been established. The major value of umbilical artery Doppler evaluation is in surveillance of fetuses with growth restriction and staging twin-to-twin transfusion syndrome. Because she does not have any signs of twin-to-twin transfusion syndrome or fetal growth restriction, this patient should not be evaluated with umbilical artery Doppler at 22 weeks of gestation, according to the American College of Obstetricians and Gynecologists and the Society for Maternal-Fetal Medicine. Although middle cerebral artery Doppler measurements may be helpful in evaluating for the presence of twin anemia–polycythemia sequence, no consensus has been reached on their role in monitoring monochorionic twin gestations. Thus, Doppler protocols for monitoring monochorionic twins vary widely among centers.

Bahtiyar MO, Dulay AT, Weeks BP, Friedman AH, Copel JA. Prevalence of congenital heart defects in monochorionic/diamniotic twin gestations: a systematic literature review. J Ultrasound Med 2007;26:1491–8. doi: 10.7863/jum.2007.26.11.1491 https://onlinelibrary.wiley.com/doi/abs/10.7863/jum.2007.26.11.1491

Emery SP, Bahtiyar MO, Dashe JS, Wilkins-Haug LE, Johnson A, Paek BW, et al. The North American Fetal Therapy Network Consensus Statement: prenatal management of uncomplicated monochorionic gestations. Obstet Gynecol 2015;125:1236–43. doi: 10.1097/AOG.0000000000000723 https://journals.lww.com/greenjournal/Fulltext/2015/05000/The_North_American_Fetal_Therapy_Network_Consensus.34.aspx

Gijtenbeek M, Shirzada MR, Ten Harkel ADJ, Oepkes D, Haak MC. Congenital heart defects in monochorionic twins: a systematic review and meta-analysis. J Clin Med 2019;8:902. doi: 10.3390/jcm8060902. https://www.mdpi.com/2077-0383/8/6/902

Hoskins IA, Combs CA. Society for Maternal–Fetal Medicine special statement: updated checklists for management of monochorionic twin pregnancy. Patient Safety and Quality Committee, Society for Maternal–Fetal Medicine. Am J Obstet Gynecol 2020;223:B16–20. doi: 10.1016/j.ajog.2020.08.066 https://www.ajog.org/article/S0002-9378(20)30947-9/fulltext

Khalil A, Rodgers M, Baschat A, Bhide A, Gratacos E, Hecher K, et al. ISUOG practice guidelines: role of ultrasound in twin pregnancy [published erratum appears in Ultrasound Obstet Gynecol 2018;52:140]. Ultrasound Obstet Gynecol 2016;47:247–63. doi: 10.1002/uog.15821 https://obgyn.onlinelibrary.wiley.com/doi/10.1002/uog.15821

Multifetal gestations: twin, triplet, and higher-order multifetal pregnancies. ACOG Practice Bulletin No. 231. American College of Obstetricians and Gynecologists. Obstet Gynecol 2021;137:e145–62. doi: 10.1097/AOG.0000000000004397 https://journals.lww.com/greenjournal/Fulltext/2021/06000/Multifetal_Gestations__Twin,_Triplet,_and.39.aspx

Panagiotopoulou O, Fouzas S, Sinopidis X, Mantagos SP, Dimitriou G, Karatza AA. Congenital heart disease in twins: the contribution of type of conception and chorionicity. Int J Cardiol 2016;218:144–9. doi: 10.1016/j.ijcard.2016.05.029 https://www.internationaljournalofcardiology.com/article/S0167-5273(16)30931-7/fulltext

Pettit KE, Merchant M, Machin GA, Tacy TA, Norton ME. Congenital heart defects in a large, unselected cohort of monochorionic twins. J Perinatol 2013;33:457–61. doi: 10.1038/jp.2012.145 https://www.nature.com/articles/jp2012145

Springer S, Mlczoch E, Krampl-Bettelheim E, Mailáth-Pokorny M, Ulm B, Worda C, et al. Congenital heart disease in monochorionic twins with and without twin-to-twin transfusion syndrome. Prenat Diagn 2014;34:994–9. doi: 10.1002/pd.4411 https://obgyn.onlinelibrary.wiley.com/doi/10.1002/pd.4411

62 Fetal growth restriction

A 36-year-old gravida 1 with chronic hypertension well-controlled on medications underwent cell-free DNA screening in the first trimester. The test result indicated a low risk of aneuploidy, and her detailed fetal anatomy survey at 20 weeks of gestation showed no abnormalities. On routine ultrasonography to evaluate fetal growth at 31 0/7 weeks of gestation, estimated fetal weight was at the 4th percentile, and the umbilical artery Doppler systolic/diastolic ratio was greater than the 95th percentile for gestational age. After the ultrasonography, she received a course of antenatal corticosteroids, and weekly surveillance including umbilical artery Doppler assessment was initiated. At 32 weeks, the umbilical artery Doppler findings are shown in Figure 62-1. The best next step in management is to admit the patient to the hospital and

(A) administer rescue course of antenatal corticosteroids
* (B) deliver
(C) initiate twice-weekly umbilical artery Doppler assessments
(D) schedule delivery at 37 weeks of gestation
(E) screen for TORCH (toxoplasmosis, syphilis, rubella, cytomegalovirus, and herpes simplex virus)

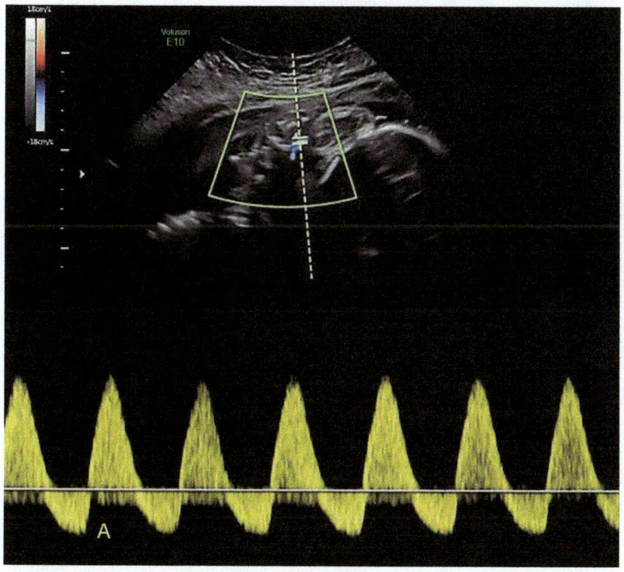

FIGURE 62-1. Ultrasonographic image of umbilical artery Doppler at 32 weeks of gestation.

Fetal growth restriction, formerly referred to as *intrauterine growth restriction*, is defined as an ultrasonographic estimated fetal weight or abdominal circumference below the 10th percentile for gestational age. Fetal growth restriction can lead to significant perinatal morbidity and mortality as well as long-term health complications, including obesity, metabolic dysfunction, and cardiovascular and renal diseases. The stillbirth rate of fetal growth restriction is approximately 1.5%, which is twice that of normally grown fetuses. The severity of the fetal growth restriction affects outcome. An estimated fetal weight less than the 3rd percentile is considered a severe form of fetal growth restriction and is associated with adverse perinatal outcomes, with a stillbirth risk approximately three times higher than that of fetuses in the 3rd to 5th percentile and four to seven times higher than that of those in the 5th to 10th percentile. Fetal growth restriction is referred to as *early* or *late* onset depending on whether the diagnosis was before or after 32 weeks of gestation. Early-onset fetal growth restriction is considered more severe and is often associated with maternal hypertension.

Fetal growth restriction can develop as a result of maternal, fetal, and placental factors. Maternal causes include vascular diseases, such as hypertensive disorders; diabetes mellitus; autoimmune conditions; diseases associated with decreased oxygen delivery, such as cyanotic heart disease or hemoglobinopathy; as well as infection, cigarette smoking, and poor nutrition. Fetal etiologies include genetic abnormalities, congenital anomalies, and multiple gestations. Placental etiologies range from abnormal placental implantation to changes in placental perfusion secondary to maternal disease.

Once fetal growth restriction has been diagnosed, fetal surveillance is recommended because of the increased risk of stillbirth. Surveillance includes standard fetal testing, such as nonstress tests and biophysical profiles, in addition to serial umbilical artery Doppler velocimetry. Umbilical artery Doppler assessment plays an integral role in managing pregnancies with fetal growth restriction. When added to standard antepartum testing, it reduces the chances of an unnecessary preterm delivery and has been shown to significantly reduce the perinatal death rate.

Abnormal findings in umbilical artery Doppler velocimetry reflect placental insufficiency and include a systolic-to-diastolic (S/D) ratio, pulsatility index, or resistance index greater than the 95th percentile for gestational age, or the finding of absent or reversed end-diastolic velocity. Absent or reversed diastolic flow is an indication of placental deterioration and is associated with adverse fetal and neonatal outcomes. Therefore, surveillance frequency is largely based on umbilical artery Doppler findings. A standardized approach to diagnosis and management of fetal growth restriction improves perinatal morbidity and mortality. The Society for Maternal-Fetal Medicine has proposed a management algorithm (Fig. 62-2).

In the described scenario, the patient has a diagnosis of early-onset fetal growth restriction with an estimated fetal weight in the 4th percentile at 31 weeks of gestation. Umbilical artery Doppler S/D ratios are abnormal (above the 95th percentile, reflecting a decrease in end-diastolic flow). Thus, according to the algorithm, weekly umbilical artery Doppler assessment in addition to standard antenatal testing is recommended. The patient also received a course of antenatal corticosteroids secondary to the potential need for preterm delivery. When she presented for her follow-up ultrasonographic evaluation the next week at 32 weeks of gestation, the umbilical artery Doppler waveforms showed reversed end-diastolic velocity. The recommended management of the growth-restricted fetus with reversed end-diastolic velocity includes delivery by 30–32 weeks of gestation. Although there may be complications of prematurity at this gestational age, they are fewer than the complications associated with reversed end-diastolic velocity. Therefore, the best next step for this patient is delivery because she has already achieved 32 0/7 weeks of gestation.

Initiating more frequent umbilical artery Doppler assessment is not indicated in this scenario secondary to the finding of reversed end-diastolic velocity and the gestational age. Administration of antenatal corticosteroids is not indicated because a course of antenatal corticosteroids was initiated when she was seen 1 week ago. If her gestational age was less than 30 weeks with the finding of reversed end-diastolic velocity, inpatient admission with frequent fetal surveillance would have been recommended until delivery at 30–32 weeks of gestation. If the Doppler results had shown absent end-diastolic velocity, continued inpatient management could be considered with increased umbilical artery Doppler surveillance (23 times weekly) and planned delivery at 33–34 weeks of gestation. Delivery at 37 0/7 weeks is recommended in women with isolated fetal growth restriction less than the 3rd percentile and in those with an estimated fetal weight between the 3rd and 10th percentile who have umbilical artery Doppler findings of decreased end-diastolic flow (ie, S/D, pulsatility index, or resistance index greater than the 95th percentile).

Although maternal infections can result in fetal growth restriction, if there are no maternal or ultrasonographic findings suggestive of infection, routine screening is not recommended. The Society for Maternal-Fetal Medicine advises against screening for TORCH because the incidence of these infections in fetal growth restriction is low. However, if the patient undergoes an amniocentesis, the amniotic fluid can be tested for cytomegalovirus by polymerase chain reaction.

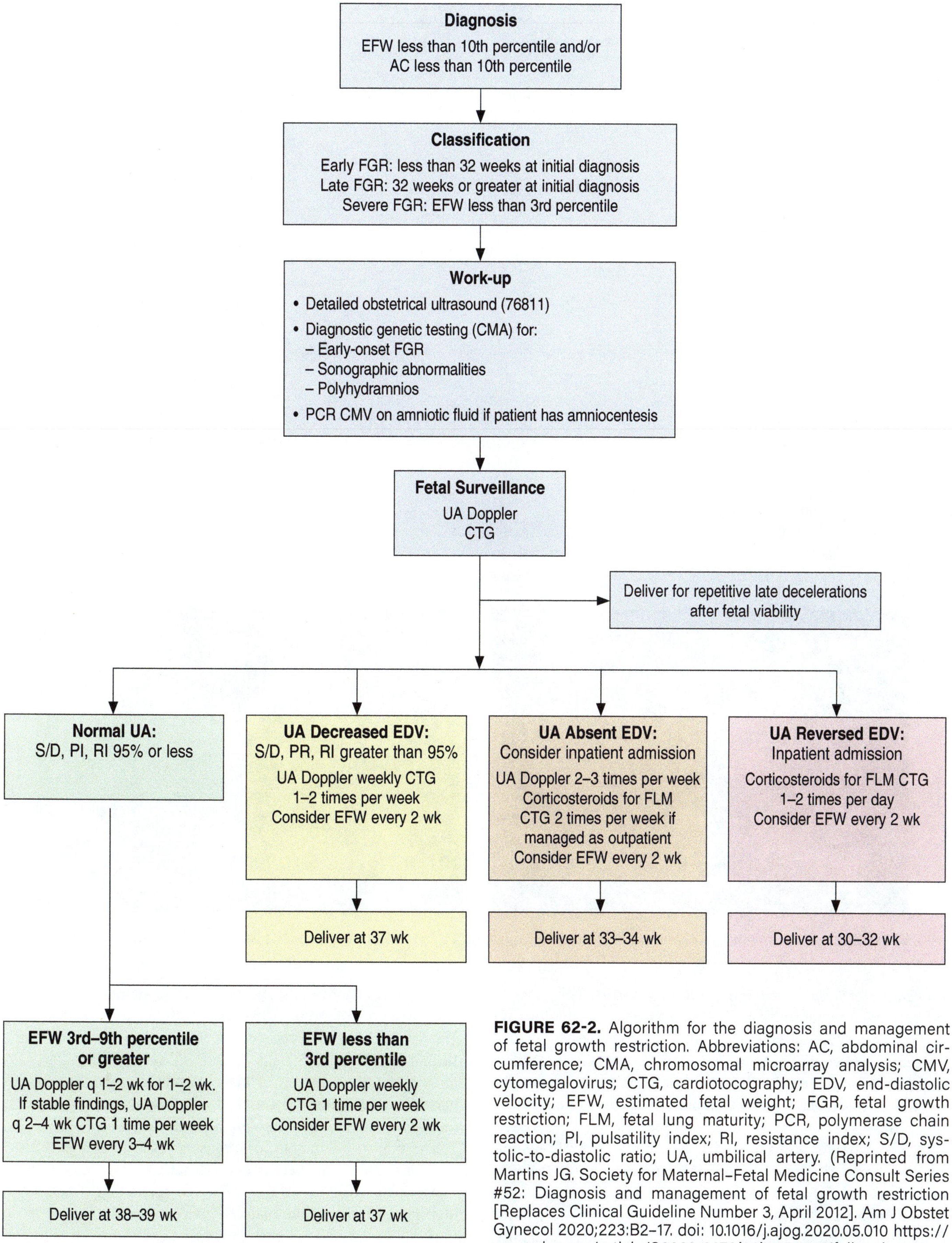

FIGURE 62-2. Algorithm for the diagnosis and management of fetal growth restriction. Abbreviations: AC, abdominal circumference; CMA, chromosomal microarray analysis; CMV, cytomegalovirus; CTG, cardiotocography; EDV, end-diastolic velocity; EFW, estimated fetal weight; FGR, fetal growth restriction; FLM, fetal lung maturity; PCR, polymerase chain reaction; PI, pulsatility index; RI, resistance index; S/D, systolic-to-diastolic ratio; UA, umbilical artery. (Reprinted from Martins JG. Society for Maternal-Fetal Medicine Consult Series #52: Diagnosis and management of fetal growth restriction [Replaces Clinical Guideline Number 3, April 2012]. Am J Obstet Gynecol 2020;223:B2–17. doi: 10.1016/j.ajog.2020.05.010 https://www.ajog.org/article/S0002-9378(20)30535-4/fulltext)

Fetal growth restriction. ACOG Practice Bulletin No. 227. American College of Obstetricians and Gynecologists. Obstet Gynecol 2021;137:e16–28. doi: 10.1097/AOG.0000000000004251 https://journals.lww.com/greenjournal/pages/articleviewer.aspx?year=2021&issue=02000&article=00043&type=Fulltext

Lees C, Marlow N, Arabin B, Bilardo CM, Brezinka C, Derks JB, et al. Perinatal morbidity and mortality in early-onset fetal growth restriction: cohort outcomes of the trial of randomized umbilical and fetal flow in Europe (TRUFFLE). TRUFFLE Group. Ultrasound Obstet Gynecol 2013;42:400–8. doi: 10.1002/uog.13190 https://obgyn.onlinelibrary.wiley.com/doi/10.1002/uog.13190

Martins JG. Society for Maternal–Fetal Medicine Consult Series #52: Diagnosis and management of fetal growth restriction (Replaces Clinical Guideline Number 3, April 2012). Am J Obstet Gynecol 2020;223:B2–17. doi: 10.1016/j.ajog.2020.05.010 https://www.ajog.org/article/S0002-9378(20)30535-4/fulltext

Medically indicated late-preterm and early-term deliveries. ACOG Committee Opinion No. 831. American College of Obstetricians and Gynecologists. Obstet Gynecol 2021;138:e35–9. doi: 10.1097/AOG.0000000000004447 https://journals.lww.com/greenjournal/Fulltext/2021/07000/Medically_Indicated_Late_Preterm_and_Early_Term.38.aspx

63 Placenta previa

A 33-year-old gravida 3, para 2, was diagnosed with a placenta previa earlier in her pregnancy. At 36 weeks of gestation, she presents for ultrasonographic reevaluation of the placental location. Her obstetric history includes one previous low transverse cesarean birth followed by a successful vaginal birth after cesarean. She desires a trial of labor if she is a candidate. After reviewing Figure 63-1, you determine that the best next step is to

(A) continue routine care
* (B) deliver with cesarean by 37 6/7 weeks of gestation
(C) perform magnetic resonance imaging (MRI)
(D) repeat ultrasonography in 2 weeks

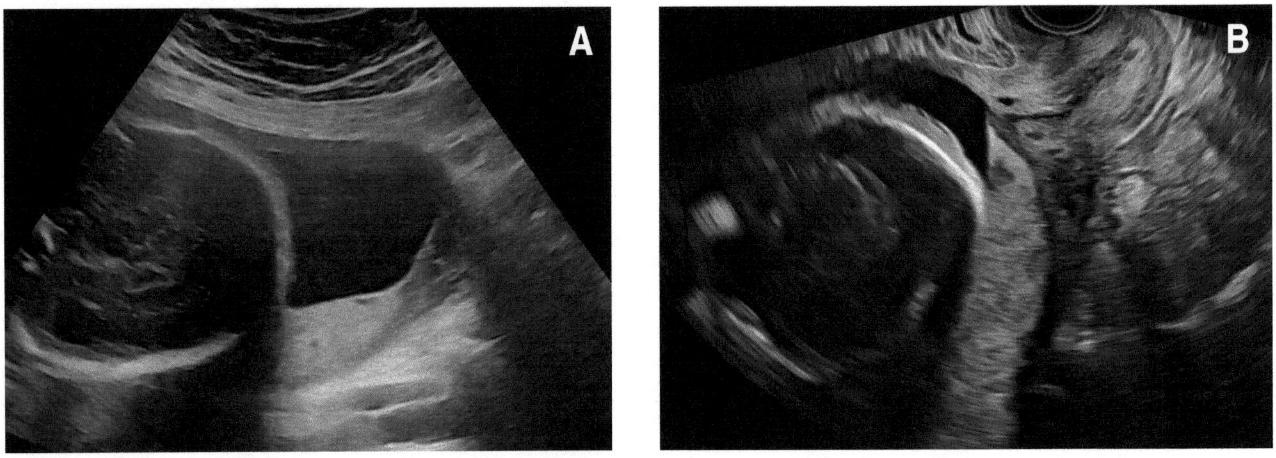

FIGURE 63-1. A. Patient's transabdominal ultrasonography. B. Patient's transvaginal ultrasonographic image.

Placenta previa is defined as the complete or partial covering of the cervical internal os by the placenta. Former terminology for describing a placenta previa included the terms *complete* and *partial*; however, this nomenclature is no longer recommended. If the inferior placental edge is within 2 cm from the internal os, but does not cover it, the diagnosis is termed *low-lying placenta*.

Placenta previa is a major risk factor for obstetric hemorrhage before and during delivery and can lead to morbidity and mortality for the woman and fetus or neonate, particularly when it is undiagnosed. Women with placenta previas are more likely to experience blood transfusions and undergo hysterectomy. Neonatal morbidity and mortality are primarily secondary to complications of prematurity. The presence of a placenta previa also increases the risk of placenta accreta spectrum, which further increases the risks of morbidity and mortality. The most common symptom of placenta previa is painless vaginal bleeding in the second or third trimester of pregnancy. The recurrence rate for placenta previa is estimated at 4–8%.

The major risk factors for a placenta previa include a previous cesarean birth, increased maternal age, previous placenta previa, use of assisted reproductive technology, history of uterine instrumentation, maternal smoking, and multiple gestation. The prevalence of placenta previa is difficult to determine because the definitions have not been consistent; however, it is thought to complicate approximately 1 of every 200 births. Rates are expected to increase as the major risk factors for previa—primarily previous cesarean birth, increasing maternal age, and use of assisted reproductive technology—continue to increase.

Determining placental location is an important component of the midtrimester ultrasonographic evaluation. To diagnose a placenta previa, the gestational age should be at least 16 weeks when the ultrasonography is performed. Transvaginal ultrasonography is considered safe and is superior to transabdominal and transperineal approaches. An overdistended maternal bladder or uterine contraction can give a false diagnosis of a previa. As a general rule, if the lower placental edge appears to be less than 2 cm from the cervical os, or if it covers the cervix during transabdominal evaluation, a transvaginal approach is suggested. Figure 63-1 depicts the transabdominal and transvaginal views of the same patient. In the transabdominal view, the placenta appears to approach and possibly cover the cervix. In contrast, the transvaginal view clearly shows the placental edge covering the cervical os, confirming the diagnosis of persistent placenta previa (Fig. 63-2).

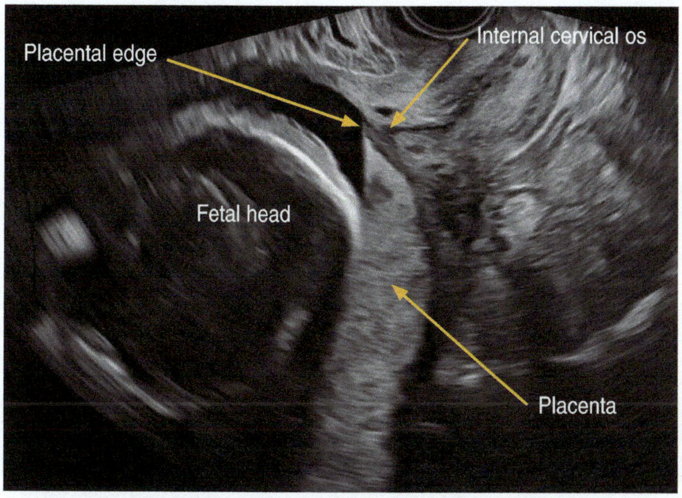

FIGURE 63-2. Transvaginal ultrasonic image of placenta previa.

If placenta previa is diagnosed, assessment for placenta accreta spectrum is necessary. Ultrasonographic markers of placenta accreta include loss of the normal retroplacental hypoechoic zone between the placenta and uterus, placental lacunae, bulging of the placenta into the posterior wall of the bladder, hypervascularity, and thinning of the myometrium. Vasa previa also should be ruled out using color and pulsed Doppler examinations in all women diagnosed with a low-lying placenta or placenta previa, even if they resolve.

If placenta previa is diagnosed at the time of the routine fetal anatomy ultrasonogram, a follow-up ultrasonographic examination is recommended at 32 weeks of gestation. As gestational age advances and the lower uterine segment develops, the distance between the placental edge and the internal os increases. Because of this phenomenon, it is estimated that more than 90% of placenta previas diagnosed in the midtrimester period resolve by term. The more the previa extends over the internal os, the more likely it is to persist. If bleeding occurs before 32 weeks of gestation, earlier follow-up is indicated. If the previa is persistent at 32 weeks of gestation, repeat evaluation at 36 weeks of gestation is recommended to determine the mode of delivery. If the placenta previa persists at the 36-week follow-up, cesarean birth should be scheduled.

Recommended delivery timing in women with a placenta previa and no other complications is 36 0/7 to 37 6/7 weeks of gestation. If a late preterm delivery is anticipated, a single course of antenatal corticosteroids is recommended within 7 days of delivery if a previous course has not been administered. In the present scenario, the patient has a persistent placenta previa and should be scheduled for cesarean birth before 37 6/7 weeks of gestation. A vaginal delivery is contraindicated in the presence of a placenta previa. Only in unique situations, such as a fetal death, is vaginal delivery considered a potentially appropriate option. Although MRI may be helpful in the management of a complicated placenta accreta, because transvaginal ultrasonography provides such clear images of the placenta and cervix and is highly accurate, MRI is not indicated to confirm the diagnosis of placenta previa. There is no utility in further ultrasonographic evaluation at this gestational age.

If the placenta continues to be low-lying at follow-up ultrasonography at 36 weeks of gestation, there is no consensus on management. Risks and benefits of a trial of labor should be discussed. With a low-lying placenta, the risk of bleeding is increased with labor and the risk of an emergency cesarean birth is increased. Vaginal birth is more likely if the placental edge is 10–20 mm from the internal os compared with within 10 mm. A systematic review reported successful vaginal birth in 85% of women with a placenta 11–20 mm from the internal os and in only 43% when the placenta is 10 mm or less from the internal os.

Jansen C, de Mooij YM, Blomaard CM, Derks JB, van Leeuwen E, Limpens J, et al. Vaginal delivery in women with a low-lying placenta: a systematic review and meta-analysis. BJOG 2019;126:1118–26. doi: 10.1111/1471-0528.15622 https://obgyn.onlinelibrary.wiley.com/doi/10.1111/1471-0528.15622

Jauniaux E, Moffett A, Burton GJ. Placental implantation disorders. Obstet Gynecol Clin North Am 2020;47:117–32. doi: 10.1016/j.ogc.2019.10.002 https://www.obgyn.theclinics.com/article/S0889-8545(19)30111-1/fulltext

Jauniaux E, Alfirevic Z, Bhide AG, Belfort MA, Burton GJ, Collins SL, et al. Placenta praevia and placenta accreta: diagnosis and management: Green-Top guideline No. 27a. Royal College of Obstetricians and Gynaecologists. BJOG 2019;126:e1–48. doi: 10.1111/1471-0528.15306 https://obgyn.onlinelibrary.wiley.com/doi/10.1111/1471-0528.15306

Medically indicated late-preterm and early-term deliveries. ACOG Committee Opinion No. 831. American College of Obstetricians and Gynecologists. Obstet Gynecol 2021;138:e35–9. doi: 10.1097/AOG.0000000000004447 https://journals.lww.com/greenjournal/Fulltext/2021/07000/Medically_Indicated_Late_Preterm_and_Early_Term.38.aspx

Ornaghi S, Vaglio Tessitore I, Vergani P. Pregnancy and delivery outcomes in women with persistent versus resolved low-lying placenta in the late third trimester. J Ultrasound Med 2022;41:123–33. doi: 10.1002/jum.15687 https://onlinelibrary.wiley.com/doi/epdf/10.1002/jum.15687

Placenta accreta spectrum. Obstetric Care Consensus No. 7. American College of Obstetricians and Gynecologists. Obstet Gynecol 2018;132:e259–75. doi: 10.1097/AOG.0000000000002983 https://journals.lww.com/greenjournal/Fulltext/2018/12000/Obstetric_Care_Consensus_No__7__Placenta_Accreta.50.aspx

Reddy UM, Abuhamad AZ, Levine D, Saade GR. Fetal imaging: executive summary of a joint Eunice Kennedy Shriver National Institute of Child Health and Human Development, Society for Maternal-Fetal Medicine, American Institute of Ultrasound in Medicine, American College of Obstetricians and Gynecologists, American College of Radiology, Society for Pediatric Radiology, and Society of Radiologists in Ultrasound Fetal Imaging Workshop. J Ultrasound Med 2014;33:745–57. doi: 10.7863/ultra.33.5.745 https://onlinelibrary.wiley.com/doi/abs/10.7863/ultra.33.5.745

Shainker SA, Coleman B, Timor-Tritsch IE, Bhide A, Bromley B, Cahill AG, et al. Special Report of the Society for Maternal–Fetal Medicine Placenta Accreta Spectrum Ultrasound Marker Task Force: consensus on definition of markers and approach to the ultrasound examination in pregnancies at risk for placenta accreta spectrum. Society for Maternal–Fetal Medicine [published erratum appears in Am J Obstet Gynecol 2021;225:91]. Am J Obstet Gynecol 2021;224:B2–14. doi: 10.1016/j.ajog.2020.09.001 https://www.ajog.org/article/S0002-9378(20)31053-X/fulltext

64 Migraine

A 34-year-old gravida 1 at 24 weeks of gestation presents to the emergency department with a headache with 8 out of 10 intensity, nausea, vomiting, and photophobia. She has tried acetaminophen and caffeine, which have helped her in the past, at home with no relief. She reports having this type of headache when not pregnant. Her blood pressure is 110/84 mm Hg, she has a normal complete metabolic profile, and her urinalysis is notable only for ketonuria. In addition to receiving intravenous fluids, the best next step in management of her headache is to administer

(A) dexamethasone
(B) ketorolac
(C) magnesium sulfate
* (D) metoclopramide
(E) sumatriptan

Headache is a common complaint during pregnancy and may have a variety of causes. Migraine is a dull, throbbing headache typically accompanied with nausea and vomiting and visual, sensory, or motor symptoms, which may be preceded by auras containing visual, sensory, or focal neurologic symptoms. Migraine often is associated with or precipitated by hormonal changes including menstruation, oral contraceptive use, pregnancy, and breastfeeding.

Migraine generally decreases in frequency during pregnancy, improving in approximately 50% of women in the first trimester and by the third trimester in up to 80–90% of women. Despite this trend, migraine does occasionally worsen or occur for the first time in pregnancy. New-onset or worsening migraine typically presents in the first trimester.

When a pregnant woman presents with headache, it is important to thoroughly evaluate the patient and rule out other causes. When a headache is accompanied by hypertension, altered mental status, fever, seizures, or an abnormal neurologic examination, this should alert the obstetrician to consider a further workup to rule out other causes of headache. Additionally, if a headache does not respond to treatment or persists despite treatment, a more comprehensive evaluation should be performed. This may include imaging, consultation, and other indicated testing.

Once the headache has been evaluated and determined to be a migraine, pregnant women can be encouraged to first try simple analgesics, including acetaminophen, and nonpharmacologic approaches including hydration, ice, sleep, caffeine, and avoidance of triggers. When migraine refractory to these initial treatment modalities is encountered, the patient may require more intensive therapy.

A simple treatment algorithm for acute migraine refractory to initial treatment modalities is shown in Figure 64-1. Volume and electrolyte status should be evaluated. The patient should then be given 1–2 L of normal saline or lactated Ringer solution. Choice of intravenous fluid can be adjusted according to electrolyte status. Several medications may be given in sequence after intravenous fluids, allowing at least 10–20 minutes between medications to evaluate response and possible adverse reactions. These medications are seen in Figure 64-1.

Generally, first-line medical treatment after initial modalities and volume resuscitation in the setting of acute migraine is dopamine antagonists, which serve as antiemetics and are effective migraine treatment. The benefits of dopamine antagonists in this situation outweigh any theoretical pregnancy risks. The dopamine antagonist metoclopramide is the best initial medical treatment choice for treatment of acute migraine in pregnancy, such as in the patient in this scenario. Patients may be pretreated with diphenhydramine to reduce the risk of acute dystonic reaction, but these reactions are rare. Although dopamine antagonists are considered highly efficacious for migraine treatment and result in partial pain relief in 65–80% of patients, they provide total relief for only 40–53% of patients. Metoclopramide is the best answer as the next treatment for the described patient.

Magnesium sulfate can be given intravenously as a second-line agent in the treatment of acute migraine. There is significant experience with magnesium sulfate use in pregnancy. Magnesium sulfate is estimated to provide partial pain relief in 40% of patients and is considered to have moderate efficacy. Magnesium sulfate does have significant adverse effects, including upset stomach, nausea, flushing, and diarrhea, and it is not the best next choice for the described patient. Furthermore, magnesium sulfate would not be given until after metoclopramide or another dopamine antagonist had been tried.

Sumatriptan may be given as a third-line agent for treatment of acute migraine. Sumatriptan has vasoconstrictive properties and, for this reason, previously has not been recommended in pregnancy. However, more recent data suggest that it is a safe option in pregnant patients. There are no human data suggesting teratogenicity in a large triptan pregnancy registry. Because of rapid elimination, high molecular weight, and poor water solubility, only small amounts of triptans will cross the placenta or into breast milk. Sumatriptan is not the best answer choice in this scenario as it would not be the best next step in management; it would only be used after other interventions had been tried.

Nonsteroidal anti-inflammatory drugs, including ketorolac, are frequently used for migraine relief outside of pregnancy. However, they are generally avoided during pregnancy because they inhibit prostaglandin synthesis, which may cause oligohydramnios or premature closure of the ductus arteriosus. However, if there are no medical contraindications to use of nonsteroidal anti-inflammatory drugs, they may be used in combination with other medications in the second trimester.

Finally, although they are considered low efficacy, corticosteroids, including dexamethasone and methylprednisolone, may be used in the treatment of acute migraine. Because dexamethasone is low efficacy, it would be considered as a treatment for migraine in pregnancy only after discussion of the risks and when other treatments do not provide relief. Therefore, dexamethasone is not the best answer choice in this scenario.

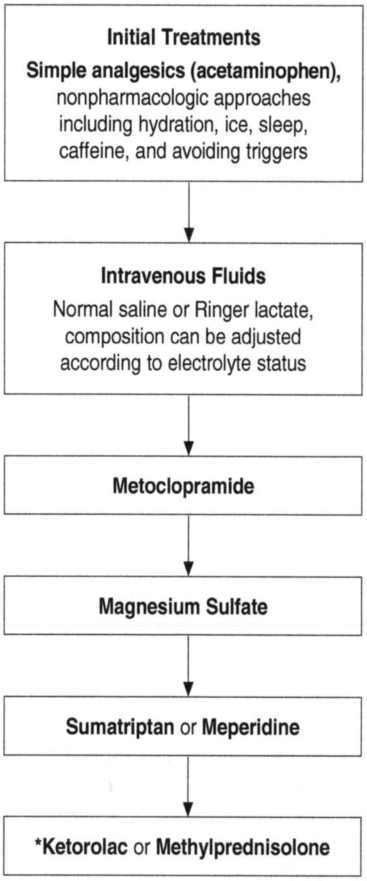

FIGURE 64-1. Medications that may be given in sequence after intravenous fluids. *Ketorolac and other nonsteroidal anti-inflammatory medications are associated with increased risk of transitory oligohydramnios and premature closure of the ductus arteriosus after 32 weeks. Ketorolac should not be used in pregnancy without discussion of risks and benefits with the patient. (Modified from Lucas S, Rawner E. Approach to the pregnant or lactating patients with headache in the emergency department. In: Orr SL, Friedman BW, Dodick DW, editors. Emergency headache: diagnosis and management. United Kingdom: Cambridge University Press; 2017. p. 125–40.)

Amundsen S, Øvrebø TG, Amble NMS, Poole AC, Nordeng H. Risk perception, beliefs about medicines and medical adherence among pregnant and breastfeeding women with migraine: findings from a cross-sectional study in Norway. BMJ Open 2019;9:e026690. doi: 10.1136/bmjopen-2018-026690 https://bmjopen.bmj.com/content/9/2/e026690.long

Lucas S. Migraine and other headache disorders. Clin Update Womens Health Care 2019;XVIII(4):1–55.

Marchenko A, Etwel F, Olutunfese O, Nickel C, Koren G, Nulman I. Pregnancy outcome following prenatal exposure to triptan medications: a meta-analysis [published erratum appears in Headache 2015;55:1478]. Headache 2015;55: 490–501. doi: 10.1111/head.12500 https://headachejournal.onlinelibrary.wiley.com/doi/10.1111/head.12500

Orr SL, Rawner E. Approach to pregnant or lactating patients with headache in the emergency department. In: Orr SL, Friedman BW, Dodick DW, editors. Emergency headache: diagnosis and management: Cambridge University Press; 2017. p. 125–40.

65 Antiphospholipid antibody syndrome

A 34-year-old multigravida presents for prepregnancy counseling. She has a history of delivery at 36 weeks of gestation with preeclampsia with severe features, a second-trimester fetal death at 13 weeks of gestation after normal 10-week ultrasonography, and an early pregnancy loss at 6 weeks of gestation. Her mother and sister have a history of venous thromboembolism (VTE). The clinical history that most supports screening for antiphospholipid antibody syndrome (APS) is

(A) family history of vascular thrombosis
(B) history of severe preeclampsia at 36 weeks of gestation
* (C) second-trimester fetal death at 13 weeks of gestation
(D) two consecutive fetal losses

Antiphospholipid antibody syndrome is an autoimmune condition that affects mostly women of reproductive age. Antiphospholipid antibodies are a large group of different antibodies that bind to negatively charged phospholipids on cell surfaces. Antiphospholipid antibody syndrome is associated with many different clinical consequences, ranging from arterial and venous thrombosis to autoimmune thrombocytopenia. Antiphospholipid antibody syndrome has a significant effect on the obstetric population and increases the risk of miscarriage, stillbirth, preeclampsia, growth restriction, placental insufficiency, and preterm birth.

The most common complication of APS is VTE, typically in a lower extremity. Among patients with VTE, approximately 2–3% have APS. In patients with APS, the risk of VTE is significantly increased during pregnancy and the postpartum period and is estimated to be as high as 12% in some studies. Women with APS also are at risk of arterial thrombosis and stroke, most commonly involving the middle cerebral artery. About 5% of strokes that occur in patients younger than 50 years are caused by APS.

Another complication of APS is pregnancy loss, with a significant portion of those losses occurring after 10 weeks of gestation. Additionally, APS can cause recurrent early pregnancy loss before 10 weeks of gestation. Studies have reported that 5–20% of women with two or more losses have APS. In one study, fetal loss after 10 weeks of gestation was more common than early pregnancy losses among women with APS.

Antiphospholipid antibody syndrome also has been implicated in a variety of adverse pregnancy outcomes related to placental pathology. Some studies report that 15–17% of women with preeclampsia have antiphospholipid antibodies, and APS can lead to severe preeclampsia before 34 weeks of gestation. Fetal growth restriction also is common among women with APS, occurring in 15–30% of pregnancies.

Antiphospholipid antibody syndrome is diagnosed by clinical criteria and the presence of antiphospholipid antibodies. These criteria are shown in Box 65-1. Although the expert consensus includes preterm severe preeclampsia as part of the clinical criteria for APS, there is not clear evidence for screening and treating women with only preterm preeclampsia. The described patient meets clinical criteria for testing for APS because of her second-trimester fetal death at 13 weeks of gestation. She has only had a single early pregnancy loss at 6 weeks of gestation, which does not meet criteria. Her preterm preeclampsia was at 36 weeks and is not an indication for testing. The American College of Obstetricians and Gynecologists recommends against testing for this reason alone. Family history of VTE is not an indication for testing.

Patients with APS and a history of a thrombotic event should be treated with prophylactic anticoagulation throughout pregnancy and for 6 weeks after delivery. Patients also generally receive low-dose aspirin, although the benefit for patients with APS who only have had thrombosis is unclear. For women with early pregnancy loss or fetal loss, prophylactic use of heparin and low-dose aspirin has been shown to reduce pregnancy loss by as much as 50%. Other treatments, such as corticosteroids and intravenous immunoglobulin, have not been shown to be cost effective or clearly efficacious.

BOX 65-1

Classification Criteria for the Diagnosis of Antiphospholipid Antibody Syndrome

Antiphospholipid antibody syndrome is present if at least one of the clinical criteria and one of the laboratory criteria that follow are met:

Clinical Criteria

1. Vascular thrombosis
   a. One or more clinical episodes of arterial, venous, or small vessel thrombosis in any tissue or organ.
   b. Thrombosis must be confirmed by objective validated criteria (ie, unequivocal findings of appropriate imaging studies).
2. Pregnancy morbidity
   a. One or more unexplained deaths of a morphologically normal fetus at or beyond the 10th week of gestation, with normal fetal morphology documented by ultrasound or by direct examination of the fetus.
   b. One or more premature births of a morphologically normal neonate before the 34th week of gestation because of severe preeclampsia or eclampsia or features consistent with placental insufficiency.
   c. Three or more unexplained consecutive spontaneous abortions before the 10th week of gestation, with maternal anatomic or hormonal abnormalities and paternal and maternal chromosomal causes excluded.

In studies of populations of patients who have more than one type of pregnancy morbidity, investigators are strongly encouraged to stratify groups of subjects according to a, b, or c above.

Laboratory Criteria

1. Lupus anticoagulant present in plasma, on two or more occasions at least 12 weeks apart.
2. Anticardiolipin antibody of IgG and/or IgM isotype in serum or plasma, present in medium or high titer (ie, 40 or greater GPL or MPL, or 99th or greater percentile), on two or more occasions, at least 12 weeks apart, measured by a standardized ELISA.
3. Anti-β_2-glycoprotein-1 antibody of IgG and/or IgM isotype in serum or plasma (in titer 99th or greater percentile), present on two or more occasions, at least 12 weeks apart, measured by a standardized ELISA, according to recommended procedures.

Abbreviations: ELISA, enzyme-linked immunosorbent assay; IgG, immunoglobulin G; IgM, immunoglobulin M.

Modified from Miyakis S, Lockshin MD, Atsumi T, Branch DW, Brey RL, Cervera R, et al. International consensus statement on an update of the classification criteria for definite antiphospholipid syndrome (APS). J Thromb Haemost 2006;4:295–306. doi: 10.1111/j.1538-7836.2006.01753.x https://onlinelibrary.wiley.com/doi/10.1111/j.1538-7836.2006.01753.x.

Antiphospholipid syndrome. Practice Bulletin No. 132. American College of Obstetricians and Gynecologists. Obstet Gynecol 2012;120:1514–21. doi: 10.1097/01.AOG.0000423816.39542.0f https://journals.lww.com/greenjournal/Abstract/2012/12000/Practice_Bulletin_No__132__Antiphospholipid.44.aspx

Branch DW, Andres R, Digre KB, Rote NS, Scott JR. The association of antiphospholipid antibodies with severe preeclampsia. Obstet Gynecol 1989;73:541–5. https://journals.lww.com/greenjournal/Abstract/1989/04000/The_Association_of_Antiphospholipid_Antibodies.1.aspx

Empson M, Lassere M, Craig JC, Scott JR. Recurrent pregnancy loss with antiphospholipid antibody: a systematic review of therapeutic trials. Obstet Gynecol 2002;99:135–44. doi: 10.1016/s0029-7844(01)01646-5 https://journals.lww.com/greenjournal/Fulltext/2002/01000/Recurrent_Pregnancy_Loss_With_Antiphospholipid.25.aspx

Miyakis S, Lockshin MD, Atsumi T, Branch DW, Brey RL, Cervera R, et al. International consensus statement on an update of the classification criteria for definite antiphospholipid syndrome (APS). J Thromb Haemost 2006;4:295–306. doi: 10.1111/j.1538-7836.2006.01753.x https://onlinelibrary.wiley.com/doi/10.1111/j.1538-7836.2006.01753.x

66 Recommended weight gain during pregnancy

A 28-year-old gravida 3, para 2, presents to your office at 28 weeks of gestation. Her prepregnancy body mass index (BMI) is 32. She lost weight during the first trimester, and although her weight has stabilized, her current BMI is 29. The most likely pregnancy complication associated with weight loss during pregnancy among women with obesity is

* (A) fetal growth restriction
(B) preeclampsia
(C) preterm labor
(D) preterm prelabor rupture of membranes
(E) stillbirth

Obesity, which is defined as having a BMI of 30 or greater, is increasingly prevalent worldwide. Obesity is the most common medical condition among pregnant women, affecting more than one-third of women of reproductive age. Prepregnancy BMI has been found to be a significant predictor of risk in pregnancy.

Obesity increases risks of pregnancy to the patient and her fetus. There is an increased risk of miscarriage and recurrent miscarriage among women with obesity. Additionally, there is increased risk of certain congenital anomalies, including neural tube defects, cardiovascular anomalies, cleft lip, and cleft palate. In addition to congenital anomalies, women with obesity are at risk of antenatal complications of pregnancy including preeclampsia, gestational diabetes mellitus, and stillbirth. The risk of stillbirth increases with increasing degree of obesity. A recent systematic review showed that the risk increases for each 5-unit increase in maternal BMI. Women with obesity also are at increased risk of indicated preterm birth, cesarean birth, and postpartum endometritis and wound complications. Finally, fetuses born to women with obesity are more likely to have macrosomia and childhood obesity. Some data also suggest that maternal obesity is associated with autism and developmental delay.

For these reasons, maternal weight should be optimized before pregnancy. Clinicians should assess patients' readiness for change and encourage them to achieve weight loss by surgical or nonsurgical methods. This can be facilitated with motivational interviewing and referral to medical weight loss programs. Even small weight reductions in women with obesity may improve pregnancy outcomes if achieved before pregnancy, and weight loss of 5–7% can significantly improve metabolic health.

In addition to prepregnancy BMI, gestational weight gain has been shown to have an important effect on pregnancy outcomes. The National Academy of Medicine (formerly Institute of Medicine) has published gestational weight gain guidelines that are based on prepregnancy BMI (Table 66-1). They recommend that women with a BMI of 26–29 gain 15–25 lb and that women with a BMI of 30 or greater gain 11–20 lb. Obstetricians can support patients by guiding them regarding appropriate gestational weight gain for pregnancy based on their prepregnancy BMI. Patients should be counseled regarding nutrition and exercise. Medication for weight loss or weight management should not be used during pregnancy. Studies have shown that the addition of metformin for pregnant patients with obesity does not improve pregnancy or birth outcomes, nor does it significantly affect gestational weight gain. Likewise, there are no data to suggest that education regarding a low-glycemic or low-calorie diet reduces the risk of excessive gestational weight gain.

The National Academy of Medicine does not delineate lower weight gain targets for women with more significant obesity. Some studies have suggested that, when women with obesity gain less than 11–20 lb, it may lead to decreased rates of cesarean birth, large-for-gestational-age newborns, gestational diabetes, preeclampsia, and postpartum weight retention. However, many studies also have demonstrated

TABLE 66-1. Recommendations for Weight Gain in Singleton Pregnancy

PREPREGNANCY WEIGHT CATEGORY	BMI	RECOMMENDED TOTAL WEIGHT GAIN IN PREGNANCY (LB)
Underweight	Less than 18.5	28–40
Normal weight	18.5–24.9	25–35
Overweight	25–29.9	15–25
Obese (includes all classes)	30 and greater	11–20

Data from Institute of Medicine, National Research Council. Weight gain during pregnancy: reexamining the guidelines. National Academies Press; 2009. Accessed March 31, 2022. https://nap.nationalacademies.org/catalog/12584/weight-gain-during-pregnancy-reexamining-the-guidelines some risks of inadequate weight gain. One study from the Pregnancy Nutrition Surveillance System suggested that women with inadequate weight gain regardless of BMI are more likely to have fetuses that are growth restricted or neonates that are small for gestational age. These findings were confirmed in a recent systematic review. Additionally, other researchers have suggested that the National Academy of Medicine guidelines may be too restrictive for women with severe obesity, placing them at increased risk of preterm birth, small-for-gestational-age newborns, and even perinatal mortality if they gain only what is recommended by the guidelines. Overall, this evidence suggests that the relationship between prepregnancy BMI, gestational weight gain, and pregnancy outcomes is complex and may be mediated by individual risk factors.

Inadequate weight gain or even weight loss should not be encouraged for pregnant women with obesity given the lack of clear evidence of benefit at this time. For the described patient, the most commonly reported complication with weight loss or inadequate weight gain is fetal growth restriction. Preterm birth has been reported but much less commonly. Inadequate gestational weight gain may be associated with decreased rates of preeclampsia and has not been shown to have an effect on prelabor rupture of membranes or stillbirth.

Beyerlein A, Lack N, von Kries R. Within-population average ranges compared with Institute of Medicine recommendations for gestational weight gain. Obstet Gynecol 2010;116:1111–8. doi: 10.1097/AOG.0b013e3181f1ad8b https://journals.lww.com/greenjournal/Fulltext/2010/11000/Within_Population_Average_Ranges_Compared_With.17.aspx

Catalano PM, Mele L, Landon MB, Ramin SM, Reddy UM, Casey B, et al. Inadequate weight gain in overweight and obese pregnant women: what is the effect on fetal growth? *Eunice Kennedy Shriver* National Institute of Child Health and Human Development Maternal-Fetal Medicine Units Network. Am J Obstet Gynecol 2014;211:137.e1–7. doi: 10.1016/j.ajog.2014.02.004 https://www.ajog.org/article/S0002-9378(14)00121-5/fulltext

Institute of Medicine, National Research Council. Weight gain during pregnancy: reexamining the guidelines. National Academies Press; 2009. Accessed March 31, 2022. https://nap.nationalacademies.org/catalog/12584/weight-gain-during-pregnancy-reexamining-the-guidelines

Kapadia MZ, Park CK, Beyene J, Giglia L, Maxwell C, McDonald SD. Weight loss instead of weight gain within the guidelines in obese women during pregnancy: a systematic review and meta-analyses of maternal and infant outcomes. PLoS One 2015;10:e0132650. doi: 10.17226/12584 https://journals.plos.org/plosone/article?id=10.1371/journal.pone.0132650

Obesity in pregnancy. ACOG Practice Bulletin No. 230. American College of Obstetricians and Gynecologists. Obstet Gynecol 2021;137:e128–44. doi: 10.1097/AOG.0000000000004395 https://journals.lww.com/greenjournal/Fulltext/2021/06000/Obesity_in_Pregnancy__ACOG_Practice_Bulletin,.38.aspx

Weight gain during pregnancy. ACOG Committee Opinion No. 548. American College of Obstetricians and Gynecologists. Obstet Gynecol 2013;121:210–2. doi: 10.1097/01.aog.0000425668.87506.4c https://journals.lww.com/greenjournal/Fulltext/2013/01000/Committee_Opinion_No__548__Weight_Gain_During.47.aspx

67 Obstetric changes in physiology

A 33-year-old patient at 29 weeks of gestation presents with burning with urination and fever. Her temperature is 39.4 °C (103 °F), pulse is 115 beats per minute, and respiratory rate is 22 respirations per minute. Her pulse oximetry is 97%, and her urine output is adequate. She has costovertebral angle tenderness, bibasilar rales, and diffuse diaphoresis. The finding in this patient that most strongly indicates a potential need for intensive care support is the

* (A) bibasilar rales
(B) diaphoresis
(C) pyrexia
(D) tachycardia
(E) tachypnea

Pulmonary physiology alterations in pregnancy include physical and functional changes. Estrogen causes the mucosa of the upper respiratory tract to be hyperemic and edematous. High progesterone concentrations result in hyperventilation. The thoracic cage expands because of the chest circumference increasing by 5–7 cm and the subcostal angle increasing from 68 to 103 degrees. The diaphragm lifts by 4 cm, reducing the total lung capacity by 5%. Inspiratory reserve and vital capacity increase from the first to the third trimester. Expiratory reserve volume remains approximately the same. Residual volume decreases slightly (from 1.2 to 1.0 L) by the third trimester. Despite the variation in lung volume and chest mechanics, the respiratory muscles do not change, and spirometry measurements in pregnancy remain the same (specifically FEV_1 [forced expiratory volume in 1 second]). Therefore, peak flow meter readings are unchanged and may be used to diagnose or monitor respiratory illnesses. Pregnancy also results in increased minute ventilation and oxygen consumption. Functional residual capacity decreases by 35%, and arterial Pco_2 (necessary for the placental CO_2 gradient between fetus and mother) and serum bicarbonate also decrease. The compensatory respiratory alkalosis and decreased buffering capacity contribute to the rapid decrease in Pao_2 in a hypoxic state. These physiologic changes form the basis for a different decompensation of pulmonary function in pregnant individuals compared with nonpregnant individuals.

Pyelonephritis, maternal varicella, influenza, and COVID-19 all increase the risk of a nonspecific pulmonary response of inflammation, greater vascular permeability, and decreased aerated lung units resulting in hypoxemia. The described patient has pyelonephritis. Eighty percent of cases of pyelonephritis occur after 20 weeks of gestation, and complications include sepsis (49%), acute respiratory distress syndrome (ARDS) (47%), acute renal injury (10%), and renal abscess (6%).

The five physical examination measurements consistent with sepsis are as follows:

- Systolic blood pressure, less than 90 or greater than 160 mm Hg, and diastolic blood pressure, greater than 100 mm Hg
- Heart rate, less than 50 or greater than 120 beats per minute
- Respiratory rate, less than 10 or greater than 30 breaths per minute
- Oxygen saturation on room air, less than 95%
- Oliguria, less than 35 mL/h for more than 2 hours

Confusion, agitation, or unresponsiveness increase the suspicion of sepsis. Each physical examination finding, taken separately, has a broad range of reversible and treatable causes. Individually, diaphoresis is a nonspecific finding and alone would not merit admission to the intensive care unit (ICU). Similarly, an isolated maternal heart rate of 115 beats per minute warrants evaluation; however, as a singular vital sign, it does not warrant ICU care. The heart rate will increase in pregnancy about 17% from the nonpregnant state. Pyrexia is not a physiologic response to pregnancy and is concerning for infection. Maternal respiratory rate increases above the nonpregnant state and alone warrants evaluation, not ICU care. Bibasilar rales are consistent with compromise of pulmonary lung function, which may potentially require ventilatory support in a critical care unit. A reported 38% of people with pyelonephritis and concomitant ARDS will require ventilatory support. The bibasilar rales noted in this scenario are most concerning for cardiac or pulmonary decompensation. Rales or crackles are adventitious lung sounds occurring when air passes over retained airway secretions or the opening of a collapsed airway—they are not a result of the physiologic changes of pregnancy. The presence of rales on examination increases the possibility of decompensation and need for additional pulmonary support to maintain maternal oxygenation. Taken as an individual finding, bibasilar rales are the most urgent of the five objective findings for sepsis and ARDS requiring intensive care admission.

There is no single diagnostic test to determine whether an individual, pregnant or not, is in sepsis. The current clinical approach is timely suspicion, initiation of antibiotic therapy, and fluid resuscitation in the first hour of care. Maternal fever may not be present, site cultures may be negative, and no clear source may be immediately apparent in a patient with sepsis. In addition, the physiologic changes in pregnancy and immediately postpartum add complexity to critical care, necessitating interpretation by the obstetrician. Specifically, these changes include dilutional anemia, increased circulation demands during cardiopulmonary resuscitation, increased third spacing, more difficult intubation, decreased buffering capacity, increased risk of aspiration, and decreased uterine perfusion with decreases in maternal blood pressure.

In a 2020 review of pyelonephritis in pregnancy, the approximate incidence was 2.5% (14 per 1,000 deliveries), which is 10-fold higher than the incidence in the nonpregnant population. When the diagnosis of pyelonephritis was delayed and aggressive therapy was not started, maternal respiratory distress requiring ventilation occurred. Additional maternal complications included sepsis, anemia, and renal compromise. Primary varicella zoster, influenza, and COVID-19 also increase the risk of developing ARDS in pregnancy. Sepsis and ARDS often are seen together. In 2012, an international expert panel developed the Berlin definition of ARDS, which is endorsed by the American Thoracic Society and the Society of Critical Care Medicine. The Berlin definition is a combination of clinical and physiologic features of ARDS:

- Respiratory failure within 1 week of clinical insult or new symptoms
- Degree of hypoxemia (mild: Pao_2/Fio_2, greater than 200 to 300 mm Hg with PEEP [positive end expiratory pressure] or CPAP [continuous positive airway pressure] greater than or equal to 5 cm H_2O; moderate: Pao_2/Fio_2, greater than 100 to 200 mm Hg; severe: Pao_2/Fio_2, less than or equal to 100 mm Hg)
- Pulmonary edema (nonhydrostatic origin)
- Radiographic findings (bilateral opacities not explained by effusions or nodularities)

Currently, there are no biomarkers for ARDS. Lung-protective ventilation support is the mainstay of treatment for ARDS with a decreased $Paco_2$ preferred to maintain maternal tidal volumes and plateau pressures. The physiologic changes affecting resuscitation are listed in Table 67-1. If maternal pulmonary function is severely compromised, mild hypercapnia (50–60 mm Hg) is acceptable in pregnancy to minimize hyperinflation and to reduce end-exhalation atelectasis. A pulmonary artery CO_2 level of greater than 60 mm Hg decreases uterine blood flow and increases fetal intracranial pressure and is not recommended. Plateau pressures are limited by the gravid uterus. A high PEEP decreases preload and cardiac output in an individual who is not pregnant; however, if PEEP beyond 10 mm Hg is required to optimize maternal status, it can be done with maternal and fetal continuous monitoring. Newer potential therapies include extracorporeal CO_2 removal, lung recruitment maneuvers, and high-frequency oscillatory ventilation. Intensive care support is recommended for treatment of ARDS in pregnancy.

TABLE 67-1. Physiologic Changes of Pregnancy That Affect Resuscitation

	CARDIOVASCULAR	**EFFECT**
Increased	Plasma volume by 40–50%, but erythrocyte volume by only 20%	Dilutional anemia results in decreased oxygen-carrying capacity
	Cardiac output by 40%	Increased CPR circulation demands
	Heart rate by 15–20 beats per min	Increased CPR circulation demands
	Clotting factors susceptible to thromboembolism	
	Dextrorotation of the heart	Increased EKG left axis deviation
	Estrogen effect on myocardial receptors	Supraventricular arrhythmias
Decreased	Supine blood pressure and venous return with aortocaval compression	Decreases cardiac output by 30%
	Arterial blood pressure by 10–15 mm Hg	Susceptible to cardiovascular insult
	Systemic vascular resistance	Sequesters blood during CPR
	Colloid oncotic pressure (COP)	Susceptible to third spacing
	Pulmonary capillary wedge pressure (PCWP)	Susceptible to pulmonary edema
	RESPIRATORY	**EFFECT**
Increased	Respiratory rate (progesterone-mediated)	Decreased buffering capacity
	Oxygen consumption by 20%	Rapid decrease of Pao_2 in hypoxia
	Tidal volume (progesterone-mediated)	Decreased buffering capacity
	Minute ventilation	Compensated respiratory alkalosis
	Laryngeal angle	Failed intubation
	Pharyngeal edema	Failed intubation
	Nasal edema	Difficult nasal intubation
Decreased	Functional residual capacity by 25%	Decreases ventilatory capacity
	Arterial Pco_2	Decreases buffering capacity
	Serum bicarbonate	Compensated respiratory alkalosis
	GASTROINTESTINAL	**EFFECT**
Increased	Intestinal compartmentalization	Susceptible to penetrating injury
Decreased	Peristalsis, gastric motility	Aspiration of gastric contents
	Gastroesophageal sphincter tone	Aspiration of gastric contents
	UTEROPLACENTAL	**EFFECT**
Increased	Uteroplacental blood flow by 30% of cardiac output	Sequesters blood in CPR
	Aortocaval compression	Decreases cardiac output by 30%
	Elevation of diaphragm by 4–7 cm	Aspiration of gastric contents
Decreased	Autoregulation of blood pressure	Uterine perfusion decreases with drop in maternal blood pressure
	BREAST	**EFFECT**
Decreased	Chest wall compliance secondary to breast hypertrophy	Requires increased CPR compression force
	RENAL/URINARY	**EFFECT**
Increased	Compensated respiratory alkalosis	Decreases buffering capacity and increases acidosis during CPR
	Ureteral dilation, especially right side	Interpretation of radiographs
Decreased	Bladder emptying	Interpretation of radiographs

Abbreviations: CPR, cardiopulmonary resuscitation; EKG, electrocardiogram.

Modified from Critical care in pregnancy. ACOG Practice Bulletin No. 211. American College of Obstetricians and Gynecologists. Obstet Gynecol 2019;133:e303–19. doi: 10.1097/AOG.0000000000003241 https://journals.lww.com/greenjournal/Fulltext/2019/05000/ACOG_Practice_Bulletin_No__211__Critical_Care_in.39.aspx

Critical care in pregnancy. ACOG Practice Bulletin No. 211. American College of Obstetricians and Gynecologists. Obstet Gynecol 2019;133:e303–19. doi: 10.1097/AOG.0000000000003241 https://journals.lww.com/greenjournal/Fulltext/2019/05000/ACOG_Practice_Bulletin_No__211__Critical_Care_in.39.aspx

Fan E, Brodie D, Slutsky AS. Acute respiratory distress syndrome: advances in diagnosis and treatment. JAMA 2018;319:698–710. doi: 10.1001/jama.2017.21907 https://jamanetwork.com/journals/jama/fullarticle/2673154

Grette K, Cassity S, Holliday N, Rimawi BH. Acute pyelonephritis during pregnancy: a systematic review of the aetiology, timing, and reported adverse perinatal risks during pregnancy. J Obstet Gynaecol 2020;40:739–48. doi: 10.1080/01443615.2019.1647524 https://www.tandfonline.com/doi/abs/10.1080/01443615.2019.1647524

Landon M, Galan H, Jauniaux E, Driscoll D, Berghella V, Grobman W, et al, editors. Gabbe's obstetrics: normal and problem pregnancies. 8th ed. Elsevier; 2020.

Neligan PJ, Laffey JG. Clinical review: special populations--critical illness and pregnancy. Crit Care 2011;15:227. doi: 10.1186/cc10256 https://ccforum.biomedcentral.com/articles/10.1186/cc10256

Snyder CC, Barton JR, Habli M, Sibai BM. Severe sepsis and septic shock in pregnancy: indications for delivery and maternal and perinatal outcomes. J Matern Fetal Neonatal Med 2013;26:503–6. doi: 10.3109/14767058.2012.739221 https://www.tandfonline.com/doi/abs/10.3109/14767058.2012.739221

Tolcher MC, McKinney JR, Eppes CS, Muigai D, Shamshirsaz A, Guntupalli KK, et al. Prone positioning for pregnant women with hypoxemia due to coronavirus disease 2019 (COVID-19). Obstet Gynecol 2020;136:259–61. doi: 10.1097/AOG.0000000000004012 https://journals.lww.com/greenjournal/Fulltext/2020/08000/Prone_Positioning_for_Pregnant_Women_With.7.aspx

68 Enhanced recovery after surgery

A gravida 2, para 1, at 36 weeks of gestation presents for her preoperative history and physical examination for her second cesarean birth. She experienced significant nausea and vomiting with her first birth. You discuss preoperative and postoperative strategies to reduce nausea. In the preoperative anesthesia care unit, she is given a scopolamine patch and ondansetron. In the operating room, after placement of a spinal anesthetic, she experiences increased nausea and hypotension. The best next intraoperative medication to treat her nausea is a

(A) dopamine antagonist
(B) gamma-aminobutyric acid analog
(C) glucocorticoid
(D) serotonin antagonist
* (E) vasopressor

Enhanced Recovery After Surgery (ERAS) programs recommend standard interventions to support and maintain normal physiology, thereby optimizing surgical outcomes and reducing health system costs. The targeted outcomes of ERAS protocols include shorter length of stay, reduced reliance on narcotics, decreased postoperative pain, a more rapid return to normal bowel function, increased patient satisfaction, and reduced readmission rates. Enhanced recovery systems are dynamic, require periodic assessment, and thrive in a multidisciplinary, growth-oriented culture in which continued quality improvement is the normal state. The general elements of an ERAS program include preprocedural counseling with expectation management, limited preprocedural fasting, regional anesthesia when appropriate, early mobilization, nonopioid combined with limited opioid analgesia, maintenance of fluid balance, normothermia, and thromboprophylaxis (Table 68-1). General success and positive outcomes using the ERAS approach in surgery have led to the development of the Enhanced Recovery After Cesarean program, which includes consideration of neonatal and maternal outcomes.

Cesarean births accounted for 31.8% of the 3,605,201 births in the United States in 2020. A 2020 study summarized the current evidence supporting standardization of the cesarean technique (Box 68-1) using surgical bundles specifically to reduce surgical site infection. Current evidence supports avoiding spinal-induced hypotension to prevent intraoperative nausea and vomiting. In addition, implementation of multimodal anesthesia, early mobilization, and narrow glycemic control are recommended.

Hypotension after spinal placement has maternal and fetal effects. It is a common cause of maternal intraoperative nausea and vomiting. Fetal perfusion is decreased with a rapid decrease in maternal mean arterial pressure and hypotension. Beginning an infusion of a direct alpha vasopressor (phenylephrine or norepinephrine) immediately after placement of the spinal medications and co-loading with a 1-L crystalloid bolus has been shown to improve maternal nausea and vomiting and maintain placental blood flow reflected in a higher fetal umbilical artery pH. An infusion of phenylephrine is the best next intraoperative medication to minimize this patient's nausea and respond to her hypotension.

Additional interventions to minimize nausea and vomiting include avoidance of uterine exteriorization, elimination of intra-abdominal saline irrigation, and multimodal antiemetic medication. Exteriorization of the uterus has been studied with 17 randomized controlled trials or systematic reviews, and although it has been shown to reduce blood loss, repair in situ reduces nausea and vomiting and facilitates a faster return of bowel function. Intra-abdominal saline irrigation

TABLE 68-1. Components of Cesarean-Section Enhanced Recovery After Surgery

GOAL	TIMING OF INTERVENTION		
	PREOPERATIVE	INTRAOPERATIVE	POSTOPERATIVE
Expectation management and planning	Patient education		Patient education
Dietary and fluid management	Limit fasting interval, clears until 2 h prior	Maintain fluid balance	Early oral intake of clears within 1 h, solid foods at 6 h
	Nonparticulate liquid carbohydrate loading until NPO	Prevention and management of nausea and vomiting	
Infection risk reduction	Chlorohexidine bathing the day before and morning of surgery	Antibiotic prophylaxis	Glycemic control
Neonatal health	Preparation for lactation and breastfeeding	Delayed cord clamping	Breastfeeding support
		Breastfeeding and initiation of skin-to-skin contact	
Hemorrhage risk reduction	Hemoglobin optimization	Maintain euthermia with goal to maintain temperature at 36 °C	Treatment of anemia
		Uterotonic administration	
Pain control	Acetaminophen orally	Multimodal analgesia, consideration of transabdominus plane block (TAP)	Multimodal analgesia and minimization of opioid use
		Prevent and treat hypotension secondary to spinal anesthesia	
Venous thromboembolism risk reduction		Venous thromboembolism prophylaxis	Early removal of urinary catheter
			Ambulation within 6 h
			Timely discharge to home

Data from Perioperative pathways: enhanced recovery after surgery. ACOG Committee Opinion No. 750. American College of Obstetricians and Gynecologists [published errata appear in Obstet Gynecol 2019;133:1288; Obstet Gynecol 2019;134:1121]. Obstet Gynecol 2018;132:e120–30. doi: 10.1097/AOG.0000000000002818 https://journals.lww.com/greenjournal/Fulltext/2018/09000/ACOG_Committee_Opinion_No__750__Perioperative.68.aspx

BOX 68-1

Recommended Standardized Cesarean Birth Surgical Technique

- Transverse skin incision 2–3 cm above the pubic symphysis
- Sharp cutaneous and fascia dissection
- Blunt subcutaneous and fascia expansion with the omission of superior and inferior fascia dissection
- Blunt peritoneal entry
- Omit bladder flap development
- Sharp 2- to 3-cm transverse uterine incision with blunt entry and cephalad–caudad expansion
- Spontaneous placenta removal
- Perform intrauterine wiping only when placental membranes are seen
- Omit routine cervical dilatation
- Uterine exteriorization during repair to minimize blood loss
- Single-layer uterine closure
- Omit intra-abdominal irrigation, peritoneal closure, rectus muscle approximation, routine glove change
- Continuous fascia closure with delayed absorbable suture
- Perform subcutaneous tissue irrigation
- Subcutaneous tissue closure if 2-cm depth or greater
- Skin closure with subcuticular, absorbable monofilament suture

Adapted from Dahlke JD, Mendez-Figueroa H, Maggio L, Sperling JD, Chauhan SP, Rouse DJ. The case for standardizing cesarean delivery technique: seeing the forest for the trees. Obstet Gynecol 2020;136:972-80. doi: 10.1097/AOG.0000000000004120.

has been shown to increase intraoperative and postoperative nausea and vomiting without reducing the rate of infection. The multimodal approach to intraoperative and postoperative nausea and vomiting includes dopamine antagonists (metoclopramide or droperidol), a glucocorticoid (dexamethasone), and a serotonin receptor antagonist (ondansetron). The combination of dexamethasone and ondansetron is more effective than ondansetron alone. The combination of metoclopramide and tropisetron has been proved highly effective. A single agent approach is not recommended. Lastly, a gamma-aminobutyric acid analog (gabapentin) has not been shown to significantly affect nausea and vomiting and would not be indicated.

Bollag L, Lim G, Sultan P, Habib AS, Landau R, Zakowski M, et al. Consensus statement and recommendations for enhanced recovery after cesarean. Society for Obstetric Anesthesia and Perinatology. Anesth Analg 2021;132:1362–77. doi: 10.1213/ANE.0000000000005257 https://journals.lww.com/anesthesia-analgesia/Abstract/2021/05000/Society_for_Obstetric_Anesthesia_and_Perinatology_.25.aspx

Dahlke JD, Mendez-Figueroa H, Maggio L, Sperling JD, Chauhan SP, Rouse DJ. The case for standardizing cesarean delivery technique: seeing the forest for the trees. Obstet Gynecol 2020;136:972–80. doi: 10.1097/AOG.0000000000004120 https://journals.lww.com/greenjournal/Fulltext/2020/11000/The_Case_for_Standardizing_Cesarean_Delivery.17.aspx

Macones GA, Caughey AB, Wood SL, Wrench IJ, Huang J, Norman M, et al. Guidelines for postoperative care in cesarean delivery: Enhanced Recovery After Surgery (ERAS) Society recommendations (part 3). Am J Obstet Gynecol 2019;221:247.e1–9. doi: 0.1016/j.ajog.2019.04.012 https://www.ajog.org/article/S0002-9378(19)30572-1/fulltext

Perioperative pathways: enhanced recovery after surgery. ACOG Committee Opinion No. 750. American College of Obstetricians and Gynecologists [published errata appear in Obstet Gynecol 2019;133:1288; Obstet Gynecol 2019;134:1121]. Obstet Gynecol 2018;132:e120–30. doi: 10.1097/AOG.0000000000002818 https://journals.lww.com/greenjournal/Fulltext/2018/09000/ACOG_Committee_Opinion_No__750__Perioperative.68.aspx

69 Pneumonia in pregnancy

A 22-year-old primipara at 32 weeks of gestation presents with shortness of breath, fever, and cough. She has had no prenatal care. Her history reveals limited access to preventive medicine, and this visit is her first interaction with the health care system. She reports fever and malaise starting 1 week ago, followed by development of a widespread pruritic, vesicular, and painful rash (Fig. 69-1). Her COVID-19 test is negative, and a chest radiograph reveals diffuse bilateral infiltrates. The best next step in her treatment is to administer

* (A) acyclovir
(B) azithromycin
(C) ceftriaxone
(D) isoniazid
(E) oseltamivir

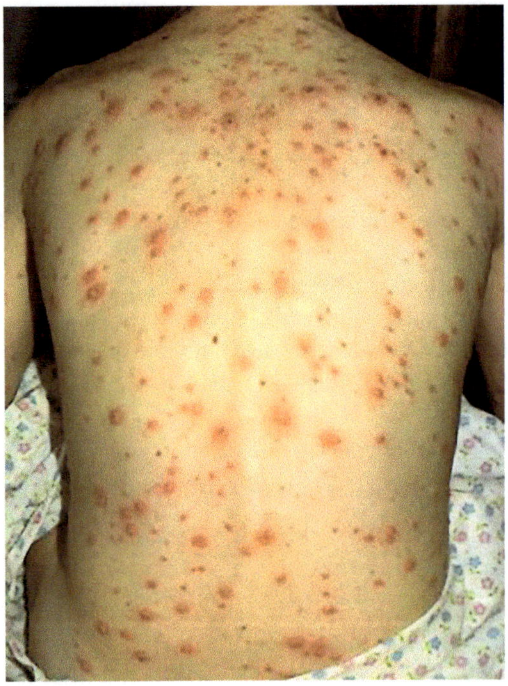

FIGURE 69-1. Varicella rash. (Reproduced with permission from American Academy of Pediatrics. Varicella-zoster virus infections. In: Kimberlin DW, Barnett ED, Lynfield R, Sawyer MH, editors. Red Book: 2021-2024 Report of the Committee on Infectious Diseases. 32nd ed. AAP; 2021. p. 831–43.)

Since the routine administration of varicella vaccine in 1995, varicella infection during pregnancy is rare. Varicella infections that occur during pregnancy are associated with maternal, fetal, and neonatal risks. Varicella is highly communicable. The virus enters the body through the respiratory tract and conjunctiva, and it replicates in the nasopharynx and regional lymph nodes. A primary viremia occurs 4–6 days after the initial infection, and many organs can be infected during the initial viremia. Secondary viremia then occurs and results in viral skin infection and lesions. Unvaccinated individuals typically have a generalized rash that starts on the trunk, scalp, or face. Adults can have up to 12 days of fever and malaise before the rash appears and are more likely to have higher complication rates than children. Serologic testing, with evaluation for increase in varicella immunoglobulin G, is a diagnosis option, but polymerase chain reaction for amplification of viral DNA obtained from scrapings of the skin lesion is the laboratory test of choice. The most common complication of varicella in adults is pneumonia, which often is viral but also may result from a bacterial superinfection.

Approximately 10–20% of pregnant individuals with varicella infection develop pneumonia. Pneumonia is diagnosed by chest radiograph findings of diffuse, patchy infiltrates or miliary or nodular infiltrates in the peribronchial region. Varicella pneumonia has a highly variable course with severe illness leading to hypoxia and respiratory failure and should be promptly treated with acyclovir or valacyclovir to mitigate risks. Acyclovir and valacyclovir have similar efficacies. Varicella pneumonia predisposes women to risk of developing acute respiratory distress syndrome in pregnancy, which carries up to a 40% maternal mortality rate. Other potential maternal complications from varicella include central nervous system infection ranging from aseptic meningitis to encephalitis. Reye syndrome occurs with less frequency given the avoidance of aspirin with viral illnesses.

All pregnant women who are varicella naive (unvaccinated or without prior exposure) should be counseled on the risks of congenital varicella syndrome and instructed to avoid exposure. Primary maternal varicella infection occurring before 20 weeks of gestation can be associated with congenital anomalies, including limb hypoplasia, skin scarring, localized muscular atrophy, encephalitis, cortical atrophy, chorioretinitis, microcephaly, and low birth weight. Collectively, this constellation of abnormalities is known as *congenital varicella syndrome.* Congenital varicella is rare and estimated to occur at a rate of 1–2% among women with infection during pregnancy. For diagnosis of acute varicella infection in a naive pregnant woman, polymerase chain reaction testing is necessary.

Varicella infections occurring after 20 weeks of gestation have lower risk of congenital varicella but when close to delivery pose different risks. Varicella infections occurring near delivery, specifically maternal disease that develops from 5 days before delivery to 48 hours postpartum, carry the highest risk of neonatal varicella zoster virus (VZV) infection and are least likely to result in passive antibody protection for the neonate. Neonatal VZV infection carries a high risk of mortality for the immune-naive neonate in the absence of treatment. Pregnancy complicated by maternal varicella infection is rare given routine vaccination and the overall reduction in disease.

Anyone at risk of serious sequelae from varicella infection with a viral exposure should be given varicella zoster immune globulin. Varicella zoster immune globulin is a purified human immune globulin preparation containing high levels of anti-varicella antibodies and is recommended for use by the U.S. Advisory Committee on Immunization Practices as indicated in Box 69-1. Varicella zoster immune globulin should be given, usually as an intramuscular dose, within 4–10 days of exposure. Studies have shown that when immune globulin is given within the recommended window, it has greater than 90% reduction in VZV infection when studied over a 28-day period. When varicella immune globulin is used outside the optimal 4- to 10-day window after exposure, VZV infection prevention rates are unknown.

BOX 69-1

Indications for Varicella Zoster Immune Globulin for Postexposure Prophylaxis

- Pregnant women without evidence of immunity to varicella
- Neonates whose mothers have signs or symptoms of varicella at or around delivery (5 days before or 2 days after)
- Immunocompromised patients without evidence of immunity to varicella

The patient described in this scenario has VZV infection and likely varicella pneumonia. Limited access to preventive care (specifically vaccinations) and her symptom pattern (malaise, rash, and then cough and shortness of breath) are most consistent with varicella. The 10–20% chance that her illness will progress to pneumonia, along with her cough, shortness of breath, and patchy infiltrates seen on chest radiograph, make varicella pneumonia the most likely diagnosis. In this scenario, acyclovir is the best treatment for varicella pneumonia.

Other causes of pneumonia in pregnancy are similar to those in nonpregnant adults and include *Streptococcus pneumoniae*, *Haemophilius influenzae*, mycoplasma, chlamydia, viruses, legionella, *Staphylococcus aureus*, and gram-negative bacilli. Most of these organisms do not present with prodromal rash as in the scenario above. Pneumonia in pregnancy is associated with increased risk of sepsis, preterm labor and delivery, and pulmonary edema. Risk factors for pneumonia during pregnancy include anemia, asthma, tobacco use, drug use, and immunosuppression (either from therapy or from human immunodeficiency virus [HIV]). The symptoms of varicella pneumonia often include fever, pleuritic chest pain, shortness of breath, and productive cough, and a chest radiograph remains the first-line choice for diagnosis. Influenza should be considered anytime, but especially when it is active in the community. Many laboratories offer testing for respiratory viral pathogens in a comprehensive panel, with use typically reserved for hospitalized patients. Chest radiograph findings for viral pneumonia often reveal more diffuse reticular or reticulonodular opacities, whereas the presence of a lobar consolidation or interstitial infiltrates is seen with bacterial pneumonia.

Treatment options for pneumonia in pregnancy depend on the causative organism and severity of illness. Outpatient therapy for pregnant women with pneumonia often consists of amoxicillin or amoxicillin-clavulanate with azithromycin. Inpatient therapy for pregnant women with pneumonia includes a β-lactam (cephalosporin) plus azithromycin, but treatment may vary depending on the patient's allergies and other risk factors. Azithromycin usually would not be used alone in the treatment of community-acquired pneumonia given the need to provide antipneumococcal treatment with a β-lactam. Antiviral agents similarly are used according to the type of virus diagnosed. Oseltamivir is used to treat influenza infection or to prevent infection in postexposure prophylaxis. Acyclovir and valacyclovir are used for treatment of varicella pneumonia.

Isonaizid would be the treatment alone or in combination with other antitubercular agents in the case of latent tuberculosis infection in pregnancy. The decision to treat a pregnant patient with latent tuberculosis depends on whether the patient has recent exposure to active, untreated tuberculosis or recent infection, even in the setting of co-infection with HIV.

Brito V, Niederman MS. Pneumonia complicating pregnancy. Clin Chest Med 2011;32:121–32. doi: 10.1016/j.ccm.2010.10.004 https://www.sciencedirect.com/science/article/pii/S0272523110001267

Cytomegalovirus, parvovirus B19, varicella zoster, and toxoplasmosis in pregnancy. Practice Bulletin No. 151. American College of Obstetricians and Gynecologists [published errata appear in Obstet Gynecol 2016;127:405; Obstet Gynecol 2016;127:405]. Obstet Gynecol 2015;125:1510–25. doi: 10.1097/01.AOG.0000466430.19823.53 https://journals.lww.com/greenjournal/Fulltext/2015/06000/Practice_Bulletin_No__151__Cytomegalovirus,.54.aspx

Duchon JM, Levin MJ, Gershon AA. Safety and varicella outcomes in in utero-exposed newborns and preterm infants treated with varicella zoster immune globulin (VARIZIG): a subgroup analysis of an expanded-access program. J Pediatric Infect Dis Soc 2020;9:449–53. doi: 10.1093/jpids/piz070 https://academic.oup.com/jpids/article/9/4/449/5644533

Fortner KB, Nieuwoudt C, Reeder CF, Swamy GK. Infections in pregnancy and the role of vaccines. Obstet Gynecol Clin North Am 2018;45:369–88. doi: 10.1016/j.ogc.2018.01.006 https://www.sciencedirect.com/science/article/abs/pii/S0889854518300068

Lopez A, Harrington T, Marin M. Varicella. In: Hall E, Wodi AP, Hamborsky J, Morelli M, Schillie S, editors. Epidemiology and prevention of vaccine-preventable diseases. 14th ed. Centers for Disease Control and Prevention; Public Health Foundation; 2021. p. 329–48. Accessed February 11, 2022. https://www.cdc.gov/vaccines/pubs/pinkbook/varicella.html

Sheffield JS, Cunningham FG. Community-acquired pneumonia in pregnancy. Obstet Gynecol 2009;114:915–22. doi: 10.1097/AOG.0b013e3181b8e76d https://journals.lww.com/greenjournal/Fulltext/2009/10000/Community_Acquired_Pneumonia_in_Pregnancy.29.aspx

Updated recommendations for use of VariZIG—United States, 2013. Centers for Disease Control and Prevention (CDC). MMWR Morb Mortal Wkly Rep 2013;62:574–6. https://www.cdc.gov/mmwr/preview/mmwrhtml/mm6228a4.htm

70 Perinatal survival

A 28-year-old nulliparous patient at 22 0/7 weeks of gestation is diagnosed with preterm prelabor rupture of membranes (PPROM). Her due date was determined with first-trimester ultrasonography concordant with her last menstrual period. On examination, she is afebrile with a nontender fundus, is 2-cm dilated on speculum examination, and has a white blood cell count of 9,000. The patient and her wife are interested in pursuing potential obstetric interventions to optimize outcomes for the pregnancy. The most appropriate intervention at this gestational age is

(A) antenatal corticosteroids
* (B) antibiotics
(C) cesarean birth
(D) magnesium sulfate
(E) tocolytic

Managing obstetric care that may result in a periviable delivery is challenging. The clinical situation can change rapidly, and informed decision making is critical. Although available data about outcomes of *periviable birth*, defined as 20 0/7 to 25 6/7 weeks of gestation, are improving, significant variation exists. Outcomes vary by birth weight, neonatal gender, exposure to antenatal corticosteroids, and neonatal intensive care unit experience. Outcome statistics are separated by "survival of the newborn" (newborns alive at discharge from the neonatal intensive care unit) compared with "intact survival" (survival without neurodevelopmental impairment). The survival of the newborn with and without neurodevelopmental impairment also varies by institution. An in-depth review of data from the *Eunice Kennedy Shriver* National Institute of Child Health and Human Development (NICHD) reveals that despite improvements over time, the incidence of death, neurodevelopmental impairment, and adverse outcomes remains high among extremely premature infants.

Discussion and counseling with the patient and the family should include literacy-appropriate information about short-term and long-term outcomes. Modifiable factors are location of delivery and level of intervention, but many factors affecting outcomes are not modifiable, including maternal comorbidities, fetal sex, birth weight, and the presence of a singleton versus a multiple gestation. Options available to the patient and family may include monitoring during labor, intervention with cesarean birth, administration of antenatal corticosteroids or magnesium sulfate, life-sustaining interventions, and postnatal management (Appendix E).

Administration of antibiotics to prolong the latency following PPROM poses the most appropriate intervention at 22 weeks of gestation in a well-dated pregnancy. There are reproducible data affirming the use of antibiotics to prolong latency after PPROM.

A prediction tool has been created by the NICHD Neonatal Research Network to estimate outcomes among newborns delivered between 22 and 25 weeks of gestation. This prediction tool is based on currently available data from several large cohorts (Vermont Oxford Network and NICHD Neonatal Research Network) and is intended to be used only as an estimate of possible outcomes. Because the tool is not individualized, it is not known if its use improves patient-centered outcomes.

The American College of Obstetricians and Gynecologists' Obstetric Care Consensus No. 6, "Periviable Birth," provides a summary of recommendations regarding potential interventions by week of gestation that are listed in Appendix E.

Antenatal corticosteroids given when preterm delivery appears imminent has been demonstrated as one of the most important antenatal therapies that improves neonatal outcomes. Antenatal corticosteroids decrease the risk of neonatal death, intraventricular hemorrhage, periventricular leukomalacia, and necrotizing enterocolitis among infants at 23–25 weeks of gestation. However, these benefits do not appear to be sustained with a decreased number of weeks of gestation. Specifically, in recent data, no differences were seen in the outcome of neonates born at 22 weeks of gestation who received antenatal care corticosteroids compared with those who did not.

Tocolytics for preterm labor, at least for the benefit of corticosteroid administration, have been shown to be effective starting at around 26 weeks of gestation through late-preterm gestation. Although delaying delivery for administration of antenatal corticosteroids improves neonatal outcomes after 26 weeks of gestation, the data demonstrating improvement in outcomes at periviable gestational ages have not consistently shown benefit.

Administration of magnesium sulfate for neuroprotection has been shown to decrease the risk of adverse neurologic outcomes among preterm newborns when given between 24 and 30 weeks of gestation. Specifically, when magnesium sulfate is administered before delivery at 30 weeks of gestation or less, reduced incidence of cerebral palsy without an increase in risk of mortality is seen. Five randomized controlled trials evaluating magnesium sulfate have started enrollment with 24 weeks of gestation, and thus specific data extrapolated to earlier periviable gestational ages are not available at this time (Appendix E).

The administration of antibiotics to prolong latency in the setting of PPROM has been shown to be effective at prolonging pregnancy and reducing newborn infections. As with other demonstrated treatments in association with preterm birth, specific guidance for antibiotic use is limited, but no adverse outcomes are reported. Given demonstrated benefit of antibiotics among women with PPROM, lack of specific data guiding management at periviable gestations, and no demonstration of harm, the administration of antibiotics can be considered following shared decision making. In contrast, antibiotic treatment of women with preterm labor and advanced cervical dilation with intact fetal membranes has not been shown to prolong the pregnancy.

Cesarean birth for fetal indications is associated with potential benefit for the fetus, especially in cases of malpresentation or decreased tolerance of labor. Preterm deliveries often require classical uterine hysterotomy, which is associated with increased maternal blood loss and perioperative morbidities, and prompts the recommendation for delivery by repeat cesarean in all subsequent pregnancies. Compounding upon consequences of the initial classical cesarean birth, increasing maternal morbidity is noted among higher-order cesarean births. Actual benefit to the fetus should be balanced with maternal risk, especially with regard to expected neonatal survival rates when considering cesarean birth at periviable gestational ages.

Periviable birth. Obstetric Care Consensus No. 6. American College of Obstetricians and Gynecologists. Obstet Gynecol 2017;130:e187–99. doi: 10.1097/AOG.0000000000002352 https://journals.lww.com/greenjournal/Fulltext/2017/10000/Obstetric_Care_Consensus_No__6__Periviable_Birth.57.aspx

Rysavy MA, Horbar JD, Bell EF, Li L, Greenberg LT, Tyson JE, et al. Assessment of an updated neonatal research network extremely preterm birth outcome model in the Vermont Oxford Network. *Eunice Kennedy Shriver* National Institute of Child Health and Human Development Neonatal Research Network and Vermont Oxford Network. JAMA Pediatr 2020;174:e196294. doi: 10.1001/jamapediatrics.2019.6294 https://jamanetwork.com/journals/jamapediatrics/fullarticle/2761306

Younge N, Goldstein RF, Bann CM, Hintz SR, Patel RM, Smith PB, et al. Survival and neurodevelopmental outcomes among periviable infants. Eunice Kennedy Shriver National Institute of Child Health and Human Development Neonatal Research Network. N Engl J Med 2017;376:617–28. doi: 10.1056/NEJMoa1605566 https://www.nejm.org/doi/10.1056/NEJMoa1605566

71 Neonatal encephalopathy

A 32-year-old gravida 2, para 1, presents in spontaneous labor at 40 weeks of gestation. She has a history of one prior cesarean birth. She is treated with antibiotics for chorioamnionitis. She develops a persistent Category II fetal heart rate tracing unresponsive to resuscitative measures. She undergoes a repeat cesarean birth. At the time of delivery, a uterine rupture is identified. Apgar scores are 3 and 7 at 1 and 5 minutes, respectively. The umbilical cord arterial pH is 6.9 with a base excess of 11 mmol/L. The neonate is subsequently diagnosed with neonatal encephalopathy. The finding most associated with an intrapartum cause of hypoxic ischemic encephalopathy is

(A) Apgar score of 7 at 5 minutes
(B) Category II fetal heart rate tracing
(C) chorioamnionitis
* (D) umbilical arterial cord pH of 6.9

Neonatal encephalopathy refers to a clinical syndrome of neurologic dysfunction manifesting in the earliest days of life in a neonate born at 35 weeks of gestation or later. It is defined by the presence of an abnormal level of consciousness or incidence of seizures, difficulty maintaining respiration, and depression of reflexes or tone. To determine whether neonatal encephalopathy occurred as a result of intrapartum events due to acute hypoxia-ischemia, several factors must be considered. An assessment should include maternal history, obstetric complications, intrapartum events, including fetal heart tracing and delivery complications, and placental pathology. Findings consistent with an intrapartum cause of neonatal encephalopathy include Apgar score less than 5 at both 5 and 10 minutes, umbilical artery acidemia with pH less than 7.0 (such as in the described case) or base deficit 12 mmol/L or greater, neuroimaging with evidence of acute brain injury consistent with hypoxia-ischemia, multisystem organ failure, and cerebral palsy of the spastic quadriplegic or dyskinetic type.

An umbilical artery pH of less than 7.0 or base deficit 12 mmol/L or greater increases the probability that neonatal encephalopathy had an intrapartum origin. The risk of neonatal encephalopathy increases with worsening fetal acidemia, as evidenced by decreasing pH. That said, most newborns with acidemia, even those with significant acidosis, will be neurologically normal.

Acute obstetric emergencies, such as uterine rupture, umbilical cord prolapse, massive placental abruption, or bleeding vasa previa, are associated with the highest risk of neonatal encephalopathy due to a peripartum event. In these conditions, the fetus is acutely deprived of blood flow and oxygen, sometimes for a prolonged period. Uterine rupture is a rare complication, occurring most commonly after a trial of labor in the setting of prior cesarean birth. Acute obstetric emergencies account for approximately 12% of cases of neonatal encephalopathy that require neonatal therapeutic hypothermia.

Low Apgar scores are associated with an increased risk of neonatal encephalopathy. The lower the Apgar score, the higher the risk of cerebral palsy. However, most infants born with low Apgar scores will not develop cerebral palsy. There are many causes for low Apgar scores. Low Apgar scores at 10, 15, or 20 minutes appear to be better predictors of cerebral palsy than low scores at 1 and 5 minutes. This is probably because persistent low Apgar scores after several minutes likely indicate a failure to respond to initial resuscitation and a higher risk of adverse outcome. If the Apgar score is 7 or greater at 5 minutes, it is unlikely that an intrapartum hypoxic-ischemic event played a major role in causing neonatal encephalopathy.

Category II fetal heart tracings are indeterminate and require further evaluation with intervention dependent on the clinical scenario. Electronic fetal monitoring was designed to prevent perinatal asphyxia, but rates of cerebral palsy have not changed since its introduction. It is important to evaluate and document fetal status upon initial presentation. For instance, a fetus that presents in a Category I pattern and then progresses to a Category III during labor may be associated with an intrapartum hypoxic-ischemic event. However, when a fetus presents in a Category II pattern and is found to be compromised at birth, it is suggestive that the compromise occurred before admission. Of the listed factors, a Category II tracing alone is not the most suggestive of an intrapartum event.

Chorioamnionitis (or intra-amniotic infection) is associated with an increased risk of neonatal encephalopathy (odds ratio [OR], 3.2; 95% CI, 1.9–5.3). However, most neonates born to women with chorioamnionitis, particularly those at term (such as the described patient) will not be encephalopathic. Of the risk factors listed, acute obstetric emergencies represent a much stronger risk. In a retrospective cohort study examining obstetric antecedents to infant whole-body cooling, catastrophic events including umbilical cord prolapse (OR, 14; 95% CI, 3–72), placental abruption (OR, 17; 95% CI, 7–44), and uterine rupture (OR, 130; 95% CI, 11–1,477) were the strongest risk factors.

American College of Obstetricians and Gynecologists, American Academy of Pediatrics. Neonatal encephalopathy and neurologic outcome. 2nd ed. ACOG; AAP; 2014. https://www.acog.org/clinical/clinical-guidance/task-force-report/articles/2014/neonatal-encephalopathy-and-neurologic-outcome

Herrera CA, Silver RM. Perinatal asphyxia from the obstetric standpoint: diagnosis and interventions. Clin Perinatol 2016;43:423–38. doi: 10.1016/j.clp.2016.04.003 https://www.sciencedirect.com/science/article/abs/pii/S0095510816300288

Nelson DB, Lucke AM, McIntire DD, Sánchez PJ, Leveno KJ, Chalak LF. Obstetric antecedents to body-cooling treatment of the newborn infant. Am J Obstet Gynecol 2014;211:155.e1–6. doi: 10.1016/j.ajog.2014.02.013 https://www.ajog.org/article/S0002-9378(14)00155-0/fulltext

72 Evaluation for thyroid disorders in pregnancy

A 35-year-old woman presents for a prenatal visit at 10 weeks of gestation. She requests a thyroid-stimulating hormone (TSH) test because of her family history of thyroid disease. Her TSH concentration is 4.3 mU/L and free thyroxine (T_4) is 0.9 ng/dL. Based on the laboratory results, the best next step in management is to

(A) initiate levothyroxine
(B) measure thyroid antibodies
(C) measure total triiodothyronine
* (D) reassure the patient
(E) repeat thyroid function tests in the second trimester

The described patient has an elevated TSH concentration and normal T_4 level. This is consistent with the diagnosis of subclinical hypothyroidism (Fig. 72-1). The treatment of subclinical hypothyroidism has not been shown to improve pregnancy outcomes nor neurocognitive function in the offspring and is not recommended. The Maternal–Fetal Medicine Units Networks' Randomized Trial of Thyroxine Therapy for Subclinical Hypothyroidism or Hypothyroxinemia Diagnosed

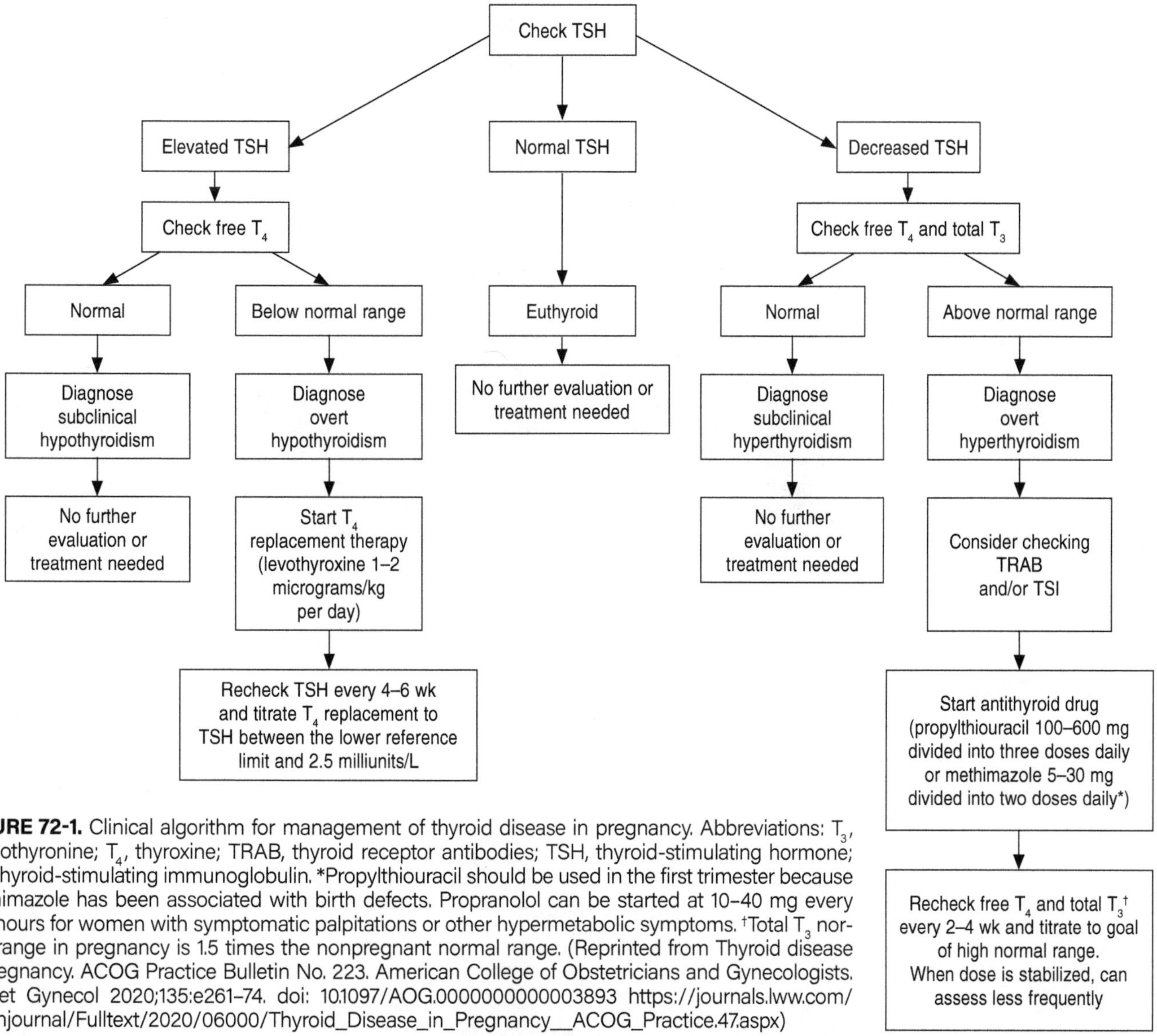

FIGURE 72-1. Clinical algorithm for management of thyroid disease in pregnancy. Abbreviations: T_3, triiodothyronine; T_4, thyroxine; TRAB, thyroid receptor antibodies; TSH, thyroid-stimulating hormone; TSI, thyroid-stimulating immunoglobulin. *Propylthiouracil should be used in the first trimester because methimazole has been associated with birth defects. Propranolol can be started at 10–40 mg every 6–8 hours for women with symptomatic palpitations or other hypermetabolic symptoms. †Total T_3 normal range in pregnancy is 1.5 times the nonpregnant normal range. (Reprinted from Thyroid disease in pregnancy. ACOG Practice Bulletin No. 223. American College of Obstetricians and Gynecologists. Obstet Gynecol 2020;135:e261–74. doi: 10.1097/AOG.0000000000003893 https://journals.lww.com/greenjournal/Fulltext/2020/06000/Thyroid_Disease_in_Pregnancy__ACOG_Practice.47.aspx)

During Pregnancy demonstrated no differences in cognitive outcomes in children through age 5 years among women treated with levothyroxine versus placebo. Rarely, there may be an indication to treat subclinical hypothyroidism. Potential indications include a TSH greater than 10 mU/L, history of thyroid irradiation or surgery, or presence of symptoms. In the described patient, the best next step would be to reassure the patient.

The initiation of levothyroxine would not be appropriate for this patient who has subclinical hypothyroidism because treatment has not been shown to improve outcomes. In women with overt hypothyroidism, monitoring of TSH concentration at least every trimester and every 4–6 weeks while adjusting thyroid replacement therapy to ensure adequate control is recommended. A goal TSH concentration less than 2.5 milliunits/L is recommended. Approximately one-third of women with hypothyroidism will have an increasing T_4 requirement during pregnancy.

Universal screening for thyroid disease in pregnancy is not recommended and treatment of subclinical hypothyroidism has not been shown to improve outcomes. Potential indications for thyroid function testing include a personal or family history of thyroid disease, type 1 diabetes mellitus (or other autoimmune disorder), or clinical symptoms.

The measurement of total triiodothyronine (T_3) is not indicated because this would not alter management. Total T_3 and total T_4 increase during normal pregnancy. Expected changes in thyroid function tests during pregnancy are found in Table 72-1. Pregnancy reference ranges should be used when interpreting laboratory studies from pregnant patients.

Screening for thyroid antibodies is not recommended in this patient because this would not alter the ultimate management. Many women who test positive for antithyroid antibodies will be euthyroid. Thyroid peroxidase antibodies have been shown to be associated with an increased risk of miscarriage and preterm birth. However, a recent randomized controlled trial demonstrated that the use of levothyroxine in euthyroid women with thyroid peroxidase antibodies and a history of infertility or miscarriage did not improve live birth rates (over 34 weeks of gestation) when compared with placebo. On the contrary, in women with Graves disease, identification of these antibodies may be helpful. The presence of thyroid receptor antibodies or thyroid-stimulating immunoglobulin may predict the risk for fetal or neonatal hyperthyroidism and adverse outcomes. Accordingly, this may alter antenatal management including ultrasonography, antenatal fetal surveillance, delivery timing, and neonatal care.

TABLE 72-1. Normal Physiologic Changes in Thyroid Function Tests During Pregnancy

THYROID TEST	EXPECTED PHYSIOLOGIC CHANGE DURING PREGNANCY
Thyroid-binding globulin (TBG)	Increases
Total thyroxine (T_4)	Increases
Total triiodothyronine (T_3)	Increases
Thyroid-stimulating hormone (TSH)	Decreases in first trimester, then returns to baseline
Free thyroxine (T_4)	No change
Free triiodothyronine (T_3)	No change

Repeating thyroid function testing is not necessary unless other indications arise, such as if the patient were to become symptomatic. Subclinical hypothyroidism is unlikely to progress to overt hypothyroidism in healthy women. It is important to acknowledge that a patient seeking fertility treatment may receive different guidance depending on the specific individual clinical circumstances.

Casey BM, Thom EA, Peaceman AM, Varner MW, Sorokin Y, Hirtz DG, et al. Treatment of subclinical hypothyroidism or hypothyroxinemia in pregnancy. *Eunice Kennedy Shriver* National Institute of Child Health and Human Development Maternal–Fetal Medicine Units Network. N Engl J Med 2017;376:81525. doi: 10.1056/NEJMoa1606205 https://www.nejm.org/doi/10.1056/NEJMoa1606205

Cooper DS, Ladenson PW. Thyroid disorders. Clin Update Womens Health Care 2013;XII(5):1–88. https://www.acog.org/clinical/journals-and-publications/clinical-updates/2013/11/thyroid-disorders

Dhillon-Smith RK, Middleton LJ, Sunner KK, Cheed V, Baker K, Farrell-Carver S, et al. Levothyroxine in women with thyroid peroxidase antibodies before conception. N Engl J Med 2019;380:1316–25. doi: 10.1056/NEJMoa1812537 https://www.nejm.org/doi/10.1056/NEJMoa1812537

Thyroid disease in pregnancy. ACOG Practice Bulletin No. 223. American College of Obstetricians and Gynecologists. Obstet Gynecol 2020;135:e261–74. doi: 10.1097/AOG.0000000000003893 https://journals.lww.com/greenjournal/Fulltext/2020/06000/Thyroid_Disease_in_Pregnancy__ACOG_Practice.47.aspx

73 Anemia

A 25-year-old gravida 1, para 0, presents for a prenatal visit at 32 weeks of gestation. Routine third-trimester laboratory results returned a hemoglobin concentration of 9.2 g/dL, a hematocrit of 28.6%, a mean corpuscular volume (MCV) of 102.8 fL, and a platelet count of 219,000/mm^3. The patient has a history of gastric bypass, but her pregnancy is otherwise uncomplicated. The laboratory test that is most likely to determine the etiology of her anemia is a (an)

(A) ferritin level
(B) hemoglobin electrophoresis
(C) iron panel
(D) peripheral smear
* (E) vitamin B_{12} level

Pregnancy is associated with a physiologic anemia because of increased expansion in plasma over red blood cell mass. In a normal singleton gestation, blood volume increases by approximately 50%, whereas red blood cell mass increases by only approximately 25%. The Centers for Disease Control and Prevention defines *anemia in pregnancy* by the following criteria: hemoglobin less than 11 g/dL or hematocrit less than 33% in the first or third trimester and hemoglobin less than 10.5 g/dL or hematocrit less than 32% in the second trimester.

The workup for anemia starts with a complete history, physical examination, complete blood count, red blood cell indices, and serum iron and ferritin levels (Fig. 73-1). *Macrocytic anemia* is defined by an MCV greater than 100 fL, whereas *microcytic anemia* is defined by an MCV of less than 80 fL. The described patient has macrocytic anemia, which is an important clue in establishing the diagnosis (Fig. 73-2). Macrocytic anemias may be further characterized as megaloblastic or nonmegaloblastic. Examples of megaloblastic etiologies include folate and vitamin B_{12} (cobalamin) deficiency or pernicious anemia. Nonmegaloblastic etiologies include alcoholism or liver dysfunction, myelodysplasia, aplastic anemia, hypothyroidism, or increased reticulocyte count. Certain medications also can cause a macrocytic anemia.

In the United States, the most common cause of macrocytic anemia during pregnancy is folic acid deficiency. However, in women with a history of gastric bypass surgery (as in the described patient), the most common cause of macrocytic anemia is vitamin B_{12} deficiency. In women with a history of gastric bypass surgery, B_{12} should be supplemented and levels monitored to maintain a normal range. Folic acid deficiency may result from lack of dietary intake (such as diets lacking leafy vegetables or animal protein). In pregnancy, the folic acid requirement increases by 50–400 micrograms per day. A folic acid supplement of 1 mg is usually sufficient to treat deficiency.

Ferritin and iron levels may be included in the diagnostic workup, but would not be the most likely test to determine the etiology of the underlying anemia. Iron deficiency anemia is characterized by low or normal MCV, decreased iron levels and iron stores, high iron-binding capacity, low serum ferritin levels, and increased free erythrocyte protoporphyrin. A serum ferritin level of less than 10–15 micrograms/dL has the highest sensitivity and specificity for the diagnosis of iron deficiency anemia.

All pregnant women should have a complete blood count with red blood cell indices to assess for anemia. A hemoglobin electrophoresis should be performed if there is concern for hemoglobinopathy based on ethnicity (African, Mediterranean, Middle Eastern, Southeast Asian, or West Indian descent) or in the presence of red blood cell indices with low mean corpuscular hemoglobin or MCV. The described patient does not have any of these risk factors and, therefore, a hemoglobin electrophoresis would not aid in determination of the cause of her anemia.

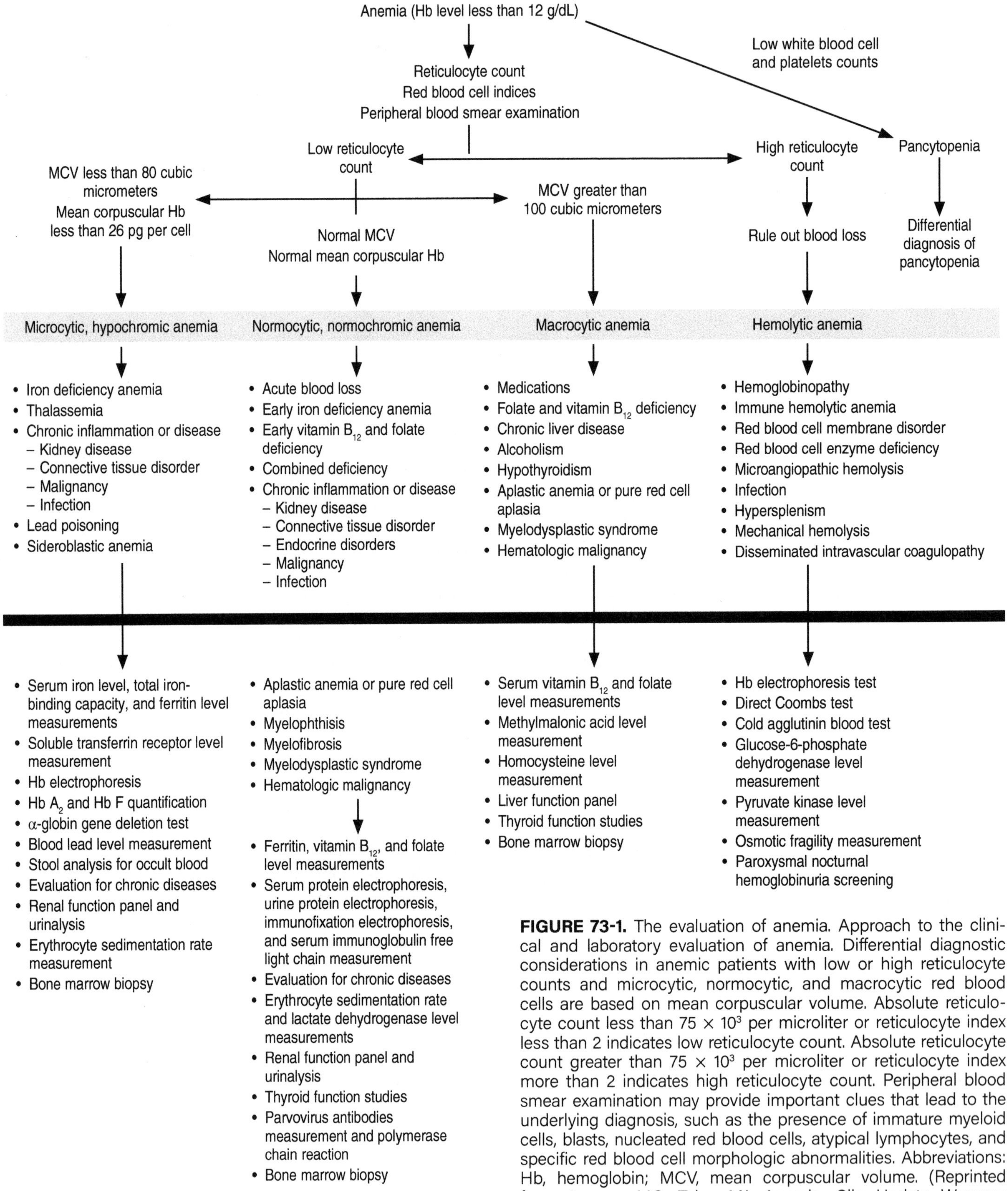

FIGURE 73-1. The evaluation of anemia. Approach to the clinical and laboratory evaluation of anemia. Differential diagnostic considerations in anemic patients with low or high reticulocyte counts and microcytic, normocytic, and macrocytic red blood cells are based on mean corpuscular volume. Absolute reticulocyte count less than 75×10^3 per microliter or reticulocyte index less than 2 indicates low reticulocyte count. Absolute reticulocyte count greater than 75×10^3 per microliter or reticulocyte index more than 2 indicates high reticulocyte count. Peripheral blood smear examination may provide important clues that lead to the underlying diagnosis, such as the presence of immature myeloid cells, blasts, nucleated red blood cells, atypical lymphocytes, and specific red blood cell morphologic abnormalities. Abbreviations: Hb, hemoglobin; MCV, mean corpuscular volume. (Reprinted from Arcasoy MO, Telen MJ. Anemia. Clin Update Womens Health Care 2012;XI(5):1–103. https://www.acog.org/clinical/journals-and-publications/clinical-updates/2012/11/anemia)

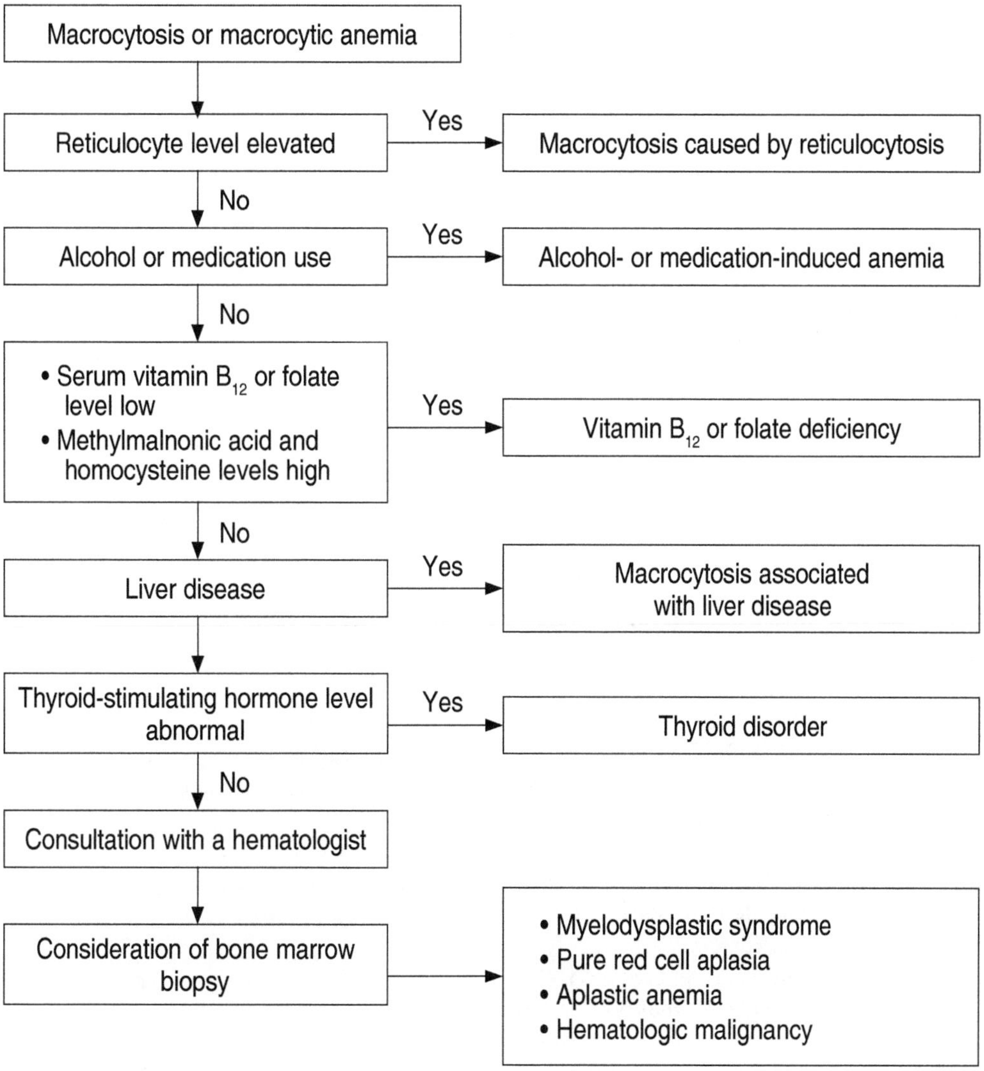

FIGURE 73-2. The evaluation of microcytic, hypochromic anemia. Abbreviation: Hb, hemoglobin. (Reprinted from Arcasoy MO, Telen MJ. Anemia. Clin Update Womens Health Care 2012;XI(5):1–103. https://www.acog.org/clinical/journals-and-publications/clinical-updates/2012/11/anemia)

Anemia in pregnancy. ACOG Practice Bulletin No. 233. American College of Obstetricians and Gynecologists. Obstet Gynecol 2021;138:e55–64. doi: 10.1097/AOG.0000000000004477 https://journals.lww.com/greenjournal/Fulltext/2021/08000/Anemia_in_Pregnancy__ACOG_Practice_Bulletin,.34.aspx

Arcasoy MO, Telen MJ. Anemia. Clin Update Womens Health Care 2012;XI(5):1–103. https://www.acog.org/clinical/journals-and-publications/clinical-updates/2012/11/anemia

Carrier screening for genetic conditions. Committee Opinion No. 691. American College of Obstetricians and Gynecologists. Obstet Gynecol 2017;129:e41–55. doi: 10.1097/AOG.0000000000001952 https://journals.lww.com/greenjournal/Fulltext/2017/03000/Committee_Opinion_No__691__Carrier_Screening_for.48.aspx

74 Fetal death in a patient with a previous cesarean birth

A 28-year-old gravida 2, para 1, presents with a fetal death at 23 0/7 weeks of gestation. Her first pregnancy was complicated by preeclampsia with severe features requiring cesarean birth by low transverse incision at 35 weeks of gestation. She has no significant medical history. The patient's vital signs are normal. She requests delivery at this time, and she would like to hold the newborn. Her fetus is presenting as a complete breech on ultrasonographic examination, and her cervix is closed with no effacement. The most appropriate initial method of induction is oral mifepristone followed by

(A) high-dose intravenous oxytocin
(B) low-dose intravenous oxytocin
(C) transcervical mechanical dilation
* (D) vaginal misoprostol
(E) vaginal prostaglandin E2

A *stillbirth* is defined as delivery of a fetus with no breathing, no heartbeat, no perceptible umbilical cord pulsation, and no definitive movement. Most cases of fetal death are identified and confirmed while in utero. Data from 2013 and 2017 demonstrate that the rate of fetal death in the United States has been relatively stable. Risk factors for fetal death include nulliparity; advanced and young maternal age; preexisting medical conditions including obesity, diabetes mellitus, and hypertension; modifiable risk factors, such as tobacco and alcohol use; nonmodifiable risks, such as multiple gestations and male fetuses; and a previous history of stillbirth.

The delivery management of a fetal death is based on gestational age, previous uterine surgery, and maternal preference. The development of coagulopathies in the setting of a retained fetal death is rare, even with prolonged time frames, and generally there is no need for expedient intervention. After 28 weeks of gestation, induction of labor is conducted based on accepted protocols for typical labor induction. In the setting of a fetal death in the second trimester, the patient should be offered the choice between a dilation and evacuation (D&E) and a medical induction of labor, although few clinicians who perform D&E will offer it beyond 24 weeks of gestation. Dilation and evacuation procedures have a 4% complication rate, compared with 29% for labor inductions. Dilation and evacuation can be accomplished faster with completion of the process on a more predictable timeline. Drawbacks to D&E include a decreasing number of obstetricians in the workforce with experience in the procedure and the inability to conduct an intact assessment and autopsy of the fetus.

Medical induction of labor is the other option. This method has the potential to avoid surgery and allow intact birth. Induction has more complications, including infections and retained placentas, when compared with D&E. The use of vaginal misoprostol is a common induction technique in this type of scenario, but high-dose oxytocin infusion is an alternative. Recent evidence shows that the use of mifepristone, a progesterone antagonist, with misoprostol decreases the time to delivery versus misoprostol alone with an equivalent rate of achieving delivery. The evidence is strongest for pregnancies at less than 20 weeks of gestation with more limited data for late second-trimester induction from 24 to 28 weeks of gestation. The oral dose of mifepristone should precede the misoprostol by 24 to 48 hours when possible.

When a patient experiences a fetal death and has a history of a previous hysterotomy, the most appropriate course in most cases will be to pursue a vaginal birth after cesarean. Evidence supports the use of misoprostol for induction of labor of stillbirths at less than 24 weeks of gestation in those with a previous cesarean birth. Data are more limited for patients at 24–28 weeks of gestation, with some sources suggesting use of lower doses of misoprostol, but more data are required to identify an optimal regimen. Overall, small case series have found the rate of uterine rupture with misoprostol-induced labor in the second trimester, including patients with a history of cesarean birth, to be less than 1%.

For those patients who experience fetal death at greater than 28 weeks of gestation and who have a history of previous cesarean birth, induction of labor should be conducted in the same manner as a typical trial of labor after cesarean birth, meaning prostaglandins should be avoided. Transcervical mechanical dilation remains a good option for patients with unfavorable cervices, with uterine rupture rates similar to those for spontaneous labor. For patients with a history of a previous classical hysterotomy or multiple cesarean births, care plans should be individualized through a shared decision-making process. In general, cesarean birth in the setting of an intrauterine death should be avoided because there is additional maternal morbidity risk without fetal benefit. The data are limited on induction methods and risks in these situations, but after appropriate counseling, a medical induction remains an option in patients at higher risk for uterine rupture.

Management of stillbirth. ACOG Obstetric Care Consensus No. 10. American College of Obstetricians and Gynecologists. Obstet Gynecol 2020;135:e110–32. doi: 10.1097/AOG.0000000000003719 https://journals.lww.com/greenjournal/Fulltext/2020/03000/Management_of_Stillbirth__Obstetric_Care_Consensus.49.aspx

Second-trimester abortion. Practice Bulletin No. 135. American College of Obstetricians and Gynecologists. Obstet Gynecol 2013;121:1394–406. doi: 10.1097/01.AOG.0000431056.79334.cc https://journals.lww.com/greenjournal/Fulltext/2013/06000/Practice_Bulletin_No__135__Second_Trimester.42.aspx

Vaginal birth after cesarean delivery. ACOG Practice Bulletin No. 205. American College of Obstetricians and Gynecologists. Obstet Gynecol 2019;133:e110–27. doi: 10.1097/AOG.0000000000003078 https://journals.lww.com/greenjournal/Fulltext/2019/02000/ACOG_Practice_Bulletin_No__205__Vaginal_Birth.40.aspx

75 Fetal acid-base assessment

A 19-year-old gravida 1 at 33 weeks of gestation arrives to the obstetric triage unit by emergency medical services. She has altered sensorium and is reporting abdominal pain. Her pregnancy is complicated by type 1 diabetes mellitus. Her blood pressure is 115/80 mm Hg, her heart rate is 105 beats per minute, her respiratory rate is 25 respirations per minute, and her temperature is 37.2 °C (99.0 °F). Her blood glucose concentration is 408 mg/dL. An arterial blood gas reveals a pH of 7.15. Her anion gap is 14 mEq/L, and her serum bicarbonate is 12 mEq/L. She is placed on continuous electronic fetal monitoring with the tracing demonstrated below (Fig. 75-1). In addition to starting intravenous fluids, the most appropriate next step in management is

(A) betamethasone
(B) cesarean birth
* (C) insulin
(D) oxytocin
(E) terbutaline

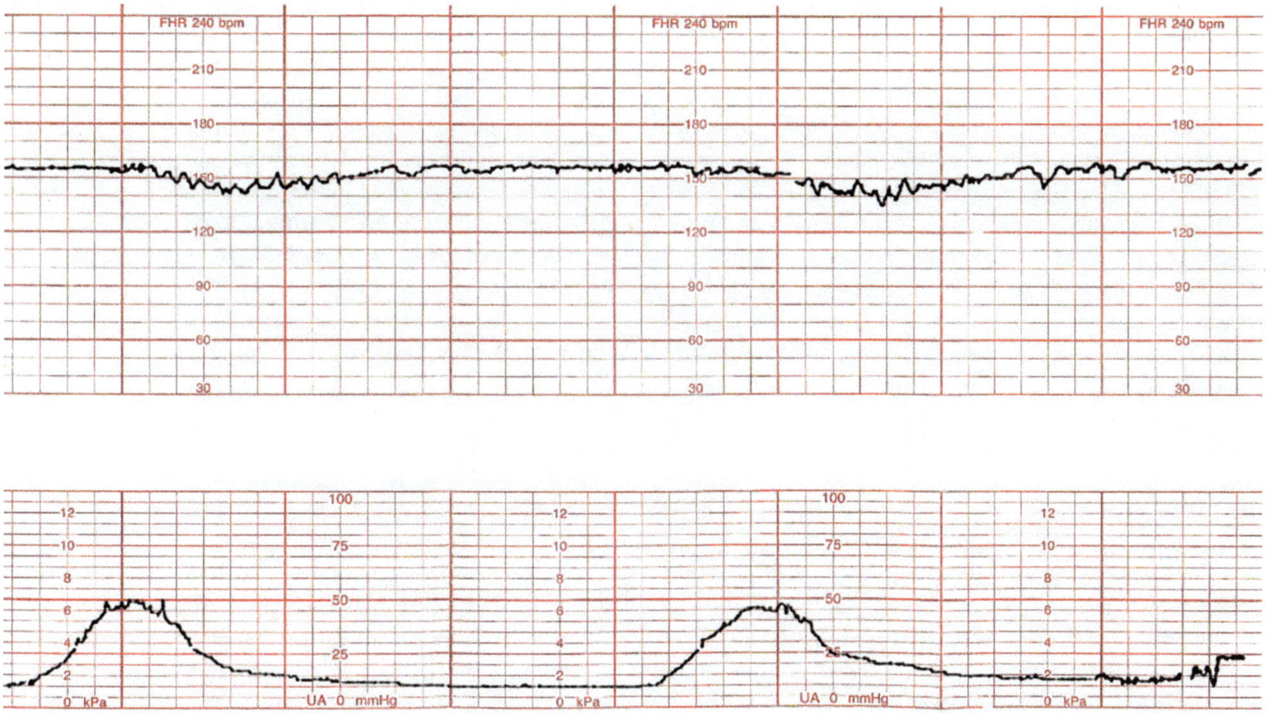

FIGURE 75-1. Patient's fetal heart rate tracing

Intrapartum fetal acid–base assessment is an evolving science in obstetrics. The fetal heart rate is controlled through sympathetic and parasympathetic forces, and the fetal heart rate pattern has been used for decades to assess fetal oxygenation and acid–base status. The fetal heart rate tracing is a snapshot of the fetal condition at one moment in time that will change based on the conditions encountered. The use of the fetal heart rate tracing for the assessment of fetal well-being has proved problematic with wide interobserver and intraobserver variability and a false-positive rate of greater than 99% for cerebral palsy, yet it is now standard medical practice in obstetrics. There are no data demonstrating a reduction in cerebral palsy with electronic fetal monitoring, but there has been an increase in cesarean births and operative vaginal deliveries with its use.

To address these deficiencies and to standardize the use and interpretation of electronic fetal heart rate patterns, the *Eunice Kennedy Shriver* National Institute of Child Health and Human Development convened a workshop in collaboration with the American College of Obstetricians and Gynecologists and the Society for Maternal-Fetal Medicine. In 2008, this panel formalized definitions of fetal heart rate patterns and classified fetal heart rate tracings into three categories. A *Category I* tracing has a baseline of 110–160 beats per minute, moderate variability, and no late or variable decelerations. Early decelerations and accelerations of the fetal heart rate may or may not be present. A Category I tracing is strongly indicative of fetal well-being and a normal acid–base status. A *Category III* fetal heart rate tracing has absent variability with either recurrent late or variable decelerations or bradycardia. A sinusoidal fetal heart rate tracing also is Category III. Category III tracings can be associated with fetal acidemia and require prompt evaluation and treatment.

Category II tracings are indeterminate patterns and are not predictive of fetal acid–base abnormalities. Category II tracings can have abnormalities of the heart rate, will show preserved beat-to-beat variability, may have or lack heart rate accelerations, and may have fetal heart rate decelerations. Bradycardia with minimal variability or greater and fetal tachycardia are considered Category II. Minimal variability, marked variability, and absent variability without recurrent decelerations also are within this category. Lack of accelerations in response to fetal scalp stimulation also is a Category II finding. Recurrent variable decelerations with minimal or absent variability, recurrent late decelerations with minimal or absent variability, and prolonged fetal heart rate decelerations are examples of Category II features.

In the setting of a Category II or III fetal heart rate tracing, the cause of the abnormality should be assessed, and appropriate intrauterine resuscitation performed. With variable decelerations, the obstetrician should ensure the umbilical cord has not prolapsed. In the absence of a prolapse, maternal position changes can relieve intrauterine cord compression, and intra-amniotic saline infusion has been shown to lower cesarean birth rates when variable decelerations are encountered. Late decelerations represent uteroplacental insufficiency. Acute causes of uteroplacental insufficiency include maternal hypotension, maternal hypoxia, and uterine tachysystole. Intrauterine resuscitation in these situations can include repositioning to reduce compression of the vena cava and improve uterine perfusion, intravenous fluid resuscitation and ephedrine administration for hypotension, oxygen supplementation for hypoxia, and uterine tocolysis for tachysystole with fetal heart rate changes. Fetal heart rate variability will change with fetal sleep cycles. Generally, reduced variability due to a sleep cycle lasts 20 minutes but can persist for up to 60 minutes. As an isolated finding, the reduced variability due to a sleep cycle can be monitored. Maternal opioid administration also can reduce fetal heart rate variability with the return of moderate variability expected within 1–2 hours.

Fetal scalp stimulation is a procedure that can help evaluate Category II fetal heart rate tracings. Methods of fetal stimulation include a vibroacoustic device or digital stimulation. An acceleration of the fetal heart rate in response to any of these stimuli is reassuring and indicative of a normal acid–base status. No data support the use of fetal pulse oximetry to assess fetal acid–base status in utero.

Of the individual parameters in the fetal heart rate tracing, there is evidence that variability is the most predictive of the fetal acid–base status. One study demonstrated that 97% of deliveries that maintained moderate variability, even when complicated by late and variable decelerations, had an umbilical arterial pH greater than 7.0. The same study noted that tracings that experienced minimal to absent variability for greater than 1 hour had significant acidemia (umbilical arterial pH less than 7.0) in 12–31% of cases.

The patient in this clinical scenario has diabetic ketoacidosis with a Category II fetal heart tracing. Approximately 5–10% of patients with pregestational diabetes will have at least one episode of diabetic ketoacidosis during pregnancy, likely due to increased insulin resistance. Other risk factors for diabetic ketoacidosis include a new diagnosis of diabetes, inability to complete therapy, insulin pump malfunctions, infections, and the use of β-mimetic tocolytic agents and corticosteroids during pregnancy. Patients with diabetic ketoacidosis will present with abdominal pain, nausea, vomiting, altered sensorium, a serum bicarbonate of less than 15 mEq/L, an increased anion gap, and serum ketones.

In pregnancy, blood glucose values may be lower than expected in patients with diabetic ketoacidosis compared with values in nonpregnant patients. The fetal heart tracing frequently demonstrates minimal variability and can be complicated by late or variable decelerations if the patient is contracting. These fetal heart rate abnormalities usually will resolve as the maternal condition improves, and delivery in these situations rarely is indicated. Aggressive intravenous hydration should be started along with intravenous insulin. One to 2 L of normal saline should be infused over the first hour, followed by another 2–4 L over the next 8 hours.

Although the patient is preterm and contracting, antenatal corticosteroid administration and terbutaline should be withheld because they can induce hyperglycemia. Her contractions will likely abate with hydration, and the abnormal fetal heart rate pattern will resolve as the maternal acidosis corrects, decreasing the chances of an indicated preterm delivery.

Intrapartum fetal heart rate monitoring: nomenclature, interpretation, and general management principles. ACOG Practice Bulletin No. 106. American College of Obstetricians and Gynecologists. Obstet Gynecol 2009;114:192–202. doi: 10.1097/AOG.0b013e3181aef106 https://journals.lww.com/greenjournal/Citation/2009/07000/ACOG_Practice_Bulletin_No__106__Intrapartum_Fetal.51.aspx

Management of intrapartum fetal heart rate tracings. Practice Bulletin No. 116. American College of Obstetricians and Gynecologists. Obstet Gynecol 2010;116:1232–40. doi: 10.1097/AOG.0b013e3182004fa9 https://journals.lww.com/greenjournal/Citation/2010/11000/Practice_Bulletin_No__116__Management_of.53.aspx

Pregestational diabetes mellitus. ACOG Practice Bulletin No. 201. American College of Obstetricians and Gynecologists. Obstet Gynecol 2018;132:e228–48. doi: 10.1097/AOG.0000000000002960 https://journals.lww.com/greenjournal/Fulltext/2018/12000/ACOG_Practice_Bulletin_No__201__Pregestational.48.aspx

Williams KP, Galerneau F. Intrapartum fetal heart rate patterns in the prediction of neonatal acidemia. Am J Obstet Gynecol 2003;188:820–3. doi: 10.1067/mob.2003.183 https://www.ajog.org/article/S0002-9378(02)71324-0/fulltext

76 Prevention of recurrent preterm birth

A patient is having an ultrasonographic examination at 19 weeks of gestation to assess fetal anatomy and cervical length. In her last pregnancy, she delivered at 28 weeks of gestation after preterm prelabor rupture of membranes (PPROM). She is receiving vaginal progesterone supplementation for prevention of preterm labor. Her examination shows normal fetal anatomy, and her transvaginal cervical length is 22 mm. The best next step in management of her pregnancy is

* (A) cervical cerclage
(B) cervical pessary
(C) fetal fibronectin
(D) repeat cervical length measurement

Preterm birth is the leading cause of neonatal morbidity and mortality in the United States, and the risk of neonatal complications increases with earlier gestational age. Preterm birth may be indicated for maternal or fetal reasons, or may be spontaneous because of complications such as preterm labor, PPROM, and cervical insufficiency. Risk factors for spontaneous preterm birth include multiple gestation, vaginal bleeding, urinary and genital tract infections, periodontal disease, maternal body mass index of less than 18.5, short interpregnancy interval, and substance use disorder and tobacco use. A history of a spontaneous preterm birth is a strong risk factor for recurrent preterm birth in future pregnancies. Women who have a history of preterm birth traditionally have been offered progesterone supplementation with weekly intramuscular 17α-hydroxyprogesterone caproate starting at 16 weeks of gestation to decrease the risk of recurrent preterm birth. Recent randomized controlled trials and meta-analyses have shown variable results on the efficacy of progesterone supplementation in decreasing preterm birth. Currently, it is recommended that patients and practitioners engage in shared decision making to determine whether progesterone supplementation should be given, as well as which type of supplementation is effective. Vaginal progesterone also may be considered for preterm birth prevention in women at risk of recurrent preterm birth, and trials comparing intramuscular and vaginal types are ongoing.

Shortened cervical length also is associated with an increased risk of preterm birth, and this risk increases as cervical length becomes shorter. The cutoff for a *shortened cervical length* usually is defined as less than 25 mm before 24 weeks of gestation. Transvaginal ultrasonography is a reliable method to measure cervical length, and it is recommended in women who have had a previous spontaneous preterm delivery, usually every 2 weeks from 16 weeks to 24 weeks of gestation. Studies have shown that cerclage placement reduces the risk of preterm birth in women who have had a previous spontaneous preterm delivery before 34 weeks of gestation and now have a cervical length of less than 25 mm before 24 weeks of gestation. In the described patient, who had a previous preterm delivery and now has a shortened cervix, a cerclage is indicated. Routine cervical length screening is not universally performed in low-risk women; however, if a shortened cervix is identified, vaginal progesterone supplementation is recommended.

Cervical pessary placement has been studied as a strategy to decrease the risk of preterm birth, but it appears to be ineffective. It is not currently recommended outside of research settings in women with a singleton or twin gestation, women who have had a previous preterm birth, or women with a shortened cervix. Fetal fibronectin is a protein present at the decidual–chorionic interface. Disruption of this interface releases fetal fibronectin into vaginal secretions, and testing for this is sometimes used to distinguish preterm labor versus preterm contractions. Fetal fibronectin screening is not recommended to assess asymptomatic women and their risk of preterm delivery.

For the described patient, waiting to repeat the cervical length would not be an appropriate next step in management, as a cerclage placement is indicated. Adding additional forms of progesterone, such as prescribing vaginal progesterone in a woman who is already receiving intramuscular progesterone, has not been appropriately studied and is not recommended even when a short cervix is identified.

Berghella V, Rafael TJ, Szychowski JM, Rust OA, Owen J. Cerclage for short cervix on ultrasonography in women with singleton gestations and previous preterm birth: a meta-analysis. Obstet Gynecol 2011;117:663–71. doi: 10.1097/AOG.0b013e31820ca847 https://journals.lww.com/greenjournal/Fulltext/2011/03000/Cerclage_for_Short_Cervix_on_Ultrasonography_in.21.aspx

Blackwell SC, Gyamfi-Bannerman C, Biggio JR, Chauhan SP, Hughes BL, Louis JM, et al. 17-OHPC to prevent recurrent preterm birth in singleton gestations (PROLONG Study): a multicenter, international, randomized double-blind trial. Am J Perinatol 2020;37:127–36. doi: 10.1055/s-0039-3400227 https://www.thieme-connect.com/products/ejournals/abstract/10.1055/s-0039-3400227

Cerclage for the management of cervical insufficiency. Practice Bulletin No. 142. American College of Obstetricians and Gynecologists. Obstet Gynecol 2014;123:372–9. doi: 10.1097/01.AOG.0000443276.68274.cc https://journals.lww.com/greenjournal/Fulltext/2014/02000/Practice_Bulletin_No__142__Cerclage_for_the.33.aspx

Evaluating Progestogens for Preventing Preterm Birth International Collaborative (EPPPIC): meta-analysis of individual participant data from randomised controlled trials. EPPPIC Group [published erratum appears in Lancet 2021;397:1446]. Lancet 2021;397:1183–94. doi: 10.1016/S0140-6736(21)00217-8 https://www.thelancet.com/journals/lancet/article/PIIS0140-6736(21)00217-8/fulltext

Prediction and prevention of spontaneous preterm birth. ACOG Practice Bulletin No. 234. American College of Obstetricians and Gynecologists. Obstet Gynecol 2021;138:e65–90. doi: 10.1097/AOG.0000000000004479 https://journals.lww.com/greenjournal/Fulltext/2021/08000/Prediction_and_Prevention_of_Spontaneous_Preterm.35.aspx

Resnik R, Lockwood CJ, Moore TR, Greene MF, Copel JA, Silver RM, editors. Creasy & Resnik's maternal–fetal medicine: principles and practice. 8th ed. Elsevier; 2019.

77 Postpartum hemorrhage

A 38-year-old gravida 1, para 1, develops heavy vaginal bleeding 4 hours after an uncomplicated primary cesarean birth of a term neonate. The uterus is massaged and uterotonics are administered, including misoprostol, oxytocin, methylergonovine, and 15-methyl prostaglandin $F_{2\alpha}$. A uterine tamponade balloon is attempted but placement is unsuccessful. The massive transfusion protocol is initiated. Her abdomen is reopened and uterine atony is identified. A B-Lynch suture is placed without a significant decrease in bleeding. Her blood pressure is 80/40 mm Hg, and her pulse is 130 beats per minute. You continue to transfuse with blood product replacement. Quantitative blood loss is 4,500 mL. The best next step is

(A) administration of tranexamic acid
* (B) hysterectomy
(C) repeat administration of methylergonovine
(D) second uterine compression suture
(E) uterine artery embolization

Postpartum hemorrhage is a common cause of maternal morbidity and mortality in the United States and worldwide. The most common cause is uterine atony, or failure of the uterus to contract after delivery. Other etiologies include vaginal, cervical, and uterine lacerations, retained adherent placenta, infection, and coagulopathy. Primary postpartum hemorrhage occurs in the first 24 hours after delivery, and secondary postpartum hemorrhage occurs between 24 hours and 12 weeks postpartum.

Once uterine atony has been identified, fundal massage along with medical management with uterotonics generally is the first-line treatment. The most commonly used agents are oxytocin, misoprostol, methylergonovine, and 15-methyl prostaglandin $F_{2\alpha}$. These medications have varying half-lives and recommended frequency of administration. Repeat methylergonovine is not recommended for this patient because it should be given every 2–4 hours. The uterotonic medication that may be given most frequently is 15-methyl prostaglandin $F_{2\alpha}$, every 15–90 minutes for a maximum of eight doses.

Tranexamic acid is an antifibrinolytic agent that has been shown to reduce obstetric blood loss when given prophylactically and as part of treatment for postpartum hemorrhage. In studies it appeared that the benefit was primarily in women treated sooner than 3 hours from the time of delivery. Although tranexamic acid can be considered in this patient 4 hours after delivery, given the degree of blood loss and unstable vital signs, treatment with hysterectomy is the most appropriate intervention. If bleeding is significant and ongoing, blood transfusion should be initiated, and a massive transfusion protocol should be activated. Massive transfusion is indicated when there is ongoing bleeding despite interventions, vital signs are unstable, or there is suspicion of disseminated intravascular coagulation.

If medical management fails to control bleeding from uterine atony, escalation to other techniques is indicated. These include tamponade with a commercially available intrauterine balloon device, Foley catheter, or uterine packing (Table 77-1). There also is a commercially available intrauterine device that

TABLE 77-1. Tamponade Techniques for Postpartum Hemorrhage

TECHNIQUE	COMMENT
Commercially available intrauterine balloon tamponade devices	Inserted transcervically or through cesarean incision; has an exit port for blood drainage
· Bakri Balloon	Inflated with 300–500 mL of saline
· ebb uterine tamponade system	Double balloon: maximum recommended fill volumes are 750 mL for the uterine balloon and 300 mL for the vaginal balloon.
Foley catheter	Insert one or more 60-mL bulbs and fill with 60 mL of saline.
Uterine packing	4-inch gauze, can be soaked with 5,000 units of thrombin in 5 mL of saline, then insert from one cornua to the other with ring forceps.

Reprinted from Postpartum hemorrhage. Practice Bulletin No. 183. American College of Obstetricians and Gynecologists. Obstet Gynecol 2017;130:e168–86. doi: 10.1097/AOG.0000000000002351 https://journals.lww.com/greenjournal/Fulltext/2017/10000/Practice_Bulletin_No__183__Postpartum_Hemorrhage.56.aspx

uses low-level vacuum to induce uterine contraction. Uterine artery embolization also may be undertaken with fluoroscopic guidance and placement of absorbable gelatin sponges, coils, or microparticles. Ideal candidates for this procedure are those who have not improved with less invasive methods to control bleeding, are hemodynamically stable, and have persistent slow bleeding. This patient is not a good candidate for uterine artery embolization given her ongoing significant bleeding and abnormal vital signs.

Surgical techniques to control bleeding from uterine atony (Fig. 77-1) include vascular ligation of the bilateral uterine arteries (O'Leary sutures), utero-ovarian ligaments, or the hypogastric artery. Uterine compression suture also is commonly used to control uterine atony, most often the B-Lynch technique. A second compression suture is not a recommended method to control bleeding if the first has been unsuccessful. In general, the treatment of postpartum hemorrhage should use the least invasive method possible, but when more conservative therapies have failed, hysterectomy is the definitive treatment and may be lifesaving. The best next step in the management of this hemodynamically unstable patient is hysterectomy.

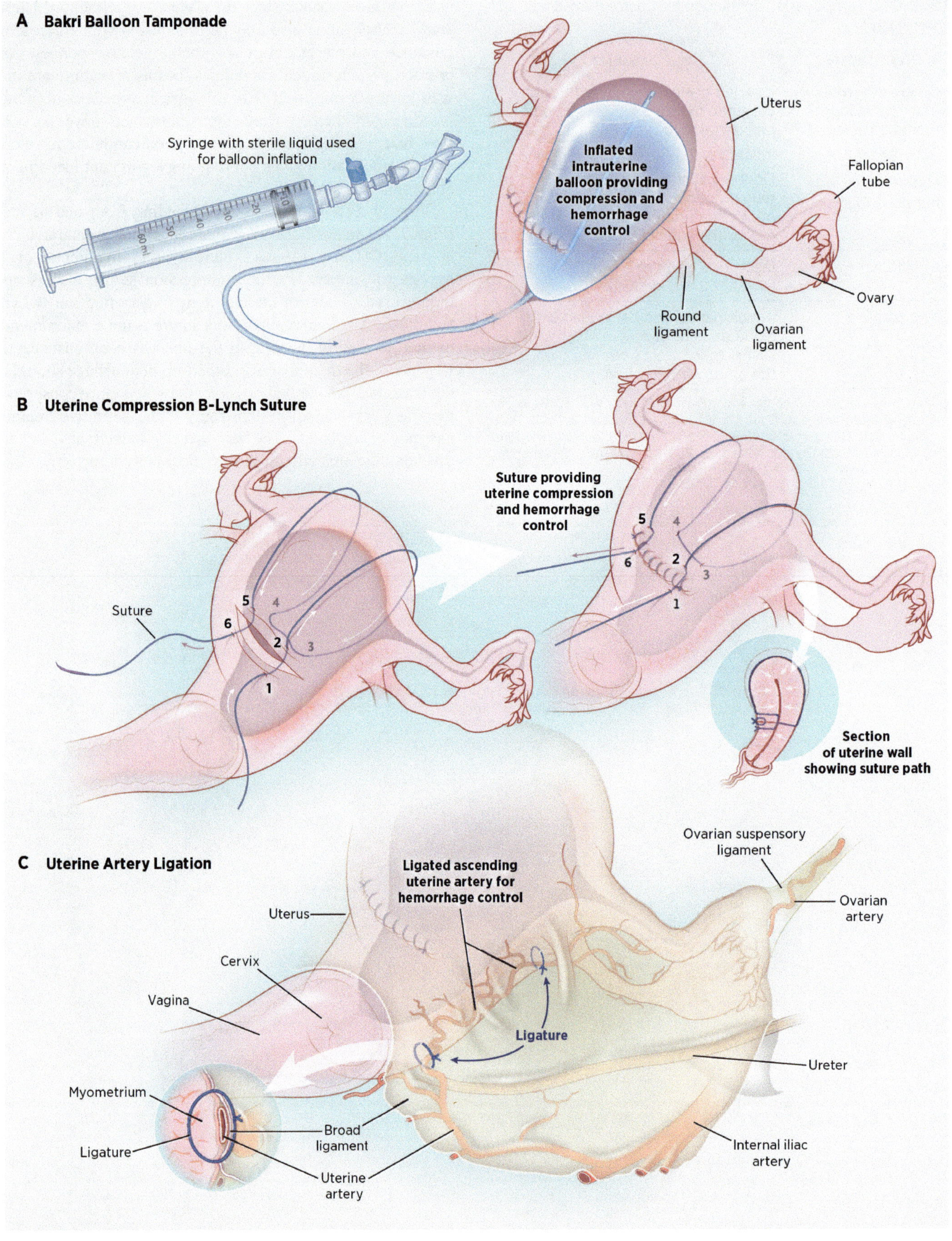

FIGURE 77-1. Mechanical methods for managing uterine atony. (Reprinted from Bienstock JL, Eke AC, Hueppchen NA. Postpartum hemorrhage. N Engl J Med 2021;384:1635–45. doi: 10.1056/NEJMra1513247 https://www.nejm.org/doi/10.1056/NEJMra1513247)

Bienstock JL, Eke AC, Hueppchen NA. Postpartum hemorrhage. N Engl J Med 2021;384:1635–45. doi: 10.1056/NEJMra1513247 https://www.nejm.org/doi/10.1056/NEJMra1513247

Landon MB, Galan HL, Jauniaux ER, Driscoll DA, Berghella V, Grobman WA, et al, editors. Gabbe's obstetrics: normal and problem pregnancies. 8th ed. Elsevier; 2021.

Mousa HA, Blum J, Abou El Senoun G, Shakur H, Alfirevic Z. Treatment for primary postpartum haemorrhage. Cochrane Database of Systematic Reviews 2014, Issue 2. Art. No.: CD003249. doi: 10.1002/14651858.CD003249.pub3 http://dx.doi.org/10.1002/14651858.CD003249.pub3

Postpartum hemorrhage. Practice Bulletin No. 183. American College of Obstetricians and Gynecologists. Obstet Gynecol 2017;130:e168–86. doi: 10.1097/AOG.0000000000002351 https://journals.lww.com/greenjournal/Fulltext/2017/10000/Practice_Bulletin_No__183__Postpartum_Hemorrhage.56.aspx

78 Dermatologic conditions in pregnancy

A 16-year-old gravida 1 presents in the third trimester for prenatal care. She reports intense itching on her abdomen that started 2 weeks ago, followed by widespread, large red plaques with areas of blistering. On physical examination, she has papules, plaques, and vesicles on her entire abdomen and trunk, involving the periumbilical area, and spreading to the proximal extremities (Fig. 78-1). The most likely diagnosis is

(A) contact dermatitis
(B) eczema
(C) intrahepatic cholestasis of pregnancy
* (D) pemphigoid gestationis
(E) polymorphic eruption of pregnancy

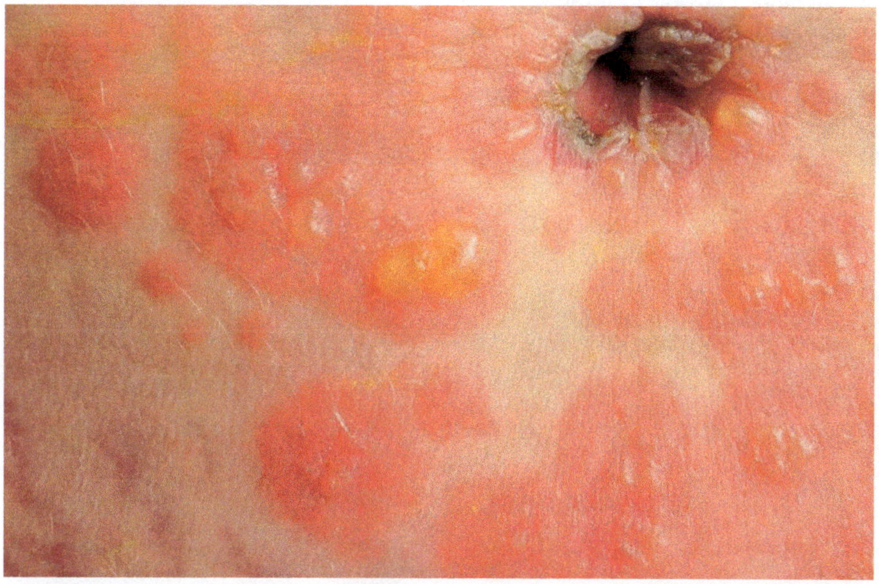

FIGURE 78-1. Periumbilical eruption. (Reprinted from Sävervall C, Sand FL, Thomsen SF. Dermatological diseases associated with pregnancy: pemphigoid gestationis, polymorphic eruption of pregnancy, intrahepatic cholestasis of pregnancy, and atopic eruption of pregnancy. Dermatol Res Pract 2015;2015:979635. doi: 10.1155/2015/979635 https://www.hindawi.com/journals/drp/2015/979635/)

Itching, or pruritis, is a common complaint in pregnancy that may be caused by a wide variety of conditions, ranging from harmless rashes to serious conditions with increased morbidity to the woman and the fetus. There are many rashes that occur in pregnancy, most of which lack specific diagnostic criteria. Most are pruritic and resolve after delivery. Pregnant women may be affected by skin disorders that occur outside pregnancy as well, such as contact dermatitis, eczema, superficial fungal infections, folliculitis, and drug eruptions.

The most likely diagnosis in this patient is pemphigoid gestationis, sometimes called herpes gestationis. This is a rare, autoimmune, blistering dermatosis of pregnancy and the postpartum period. It is thought to result from an autoimmune response to a placental antigen. Onset usually occurs in the second or third trimester with lesions around the umbilicus, and other commonly affected areas include the trunk, buttocks, and extremities. Lesions may include vesicles, bullae, and erythematous plaques.

An increased incidence of preterm birth and fetal growth restriction in patients with this disease has been reported. Infants born to affected women have an increased mortality rate and may have mild lesions after birth. Treatment should be given to relieve pruritus symptoms and suppress the appearance of new lesions and may include potent topical corticosteroids, systemic corticosteroids, or both.

Contact dermatitis is a localized skin response to an irritant or allergen and may occur in pregnant or nonpregnant individuals. Common causes include cleaners and detergents, oils and solvents, plants, metals, cosmetics, and personal care products. Treatment includes removal and avoidance of the cause and use of topical corticosteroids. Systemic corticosteroids, phototherapy, and immunosuppressive agents also may be used in unresponsive or severe cases.

Eczema, or atopic dermatitis, is a chronic inflammatory skin disease that causes skin itching, dryness, erythema, and crusting. It is common in children but also occurs in adults and may occur during pregnancy. Management of atopic dermatitis includes elimination of exacerbating factors, skin hydration, and restoration of the skin's barrier function, and may include topical corticosteroids. Patients with moderate to severe eczema may be treated with phototherapy or immunosuppressive agents.

Another possible cause of itching in pregnancy is intrahepatic cholestasis of pregnancy. In women with this condition, the itching is worse on the palms and soles, often worse at night, and not accompanied by a rash. The diagnosis can be confirmed by an elevated level of serum bile acids (greater than or equal to 10 micromoles/L). The usual treatment is oral ursodeoxycholic acid and also may include antihistamines for symptomatic relief. In patients with this disease, there is an increased risk of stillbirth in the third trimester, and late-preterm or early-term delivery is recommended. Intrahepatic cholestasis of pregnancy has a high recurrence risk in future pregnancies.

Polymorphic eruption of pregnancy, previously called PUPP (pruritic and urticarial papules and plaques of pregnancy), often is seen in the third trimester in primigravid women. It is associated with increased weight gain and multifetal gestation causing skin stretching. Symptoms usually begin in the abdominal striae with pruritic papules that may form plaques and vesicles and may spread to the buttocks and thighs. The periumbilical skin usually is spared. Treatment includes topical corticosteroids and antihistamines. Pregnancy outcomes are not negatively affected by this disorder. It is important to differentiate this disorder from pemphigoid gestationis, and biopsy should be considered. Tissue sampling submitted in Michel's or Zeus medium is recommended for direct immunofluorescent testing for pemphigoid gestationis.

Khorsand KO, Iyer JG, Abson KG. Common dermatologic conditions. Clin Update Womens Health Care 2018;XVII(1):1–84. https://www.acog.org/clinical/journals-and-publications/clinical-updates/2018/01/common-dermatologic-conditions

Landon MB, Galan HL, Jauniaux ER, Driscoll DA, Berghella V, Grobman WA, et al, editors. Gabbe's obstetrics: normal and problem pregnancies. 8th ed. Elsevier; 2021.

Resnik R, Lockwood CJ, Moore TR, Greene MF, Copel JA, Silver RM, editors. Creasy & Resnik's maternal–fetal medicine: principles and practice. 8th ed. Elsevier; 2019.

79 Immunization in pregnancy

A 27-year-old gravida 2, para 1, at 23 weeks of gestation presents for a prenatal visit in October. She has a history of mild intermittent asthma without recent exacerbation. She has received vaccination for COVID-19. She is concerned about respiratory illness in her newborn. The immunization most appropriate at this visit to decrease the risk of respiratory illness in both the woman and her newborn is

* (A) influenza
(B) measles–mumps–rubella
(C) pneumococcal
(D) respiratory syncytial virus
(E) tetanus toxoid, reduced diphtheria toxoid, and acellular pertussis (Tdap)

All pregnant and postpartum patients, as well as patients planning to become pregnant, should be immunized against seasonal influenza to protect themselves and their newborns, and this is the best next step for this patient. Influenza carries significant risk in pregnancy, including hospitalization, severe respiratory illness, intensive care unit admission, and other adverse maternal and perinatal outcomes. Currently, the most effective form of prevention of seasonal influenza is vaccination.

In addition to the protective effects of immunization for pregnant patients, significant benefit is conferred to the newborn and infant. Multiple studies have shown neonatal protection from maternal immunization, and newborns and infants of vaccinated mothers are less likely to be hospitalized than those of unvaccinated mothers. Because there currently is no influenza vaccine available to infants less than 6 months of age, maternal immunization allows the best protection for newborns and young infants.

All inactivated influenza vaccinations are appropriate for use in pregnancy and should be withheld only from individuals with a history of severe allergic reaction to previous influenza immunization. Those with an allergy to eggs can receive the vaccine; however, if they have had a reaction more severe than hives, they should receive their vaccine in an inpatient or outpatient medical setting. Influenza vaccination can be administered in any trimester, concomitantly with the Tdap and COVID vaccines, and is safe in breastfeeding women.

The Tdap vaccine also is recommended to all pregnant women. This vaccine decreases the risk of respiratory disease in pregnant women and their newborns and infants. It should be administered between 27 and 36 weeks of gestation to allow maternal antibody response and transfer to the fetus. This patient is at 23 weeks of gestation, so administering the Tdap vaccine is not the best next step in her prenatal care.

The measles–mumps–rubella vaccine is an attenuated live vaccine and is contraindicated in pregnancy because of the risk of congenital rubella. Pneumococcal immunization is safe in pregnancy but has not specifically been shown to have neonatal benefit. Although respiratory syncytial virus is a significant cause of respiratory morbidity in infants, currently there is no maternal vaccine for this virus. Appendix F gives a summary of recommendations regarding immunization in pregnancy.

Grohskopf LA, Alyanak E, Broder KR, Blanton LH, Fry AM, Jernigan DB, et al. Prevention and control of seasonal influenza with vaccines: recommendations of the advisory committee on immunization practices - United States, 2020-21 influenza season. MMWR Recomm Rep 2020;69:1–24. doi: 10.15585/mmwr.rr6908a1 https://www.cdc.gov/mmwr/volumes/69/rr/rr6908a1.htm

Influenza vaccination during pregnancy. ACOG Committee Opinion No. 732. American College of Obstetricians and Gynecologists Obstet Gynecol 2018;131:e109–14. doi: 10.1097/AOG.0000000000002588 https://journals.lww.com/greenjournal/Fulltext/2018/04000/ACOG_Committee_Opinion_No__732__Influenza.45.aspx

Maternal immunization. ACOG Committee Opinion No. 741. American College of Obstetricians and Gynecologists. Obstet Gynecol 2018;131:e214–7. doi: 10.1097/AOG.0000000000002662 https://journals.lww.com/greenjournal/Fulltext/2018/06000/Maternal_Immunization__ACOG_Committee_Opinion,.60.aspx

80 Differential diagnosis for postpartum fever

A 28-year-old gravida 1, para 1, presents to your office at 5 days postpartum with a report of fever. She underwent primary cesarean birth for arrest of dilation after a labor complicated by presumed intra-amniotic infection. She received intravenous antibiotic therapy intrapartum and remained afebrile during the remainder of her hospitalization. The patient had an indwelling catheter during labor and cesarean birth that was removed on the first postoperative day. She has no dysuria, urinary frequency, or back pain. Her fever started yesterday along with incisional pain. Breastfeeding is going well, and she has no breast tenderness other than engorgement. Her vital signs are normal. On examination, the incision is intact with surrounding erythema and induration without drainage or fluctuance. Her examination is otherwise normal. The most likely diagnosis is

* (A) cellulitis
(B) endometritis
(C) mastitis
(D) urinary tract infection

The differential diagnosis for postpartum fever is broad. It includes wound infection, breast infection, uterine infection, urinary tract infection, septic pelvic thrombophlebitis, and other infectious causes. Workup should include evaluation of symptoms and physical examination, with laboratory evaluation and imaging guided by findings.

Wound infection is a common complication of cesarean birth after intra-amniotic infection. It usually presents with fever and incisional pain around day 4 after surgery. In this clinical scenario, the most likely diagnosis is wound cellulitis without abscess based on the physical examination findings of erythema and induration of the wound. Antibiotic choice should be tailored to skin flora and those usually isolated in amniotic fluid. First-generation cephalosporins are appropriate for initial treatment of cellulitis. If methicillin-resistant *Staphylococcus aureus* is suspected, trimethoprim-sulfamethoxazole is appropriate; however, this medication should be avoided in breastfeeding women with newborns less than 1 month of age.

Uterine infection, or endometritis, can be seen in all patients after delivery and can in particular be seen after intrapartum treatment for intra-amniotic infection. Fever often is the presenting symptom, and an alteration in bleeding pattern also may be seen. Uterine tenderness is generally noted. Mild endometritis can be treated with oral antibiotics, such as amoxicillin-clavulanate, but moderate to severe cases should be treated with intravenous antibiotics. In the above scenario, there are no specific findings in the patient's history or physical examination that are suspicious for endometritis because her bleeding pattern is normal, and her uterus is nontender.

Breast infection usually presents later in the postpartum course, generally 3–4 weeks after birth. Patients present with fever, unilateral pain, and erythema. Mastitis can be treated with dicloxacillin unless methicillin-resistant *S aureus* is suspected, and if no improvement is seen within 48–72 hours, abscess should be ruled out. Mastitis is unlikely in the clinical scenario above, because the patient is close to delivery and has no breast symptoms.

This patient's other risk factors include recent catheter use, and catheter-associated urinary tract infection should be ruled out; however, she has no urinary symptoms, making this an unlikely diagnosis. Overall incidence of catheter-associated urinary tract infection after cesarean birth is low, but the possibility should remain on the differential diagnosis.

Cunningham FG, Leveno KJ, Bloom SL, Dashe JS, Hoffman BL, Casey BM, et al. Williams obstetrics. 25th ed. McGraw-Hill Education; 2018.

Intrapartum management of intraamniotic infection. Committee Opinion No. 712. American College of Obstetricians and Gynecologists. Obstet Gynecol 2017;130:e95–e101. doi: 10.1097/AOG.0000000000002236 https://journals.lww.com/greenjournal/Fulltext/2017/08000/Committee_Opinion_No__712__Intrapartum_Management.58.aspx

81 Preeclampsia with severe features and its imitators

A 23-year-old primigravida at 29 weeks of gestation is admitted to labor and delivery with persistent vaginal bleeding. On admission, her blood pressure is 167/115 mm Hg, and repeat blood pressure 4 hours later was 172/112 mm Hg. She receives oral nifedipine, and her blood pressure decreases to 142/87 mm Hg. Her hematocrit is 36%, platelet count is 112 × 10^9/L, creatinine is 0.67 mg/dL, aspartate transaminase concentration is 31 units/L, and alanine transaminase concentration is 34 units/L. Baseline fetal heart rate is 150 beats per minute with moderate variability and accelerations. Fetal growth ultrasonography shows an estimated fetal weight at the 5th percentile, with normal umbilical artery Doppler velocimetry and placentation. The clinical finding that indicates the need for expedited delivery rather than expectant management is

(A) blood pressure greater than 160/110 mm Hg that responds to nifedipine
(B) fetal growth at the 5th percentile
(C) platelet count
* (D) vaginal bleeding in the absence of placenta previa

Hypertensive disorders of pregnancy, including preeclampsia and gestational hypertension, are a significant cause of maternal morbidity and mortality in the United States and worldwide. Many risk factors for preeclampsia have been identified, including nulliparity, advanced maternal age, multifetal gestation, antiphospholipid syndrome, and diabetes mellitus (gestational and pregestational). To prevent preeclampsia, patients at increased risk of preeclampsia may be given low-dose aspirin in the second and third trimesters of pregnancy.

Preeclampsia is defined as new-onset hypertension after 20 weeks of gestation in a patient with previously normal blood pressure, with associated proteinuria or other features. The lower threshold for diagnosing hypertension is a systolic blood pressure of 140 mm Hg, a diastolic blood pressure of 90 mm Hg, or both. The patient in the above scenario meets criteria for preeclampsia with severe features because her blood pressure was greater than 160/110 mm Hg on two occasions that were more than 4 hours apart (Appendix C). Proteinuria is not required for the diagnosis of preeclampsia with severe features. Other features that are diagnostic for severe preeclampsia include thrombocytopenia (platelet count less than 100 × 10^9/L), liver dysfunction (transaminase elevation twice the upper limit of normal), renal insufficiency (creatinine greater than 1.1 mg/dL or twice the patient's baseline), pulmonary edema, and visual disturbances.

In patients with preeclampsia or gestational hypertension without severe features, delivery is recommended at 37 weeks of gestation or at diagnosis if after 37 weeks. These patients often can be treated in an outpatient setting, with frequent blood pressure monitoring, laboratory measurements, fetal growth ultrasound monitoring, and antenatal testing. Expectant management carries an increased risk of abruption, intrauterine growth restriction, development of severe hypertension, eclampsia, and HELLP (hemolysis, elevated liver enzymes, and low platelet count) syndrome, but these risks are generally outweighed by the decreased risk of prematurity to the fetus. In patients with preeclampsia with severe features, delivery is recommended at 34 weeks of gestation at the latest. These patients should be treated in a hospital setting from diagnosis until delivery.

Indications that preclude expectant management of preeclampsia with severe features include uncontrolled severe hypertension that is not responsive to antihypertensive medication, persistent headache, epigastric pain unresponsive to medication, stroke, myocardial infarction, HELLP syndrome, new or worsening renal dysfunction, pulmonary edema, eclampsia, placental abruption, or vaginal bleeding without placenta previa. Fetal indications for delivery include abnormal fetal testing, persistent reversed end-diastolic flow in the umbilical artery, extreme prematurity, and fetal death. Depending on the overall clinical picture, delay of delivery to allow administration of antenatal corticosteroids may be permissible. In the clinical scenario above, vaginal bleeding without previa is an indication for delivery because of the concern for placental abruption.

Patients whose blood pressure can be controlled with antihypertensives are candidates for continued expectant management until 34 weeks of gestation, in the absence of other indications for delivery. A platelet count of 112 × 10^9/L is not a contraindication to expectant management, but ongoing laboratory evaluation should be performed to rule out the development of HELLP syndrome. Delivery for fetal growth restriction is indicated when Doppler velocimetry shows reversed end-diastolic flow in the umbilical artery. Individual clinical scenarios are often complicated, and multiple factors must be considered.

Cunningham FG, Leveno KJ, Bloom SL, Dashe JS, Hoffman BL, Casey BM, et al. Williams obstetrics. 25th ed. McGraw-Hill Education; 2018.

Gestational hypertension and preeclampsia. ACOG Practice Bulletin No. 222. American College of Obstetricians and Gynecologists. Obstet Gynecol 2020;135:e237–60. doi: 10.1097/AOG.0000000000003891 https://journals.lww.com/greenjournal/Fulltext/2020/06000/Gestational_Hypertension_and_Preeclampsia__ACOG.46.aspx

82 Management of second-trimester fetal death

A 33-year-old gravida 3, para 2, presents at 21 weeks of gestation for anatomical survey. A fetal death is noted on ultrasonography, with the composite measurements showing a fetal size of 20 weeks of gestation. She desires a dilation and evacuation (D&E). In addition to osmotic dilators, the most effective cervical preparation is

* (A) mifepristone
(B) misoprostol
(C) oxytocin
(D) prostaglandin E2

In the second trimester, the surgical management of fetal death in utero is based on the recommendations for managing termination of pregnancy at a comparable gestational age.

Data suggest that most second-trimester abortions (95%) are performed by a D&E procedure. All women undergoing a D&E should have preoperative ultrasonography to confirm gestational age (or fetal size in the setting of a fetal death in utero), and a baseline hemoglobin or hematocrit assessment. Cervical ripening before a second-trimester procedure is indicated to reduce the risk of cervical laceration or trauma and can be accomplished either with osmotic dilators or with cervical ripening medications. Use of osmotic dilators reduces the risk of cervical lacerations and hemorrhage.

In cases with a high risk of perforation or placental abnormalities, performing the procedure in a facility with access to blood transfusion, interventional radiology, and ability to convert to hysterectomy is recommended. For all D&E procedures with moderate to high risk of hemorrhage, uterotonic medications should be available and intraoperative ultrasound guidance should be used. Women who are Rh negative should receive anti-D immunoglobulin after abortion in either the first or second trimester.

In the described patient, after placement of osmotic dilators, the most effective pharmacologic agent is mifepristone. Mifepristone is an antiprogesterone synthetic steroid. It strongly binds to progesterone receptors, leading to significant cervical ripening. When compared with misoprostol, mifepristone is associated with decreased gastrointestinal symptoms, decreased cramping, and decreased risk of fever. Use of mifepristone before D&E is associated with easier dilatation, shorter procedure time, and the need for only one night of dilator administration.

Adjuvant misoprostol for patients who receive uncomplicated dilator insertions the day before D&E does not appear to significantly decrease procedure time or decrease the need for initial dilation. In addition, it increases adverse effects such as pain, cramping, nausea, and fever.

Using mifepristone and misoprostol without osmotic dilators at 20–24 weeks of gestation increases D&E procedure time and appears to increase occurrence of immediate complications. Pharmacologic regimens without adjuvant osmotic dilators should not be implemented.

Oxytocin is a peptide hormone that stimulates uterine contractions. It is used for labor induction or augmentation in the third trimester and to reduce the risk of hemorrhage in the postpartum period. Prostaglandin E2 (dinoprostone) is used for cervical ripening as a component of labor induction and historically was used as cervical preparation for second-trimester abortion. Administration of this agent is associated with a higher risk of adverse effects, including nausea, vomiting, diarrhea, and fever, when compared with mifepristone, and is not the best option for this patient.

Second-trimester abortion. Practice Bulletin No. 135. American College of Obstetricians and Gynecologists. Obstet Gynecol 2013;121:1394–406. doi: 10.1097/01.AOG.0000431056.79334.cc https://journals.lww.com/greenjournal/Fulltext/2013/06000/Practice_Bulletin_No__135__Second_Trimester.42.aspx

Society of Family Planning clinical recommendations: Cervical preparation for dilation and evacuation at 20–24 weeks' gestation. Diedrich JT, Drey EA, Newmann SJ. Society of Family Planning clinical recommendations: cervical preparation for dilation and evacuation at 20–24 weeks' gestation. Contraception 2020;101:286–92. doi: 10.1016/j.contraception.2020.01.002 https://www.contraceptionjournal.org/article/S0010-7824(20)30002-0/fulltext

83 Successful external cephalic version

A 29-year-old gravida 4, para 2, at 37 weeks of gestation is noted to have a fetus in breech presentation. She has a history of two prior vaginal deliveries and opts for external cephalic version (ECV). She has an anxiety disorder and poor pain tolerance, and she receives epidural anesthesia. To improve the chance of successful ECV, the most appropriate medication to administer is

(A) diazepam
(B) morphine
(C) nitroglycerin
(D) nitrous oxide
* (E) terbutaline

Approximately 3–4% of pregnancies at term are in breech presentation and contribute to the growing cesarean birth rate. A successful ECV increases the opportunity for a term vaginal delivery. A patient who does not otherwise have contraindications for vaginal delivery should be offered the option of an ECV when she is at or beyond 37 weeks of gestation. External cephalic version before 37 weeks of gestation is associated with a higher reversion rate.

External cephalic version is considered a safe procedure with an overall success rate above 50%. Complications include placental abruption, fetal maternal hemorrhage, rupture of membranes, and stillbirth. Fetal heart rate changes commonly occur and typically resolve spontaneously. Overall, the risk of a serious adverse event is rare. One large meta-analysis of 12,955 attempted ECVs reported a serious complication in 0.24% of the participants and the need for emergency cesarean birth in 0.35% of the participants. Figure 83-1 shows an algorithm for ECV management.

Contraindications to ECV include conditions in which vaginal delivery is not advisable, such as placenta previa and previous classical cesarean birth. Factors that may increase the chance for a successful ECV include multiparity, posterior placenta, increased amniotic fluid, unengaged presenting part, and relaxed uterus. Information concerning ECV attempts in patients with a previous uterine scar are from retrospective case–control analyses. The overall success rate ranged from 50% to 84% in the setting of a previous uterine scar, and there were no cases of uterine rupture reported.

Most ECVs are performed using terbutaline, a β-adrenergic receptor agonist, to relax the uterus. One randomized trial showed that the use of terbutaline almost doubled the success rate when compared with a placebo.

For the described patient, administering terbutaline would improve her chance for a successful ECV. Although the patient reports anxiety and a low pain threshold, anxiolytics or parenteral analgesia has not been evaluated for use in ECV. A meta-analysis of nine studies investigating the use of regional anesthesia for ECV found that the use of neuraxial anesthesia in combination with tocolysis had a higher incidence of successful ECV, vertex presentation in labor, and vaginal birth after successful ECV. Data for the use of nitric oxide gas or nitroglycerin are limited and inadequate to support their use in this clinical scenario.

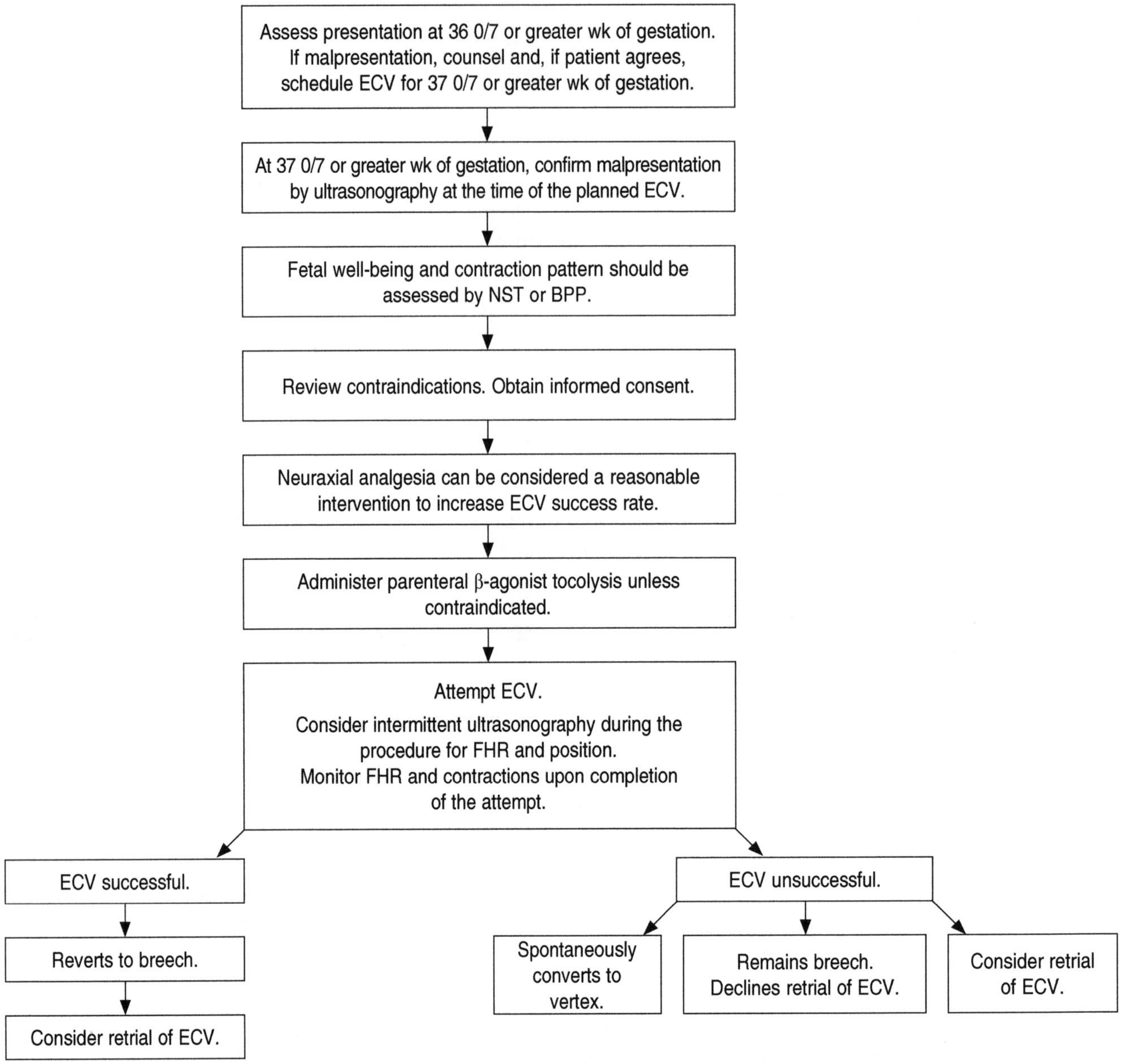

FIGURE 83-1. Algorithm for patient management for external cephalic version. Note: All Rh-negative women who undergo an ECV attempt, whether successful or not, should receive Rh-immune globulin unless they are known to have an Rh-negative fetus, are already sensitized, or will be delivered in less than 72 hours and can have an assessment for risk of sensitization Abbreviations: BPP, biophysical profile; ECV, external cephalic version; FHR, fetal heart rate; NST, nonstress test. (Reprinted from External cephalic version: ACOG Practice Bulletin No. 221. American College of Obstetricians and Gynecologists. Obstet Gynecol 2020;135:e203–12. doi: 10.1097/AOG.0000000000003837 https://journals.lww.com/greenjournal/Fulltext/2020/05000/External_Cephalic_Version__ACOG_Practice_Bulletin,.54.aspx)

External cephalic version: ACOG Practice Bulletin No. 221. American College of Obstetricians and Gynecologists. Obstet Gynecol 2020;135:e203–12. doi: 10.1097/AOG.0000000000003837 https://journals.lww.com/greenjournal/Fulltext/2020/05000/External_Cephalic_Version__ACOG_Practice_Bulletin,.54.aspx

Magro-Malosso ER, Saccone G, Di Tommaso M, Mele M, Berghella V. Neuraxial analgesia to increase the success rate of external cephalic version: a systematic review and meta-analysis of randomized controlled trials [published erratum appears in Am J Obstet Gynecol 2017;216:315]. Am J Obstet Gynecol 2016;215:276–86. doi: 10.1016/j.ajog.2016.04.036 https://www.ajog.org/article/S0002-9378(16)30134-X/fulltext.

84 Antiemetic drug metabolism

A patient presents at 10 weeks of gestation with nausea and vomiting. She has been unable to tolerate food for 2 days and fluids for 1 day. She has lost 4 kg in the past week and her prepregnancy weight was 79 kg. To treat her nausea at home, she has tried ginger supplements and replaced her prenatal vitamin with a folic acid supplement. Urinalysis shows 4+ ketones. Her medical history is significant for inherited prolonged QT interval, and she is taking nadolol and has an implantable defibrillator in place. The best antiemetic to administer for immediate relief is

* (A) lorazepam
(B) ondansetron
(C) promethazine
(D) scopolamine
(E) corticosteroids

Nausea and vomiting are common symptoms during the first trimester of pregnancy and may affect 50–80% of patients with varying degrees of severity. Hyperemesis gravidarum is a severe form of nausea and vomiting of pregnancy, usually accompanied by some measure of acute starvation, evident by ketonuria and at least 5% of prepregnancy weight loss. It is considered a diagnosis of exclusion, and other etiologies of severe nausea and vomiting should be ruled out.

First-line treatment of nausea and vomiting of pregnancy includes nonpharmacologic and pharmacologic treatment. Nonpharmacologic methods include ginger capsules and substituting prenatal vitamins with a folic acid-only supplement. First-line pharmacologic therapy includes vitamin B_6 (pyridoxine) and doxylamine. These oral medications are not appropriate for this patient who cannot tolerate oral intake, and they will not act immediately to resolve her symptoms.

Persistent nausea and vomiting symptoms combined with dehydration, as this patient has, require intravenous fluid replacement and medication treatment given in a nonoral route. Dimenhydrinate, metoclopramide, ondansetron, and promethazine all can be considered for treatment of hyperemesis gravidarum without complicating clinical factors. Many antiemetics used to treat hyperemesis gravidarum are used off-label because they have been approved by the U.S. Food and Drug Administration only for use in nonpregnant patients.

Treatment of nausea or hyperemesis gravidarum in patients with a prolonged QT interval can be difficult, and special consideration is needed for this group of patients. A prolonged QT interval may be caused by medications or electrolyte abnormalities or can be an inherited condition. A normal QT interval is less than 460 milliseconds in women. Many standard and second-line antiemetics are known to prolong the QT interval, which can lead to fatal arrhythmias in patients with inherited prolonged QT syndrome. Common medications used in the obstetric field that prolong QT interval are listed in Box 84-1. A medication that prolongs the QT interval should be used with caution in these patients, particularly in the setting of electrolyte abnormalities (eg, hypokalemia, hypomagnesemia, and hypocalcemia). With the degree of vomiting and starvation this patient has, electrolyte abnormalities would be expected, and standard antiemetics used to treat hyperemesis should not be given. These include antihistamines, such as doxylamine, which are commonly used for nausea and vomiting in pregnancy.

BOX 84-1

Common Obstetric Medications That Prolong QT Interval

- Antibiotics (azithromycin, erythromycin)
- Antidepressants (amitriptyline, escitalopram)
- Antiemetics (promethazine, ondansetron, metoclopramide)
- Antihistamines (dimenhydrinate, diphenhydramine)
- Antipsychotics (haloperidol)
- Methadone

Benzodiazepines can provide relief of nausea, may be given intravenously, and are the best option for patients with inherited prolonged QT interval, given that they do not further increase the risk of prolongation and eventual torsade de pointe. A benzodiazepine is not a good long-term choice but can provide immediate relief while the patient begins treatment for dehydration and potential electrolyte abnormalities.

Treatment with methylprednisolone may be considered, with a taper of 2 weeks if found to be effective, but it would not be expected to provide immediate relief to this patient. Patients may take up to 3 days to respond to treatment. If they are not responsive by that time, treatment with corticosteroids is unlikely to be effective and should be stopped. Methylprednisolone has a weak teratogenic effect when used in the first trimester (two cases of oral clefts per 1,000 women treated). It should be used after other treatment options are exhausted and with caution before 10 weeks of gestation because of the increased risk of oral clefting.

Scopolamine may be used as a transdermal patch to treat nausea associated with motion sickness or placed at least

4 hours preoperatively to prevent postoperative nausea. The exception is cesarean birth, in which postoperative placement is preferred to limit fetal exposure. Scopolamine is not considered to increase the risk of congenital anomalies or prolong the QT interval. However, drug levels are detectable only at 4 hours and would not provide immediate benefit to relieve the nausea and vomiting in this patient. The medication that will provide immediate relief without the risk of QT prolongation is lorazepam.

Congenital long QT (LQT) syndrome is an autosomal dominant condition with three main subtypes (LQT-1, LQT-2, and LQT-3) that normally presents with syncope or cardiac arrest during childhood. Other patients may be identified through familial screening efforts or screening electrocardiogram. Patients with LQT-1 may become symptomatic with exertion, whereas LQT-2 may be provoked with sudden auditory stimuli or an emotional event. Sudden death during sleep can present in LQT-3. Nonselective β-blockers, such as nadolol or propranolol, are used to treat LQT syndrome, and these should be continued during pregnancy.

Obstetric teams should be prepared to treat symptomatic prolonged QT interval patients on the labor unit. First-line therapy includes an oral or intravenous β-blocker, followed by magnesium sulfate, lidocaine, or mexiletine if β-blockers are ineffective. Continuous telemetry should be considered for high-risk patients (eg, those with a recent event). CredibleMeds.org lists contraindicated medications for patients with LQT syndrome.

Although elective cesarean birth has been suggested for LQT syndrome, there is no clear evidence this is protective, and it can be reserved for routine obstetric indications. In the 9 months after birth, there is a 2.7-fold increase in the risk of a cardiac event and a 4.1-fold increase in the risk of a life-threatening event, such as sudden cardiac death or aborted cardiac arrest. Although cardiac events, such as syncope, increase slightly during pregnancy itself, the antepartum, intrapartum, and immediate postpartum period of 24 hours does not appear to increase the risk of life-threatening events. Cardiac events are most common in women with LQT-2 syndrome. Hormonal changes, postpartum cardiovascular remodeling, and sleep deprivation may influence the QT interval and possibly explain the increased postpartum risk.

Farzam K, Tivakaran VS. QT prolonging drugs. In: StatPearls [Internet]; 2022. Accessed March 16, 2022. https://www.ncbi.nlm.nih.gov/books/NBK534864/

Loscalzo J, Fauci AS, Kasper DL, Hauser S, Longo D, Jameson JL. Harrison's principles of internal medicine. 21st ed. McGraw-Hill Companies; 2022.

Nausea and vomiting of pregnancy. ACOG Practice Bulletin No. 189. American College of Obstetricians and Gynecologists. Obstet Gynecol 2018;131:e15–30. doi: 10.1097/AOG.0000000000002456 https://journals.lww.com/greenjournal/Fulltext/2018/01000/ACOG_Practice_Bulletin_No__189__Nausea_And.39.aspx

Roston TM, van der Werf C, Cheung CC, Grewal J, Davies B, Wilde AA, et al. Caring for the pregnant woman with an inherited arrhythmia syndrome. Heart Rhythm 2020;17:341–8. doi: 10.1016/j.hrthm.2019.08.004 https://www.heartrhythmjournal.com/article/S1547-5271(19)30725-8/fulltext

Scopolamine transdermal. In: Facts and Comparisons [after login]. Wolters Kluwer Health, Inc.; 2022. Accessed March 16, 2022. https://fco.factsandcomparisons.com/lco/action/doc/retrieve/docid/fc_dfc/5549257

Seth R, Moss AJ, McNitt S, Zareba W, Andrews ML, Qi M, et al. Long QT syndrome and pregnancy. J Am Coll Cardiol 2007;49:1092–8. doi: 10.1016/j.jacc.2006.09.054 https://www.sciencedirect.com/science/article/pii/S0735109706031184

85 Third-trimester bleeding

A 38-year-old gravida 3, para 2, who has not initiated prenatal care presents to the emergency department with acute vaginal bleeding. Her last menstrual period is unknown because she has experienced intermittent vaginal bleeding for months. She reports constant abdominal pain and intermittent low back pain. She has a history of substance use and reports cocaine use during the last 36 hours. Her blood pressure is 105/75 mm Hg, heart rate is 115 beats per minute, and her temperature is 37.5 °C (99.5 °F). On physical examination, her abdomen is firm and tender, and her fundal height is 35 cm. Her cervix is visually closed with 30 cc of fresh blood in the vaginal vault and active bleeding from the cervical os. Obstetric ultrasonography is performed at the bedside. The placental location is fundal, and the fetus is in cephalic presentation. Electronic fetal heart tracing is Category III. She is contracting every 2 minutes. Her hemoglobin is 5.4 g/dL, and her fibrinogen is 150 mg/dL. In addition to initiating blood product transfusion, the best next step in management is

* (A) cesarean birth
(B) fetal monitoring with intrauterine resuscitation
(C) intramuscular betamethasone
(D) intravenous magnesium sulfate
(E) nifedipine tocolysis

Placental abruption, also known by the Latin term *abruptio placentae*, is the premature partial or complete separation of the placenta from the underlying decidua basalis. Placental abruptions are classified as acute or chronic depending on how rapidly they develop and how long the pregnancy is maintained. They are referred to as "concealed" when no outward signs of bleeding are evident. Clinically apparent abruptions occur in approximately 1% of pregnancies, but 2.1–3.8% of placentas will demonstrate evidence of abruption on pathologic examination. Placental abruption is the most common cause of pathologic bleeding in the third trimester.

Risk factors for placental abruption include maternal comorbidities, obstetric conditions, and fetal conditions. The greatest risk factor for an abruption is a history of a previous placental abruption, which confers a 10- to 20-fold increased risk in the subsequent gestation. Maternal conditions that increase the risk of placental abruption include hypertensive disorders, thrombophilia disorders, uterine leiomyomata, advanced maternal age, increased parity, tobacco use, and cocaine use. Hypertensive disorders are the most common maternal risk factor for placental abruption, including chronic hypertension and pregnancy-specific hypertensive disorders, such as gestational hypertension and preeclampsia. Obstetric complications that increase the risk of abruption include traumatic injury, multifetal gestation, polyhydramnios, intrauterine infection, and preterm prelabor rupture of membranes (PPROM). Approximately 5% of patients who experience PPROM will subsequently experience a placental abruption. Polyhydramnios is associated with an eightfold increased risk of abruption. A finding of a single-umbilical artery or an isolated elevation of maternal serum α-fetoprotein during second-trimester screening are associated with increased risk of placental abruption later in pregnancy.

The mechanism of placental separation is not uniform for all placental abruptions. Physical shearing of the tissue planes does occur with traumatic abruptions, but others are related to uteroplacental insufficiency with impaired trophoblastic invasion such as in hypertensive disorders. Acute vasoconstriction is the likely genesis of placental abruption with cocaine use. Regardless of the pathogenesis, the abruption begins with bleeding that creates a decidual hematoma. The bleeding can expand from beneath the placenta to under the membranes, and in some cases through the cervix with vaginal bleeding. Concealed hemorrhages can expand to great extents without vaginal bleeding becoming evident. The amount of vaginal bleeding noted during a placental abruption does not correlate with the severity of the abruption.

The maternal morbidity associated with a placental abruption is proportional to the severity of the bleeding. The patient is at risk of hemorrhage with subsequent anemia, hypovolemia, acute renal injury, and disseminated intravascular coagulopathy. Even with delivery, impairment in myometrial contractility after the abruption can lead to atony, postpartum hemorrhage, and the possible need for hysterectomy.

For the fetus, morbidity and mortality are related not only to the severity of the abruption but also to the gestational age at which it occurs. A cohort study based in the United States evaluated more than 7.5 million births and found that perinatal mortality in those complicated by abruption was 119 per 1,000 births versus 8.2 per 1,000 births for those without abruptions. Prematurity is the primary cause of mortality in births complicated by abruption.

Placental abruptions can lead to PPROM and preterm labor. Ten percent of preterm deliveries have some degree of placental abruption. Fetal blood usually is not lost with placental abruptions because the chorionic villi rarely are disrupted. When villous disruption does occur, it often is due to traumatic injuries. Partial placental abruptions will decrease oxygen and nutrient delivery to the fetus. Chronic, partial abruptions are linked to fetal growth restriction and adverse neurologic outcomes, but most abruptions that result in fetal death have greater than 50% of the placental surface separated.

Patients experiencing a placental abruption will demonstrate a wide spectrum of symptoms. The classical presentation is a patient with abdominal pain, bleeding, and evidence of fetal compromise. One prospective study noted that in women experiencing an abruption, 78% had vaginal bleeding, 66% reported uterine tenderness or back pain, and 60% had a nonreassuring fetal status. The degree of placental separation and the rate of bleeding will affect presentation. Small, nonexpanding abruptions may have no clinical consequences for the pregnancy. Uterine activity suggestive of an abruption is high-frequency but low-amplitude contractions. The fetal heart tracing in a severe abruption can demonstrate decreased variability with recurrent variable or late decelerations and bradycardia. Patients who present with acute abruptions often also labor and tend to progress rapidly.

The diagnosis of a placental abruption most often is made clinically. Studies vary widely on the sensitivity and specificity of obstetric ultrasonography in the diagnosis of an abruption. This imaging method seems to perform better at detecting chronic, more evolved hematomas than with acute abruptions, but overall, ultrasonography will identify only 50% of abruptions at best.

The management of a placental abruption in a patient should be individualized based on severity, the gestational age, and the resources available. Patients presenting with an acute abruption should be assessed for stability. Two large-bore intravenous lines should be placed. A complete blood count, coagulation profile, and blood type and cross-match should be included in the laboratory evaluation. Urine output should be monitored. Fetal well-being should be assessed. In the setting of an abruption with a fetal death, immediate delivery is indicated. A vaginal delivery is preferred if the rate of bleeding allows for conservative treatment, which can include blood product transfusion to allow labor to continue. Cesarean birth in the setting of a fetal death should be reserved for severe hemorrhages.

When a placental abruption is encountered at term, immediate delivery is indicated. If the woman and fetus are both stable, labor can be induced or allowed to progress. Labor is known to progress rapidly in the setting of a placental abruption. Maternal blood loss should be continuously evaluated. Maternal vital signs should be closely observed, and continuous fetal electronic heart rate monitoring maintained. Cesarean birth should be conducted if the woman or fetus, or both, become unstable or demonstrate a compromised state and vaginal birth is not imminent.

When a placental abruption is diagnosed in the preterm period with a live fetus, conservative management with continuation of the pregnancy should be considered. Before viability, the clinician should assess maternal stability. If the patient is stable, conservative management is appropriate. Consultation with an obstetrician with experience in high-risk cases should be obtained and transfer to a facility with appropriate neonatal services should be discussed.

With a placental abruption at a viable preterm gestational age, both maternal and fetal status will contribute to the care plan. If either the woman or the fetus demonstrates a compromised state, delivery should be initiated. Depending on the stability of the patients, there may be time for transfer to facilities with Level III or higher neonatal intensive care units. When the patient is hemodynamically stable and the preterm fetus demonstrates well-being, the pregnancy can be continued with close surveillance. Corticosteroid administration should be administered for fetal lung maturation, and intravenous magnesium sulfate can be considered for neuroprotective benefit. The use of tocolytic agents is controversial in the setting of a suspected abruption for fear of potentiating bleeding, or in the case of terbutaline, having the accompanying tachycardia complicate the evaluation of maternal status. Small studies have found no adverse effects with administration of tocolytics in these situations. Because most of the perinatal mortality in a case of placental abruption is due to prematurity, conservative management to achieve a more mature gestational age should be considered.

Women with a history of placental abruption have an increased risk of placental abruption in subsequent pregnancies; however, there are no proven interventions to prevent recurrence. Hypertensive patients should maintain good blood pressure control. Patients who use tobacco or cocaine should be counseled about cessation. For patients with diagnosed thrombophilia disorders, anticoagulation should be prescribed during pregnancy. Some experts also recommend serial obstetric ultrasonography to assess fetal growth throughout the pregnancy.

The described patient has demonstrated evidence of a severe placental abruption based on her presentation, initial laboratory evaluation, and fetal compromise. In the setting of both maternal and fetal compromise, emergent delivery should be achieved. Her cervix is closed, and vaginal birth is not imminent. When planning for an emergent cesarean birth, the administration of corticosteroids and intravenous magnesium will not achieve a therapeutic effect. Similarly, delivery should proceed immediately and not be delayed for the administration of a tocolytic agent.

Ananth CV, Wilcox AJ. Placental abruption and perinatal mortality in the United States. Am J Epidemiol 2001;153:332–7. doi: 10.1093/aje/153.4.332 https://academic.oup.com/aje/article/153/4/332/129008

Cunningham FG, Leveno KJ, Bloom SL, Dashe JS, Hoffman BL, Casey BM, et al. Williams obstetrics. 25th ed. McGraw-Hill Education; 2018.

Oyelese Y, Ananth CV. Placental abruption. Obstet Gynecol 2006;108:1005–16. doi: 10.1097/01.AOG.0000239439.04364.9a https://journals.lww.com/greenjournal/Fulltext/2006/10000/Placental_Abruption.26.aspx

86 Cerebral palsy

A patient presents at 24 weeks of gestation and is admitted for preeclampsia with severe features (Appendix C) and fetal growth restriction. During cesarean birth for nonreassuring fetal testing, a placental abruption is identified. Apgar scores are 4 and 6 at 1 and 5 minutes, respectively. The neonatal birth weight is 505 g. The factor most strongly associated with the risk of cerebral palsy in this neonate is

(A) Apgar scores
(B) birth weight
* (C) gestational age
(D) placental abruption
(E) preeclampsia

Cerebral palsy is broadly defined as a group of conditions involving motor disabilities of varying degrees. It is the most common physical disability in childhood. Cerebral palsy usually results from injury to the developing brain before, during, or after delivery. The following criteria are suggested for the diagnosis:

- Presence of motor disorder (eg, spasticity, dyskinesia, ataxia, mixed motor abnormalities, hypotonia)
- Result of a cerebral abnormality
- Occurrence early in development
- Nonprogressive or degenerative course

Patients with cerebral palsy can have associated impairments including vision, hearing, cognitive, speech, and behavioral disorders. Cerebral palsy is a lifelong condition without a cure.

The most significant risk factor for cerebral palsy is prematurity. Prematurity results in vulnerability to cerebral white matter injury that can lead to periventricular leukomalacia and intraventricular hemorrhage. The risk of cerebral palsy is inversely related to the gestational age at delivery and substantially increases with preterm delivery before 32 weeks of gestation (very preterm). The global prevalence of cerebral palsy is approximately 112 per 1,000 live births in neonates at less than 28 weeks of gestation versus 1.4 per 1,000 live births in neonates at greater than 36 weeks of gestation. Efforts to reduce preterm birth remain paramount to the prevention of cerebral palsy.

The only antenatal intervention that has been shown to reduce the risk of cerebral palsy is magnesium sulfate. In a large, randomized controlled trial, magnesium sulfate was shown to reduce the risk of moderate or severe cerebral palsy (1.9% versus 3.5%; relative risk, 0.55; 95% CI, 0.32–0.95). The American College of Obstetricians and Gynecologists supports the use of magnesium sulfate for fetal neuroprotection before an anticipated preterm birth at less than 32 weeks of gestation. Magnesium sulfate for neuroprotection should be reserved for cases with delivery anticipated within the next 12–24 hours.

Postnatally, therapeutic hypothermia improves neurologic outcomes for infants with hypoxic ischemic encephalopathy. This intervention has become a major milestone in the treatment of neonatal encephalopathy. Cooling results in neuronal rescue by reducing the rate of brain metabolism. The goal is to cool the neonate to 33–34 °C (91–93 °F). Criteria for therapeutic hypothermia vary by institution, but in general, the following are used:

- Gestational age of 36 or more weeks of gestation
- Initiation within 6 hours of delivery
- Evidence of encephalopathy
- One of the following:
  - — Neonatal acidosis
  - — 10-minute Apgar score of 5 or less
  - — Ongoing resuscitation efforts

The Apgar score is an assessment of the neonate's physiologic condition at birth and is used to assess the effectiveness of resuscitation. It contains both subjective components and certain clinical components, such as reflex irritability, that are dependent on the neurologic maturity of the neonate. Although a low Apgar score may be associated with adverse neonatal outcomes, it was not designed to predict long-term outcomes. Low 5- and 10-minute Apgar scores are associated with an increased relative risk of cerebral palsy. However, most infants with low Apgar scores will not develop cerebral palsy.

Low birth weight, particularly less than that of the 3rd percentile (as in this scenario), is associated with an increased risk of cerebral palsy. Preeclampsia and placental abruption also are risk factors for cerebral palsy. All of the listed answer choices are risk factors for cerebral palsy, but early gestational age is by far the strongest risk factor.

American College of Obstetricians and Gynecologists, American Academy of Pediatrics. Neonatal encephalopathy and neurologic outcome. 2nd ed. ACOG; AAP; 2014. https://www.acog.org/clinical/clinical-guidance/task-force-report/articles/2014/neonatal-encephalopathy-and-neurologic-outcome

Oskoui M, Coutinho F, Dykeman J, Jetté N, Pringsheim T. An update on the prevalence of cerebral palsy: a systematic review and meta-analysis [published erratum appears in Dev Med Child Neurol 2016;58:316]. Dev Med Child Neurol 2013;55:509–19. doi: 10.1111/dmcn.12080 https://onlinelibrary.wiley.com/doi/10.1111/dmcn.12080

Rouse DJ, Hirtz DG, Thom E, Varner MW, Spong CY, Mercer BM, et al. A randomized, controlled trial of magnesium sulfate for the prevention of cerebral palsy. *Eunice Kennedy Shriver* NICHD Maternal–Fetal Medicine Units Network. N Engl J Med 2008;359:895–905. doi: 10.1056/NEJMoa0801187 https://www.nejm.org/doi/10.1056/NEJMoa0801187

Shepherd E, Salam RA, Middleton P, Makrides M, McIntyre S, Badawi N, Crowther CA. Antenatal and intrapartum interventions for preventing cerebral palsy: an overview of Cochrane systematic reviews. Cochrane Database of Systematic Reviews 2017, Issue 8. Art. No.: CD012077. doi: 10.1002/14651858.CD012077.pub2 http://dx.doi.org/10.1002/14651858.CD012077.pub2

87 Amniotic fluid

A patient at 24 weeks of gestation has a fundal height of 30 cm at a routine obstetric visit. All maternal testing, including noninvasive prenatal screening and 18 weeks of gestation anatomy ultrasonography, has yielded normal results. Ultrasonography is performed and fetal growth is at the 50th percentile. Figure 87-1 represents the deepest vertical pocket. In addition to a glucose challenge, the best next step is

(A) amniocentesis with fluid reduction
* (B) detailed fetal anatomic survey
(C) fetal magnetic resonance imaging (MRI)
(D) maternal cytomegalovirus (CMV) serology
(E) reassurance

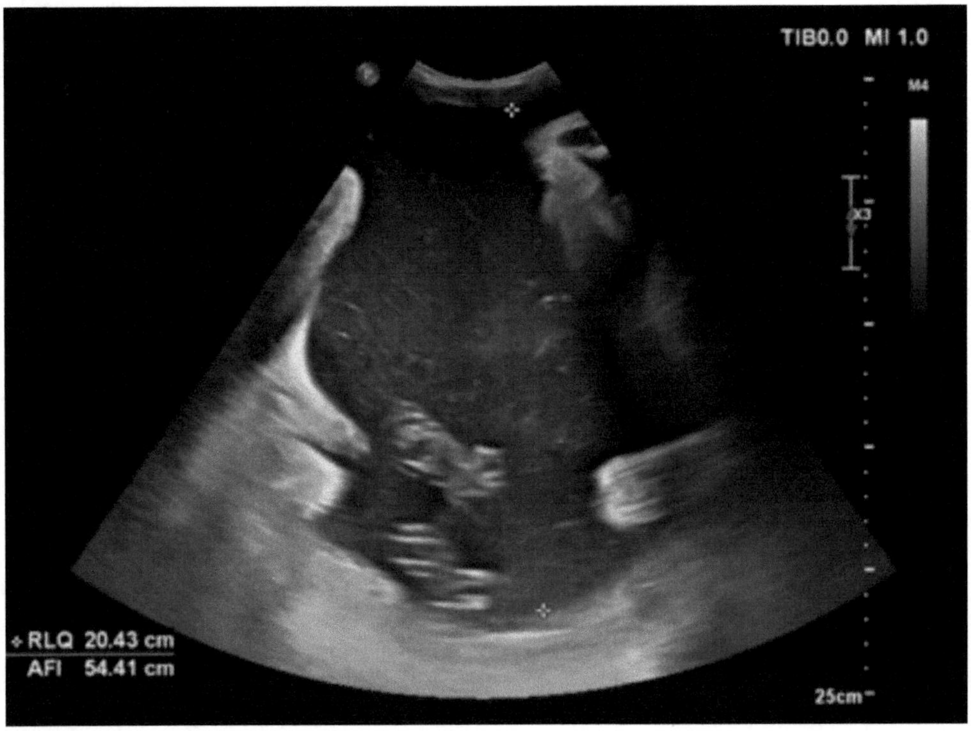

FIGURE 87-1. Maximal vertical pocket. (Image courtesy of Dr. Marcie Treadwell.)

Amniotic fluid is measured after 20 weeks of gestation by one of two recommended methods: amniotic fluid index (AFI) or maximal vertical pocket (deepest vertical pocket). The AFI is measured by dividing the gravid uterus into four quadrants. With the abdominal transducer held perpendicular to the floor and in the sagittal plane, the largest vertical pocket in each quadrant, void of umbilical cord or fetal parts, is measured and added together. Evaluating fluid volume by deepest vertical pocket is accomplished similarly, by selecting the single deepest pocket measured in the same way. These two methods are uniform and reproducible, allowing communication among clinicians. For multiple gestations, the deepest vertical pocket method is preferred to assess amniotic fluid.

Polyhydramnios is defined by a maximal vertical pocket greater than 8 cm or an AFI of 24 cm or more. *Mild*, *moderate*, and *severe* polyhydramnios are defined in Table 87-1.

Pregnancies complicated by polyhydramnios occur in 1–2% of singleton gestations, are mostly detected in the third trimester, are mild, and have an idiopathic etiology. In all pregnancies with polyhydramnios, women are more likely to have a cesarean birth. As polyhydramnios increases in severity, so does the risk of preterm birth, perinatal mortality, and small-for-gestational-age newborns. In 15–30% of cases of polyhydramnios, the fetal weight is above 4,000 g, compared with a population rate of 8%. Progressively worsening polyhydramnios over the course of a trimester is more likely related to a structural or genetic cause. Polyhydramnios warrants evaluation. Reassurance would not be appropriate, especially in cases of severe polyhydramnios, which are more likely to have a genetic or structural etiology.

Idiopathic polyhydramnios is the most common cause of mild polyhydramnios; however, this is a diagnosis of exclusion. Evaluation with ultrasonography for structural causes (Table 87-2) and screening for maternal diabetes mellitus are first steps. When the maximal vertical pocket is less than 16, as in the described patient, there is a strong association with fetal anomalies. Only approximately 15% of cases of polyhydramnios will be severe, and of those, 20–40% will have a cause identified before birth. Therefore, in addition to a glucose challenge test, the next step at 24 weeks of gestation would be a detailed ultrasound examination, including

- fetal growth
- fetal movement (to detect neurologic disorders)
- cardiac anatomy (to detect congenital heart disease leading to high-output cardiac failure, polyhydramnios, and edema)
- fetal hands and feet (to detect arthrogryposis syndromes)
- fetal stomach (to detect tracheoesophageal fistula or esophageal or duodenal atresia)
- facial anatomy (to detect cleft lip and palate)
- masses in the neck, thorax, abdomen (to detect obstruction to swallowing)
- masses in the pelvis, spine, and kidney (to detect ureteropelvic junction obstruction)

Should this evaluation be normal, consultation with a genetic counselor about possible neurologic causes, such as congenital myotonic dystrophy, would be indicated. When a cause is not

TABLE 87-1. Outcomes of Polyhydramnios Based on Severity

	AMNIOTIC FLUID INDEX	DEEPEST VERTICAL POCKET	INCIDENCE	RISK OF FETAL ABNORMALITY*	RISK OF NEONATAL ABNORMALITY†
Polyhydramnios, overall, cm	24.0 or lower	8.0 or lower	0.3–1.0%		
Mild, cm	24.0–29.9	8–11	65–70% of total	6–10%	1%
Moderate, cm	30.0–34.9	12–15	20% of total	10–15%	2%
Severe, cm	35.0 or lower	16 or lower	Less than 15% of total	20–40%	10%

*Chance that fetal anomaly will be identified prenatally.

†Chance that neonatal abnormality will be identified in cases without a detected prenatal anomaly.

Reprinted from Dashe JS, Pressman EK, Hibbard JU. SMFM Consult Series #46: evaluation and management of polyhydramnios. Society for Maternal-Fetal Medicine (SMFM). Am J Obstet Gynecol 2018;219:B2-8. doi: 10.1016/j.ajog.2018.07.016 https://www.ajog.org/article/S0002-9378(18)30589-1/fulltext

TABLE 87-2. Fetal and Neonatal Etiologies of Polyhydramnios

IMPAIRED SWALLOWING			EXCESS URINE PRODUCTION		
GI OBSTRUCTION	NEUROMUSCULAR	CRANIOFACIAL	RENAL/URINARY	CARDIAC	OSMOTIC DIURESIS/OTHER
Duodenal atresia	Myotonic dystrophy	Cleft lip/palate	UPJ obstruction	Cardiac structural anomaly	Diabetes
TE fistula	Arthrogryposis	Micrognathia	Mesoblastic nephroma	Tachyarrhythmia	Hydrops
Thoracic mass	Intracranial anomaly	Neck mass	Bartter syndrome	Sacrococcygeal teratoma	Idiopathic
Diaphragmatic hernia				Chorioangioma	

Abbreviations: GI, gastrointestinal; TE, tracheoesophageal; UPJ, ureteropelvic junction.

Reprinted from Dashe JS, Pressman EK, Hibbard JU. SMFM Consult Series #46: evaluation and management of polyhydramnios. Society for Maternal-Fetal Medicine (SMFM). Am J Obstet Gynecol 2018;219:B2-8. doi: 10.1016/j.ajog.2018.07.016 https://www.ajog.org/article/S0002-9378(18)30589-1/fulltext

determined antenatally, the neonatal period is the next appropriate time to evaluate, with a cause determined in 10% of cases. An amnioreduction may be performed in the setting of severe polyhydramnios if significant maternal dyspnea or discomfort is present.

Despite limited evidence for CMV causing polyhydramnios, testing for CMV is commonly performed. A 2019 retrospective study reviewed 1,266 CMV tests out of 21,102 pregnancies. The rate of polyhydramnios in the CMV-positive group was 3% (2 cases) compared with 4% (13 cases) in the non-CMV group. Screening for CMV is not recommended based on the finding of polyhydramnios alone.

Magnetic resonance imaging has been studied and improves the detection of central nervous system abnormalities in cases of polyhydramnios. Focused use of MRI can clarify central nervous system lesions associated with polyhydramnios; however, general application is limited by its clinical value and cost effectiveness. For this patient, starting with an MRI would not be the best next step given the normal fetal survey in the second trimester.

Antepartum fetal surveillance. ACOG Practice Bulletin No. 229. American College of Obstetricians and Gynecologists. Obstet Gynecol 2021;137:e116–27. doi: 10.1097/AOG.0000000000004410 https://journals.lww.com/greenjournal/Fulltext/2021/06000/Antepartum_Fetal_Surveillance__ACOG_Practice.37.aspx

Dashe JS, Pressman EK, Hibbard JU. SMFM Consult Series #46: evaluation and management of polyhydramnios. Society for Maternal–Fetal Medicine (SMFM). Am J Obstet Gynecol 2018;219:B2–8. doi: 10.1016/j.ajog.2018.07.016 https://www.ajog.org/article/S0002-9378(18)30589-1/fulltext

Erfani H, Diaz-Rodriguez GE, Aalipour S, Nassr A, Rezaei A, Gandhi M, et al. Amnioreduction in cases of polyhydramnios: indications and outcomes in singleton pregnancies without fetal interventions. Eur J Obstet Gynecol Reprod Biol 2019;241:126–8. doi: 10.1016/j.ejogrb.2019.05.019 https://www.ejog.org/article/S0301-2115(19)30240-4/fulltext

Fishel-Bartal M, Watad H, Hoffmann C, Achiron R, Barzilay E, Katorza E. Fetal brain MRI in polyhydramnios: is it justified? J Matern Fetal Neonatal Med 2019;32:3986–92. doi: 10.1080/14767058.2018.1480605 https://www.tandfonline.com/doi/abs/10.1080/14767058.2018.1480605

Mangels R, Blumenfeld YJ, Homeyer M, Mrazek-Pugh B, Hintz SR, Hudgins L. RASopathies: a significant cause of polyhydramnios? Prenat Diagn 2021;41:362–7. doi: 10.1002/pd.5862 https://obgyn.onlinelibrary.wiley.com/doi/10.1002/pd.5862

Yefet E, Ben Shmuel Y, Nachum Z. The association between polyhydramnios and CMV infection—retrospective cohort study. J Matern Fetal Neonatal Med 2021;34:3716–22. doi: 10.1080/14767058.2019.1691164 https://www.tandfonline.com/doi/abs/10.1080/14767058.2019.1691164

88 Tuberculosis in a pregnant patient

A 19-year-old is seen at 12 weeks of gestation for their first prenatal visit and they report feeling well. They have been living in a homeless shelter for 6 months. The patient has a history of prior bacillus Calmette-Guérin (BCG) vaccination. In addition to routine prenatal care, the best next test in evaluation of latent tuberculosis (TB) infection is

(A) chest X-ray
* (B) interferon-gamma release assay (IGRA)
(C) pulmonary function tests
(D) sputum culture
(E) tuberculin skin testing

In the United States, TB most commonly is caused by *Mycobacterium tuberculosis*. *M tuberculosis* is one of seven acid-fast bacilli linked to TB and transmitted by droplets after an infected person coughs, sneezes, or sings. The bacilli infect the lungs and travel throughout the body through the lymphatic system or bloodstream.

The World Health Organization estimates that 25% of the world's population is infected with TB, resulting in 1.5 million deaths annually. In 2019, of 10 million individuals affected with TB, 1.2 million were children. Tuberculosis was the leading infectious cause of death worldwide until 2020, when it was surpassed by COVID-19. There are few national programs that track pregnant women with TB, making exact numbers difficult to determine. Between 14% and 47% of pregnant individuals do not know they are positive for TB.

Tuberculosis is a curable and preventable disease largely found in low-resource communities. Fever, night sweats, fatigue, chest pain, cough, hemoptysis, decreased appetite, and weight loss are the symptoms of active TB. In the latent phase of TB, an individual may not have symptoms but will have risk factors (Table 88-1). Screening for social determinants of health is one way to identify persons at risk of TB. Homelessness is an important risk factor. Individuals experiencing homelessness are more likely to be in an overcrowded living arrangement. Non-cisgendered individuals comprise up to 20% of homeless youth, who are also at risk of intimate partner violence. Understanding the social determinants that increase the risk of homelessness helps the obstetrician–gynecologist offer resources. Patients at risk should undergo serial annual screening for TB infection.

Tuberculosis infections can be latent or active. Latent TB confers a 4–6% lifetime risk of progression to active disease, which is unchanged in pregnancy. Treatment of latent TB reduces the risk of progression in high-risk populations. Active TB in pregnancy has maternal and fetal consequences

TABLE 88-1. Risk Factors for Tuberculosis for Acquisition, Transmission, Progression, and Success of Treatment

	RISK FACTORS
General risk factors	• Exposure to *M tuberculosis* • HIV-positive status • Immunosuppressive drug use • Younger age • Homelessness • Overcrowded living conditions • Active or passive tobacco smoke exposure
Specific factors affecting transmission	• Infectiousness of the individual • The specific strain • The host's susceptibility of infection • The duration of exposure • The environment of exposure
Risk factors for progression from latent to active disease	• HIV-positive status • Acquisition of TB within the last 2 y • Intravenous drug use • Immunocompromised status
The highest likelihood of a latent TB infection, for which treatment has been shown to have benefit	• Individuals with recent exposure or household contacts • Age less than 5 y • HIV infection • Immunosuppressive therapy • Silicosis • Residence in high-risk congregate settings

Data from Lewinsohn DM, Leonard MK, LoBue PA, Cohn DL, Daley CL, Desmond E, et al. Official American Thoracic Society/Infectious Diseases Society of America/Centers for Disease Control and Prevention clinical practice guidelines: diagnosis of tuberculosis in adults and children. Clin Infect Dis 2017;64:e1–33. doi: 10.1093/cid/ciw694 https://academic.oup.com/cid/article/64/2/e1/2629583

with higher rates of miscarriage, antenatal admission, anemia, and cesarean birth (Table 88-2). There is a fourfold increased risk of perinatal death and a 1.6-fold increased risk of preterm birth, underscoring the importance of identification of TB in pregnancy. For all metrics evaluated, diagnosis and treatment in the first trimester have better outcomes and fewer complications compared with treatment initiation in the second or third trimester (Table 88-3). Screening and diagnosis in pregnancy allow timely treatment of TB, reducing the maternal and fetal risks from active infection.

The described asymptomatic patient is at risk of TB and should be offered screening. There are two common screening tests: 1) the Mantoux tuberculin skin test and 2) the IGRA blood test. The Mantoux tuberculin skin test screens for cell-mediated immunity by a delayed-type hypersensitivity response with purified protein derivative. Although the test is simple and inexpensive, it requires trained individuals to place the test and a second visit to interpret the test. The tuberculin skin test will be positive 2–12 weeks after exposure to TB. For individuals with a history of the BCG vaccination, such as the above-described patient, the tuberculin skin test may be falsely positive, and an IGRA is recommended as the best initial test. The assay measures interferon-gamma released by sensitized T cells, primarily CD4 cells. This test is more specific for mycobacterium and is not affected by previous BCG vaccination. After a positive screen, the patient should have a chest radiograph to evaluate for active TB. Chest radiographs are not used for primary screening.

A sputum culture positive for *M tuberculosis*, while diagnostic for active TB, is not used as an initial screening test. The Centers for Disease Control and Prevention recommends that both liquid and solid cultures be performed for patients suspected of active TB. The two liquid culture tests have a sensitivity of 88–90% (13–15 days to complete), and the solid culture test has a sensitivity of 76% (25 days to complete). All three tests together have a 99% specificity.

Pulmonary function tests are useful in pregnancy for chronic respiratory disease, such as asthma, but are not indicated in the screening for latent TB or confirmation of active TB.

TABLE 88-2. Odds Ratios for Maternal Morbidity With Active Tuberculosis in Pregnancy

	INCREASE	OR/95% CI
Miscarriage	Ninefold increase	OR, 9.0; 95% CI, 4.93–16.67
Maternal morbidity	Threefold increase	OR, 2.8; 95% CI, 1.17–4.6
Antenatal admission	Ninefold increase	OR, 9.6; 95% CI, 2.3–40.6
Anemia	Fourfold increase	OR, 3.85; 95% CI, 2.21–6.71
Cesarean birth	Twofold increase	OR, 2.10; 95% CI, 1.17–3.79

Abbreviation: OR, odds ratio.

Data from Sobhy S, Babiker Z, Zamora J, Khan KS, Kunst H. Maternal and perinatal mortality and morbidity associated with tuberculosis during pregnancy and the postpartum period: a systematic review and meta-analysis. BJOG 2017;124:727-33. doi: 10.1111/1471-0528.14408 https://obgyn.onlinelibrary.wiley.com/doi/10.1111/1471-0528.14408

TABLE 88-3. Perinatal Morbidity Based on the Trimester in Which Treatment for Tuberculosis Was Initiated

METRIC	FIRST-TRIMESTER TREATMENT	SECOND- OR THIRD-TRIMESTER TREATMENT
Perinatal death	0/9	3/13 (23%)
Low birth weight	0/23	33/54 (61%)
Preterm birth	0/9	4/12 (33%)

Data from Sobhy S, Babiker Z, Zamora J, Khan KS, Kunst H. Maternal and perinatal mortality and morbidity associated with tuberculosis during pregnancy and the postpartum period: a systematic review and meta-analysis. BJOG 2017;124:727-33. doi: 10.1111/1471-0528.14408 https://obgyn.onlinelibrary.wiley.com/doi/10.1111/1471-0528.14408

Health care for homeless women. Committee Opinion No. 576. American College of Obstetricians and Gynecologists. Obstet Gynecol 2013;122:936–40. doi: 10.1097/01.AOG.0000435417.29567.90 https://journals.lww.com/greenjournal/Fulltext/2013/10000/Committee_Opinion_No__576__Health_Care_for.43.aspx

Lewinsohn DM, Leonard MK, LoBue PA, Cohn DL, Daley CL, Desmond E, et al. Official American Thoracic Society/Infectious Diseases Society of America/Centers for Disease Control and Prevention clinical practice guidelines: diagnosis of tuberculosis in adults and children. Clin Infect Dis 2017;64:e1–33. doi: 10.1093/cid/ciw694 https://academic.oup.com/cid/article/64/2/e1/2629583

Miele K, Bamrah Morris S, Tepper NK. Tuberculosis in pregnancy. Obstet Gynecol 2020;135:1444–53. doi: 10.1097/AOG.0000000000003890 https://journals.lww.com/greenjournal/Fulltext/2020/06000/Tuberculosis_in_Pregnancy.26.aspx

Sobhy S, Babiker Z, Zamora J, Khan KS, Kunst H. Maternal and perinatal mortality and morbidity associated with tuberculosis during pregnancy and the postpartum period: a systematic review and meta-analysis. BJOG 2017;124:727–33. doi: 10.1111/1471-0528.14408 https://obgyn.onlinelibrary.wiley.com/doi/10.1111/1471-0528.14408

U.S. Department of Housing and Urban Development. The 2020 Annual Homeless Assessment Report (AHAR) to Congress. part 1: point-in-time estimates of homelessness. HUD; 2021. Accessed February 4, 2022. https://www.huduser.gov/portal/datasets/ahar/2020-ahar-part-1-pit-estimates-of-homelessness-in-the-us.html

World Health Organization. Tuberculosis. WHO; 2021. Accessed February 4, 2022. https://www.who.int/news-room/fact-sheets/detail/tuberculosis

89 Intra-amniotic infection

A 25-year-old primigravida at 39 weeks of gestation is admitted with prelabor rupture of membranes and undergoes an induction of labor. The patient has a history of insulin-dependent diabetes mellitus and obesity. Maternal vital signs include a temperature of 39.1 °C (102.4 °F), a pulse of 138 beats per minute, and blood pressure of 118/76 mm Hg. Fetal tachycardia is noted. Ampicillin and gentamicin are initiated. After a prolonged induction of labor, she undergoes a cesarean birth. The best next step in her antibiotic therapy is to

(A) add cefazolin
* (B) add clindamycin
(C) change antibiotics to piperacillin–tazobactam
(D) discontinue antibiotics

Intra-amniotic infection, previously referred to as chorioamnionitis, continues to be a relatively common obstetric complication, occurring at a frequency estimated at 5–10% of term deliveries and up to 25% of preterm deliveries.

Intra-amniotic infection often is polymicrobial, involving aerobic, anaerobic, and atypical bacteria that typically are found among vaginal flora. More rarely, intra-amniotic infection can occur following invasive procedures or in the absence of rupture of membranes, such as with *Listeria monocytogenes*, and in these cases often is not polymicrobial. The American College of Obstetricians and Gynecologists' Committee Opinion No. 712, "Intrapartum Management of Intraamniotic Infection," defines the diagnosis of *suspected intra-amniotic infection* as a maternal temperature of 39.0 °C (102.2 °F) or greater or a maternal temperature of 38.0 to 38.9 °C (100.4 to 102.2 °F) combined with the presence of one additional clinical risk factor. An isolated maternal fever between 38.0 and 38.9 °C (100.4 to 102.2 °F) without additional risk factors does not constitute a diagnosis of intra-amniotic infection by current definitions.

Once intra-amniotic infection is diagnosed, initiation of antibiotics and either augmenting labor or proceeding toward delivery are recommended. Antibiotics have been shown to decrease maternal febrile morbidity and hospital length of stay and reduce neonatal morbidity. Broad-spectrum antibiotics, such as ampicillin plus gentamicin, are the most frequently used intrapartum. In the case of a mild penicillin allergy, the current recommendation for treatment of intra-amniotic infection includes cefazolin and gentamicin, whereas severe penicillin allergy prompts treatment with clindamycin or vancomycin plus gentamicin. Additional alternative regimens are listed in Table 89-1. If *L monocytogenes* is suspected, then the chosen antibiotic regimen should include ampicillin.

Surgery in the setting of an active infection increases the risk of postoperative infectious complications, such as surgical site infection, endometritis, and pelvic abscess. As in the described patient, when cesarean birth is performed with suspected intra-amniotic infection, at least one additional dose of antimicrobial agents following delivery is recommended. Intrapartum ampicillin and gentamicin should be continued and clindamycin or metronidazole added for further anaerobic coverage. Continuation of these intravenous antibiotics, as either one additional dose or for 24–48 hours, has been shown to decrease the risk of additional infectious complications. Institutional or local protocols vary in length of antibiotic treatment and may be dependent on the presence of additional risk factors, such as positive blood cultures, persistent fever in the postpartum period, or cesarean birth. With vaginal birth in the absence of other risk factors, there is no additional benefit of extending antibiotic treatment based on available data.

When intra-amniotic infection is present and cesarean birth is indicated, coverage for skin flora still is appropriate with a preoperative dose of cefazolin. However, a single additional dose of cefazolin does not adequately treat suspected intra-amniotic infection or reduce associated postoperative infectious risks. Azithromycin often is added for cesarean birth performed without labor to reduce postoperative infectious outcomes (wound infection and endometritis) but also is not sufficient for postoperative treatment of intra-amniotic infection. Piperacillin–tazobactam is an antibiotic option for the intrapartum treatment of suspected intra-amniotic infection but is not one of the recommended postpartum alternatives if given alone. In summary, doses of ampicillin and gentamicin should be continued following delivery along with clindamycin or metronidazole when clinical risk factors, such as cesarean birth, are present.

TABLE 89-1. Recommended Antibiotic Regimens for Treatment of Intra-amniotic Infection*

PRIMARY REGIMEN	
RECOMMENDED ANTIBIOTICS	**DOSAGE**
Ampicillin	2 g IV every 6 h
and	
Gentamicin	2 mg/kg IV load followed by 1.5 mg/kg every 8 h *or* 5 mg/kg IV every 24 h
RECOMMENDED ANTIBIOTICS (MILD PENICILLIN ALLERGY)	**DOSAGE**
Cefazolin	2 g IV every 8 h
and	
Gentamicin	2 mg/kg IV load followed by 1.5 mg/kg every 8 h *or* 5 mg/kg IV every 24 h
RECOMMENDED ANTIBIOTICS (SEVERE PENICILLIN ALLERGY)	**DOSAGE**
Clindamycin	900 mg IV every 8 h
or	
Vancomycin†	1 g IV every 12 h
and	
Gentamicin	2 mg/kg IV load followed by 1.5 mg/kg every 8 h *or* 5 mg/kg IV every 24 h
Postcesarean delivery: One additional dose of the chosen regimen is indicated. Add clindamycin at 900 mg IV or metronidazole at 500 mg IV for at least one additional dose. *Postvaginal delivery*: No additional doses required; but if given, clindamycin is not indicated.	
ALTERNATIVE REGIMENS	
• Ampicillin–sulbactam	3 g IV every 6 h
• Piperacillin–tazobactam	3.375 g IV every 6 h or 4.5 g IV every 8 h
• Cefotetan	2 g IV every 12 h
• Cefoxitin	2 g IV every 8 h
• Ertapenem	1 g IV every 24 h
Postcesarean delivery: One additional dose of the chosen regimen is indicated. Additional clindamycin is not required. *Postvaginal delivery*: No additional doses required, but if given, clindamycin is not indicated.	

Abbreviation: IV, intravenous.

*The dosages in the table were published by ACOG in 2017. For the most up-to-date dosing information, please review ACOG's guidance at acog.org.

†Vancomycin should be used if the woman is colonized with group B streptococci resistant to either clindamycin or erythromycin (unless clindamycin-inducible resistance testing is available and is negative) or if the woman is colonized with group B streptococci and antibiotic sensitivities are not available.

Reprinted from Intrapartum management of intraamniotic infection. Committee Opinion No. 712. American College of Obstetricians and Gynecologists. Obstet Gynecol 2017;130:e95–101. doi: 10.1097/AOG.0000000000002236 https://journals.lww.com/greenjournal/Fulltext/2017/08000/Committee_Opinion_No__712__Intrapartum_Management.58.aspx

Black LP, Hinson L, Duff P. Limited course of antibiotic treatment for chorioamnionitis. Obstet Gynecol 2012;119:1102–5. doi: 10.1097/AOG.0b013e31824b2e29 https://journals.lww.com/greenjournal/Fulltext/2012/06000/Limited_Course_of_Antibiotic_Treatment_for.5.aspx

Intrapartum management of intraamniotic infection. Committee Opinion No. 712. American College of Obstetricians and Gynecologists. Obstet Gynecol 2017;130:e95–101. doi: 10.1097/AOG.0000000000002236 https://journals.lww.com/greenjournal/Fulltext/2017/08000/Committee_Opinion_No__712__Intrapartum_Management.58.aspx

Management of pregnant women with presumptive exposure to *Listeria monocytogenes*. Committee Opinion No. 614. American College of Obstetricians and Gynecologists. Obstet Gynecol 2014;124:1241–4. doi: 10.1097/01.AOG.0000457501.73326.6c https://journals.lww.com/greenjournal/Fulltext/2014/12000/Committee_Opinion_No__614__Management_of_Pregnant.32.aspx

Tita AT, Szychowski JM, Boggess K, Saade G, Longo S, Clark E, et al. Adjunctive azithromycin prophylaxis for cesarean delivery. C/SOAP Trial Consortium. N Engl J Med 2016;375:1231–41. doi: 10.1056/NEJMoa1602044 https://www.nejm.org/doi/10.1056/NEJMoa1602044

90 Influenza exposure

A 33-year-old multiparous patient at 29 weeks of gestation calls your office to report that her two young children have tested positive for influenza. She has no fever, cough, or other symptoms. She is without significant medical history and is up to date with her routine prenatal care. In addition to providing education on transmission risk reduction strategies, the best next step is to

(A) perform a physical examination
(B) perform influenza testing
* (C) prescribe oseltamivir
(D) recommend peramivir
(E) recommend temperature monitoring

Pregnant and postpartum patients are at increased risk of serious complications of both seasonal and pandemic influenza infections. According to the Centers for Disease Control and Prevention (CDC), pregnancy is a high-risk condition that increases the risk of serious sequelae of influenza, including higher rates of hospital admission, critical care admission, and development of complications. During the 2009 H1N1 influenza pandemic, pregnant women accounted for 6% of hospitalizations and 5% of deaths, despite representing only 1% of the U.S. population. Furthermore, in the setting of additional comorbid conditions, pregnant patients have an even higher risk of complications from influenza illness. The increase in severity of infection appears to be related to normal physiologic changes that occur during pregnancy. Influenza infection also increases the risk of adverse obstetric outcomes, such as miscarriage, preterm birth, and fetal death. Finally, newborns of pregnant people with influenza have an increased risk of adverse outcomes, including preterm birth, low birth weight, and small size for gestational age.

Influenza vaccination is a core CDC prevention strategy to reduce risks among pregnant individuals. Vaccination reduces the risk of influenza infection and mitigates severe disease in the woman while offering protection to the neonate through passive antibody transfer to the fetus. Receipt of the influenza vaccine can reduce the risk of hospitalization from influenza illness by as much as 40%, according to the Pregnancy Influenza Vaccine Effectiveness Network (PREVENT). Seasonal influenza vaccination is as effective in pregnant individuals when compared with nonpregnant counterparts and varies from season to season.

Because of the high potential for complications and death among pregnant and postpartum women, the CDC advises postexposure chemoprophylaxis even in the absence of confirmed infection. Oseltamivir is an oral medication and is the preferred treatment in pregnancy assuming sufficient supply and low incidence of resistant viruses. In addition, oseltamivir is an antiviral medication that works as a neuraminidase inhibitor. Neuraminidase is the enzyme that enables cleaving of the budding viral progeny from its cellular envelope attachment. Oseltamivir is recommended in patients who are pregnant and in those who are up to 2 weeks postpartum and have had close contact with an individual with a confirmed infection. Medication is most effective in reducing severe illness when given within 48 hours of exposure. Additional members of the household are at risk of influenza and should be referred to their primary care physician for consideration of antivirals.

Zanamivir and peramivir are alternative agents approved for treatment of influenza, and pregnancy is not a contraindication to these medications. These agents, depending on availability, can be used for patients who cannot tolerate oral therapy. Zanamivir is an inhaled antiviral medication that is a neuraminidase inhibitor and can be used for both postexposure prophylaxis and treatment. Peramivir also is a neuraminidase inhibitor that can be administered through an intravenous route for treatment of infection.

This pregnant patient has an increased risk of influenza infection given household contacts with a confirmed diagnosis. Although the patient in this scenario is healthy, she should be started on antiviral medication, even in the absence of symptoms, findings, or confirmatory testing. She should monitor for signs and symptoms of influenza, which include, but are not limited to, fever greater than 38.0 °C (100.4 °F), cough, fatigue, headache, and myalgias. If symptoms develop, the patient can be triaged during a telehealth visit and treated without having an office visit. Following symptom assessment, the patient should be encouraged to monitor the severity of her illness. She should present for further care if she cannot maintain oral fluid intake, has difficulty breathing or chest pain, or exhibits any sign of an obstetric complication, such as preterm labor. Early treatment of influenza infection with oseltamivir, at a different regimen than with prophylactic use, appears to reduce hospital length of stay even among those with severe illness.

Assessment and treatment of pregnant women with suspected or confirmed influenza. ACOG Committee Opinion No. 753. American College of Obstetricians and Gynecologists [published erratum appears in Obstet Gynecol 2020;135:734]. Obstet Gynecol 2018;132:e169–73. doi: 10.1097/AOG.0000000000002872 https://journals.lww.com/greenjournal/Fulltext/2018/10000/ACOG_Committee_Opinion_No__753__Assessment_and.59.aspx

Oboho IK, Reed C, Gargiullo P, Leon M, Aragon D, Meek J, et al. Benefit of early initiation of influenza antiviral treatment to pregnant women hospitalized with laboratory-confirmed influenza. J Infect Dis 2016;214:507–15. doi: 10.1093/infdis/jiw033 https://academic.oup.com/jid/article/214/4/507/2237788

Thompson MG, Kwong JC, Regan AK, Katz MA, Drews SJ, Azziz-Baumgartner E, et al. Influenza vaccine effectiveness in preventing influenza-associated hospitalizations during pregnancy: a multi-country retrospective test negative design study, 2010–2016. PREVENT Workgroup. Clin Infect Dis 2019;68:1444–53. doi: 10.1093/cid/ciy737 https://academic.oup.com/cid/article/68/9/1444/5126390

91 Antepartum fetal surveillance

A 32-year-old gravida 1, para 0, presents at 37 weeks of gestation with decreased fetal movement. Her pregnancy has been uncomplicated. She has a reactive nonstress test, and her vital signs are within normal limits. The amniotic fluid index (AFI) is 4 cm, and the deepest vertical pocket is shown in Figure 91-1. The best next step in management is

(A) biophysical profile (BPP)
(B) contraction stress test
* (C) discharge to home
(D) induction of labor
(E) prolonged fetal monitoring

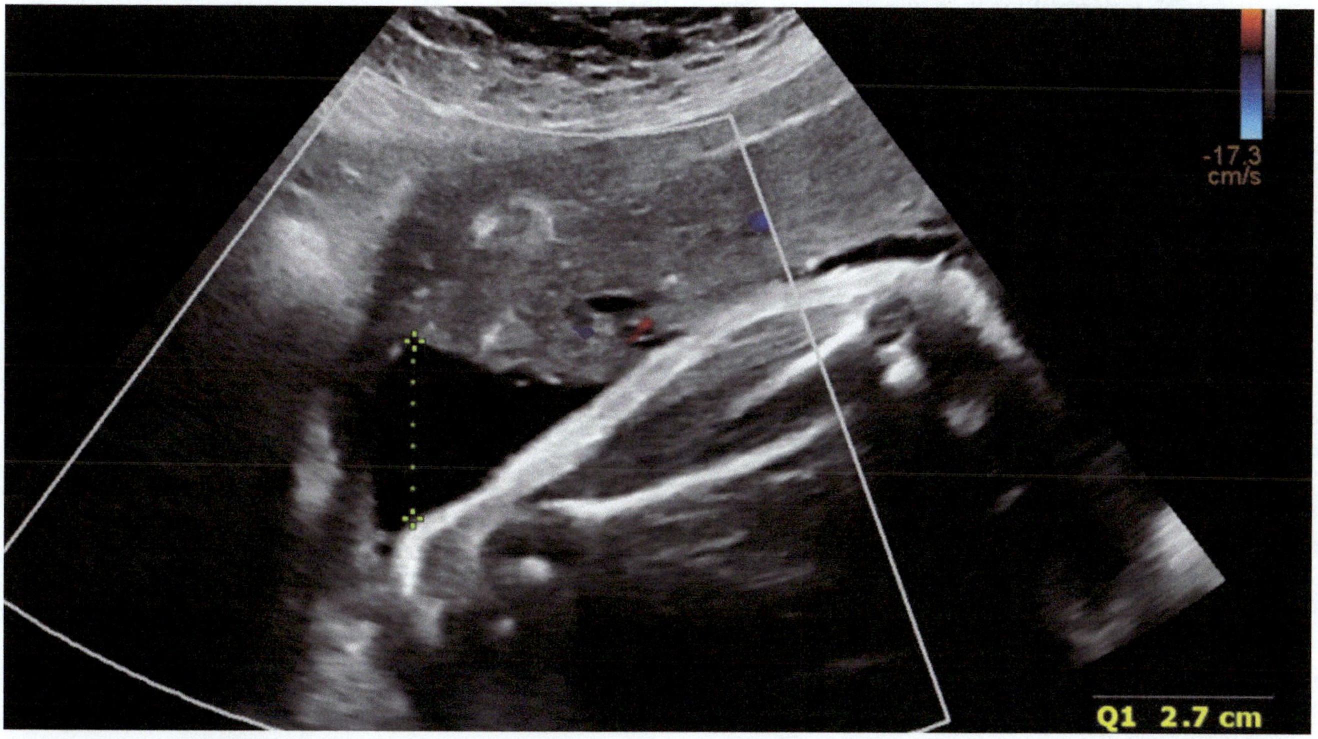

FIGURE 91-1. Deepest vertical pocket measurement.

The amniotic fluid volume is a critical ultrasonographic assessment of pregnancy. Amniotic fluid provides a supportive and protective environment for the fetus and promotes lung development. *Oligohydramnios* (or reduced fluid) is defined as an AFI of less than 5 cm or a single deepest vertical pocket of less than 2 × 1 cm. Oligohydramnios may develop as a result of fetal structural or chromosomal abnormalities, growth restriction, prolonged pregnancy, or placental insufficiency. It is associated with increased perinatal morbidity and mortality and cesarean birth, neonatal intensive care unit admission, meconium aspiration syndrome, low Apgar scores, acidosis, low birth weight, and respiratory distress syndrome. An accurate diagnosis is important in the evaluation and management of suspected oligohydramnios. To reduce the risk of perinatal morbidity and mortality, the American College of Obstetricians and Gynecologists recommends delivery at 36 0/7 to 37 6/7 weeks of gestation (or at diagnosis if diagnosed later) in pregnancies complicated by oligohydramnios.

A Cochrane systematic review including five randomized trials involving 3,226 women with singleton pregnancies demonstrated that use of the deepest vertical pocket is a better choice when compared with the AFI. When the AFI was used, this resulted in an increased number of women being diagnosed and delivered for oligohydramnios. However, it did not change the rate of neonatal intensive care unit admissions or neonatal acidosis. In addition, it increased the rate of cesarean birth for indications described as fetal distress. The other perinatal outcomes examined also were similar between the two groups, including nonreassuring fetal heart rate tracing, presence of meconium staining, or Apgar score of less than 7 at 5 minutes. Thus, the authors concluded that the single deepest vertical pocket should be used to diagnose oligohydramnios, because the AFI increases the rate of the diagnosis without improvement in peripartum outcomes. The described patient has oligohydramnios by AFI criteria, but not by single deepest vertical pocket criteria, and, therefore, discharge to home is appropriate.

Although a BPP may be indicated as part of an antepartum fetal surveillance schedule, it is not indicated in the described patient who has a reactive nonstress test and fluid assessment. Many experts prescribe weekly or twice-weekly antenatal testing with a nonstress test or modified BPP to reduce the risk of perinatal morbidity and mortality in patients with oligohydramnios. In addition, regular assessment of fetal growth is indicated because of the increased risk of fetal growth restriction in these fetuses. A contraction stress test may be useful when determining whether a fetus will tolerate labor. A contraction stress test procedure involves the administration of three contractions within 10 minutes. A negative/normal test is indicated by the absence of late or significant variable decelerations. In the described patient, delivery is not recommended, and a contraction stress test would not be necessary.

Prolonged fetal monitoring may be considered in a fetus with an abnormal nonstress test or BPP or with a concerning maternal status related to sepsis, diabetic ketoacidosis, or bleeding. The described patient has a presumably healthy fetus with a reactive nonstress test and prolonged monitoring is not indicated.

Medically indicated late-preterm and early-term deliveries. ACOG Committee Opinion No. 831. American College of Obstetricians and Gynecologists. Obstet Gynecol 2021;138:e35–9. doi: 10.1097/AOG.0000000000004447 https://journals.lww.com/greenjournal/Fulltext/2021/07000/Medically_Indicated_Late_Preterm_and_Early_Term.38.aspx

Nabhan AF, Abdelmoula YA. Amniotic fluid index versus single deepest vertical pocket as a screening test for preventing adverse pregnancy outcome. Cochrane Database of Systematic Reviews 2008, Issue 3. Art. No.: CD006593. doi: 10.1002/14651858.CD006593.pub2 http://dx.doi.org/10.1002/14651858.CD006593.pub2

92 Induction of labor

A 30-year-old gravida 2, para 1, presents for her prenatal visit at 39 weeks of gestation. Her first delivery was a cesarean birth because of an arrest of active labor at 41 weeks of gestation. She requests induction of labor, preferring to avoid another cesarean birth. Her cervix is 1-cm dilated and 20% effaced. The presenting fetal part is at –3 station. The fetus has a cephalic presentation on ultrasonographic examination. The most appropriate initial step of labor induction is

(A) amniotomy
(B) dinoprostone
(C) misoprostol
(D) oxytocin
* (E) transcervical Foley catheter

An induction of labor is performed when the risks of continuing the pregnancy appear to outweigh the risks of immediate delivery. Inductions of labor are performed for conditions of the woman in pregnancy, conditions of the fetus, and other obstetric indications. Maternal conditions requiring induction of labor at certain gestational ages include hypertensive disorders, preexisting and gestational diabetes mellitus, and intrahepatic cholestasis of pregnancy. Fetal conditions that may prompt an induction of labor include oligohydramnios, polyhydramnios, intrauterine growth restriction, multiple gestations, and alloimmunization. Obstetric conditions may include rupture of membranes and late-term or postterm pregnancies.

The 2018 ARRIVE trial (A Randomized Trial of Induction Versus Expectant Management) examined induction of labor at 39 weeks of gestation versus expectant management in 6,106 low-risk nulliparous patients. Among patients in the induction cohort, 62.7% had a Bishop score of less than 5 (Appendix B), whereas the rate in the expectant-management cohort was 64.2% at the time of random assignment. The study found no statistical difference in composite perinatal mortality or severe perinatal morbidity. The trial did find a statistical difference in the cesarean birth rate, with the induction cohort at 18.6% versus 22.2% for the expectant-management cohort. The induction cohort also had lower rates of gestational hypertension and preeclampsia (9.1% versus 14.1%). In addition, there was a statistical difference regarding the need for neonatal respiratory support within the first 72 hours of life: 3.0% for the induction cohort versus 4.2%. Based on this evidence, elective induction of labor may be considered at 39 weeks of gestation and beyond.

Cervical ripening often is performed before the induction of labor commences. The patient is assessed with a Bishop score, which is used to help guide clinical care. The Bishop score considers the cervical position, consistency, dilation, and effacement, as well as the station of the presenting fetal part. Generally, a score of less than 6 is considered unfavorable for induction of labor, and a score of greater than 8 is associated with vaginal delivery rates equivalent to those for spontaneous labor.

Cervical ripening techniques include transcervical dilation techniques and synthetic prostaglandins. Mechanical transcervical dilation can be achieved with Foley catheters or with commercially available double balloons. The transcervical Foley catheter for cervical ripening costs less than prostaglandins and is associated with less tachysystole with fetal heart rate changes. Additionally, when the cervix is unfavorable, the use of a transcervical Foley catheter lowers the cesarean birth rate compared with the use of oxytocin alone. The concomitant use of intravenous oxytocin with the transcervical Foley has not been definitively shown to shorten the time to delivery. *Laminaria japonica* osmotic dilators are another form of transcervical dilation for cervical ripening. These are used infrequently for cervical ripening in modern practice and may be associated with increased peripartum infections.

Synthetic prostaglandins used for cervical ripening include misoprostol and dinoprostone. Misoprostol is a synthetic prostaglandin-E_1 analogue that can be administered vaginally, orally, sublingually, or buccally. Although data suggest better clinical efficacy with vaginal administration, oral administration is associated with fewer tachysystole with fetal heart rate changes. The U.S. Food and Drug Administration labels misoprostol for cervical ripening and induction of labor but avoids reporting its risks, efficacy, and dosing. Complications, most notably tachysystole with fetal heart rate changes, are most often noted in doses greater than 25 micrograms. Administration is generally at intervals of 3–6 hours with longer intervals associated with fewer complications. Oxytocin infusion should not start until 4 hours after the last misoprostol administration. Dinoprostone is a prostaglandin-E_2 analogue that is commercially available as a gel and as a vaginal insert. The gel comes with a 2.5-mL syringe that contains 0.5 mg of dinoprostone. Vaginal application can be repeated every 6–12 hours with a maximum of 7.5 mL in a 24-hour period. Oxytocin infusion should be held for 6–12 hours after the last application of dinoprostone gel. The dinoprostone vaginal insert contains 10 mg of prostaglandin-E_2 analogue but releases at a rate of 0.3 mg per hour. Oxytocin infusion can commence 30–60 minutes after the insert is removed from the vagina. When compared with oxytocin alone in patients with unfavorable cervices, prostaglandins increase the rate of delivery within 24 hours. They also increase the rate of tachysystole with fetal heart rate changes. Unlike transcervical Foley catheters, prostaglandins do not decrease cesarean birth rates.

Labor induction can be initiated after cervical ripening or immediately in patients with favorable cervical examinations. Intravenous oxytocin, membrane stripping, and amniotomy are methods of labor induction. Generally, membrane stripping, performed by digitally sweeping exposed amniotic membranes on vaginal examination, is completed in the outpatient setting. Membrane stripping is shown to increase the rate of labor onset within 48 hours. Amniotomy is performed in the inpatient setting but usually is performed in combination with oxytocin infusion to avoid long delays in achieving contractions. Synthetic oxytocin infusion is the most common method of labor induction. The uterine response steadily increases from 20 weeks of gestation, eventually plateauing at 34 weeks of gestation. When endogenous oxytocin and synthetic oxytocin are used for induction of labor, patients with lower body mass indices, greater cervical dilation, and greater gestational age have the highest rates of successful vaginal birth. Low-dose and high-dose protocols are available. Low-dose protocols have a lower initial dose of intravenous oxytocin and a longer interval between rate increases. The low-dose regimens are associated with less tachysystole with fetal heart rate changes. High-dose regimens have higher initial infusion rates and more frequent rate increases. High-dose regimens have higher rates of tachysystole with fetal heart rate changes, but shorter labors, lower rates of chorioamnionitis, and fewer cesarean births for labor dystocia. No maximum safe rate of oxytocin infusion has been established, but in routine practice, institutional safety limits may provide guidance for dosing.

Cervical ripening and labor induction can be performed in appropriate candidates who have had a previous cesarean birth. In numerous small studies, prostaglandin E_1 has been found to increase the risk of uterine rupture when used for cervical ripening in patients with a previous cesarean birth, and its use is not recommended. There are very limited data on the use of prostaglandin E_{2a} analogues in trials of labor after cesarean birth. There is no compelling evidence that transcervical Foley catheter cervical ripening is associated with increased risks of uterine rupture, and its use may be considered in patients with a history of a previous cesarean birth, such as the described patient. Intravenous synthetic oxytocin also is used for induction of labor in those with a previous cesarean birth, but when the cervix is unfavorable, as in this scenario, the use of a transcervical Foley catheter lowers the cesarean birth rate compared with the use of oxytocin alone.

The described patient has an unfavorable cervical examination, and amniotomy would be an inappropriate next step. This patient has a history of cesarean birth, and dinoprostone and misoprostol are contraindicated. Low-dose oxytocin infusion alone in this clinical scenario has a higher rate of cesarean birth versus the use of a transcervical Foley catheter. The patient expresses a desire to avoid another cesarean birth; thus, the most appropriate method for cervical ripening is the transcervical Foley catheter.

American College of Obstetricians and Gynecologists. Clinical guidance for integration of the findings of the ARRIVE trial: labor induction versus expectant management in low-risk nulliparous women. Practice Advisory. ACOG; 2018. Accessed March 2, 2022. https://www.acog.org/clinical/clinical-guidance/practice-advisory/articles/2018/08/clinical-guidance-for-integration-of-the-findings-of-the-arrive-trial

Grobman WA, Rice MM, Reddy UM, Tita AT, Silver RM, Mallett G, et al. Labor induction versus expectant management in low-risk nulliparous women. *Eunice Kennedy Shriver* National Institute of Child Health and Human Development Maternal–Fetal Medicine Units Network. N Engl J Med 2018;379:513–23. doi: 10.1056/NEJMoa1800566 https://www.nejm.org/doi/10.1056/NEJMoa1800566

Induction of labor. ACOG Practice Bulletin No. 107. American College of Obstetricians and Gynecologists. Obstet Gynecol 2009;114:386–97. doi: 10.1097/AOG.0b013e3181b48ef5 https://journals.lww.com/greenjournal/Citation/2009/08000/ACOG_Practice_Bulletin_No__107__Induction_of_Labor.30.aspx

Medically indicated late-preterm and early-term deliveries. ACOG Committee Opinion No. 831. American College of Obstetricians and Gynecologists. Obstet Gynecol 2021;138:e35–9. doi: 10.1097/AOG.0000000000004447 https://journals.lww.com/greenjournal/Fulltext/2021/07000/Medically_Indicated_Late_Preterm_and_Early_Term.38.aspx

Vaginal birth after cesarean delivery. ACOG Practice Bulletin No. 205. American College of Obstetricians and Gynecologists. Obstet Gynecol 2019;133:e110–27. doi: 10.1097/AOG.0000000000003078 https://journals.lww.com/greenjournal/Fulltext/2019/02000/ACOG_Practice_Bulletin_No__205__Vaginal_Birth.40.aspx

93 Use of corticosteroids in late-preterm pregnancy

A 29-year-old presents with preterm prelabor rupture of membranes at 35 weeks of gestation. Her pregnancy had previously been uncomplicated with no hospitalizations. Her vital signs are normal. You discuss administration of antenatal corticosteroids and counsel her that the administration of late-preterm corticosteroids increases the risk of neonatal

(A) hyperbilirubinemia
* (B) hypoglycemia
(C) necrotizing enterocolitis
(D) respiratory distress
(E) sepsis

Administration of corticosteroids before preterm delivery is known to improve newborn outcomes with a decrease in, and reduced severity of, respiratory distress, intracranial hemorrhage, and necrotizing enterocolitis, and a reduction in mortality. Antenatal corticosteroids (betamethasone or dexamethasone) are commonly administered to women at risk of imminent preterm birth between 24 0/7 and 33 6/7 weeks of gestation, and in some cases can be started before 24 weeks of gestation.

The Antenatal Late Preterm Steroids (ALPS) trial was a large, double-blind, placebo-controlled randomized clinical trial performed by the National Institute of Child Health and Human Development Maternal–Fetal Medicine Units Network that evaluated the use of antenatal corticosteroids (betamethasone) in the late-preterm period (34 0/7 to 36 6/7 weeks of gestation). Neonates born in this time frame are at risk of respiratory morbidity and other adverse outcomes. The study showed a significant reduction in the primary outcome (a composite score of newborn respiratory treatment) as well as several secondary outcomes (severe respiratory complications, transient tachypnea of the newborn, surfactant use, and bronchopulmonary dysplasia) with the administration of corticosteroids in the late-preterm period. There were no differences in the rates of respiratory distress syndrome, apnea, pneumonia, hyperbilirubinemia, necrotizing enterocolitis, intraventricular hemorrhage, chorioamnionitis, or neonatal sepsis. The group of neonates whose mothers received antenatal betamethasone had a higher risk of neonatal hypoglycemia compared with the control group, but adverse events related to hypoglycemia were not noted, and hospital stay was not increased in this group. Therefore, the described patient should be counseled about the risk of neonatal hypoglycemia with late-preterm corticosteroids.

Because administration of corticosteroids in the late-preterm period is recommended on the basis of the ALPS trial alone, some exclusions should be considered because of criteria and methodologies used in the trial. Late-preterm corticosteroid administration is not recommended in women who have already received a course of corticosteroids or in women who have a diagnosis of intra-amniotic infection. Indicated late-preterm deliveries should not be delayed for the administration of corticosteroids, and tocolysis should not be used to attempt to delay spontaneous preterm delivery. It is unknown whether corticosteroids administered in the late-preterm period benefit certain groups of patients who were not studied by the trial, including those with multifetal gestations, those with pregestational diabetes mellitus, women who had previously received a course of corticosteroids, and women who had term cesarean birth. Long-term pediatric outcomes for patients exposed to late-preterm corticosteroids have not been established, and the Society for Maternal-Fetal Medicine recommends shared decision making when deciding whether to administer betamethasone between 34 0/7 and 36 6/7 weeks.

Antenatal corticosteroid therapy for fetal maturation. Committee Opinion No. 713. American College of Obstetricians and Gynecologists. Obstet Gynecol 2017;130:e102–9. doi: 10.1097/AOG.0000000000002237 https://journals.lww.com/greenjournal/Fulltext/2017/08000/Committee_Opinion_No__713__Antenatal.59.aspx

Gyamfi-Bannerman C, Thom EA, Blackwell SC, Tita AT, Reddy UM, Saade GR, et al. Antenatal betamethasone for women at risk of late preterm delivery. NICHD Maternal–Fetal Medicine Units Network. N Engl J Med 2016;374:1311–20. doi: 10.1056/NEJMoa1516783 https://www.nejm.org/doi/10.1056/NEJMoa1516783

Implementation of the use of antenatal corticosteroids in the late preterm birth period in women at risk of preterm delivery. Society for Maternal–Fetal Medicine (SMFM) Publications Committee [published erratum appears in Am J Obstet Gynecol 2017;216:180]. Am J Obstet Gynecol 2016;215:B13–5. doi: 10.1016/j.ajog.2016.03.013 https://www.ajog.org/article/S0002-9378(16)00475-0/fulltext

94 Gestational trophoblastic disease

A 39-year-old gravida 3, para 1, at 10 weeks of gestation is seen for an initial prenatal visit, during which ultrasonography is performed. The ultrasonography shows a fetus with no cardiac activity and placental tissue with multiple cystic areas. The patient undergoes dilation and suction curettage. Chromosomal evaluation of the retained fetal tissue identifies a 69,XXY karyotype. The most appropriate frequency of human chorionic gonadotropin (β-hCG) monitoring for this patient is

(A) monthly until negative
(B) weekly until negative for three consecutive tests
* (C) weekly until negative, then confirmed 1 month later
(D) weekly until negative, then monthly for 6 months

Hydatidiform mole, commonly known as *molar pregnancy*, has an incidence of approximately 1 to 2 per 1,000 deliveries. Molar pregnancy is characterized by edematous immature placental tissue. Complete molar pregnancy lacks a fetus and has diploid chromosome makeup. The chromosomes are entirely made up of paternal chromosomes. In partial molar pregnancy, a fetus and triploid chromosomes due to dispermy are present. Ultimately, fetal death occurs. Molar pregnancies can sometimes be diagnosed by ultrasonography, with characteristic findings of an echogenic uterine mass with cystic spaces. Partial molar pregnancy has similar findings, but a fetus or fetal tissue also is present.

In many cases, molar or partial molar pregnancy will be diagnosed by pathologic evaluation after dilation and curettage for incomplete abortion. In cases in which the diagnosis is suspected before treatment, a workup is recommended. Evaluation should include serum β-hCG, complete blood count, prothrombin time, partial thromboplastin time, renal function, liver function, blood type, and antibody screen. Additionally, a chest radiograph should be obtained, as well as a pelvic ultrasonogram if not previously obtained. In patients with uterine enlargement greater than 14 to 16 weeks of gestation, baseline arterial blood gas and oxygen saturation may be helpful, because these patients are at increased risk of pulmonary complications.

When molar pregnancy or partial molar pregnancy is diagnosed, surgical management with suction dilation and curettage is indicated. There often is a larger amount of tissue than would be found in a normal pregnancy at the same gestational age, and a larger cannula often is necessary. The risk of bleeding is increased, and oxytocin or other uterotonic agents should be readily available. In patients who have completed childbearing, hysterectomy may be considered instead of curettage. Although feto-maternal hemorrhage is unlikely with a molar pregnancy, administration of Rho(D) immune globulin is recommended in Rh-negative patients. Patients with uterine enlargement greater than 14 to 16 weeks of gestation should be closely monitored for pulmonary complications with serial oxygen saturation measurements.

Because molar pregnancy is a benign condition with malignant potential, posttreatment monitoring is necessary. To evaluate for persistent gestational neoplasia after evacuation or hysterectomy, serial β-hCG measurements should be evaluated. In the setting of partial molar pregnancy, the risk of postmolar gestational trophoblastic neoplasia is 1:3,195. Data suggest that β-hCG should be monitored weekly until normalized, and checked again 1 month later, which is the correct strategy in this patient. If the β-hCG remains negative, monitoring can be discontinued. In the setting of complete molar pregnancy, β-hCG should be monitored monthly after normalization for 6 months. Reliable contraception is important during this monitoring period, because a new pregnancy makes it difficult to monitor for persistent gestational trophoblastic disease.

Molar pregnancy carries the risk of invasive mole, gestational choriocarcinoma, placental site trophoblastic disease, and epithelioid trophoblastic disease. Risk factors for development of neoplasia include age greater than 40 years, pre-evacuation β-hCG greater than 100,000 milli-international units/mL, excessive uterine enlargement, and theca lutein cysts greater than 6 cm. Prophylactic chemotherapy reduces the risk of gestational trophoblastic neoplasia but has been associated with cases of fatality. It is not currently recommended except in patients with high-risk features who cannot complete β-hCG monitoring.

Postmolar gestational trophoblastic neoplasia is diagnosed when β-hCG levels have a sustained rise or plateau. The diagnostic criteria include sustained plateau, increase greater than 10%, and persistent β-hCG 6 months after evacuation, metastatic disease, or histologic diagnosis. The specific criteria can be seen in Box 94-1. These patients should be referred to a gynecologic oncologist for treatment, which may include further surgery and chemotherapy.

BOX 94-1

Diagnostic Criteria for Gestational Trophoblastic Neoplasia

Laboratory criteria

- β-hCG level plateau of ±10% of 4 values over 3 weeks
- β-hCG level rise of greater than 10% of 3 values over 2 weeks
- Persistent detectable β-hCG greater than 6 months after evacuation
- Presence of metastatic disease

Histologic diagnosis

- Invasive mole
- Gestational choriocarcinoma
- Placental site trophoblastic disease
- Epithelioid trophoblastic disease

Data from Ngan HY, Bender H, Benedet JL, Jones H, Montruccoli GC, Pecorelli S. Gestational trophoblastic neoplasia, FIGO 2000 staging and classification. FIGO Committee on Gynecologic Oncology [published erratum appears in Int J Gynaecol Obstet 2021;155:563]. Int J Gynaecol Obstet 2003;83(suppl 1):175-7. doi: 10.1016/s0020-7292(03)90120-2 https://obgyn.onlinelibrary.wiley.com/doi/abs/10.1016/S0020-7292(03)90120-2

Cunningham FG, Leveno KJ, Bloom SL, Dashe JS, Hoffman BL, Casey BM, et al. Williams obstetrics. 25th ed. McGraw-Hill Education; 2018.

Ngan HY, Seckl MJ, Berkowitz RS, Xiang Y, Golfier F, Sekharan PK, et al. Update on the diagnosis and management of gestational trophoblastic disease. Int J Gynaecol Obstet 2018; 143(suppl 2):79–85. doi: 10.1002/ijgo.12615 https://obgyn.onlinelibrary.wiley.com/doi/10.1002/ijgo.12615

Soper JT. Gestational trophoblastic disease: current evaluation and management [published erratum appears in Obstet Gynecol 2022;139:149]. Obstet Gynecol 2021;137:355–70. doi: 10.1097/AOG.0000000000004240 https://journals.lww.com/greenjournal/Fulltext/2021/02000/Gestational_Trophoblastic_Disease__Current.22.aspx

95 Operative complications of obesity

A 34-year-old gravida 2, para 0, is undergoing primary cesarean birth for arrest of dilation in labor. Her prenatal course was complicated by class III obesity, with a prepregnant body mass index (BMI) of 51. She received preoperative antibiotics at an appropriate dose for her weight. The surgical team replaces their sterile gloves after hysterotomy closure. The intervention at surgical closure that is most likely to decrease the risk of postoperative infectious morbidity is use of

(A) delayed absorbable braided suture to close the fascial layer
(B) irrigation of the subcutaneous layer
(C) negative pressure wound dressing
(D) subcutaneous drain
* (E) suture approximation of the subcutaneous layer

Obesity carries an increased risk of multiple complications of pregnancy, including miscarriage, birth defects, cesarean birth, preeclampsia, gestational diabetes mellitus, and stillbirth. Risks associated with both cesarean birth and vaginal birth include endometritis, venous thromboembolism, and wound infections.

Closure of the subcutaneous layer if it measures more than 2 cm in depth is the one surgical intervention that can decrease wound infection risk. Multiple randomized controlled trials have demonstrated that closure of the subcutaneous layer when it is greater than 2 cm decreases the risk of wound infection and seroma formation. In the clinical scenario above, this is the intervention most likely to decrease the risk of infection.

The use of delayed absorbable suture for closure of the fascial layer is recommended rather than permanent suture; however, its use does not specifically decrease risk of infection. Irrigation of the subcutaneous layer is recommended to decrease the risk of hematoma and seroma formation, but this does not decrease the risk of infection. Although prophylactic use of negative pressure wound dressings has been proposed for prevention of wound infection in women with obesity, multiple studies have failed to show a decrease in wound complications and the dressings may increase cost of care. Subcutaneous drains do not decrease infectious morbidity and may increase the rate of wound complications; thus, they should not be used regardless of the depth of the subcutaneous layer.

Other surgical considerations for patients with obesity include operating room equipment and positioning. Care should be taken to ensure that appropriate operating tables are available that can accommodate patients up to at least 500 lb. Patients with obesity are at increased risk of venous thromboembolism, and prophylactic sequential compression devices should be used before, during, and after cesarean birth, and early ambulation should be encouraged. In patients who require chemoprophylaxis, weight-based dosing of low-molecular-weight heparin may be more effective than BMI-based dosing. Increasing the dose of prophylactic antibiotics has not been shown to significantly increase concentration in the subcutaneous layer. Increasing antibiotics does not appear to decrease surgical site infections, and current data do not support use of cefazolin of greater than 2 g in the obstetric population. There is emerging evidence for the addition of 48 hours of oral antibiotics (cephalexin and metronidazole) after cesarean birth in patients with obesity who do not receive azithromycin prophylaxis (as indicated for cesarean birth in patients who are laboring or have ruptured membranes).

Dahlke JD, Mendez-Figueroa H, Maggio L, Sperling JD, Chauhan SP, Rouse DJ. The case for standardizing cesarean delivery technique: seeing the forest for the trees. Obstet Gynecol 2020;136:972–80. doi: 10.1097/AOG.0000000000004120 https://journals.lww.com/greenjournal/Fulltext/2020/11000/The_Case_for_Standardizing_Cesarean_Delivery.17.aspx

Hussamy DJ, Wortman AC, McIntire DD, Leveno KJ, Casey BM, Roberts SW. Closed incision negative pressure therapy in morbidly obese women undergoing cesarean delivery: a randomized controlled trial. Obstet Gynecol 2019;134:781–9. doi: 10.1097/AOG.0000000000003465 https://journals.lww.com/greenjournal/Fulltext/2019/10000/Closed_Incision_Negative_Pressure_Therapy_in.18.aspx

Obesity in pregnancy. ACOG Practice Bulletin No. 230. American College of Obstetricians and Gynecologists. Obstet Gynecol 2021;137:e128–44. doi: 10.1097/AOG.0000000000004395 https://journals.lww.com/greenjournal/Fulltext/2021/06000/Obesity_in_Pregnancy__ACOG_Practice_Bulletin,.38.aspx

Smid MC, Dotters-Katz SK, Grace M, Wright ST, Villers MS, Hardy-Fairbanks A, et al. Prophylactic negative pressure wound therapy for obese women after cesarean delivery: a systematic review and meta-analysis. Obstet Gynecol 2017;130:969–78. doi: 10.1097/AOG.0000000000002259 https://journals.lww.com/greenjournal/Fulltext/2017/11000/Prophylactic_Negative_Pressure_Wound_Therapy_for.6.aspx

Tuuli MG, Liu J, Tita AT, Longo S, Trudell A, Carter EB, et al. Effect of prophylactic negative pressure wound therapy vs standard wound dressing on surgical-site infection in obese women after cesarean delivery: a randomized clinical trial. JAMA 2020;324:1180–9. doi: 10.1001/jama.2020.13361 https://jamanetwork.com/journals/jama/fullarticle/2770848

Use of prophylactic antibiotics in labor and delivery. ACOG Practice Bulletin No. 199. American College of Obstetricians and Gynecologists [published erratum appears in Obstet Gynecol 2019;134:883–884]. Obstet Gynecol 2018;132:e103-19.doi: 10.1097/AOG.0000000000002833 https://journals.lww.com/greenjournal/Fulltext/2018/09000/ACOG_Practice_Bulletin_No__199__Use_of.67.aspx

96 Screening in twin pregnancies

A 40-year-old gravida 1 at 12 weeks of gestation presents for counseling on aneuploidy screening. She had multiple previous unsuccessful in vitro fertilization cycles, and after careful counseling and shared decision making, two embryos were transferred after preimplantation genetic screening for aneuploidy was performed. She has a dichorionic pregnancy following in vitro fertilization. The best next step in aneuploidy screening is

* (A) cell-free DNA (cfDNA) screening
(B) fetal anatomic survey
(C) first-trimester screening
(D) no further screening
(E) nuchal translucency

There is a risk of aneuploidy at all maternal ages, and aneuploidy screening should be recommended to all obstetric patients. Although the risk of a chromosomal disorder is higher for patients of advanced maternal age, most aneuploid fetuses are born to women younger than age 35 years, given the higher number of births in this cohort. In vitro fertilization has offered many patients the opportunity to prescreen embryos before implantation with preimplantation genetic screening. This can be done for aneuploidy or monogenetic disorders.

In the most commonly used method for preimplantation genetic screening, a group of cells is sampled from the trophectoderm at the blastocyst stage. This technology allows 5–10 cells to be tested from the layer that will become the placenta and leaves the inner cell mass (ie, the future embryo) undisturbed. However, because both false-positive and false-negative results are possible, aneuploidy screening is still recommended during the pregnancy.

Patients who choose preimplantation genetic screening of their embryos should be counseled that it is a screening test with the most updated test performance for the individual laboratory. Transfer of an embryo with a false-negative preimplantation genetic screening would lead to pregnancy affected by aneuploidy, whereas a false-positive preimplantation genetic screening may mean a healthy euploid embryo is never transferred, potentially limiting pregnancy options for couples with infertility. Not performing further screening would not be the best next step in the setting of maternal age and twin gestation, which increases the likelihood that at least one fetus may have aneuploidy. Likewise, because aneuploidy screening within the first trimester is recommended, waiting for an anatomy survey in the second trimester is not the best next step. The second-trimester anatomy survey can be used to change the a priori risk of aneuploidy based on presence or absence of soft markers or anomalies, and ultrasonography without markers or anomalies has a likelihood ratio of 0.4 for trisomy 21. However, patients should understand that approximately one-third of fetuses with trisomy 21 will not have any markers or anomalies, making it a less ideal solo screening method.

There are several options for aneuploidy testing for twin gestations that can be altered based on certain clinical scenarios. In general, nuchal translucency screening can be considered a piece of the aneuploidy screening strategy for twins, because this will apply an individual risk to each fetus. However, it is recommended in isolation only in cases in which serum testing would have a high risk of false-positive results, such as an early co-twin death during the first trimester.

Because this is an ongoing twin pregnancy, nuchal translucency screening only is not recommended, and the detection rate is approximately 75% with a 9% false-positive rate. The first-trimester screen can be offered to twin gestations. The nuchal translucency portion of the test will assess the individual fetal risk, and serum markers are used to increase the detection rate of trisomy 21 for the entire pregnancy (in monochorionic twins) or per fetus (in dichorionic twins). Although the detection rate for trisomy 21 is lower in twin gestations, it is still comparable with singleton screening (86% versus 89%, respectively) with a similar false-positive rate of 5%. However, the patient's age should be considered when choosing the most appropriate screening method.

Cell-free DNA screening is recommended for patients at high risk of aneuploidy, including patients older than age 35 and with a previous history of a pregnancy complicated by aneuploidy. Recent data have shown the detection rate for trisomy 21 is 94% in twin gestations, which is higher than that achieved with first-trimester screen. Testing platforms that used single-nucleotide polymorphism-based screening are further able to identify zygosity of the fetuses and may be used preferentially over those using massive-parallel sequencing. Because this pregnancy is at high risk of aneuploidy, cfDNA screening is the best next option.

Khalil A, Rodgers M, Baschat A, Bhide A, Gratacos E, Hecher K, et al. ISUOG Practice Guidelines: role of ultrasound in twin pregnancy [published erratum appears in Ultrasound Obstet Gynecol 2018;52:140]. Ultrasound Obstet Gynecol 2016;47:247–63. doi: 10.1002/uog.15821 https://obgyn.onlinelibrary.wiley.com/doi/10.1002/uog.15821

Preimplantation genetic testing. ACOG Committee Opinion No. 799. American College of Obstetricians and Gynecologists. Obstet Gynecol 2020;135:e133–7. doi: 10.1097/AOG.0000000000003714 https://journals.lww.com/greenjournal/Fulltext/2020/03000/Preimplantation_Genetic_Testing__ACOG_Committee.50.aspx

Resnik R, Lockwood CJ, Moore TR, Greene ME, Copel JA, Silver RM, editors. Creasy and Resnik's maternal–fetal medicine: principles and practice. 8th ed. Elsevier; 2018.

Screening for fetal chromosomal abnormalities: ACOG Practice Bulletin No. 226. American College of Obstetricians and Gynecologists. Obstet Gynecol 2020;136:e48–69. doi: 10.1097/AOG.0000000000004084 https://journals.lww.com/greenjournal/Fulltext/2020/10000/Screening_for_Fetal_Chromosomal_Abnormalities_.44.aspx

Shitara A, Takahashi K, Goto M, Takahashi H, Iwasawa T, Onodera Y, et al. Cell-free DNA in spent culture medium effectively reflects the chromosomal status of embryos following culturing beyond implantation compared to trophectoderm biopsy. PLoS One 2021;16:e0246438. doi: 10.1371/journal.pone.0246438 https://journals.plos.org/plosone/article?id=10.1371/journal.pone.0246438

97 Massive transfusion

A 37-year-old gravida 7, para 6, presents at 38 weeks of gestation in active labor. Her pulse is 98 beats per minute (bpm), and her blood pressure is 104/68 mm Hg. She delivers within 1 hour of admission, and oxytocin is administered after delivery of the fetus. Continued bleeding due to uterine atony is noted after placental delivery. Her intravenous fluids are increased, and tranexamic acid and methylergonovine are given. You have emptied her bladder and are preparing to insert an intrauterine balloon tamponade because of continued hemorrhage. You have estimated the blood loss to be 1,100 mL. The patient's heart rate is 130 bpm, her blood pressure is 90/54 mm Hg, and she has had no urine output in the past 15 minutes. The nurse notifies you that the quantitative blood loss is 2,440 mL. Laboratory studies are obtained, and you note that the phlebotomy site is bleeding significantly. The most appropriate method to estimate this patient's blood loss in preparation for a massive transfusion protocol is the

(A) hematocrit
(B) qualitative blood loss
* (C) quantitative blood loss
(D) vital signs with urine output

This patient is experiencing a life-threatening postpartum hemorrhage and has clinical signs of coagulopathy in addition to vital sign changes that begin to occur with stage 3 obstetric hemorrhage (Table 97-1). She is not yet in hypovolemic shock because she is maintaining her blood pressure without additional intravenous pressor support. Transfusion timing typically is based on estimated blood loss, but quantitative blood loss can lead to a quicker decision to start transfusion and should be used to guide initiation of a massive transfusion in the described patient. Visual estimates of blood loss are more prone to error, particularly when the blood loss is high. Quantitative blood loss is a means to obtain a higher degree of accuracy in determining blood loss, and may lead to identifying more patients who experience a postpartum hemorrhage. However, studies have not shown that quantitative blood loss changes the incidence of blood transfusion or prevention of postpartum hemorrhage. Box 97-1 provides a guide for quantified blood loss.

Relying on changes in maternal vital signs (blood pressure and heart rate) or changes in hematocrit should not be the main criteria for transfusion, because maternal vital signs do not change until there has been significant blood loss, and hematocrit will not accurately show the degree of blood loss during the

TABLE 97-1. Stages of Obstetric Hemorrhage

STAGE OF HEMORRHAGE	DIAGNOSTIC CRITERIA
Stage 1	Blood loss less than 1,000 mL after delivery with normal vital signs and laboratory values
Stage 2	Continued bleeding with EBL greater than 1,500 mL OR two or more uterotonics (in addition to routine oxytocin) with normal vital signs and laboratory values
Stage 3	Continued bleeding with EBL greater than 1,500 mL OR greater than 2 units packed RBC given OR risk of occult bleeding/coagulopathy OR abnormal vital signs/laboratory values/oliguria
Stage 4	Cardiovascular collapse (massive hemorrhage, profound hypovolemic shock, amniotic fluid embolism)

Abbreviations: EBL, estimated blood loss; RBC, red blood cells.

Modified from American College of Obstetricians and Gynecologists. Safe motherhood initiative. Obstetric hemorrhage. ACOG; 2022. Accessed March 16, 2022. https://www.acog.org/community/districts-and-sections/district-ii/programs-and-resources/safe-motherhood-initiative/obstetric-hemorrhage

BOX 97-1

Quantification of Blood Loss During Delivery

For vaginal deliveries

- Create a list of dry weights for delivery items that may become blood soaked
- Begin quantification of blood loss after delivery of neonate and before delivery of placenta using calibrated under-buttock drape
- Record total volume of fluid collected in calibrated drape, subtracting preplacental fluid volume
- Weigh blood-soaked items and determine volume of blood by subtracting dry weight of each item weight (1 g weight = 1 mL blood loss)
- Add fluid volume in calibrated drape to calculated blood loss from soaked items to determine total quantitative blood loss

For cesarean births

- Begin quantification after delivery of infant
- Suction drapes of amniotic fluid and record starting volume
- Record volume in suction canister prior to irrigation use and subtract the amniotic fluid volume prior to placenta delivery
- Weigh blood-soaked items and subtract dry weight (including items under patient at the end of the case if needed)
- Add converted volume of soaked item (1 g = 1 mL blood loss) to the cumulative volume in suction canister

Modified from Quantitative blood loss in obstetric hemorrhage. ACOG Committee Opinion No. 794. American College of Obstetricians and Gynecologists. Obstet Gynecol 2019;134:e150–6. doi: 10.1097/AOG.0000000000003564 https://journals.lww.com/greenjournal/Fulltext/2019/12000/Quantitative_Blood_Loss_in_Obstetric_Hemorrhage_.40.aspx.

acute hemorrhage. Delayed or inadequate treatment can lead to lactic acidosis, multiorgan dysfunction, and coagulopathy.

Patients with a blood loss greater than 1,500 mL or who have abnormal vital signs should be treated with transfusion. It is not only the oxygen-carrying capacity of red blood cells that is lost during severe hemorrhage; the coagulation factors necessary to prevent coagulopathy also are reduced. Therefore, other components, such as platelets and fresh frozen plasma, may need to be given, depending on the degree of blood loss and the clinical situation. A *massive transfusion* is defined as 10 or more units of packed red blood cells transfused within a 24-hour period. In settings in which disseminated intravascular coagulopathy is suspected or diagnosed, a low fibrinogen should be suspected, and consideration should be given for cryoprecipitate.

Based on bleeding from her intravenous access sites, this patient has a significant blood loss that is ongoing, and she likely has coagulopathy. The patient may require more than 4 units of packed red blood cells and coagulation factor repletion, and the best choice would be multicomponent therapy given through a massive transfusion protocol. Although crystalloid infusions are a part of the treatment algorithm for obstetric hemorrhage, large boluses of crystalloid can lead to a dilutional coagulopathy, further aggravating the clinical problem. Multicomponent therapy through a massive transfusion protocol will give a patient packed red blood cells, fresh frozen plasma, and platelets in a 1:1:1 ratio, which attempts to approximate a whole-blood transfusion. These ratios may be altered slightly from institution to institution, but they maintain a similar ratio between oxygen-carrying red blood cells and coagulation factors. An example of a massive transfusion protocol is given in Table 97-2.

TABLE 97-2. Sample Massive Transfusion Protocol

MTP PACK 1	MTP PACK 2	MTP PACK 3 UNTIL STOP
4 units of PRBC	4 units of PRBC	4 units of PRBC
4 units of FFP	4 units of FFP	4 units of FFP
1 unit of platelets	1 unit of platelets and 1 unit of cryoprecipitate	1 unit of platelets and 2 units of cryoprecipitate

- Use a Level I infuser with warmer
- TEG will be used to monitor resuscitation and product usage; repeat as needed
- Tranexamic acid to be used at discretion of physician (indicated for low systolic blood pressure, obvious significant bleeding, hyperfibrinolysis on TEG)
- Cessation of MTP include any of the following indications:
  - — Patient expiration
  - — Hemodynamic stability
  - — Attending physician discretion

Abbreviations: FFP, fresh frozen plasma; MTP, massive transfusion protocol; PRBC, packed red blood cells; TEG, thromboelastography.

Modified from Baystate Medical Center Massive Transfusion Protocol.

American College of Obstetricians and Gynecologists. Safe motherhood initiative. Obstetric hemorrhage. ACOG; 2022. Accessed March 16, 2022. https://www.acog.org/community/districts-and-sections/district-ii/programs-and-resources/safe-motherhood-initiative/obstetric-hemorrhage

Cunningham FG, Leveno KJ, Bloom SL, Dashe JS, Hoffman BL, Casey BM, et al. Williams obstetrics. 25th ed. McGraw-Hill Education; 2018.

Postpartum hemorrhage. Practice Bulletin No. 183. American College of Obstetricians and Gynecologists. Obstet Gynecol 2017;130:e168–86. doi: 10.1097/AOG.0000000000002351 https://journals.lww.com/greenjournal/Fulltext/2017/10000/Practice_Bulletin_No__183__Postpartum_Hemorrhage.56.aspx

Quantitative blood loss in obstetric hemorrhage. ACOG Committee Opinion No. 794. American College of Obstetricians and Gynecologists. Obstet Gynecol 2019;134:e150–6. doi: 10.1097/AOG.0000000000003564 https://journals.lww.com/greenjournal/Fulltext/2019/12000/Quantitative_Blood_Loss_in_Obstetric_Hemorrhage_.40.aspx

98 Autoimmune disorders in pregnancy

A 23-year-old gravida 1, para 1, presents 6 weeks after delivery for an office visit. Her pregnancy was complicated by systemic lupus erythematosus (SLE), Sjögren syndrome type A (Ro or SS-A) antibodies, and intrapartum preeclampsia with thrombocytopenia. She cannot tolerate hydroxychloroquine and is currently taking azathioprine and low-dose prednisone to control lupus flares. She delivered a small-for-gestational-age neonate at 37 weeks of gestation and is currently breastfeeding. Her blood pressure is 120/68 mm Hg. She talks with you about a skin rash her infant has had on the head and neck for the past month (Fig. 98-1). The most likely maternal cause of the infant's rash is

(A) azathioprine
(B) corticosteroids
(C) preeclampsia
* (D) SS-A antibodies

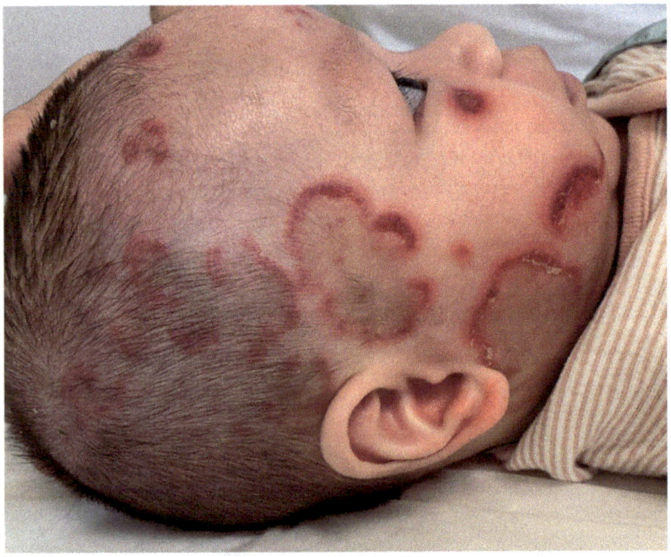

FIGURE 98-1. Neonatal rash. (Reprinted from Wu J, Berk-Krauss J, Glick SA. Neonatal lupus erythematosus. JAMA Dermatol 2021;157:590. doi: 10.1001/jamadermatol.2021.0041 https://jamanetwork.com/journals/jamadermatology/article-abstract/2777663)

Systemic lupus erythematosus affects approximately 1 in 1,250 pregnancies in the United States and is associated with increased obstetric morbidities, including preeclampsia, fetal growth restriction, preterm birth, and stillbirth. More uncommon outcomes are also possible, including congenital heart block and neonatal lupus syndrome. Sjögren syndrome type A (Ro) and Sjögren syndrome type B (La) antibodies are frequently found in rheumatologic conditions, particularly SLE and Sjögren syndrome. These autoantibodies can cross the placenta and cause fetal and neonatal complications. Adverse outcomes are more common with antiphospholipid antibodies, anti-SSA and anti-SSB antibodies, hypertension, and renal disease. Pregnancy management is aimed at surveillance and reduction of potential maternal complications (preeclampsia, thrombus, or worsening renal function) as well as fetal and neonatal diagnoses (congenital heart block, fetal growth restriction, stillbirth, and neonatal lupus).

Pregnant women with SLE should have a baseline assessment of renal function and lupus activity in the first trimester, including a complete blood count, antiphospholipid antibodies, anti-SSA and anti-SSB antibodies, anti-double-stranded DNA antibody, complement levels (C3 and C4), and assessment for proteinuria (urine protein/creatinine ratio). These may need to be repeated each trimester (or more frequently) for those with active disease, especially with renal involvement.

Preeclampsia is a known obstetric complication for these patients; a daily low-dose aspirin is recommended for risk reduction. Patients are commonly treated with hydroxychloroquine to manage symptoms. This medication should be continued throughout the pregnancy, and the patient should be encouraged to continue yearly retinal examinations because of the risk of retinopathy with long-term use. The addition of low-molecular-weight or unfractionated heparin would be recommended in the setting of antiphospholipid syndrome.

Other factors in pregnancy management are directed toward improving fetal and neonatal outcomes through early diagnosis of fetal complications. Congenital heart block may affect 1–2% of pregnancies with anti-SSA or anti-SSB antibodies. Hydroxychloroquine can reduce the risk of congenital heart block, and this is one of the reasons it is advised to continue throughout a pregnancy. Systemic lupus erythematosus increases the risk of growth restriction, and ultrasonographic assessment for fetal growth can be considered in the third trimester. This is usually performed every 4 weeks, with the addition of weekly antenatal surveillance starting at approximately 32 weeks of gestation because of the increased risk of stillbirth for uncomplicated SLE.

Even if there have been no fetal or maternal complications in the antepartum period, neonatal lupus still may occur in patients who are anti-SSA or anti-SSB antibody positive. Cutaneous findings of lupus dermatitis may be present in 30–40% of infants. Figure 98-1 depicts an infant with annular erythematous plaques with central clearing, consistent with cutaneous findings of neonatal lupus erythematosus. Affected infants may demonstrate a cutaneous rash that is sun sensitive within the first few weeks of life. The rash is thought to be benign and usually resolves within a few weeks to 9 months of life as maternal antibodies are cleared from the infant circulation. Thrombocytopenia and hepatic involvement may be seen in as many as 10% of cases, so full evaluation of the neonate is necessary.

The use of hydroxychloroquine during pregnancy also is thought to reduce the risk of neonatal lupus. Because this patient was intolerant to hydroxychloroquine, azathioprine was prescribed to control her SLE symptoms. Azathioprine is considered safe in pregnancy and breastfeeding, and it is not associated with neonatal rash, although there is an increased risk of preterm birth and growth restriction associated with its use. Small-for-gestational-age size and preeclampsia are not associated with the neonatal skin findings on examination.

Corticosteroids also may be used in patients with SLE, particularly to control flares. Long-term use and high doses have increased risks that require monitoring, including hypertension, hyperglycemia, immunosuppression, and fetal growth restriction. Corticosteroids also are compatible with breastfeeding and would not cause neonatal rash.

Cunningham FG, Leveno KJ, Bloom SL, Dashe JS, Hoffman BL, Casey BM, et al. Williams obstetrics. 25th ed. McGraw-Hill Education; 2018.

Fetal growth restriction. ACOG Practice Bulletin No. 227. American College of Obstetricians and Gynecologists. Obstet Gynecol 2021;137:e16–28. doi: 10.1097/AOG.0000000000004251 https://journals.lww.com/greenjournal/pages/articleviewer.aspx?year=2021&issue=02000&article=00043&type=Fulltext

Immune modulating therapies in pregnancy and lactation. ACOG Committee Opinion No. 776. American College of Obstetricians and Gynecologists. Obstet Gynecol 2019;133:e287–95. doi: 10.1097/AOG.0000000000003176 https://journals.lww.com/greenjournal/Fulltext/2019/04000/ACOG_Committee_Opinion_No__776__Immune_Modulating.61.aspx

Petri M. Systemic lupus erythematosus. American College of Obstetricians and Gynecologists; 2020. Accessed March 16, 2022. https://www.acog.org/clinical/journals-and-publications/clinical-updates/2020/07/systemic-lupus-erythematosus

Resnik R, Lockwood CJ, Moore TR, Greene ME, Copel JA, Silver RM, editors. Creasy and Resnik's maternal–fetal medicine: principles and practice. 8th ed. Elsevier; 2018.

Wu J, Berk-Krauss J, Glick SA. Neonatal lupus erythematosus. JAMA Dermatol 2021;157:590. doi: 10.1001/jamadermatol.2021.0041 https://jamanetwork.com/journals/jamadermatology/article-abstract/2777663

99 Seizure disorder medications

A 26-year-old gravida 1 with a history of epilepsy presents to the emergency department after experiencing a tonic-clonic seizure. She is at 7 weeks of gestation. She discontinued her antiepileptic medication therapy 6 months ago for financial reasons. Since her epilepsy diagnosis 10 years ago, she has been on numerous antiepileptic medications, including carbamazepine, levetiracetam, phenytoin, topiramate, and valproic acid, all of which have been effective in managing her seizures. Of the antiepileptic medications that she has previously taken, you recommend that she restart

(A) carbamazepine
* (B) levetiracetam
(C) phenytoin
(D) topiramate
(E) valproic acid

Epilepsy is a common neurologic condition affecting reproductive-aged women that presents unique management challenges during pregnancy. Most women with epilepsy will have uncomplicated pregnancies; however, potential risks include increased seizure activity and congenital malformations caused by the medications that control seizures (Fig. 99-1).

Antiepileptic medications historically have been linked to major congenital anomalies. Antiepileptic medications also have been associated with fetal growth restriction and may adversely affect neurocognitive development. Reports on the incidence of antiepileptic medications causing minor and major malformations vary secondary to the type of antiepileptic medication, dosage, and number of medications being administered. The rate of congenital malformation has been reported as high as 10%, which is twofold to fourfold higher than that of the general population risk. Anomalies primarily linked to antiepileptic medications include neural tube defects, congenital heart defects, cleft palate, and urinary tract and skeletal abnormalities. The newer, second- and third-generation antiepileptic medications have significantly better safety profiles compared with the traditional, first-generation medications. Table 99-1 lists examples of traditional and newer antiepileptic medications.

Seizures during pregnancy, particularly those that are tonic-clonic in nature, can adversely affect both maternal and fetal health. Seizures may result in fetal hypoxia secondary to decreased placental blood flow and may cause maternal trauma. It has been estimated that 25–30% of women with epilepsy experience increased seizure frequency during pregnancy. Seizure frequency before pregnancy is an important predictor of seizures during pregnancy. Prescribing the appropriate

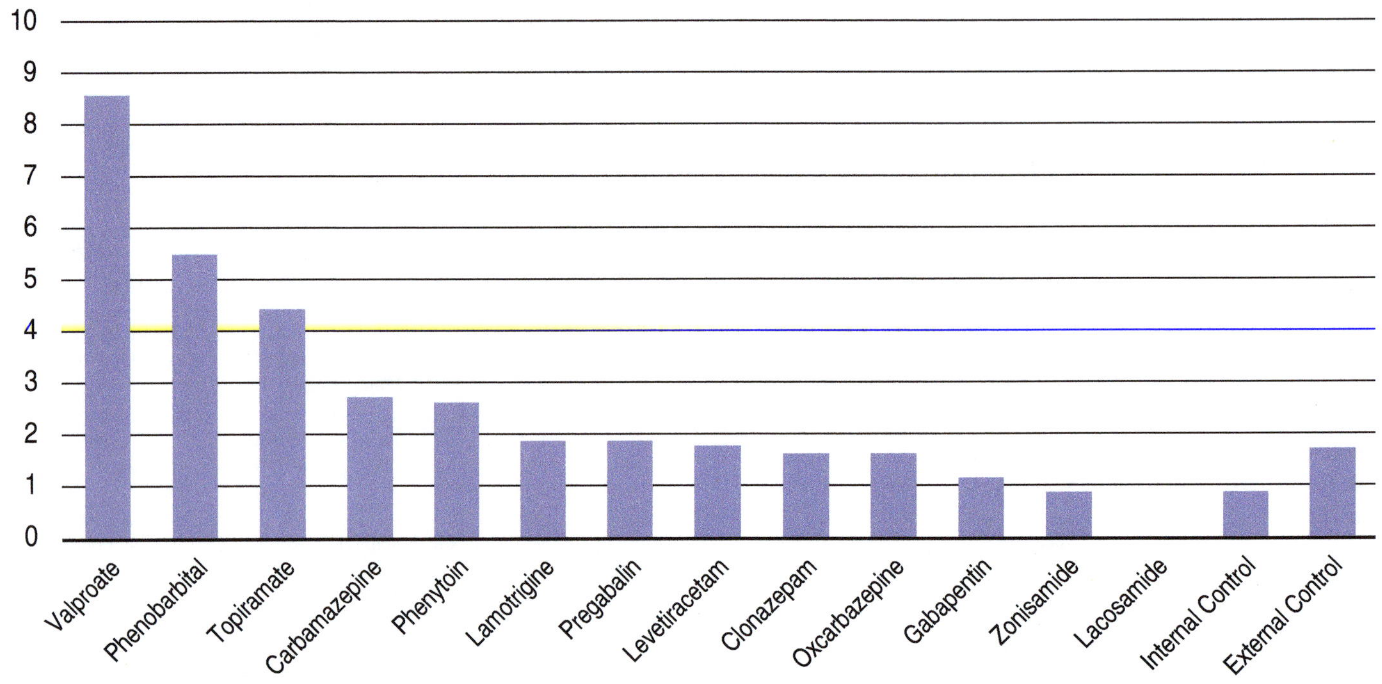

FIGURE 99-1. Major congenital abnormalities by antiepileptic drug (in percentage). (Data from North American Antiepileptic Drug Pregnancy Registry. Risk of malformations for specific AED in monotherapy and the control groups. In: Latest study data—October 2021. North American AED 2021. https://www.aedpregnancyregistry.org/wp-content/uploads/2021/08/The-NA-AED-Pregnancy-Registry-AES-2020.pdf)

TABLE 99-1. Traditional and Newer Antiepileptic Medications

TRADITIONAL ANTIEPILEPTIC MEDICATIONS	NEWER ANTIEPILEPTIC MEDICATIONS
Carbamazepine	Felbamate
Ethosuximide	Gabapentin
Phenobarbital	Lacosamide
Phenytoin	Lamotrigine
Primidone	Levetiracetam
Valproic acid	Oxcarbazepine
	Pregabalin
	Tiagabine
	Topiramate
	Vigabatrin
	Zonisamide

antiepileptic medication therapy is important to control seizure activity and reduce the risk of teratogenesis.

Ideally, women with epilepsy should have counseling to discuss medication management and optimize their antiepileptic medication regimen before becoming pregnant. This is especially important because a significant number of pregnancies are unplanned, and women may not know they are pregnant until after the critical periods of organogenesis have occurred. Many women are either counseled to discontinue their antiepileptic medications or they decide to self-discontinue them once they are pregnant because of concern regarding congenital anomalies.

In the described scenario, the patient previously has taken various antiepileptic medications to manage her seizures. When restarting antiseizure medications, it is preferable to use a medication that has been effective and well tolerated in the past. In this case, levetiracetam is the best option because it provides the best safety profile in pregnancy. Data have consistently shown that levetiracetam and lamotrigine, both second-generation antiepileptic medications, have a low risk of causing major fetal anomalies. Some reports have shown a greater prevalence of cleft lip and palate in fetuses exposed to lamotrigine; however, this is not a consistent finding.

Carbamazepine, phenytoin, and valproic acid are first-generation antiepileptic medications and have been associated with higher rates of major congenital anomalies. Valproic acid consistently has been shown to have the highest risk of teratogenesis compared with other antiepileptic medications, and the risk appears to be dose dependent; therefore, valproic acid is discouraged in reproductive-aged women. Topiramate, although a second-generation antiepileptic medication, has been associated with increased risk of oral clefts. Figure 99-1 summarizes the teratogenic risks of the various antiepileptic medications.

As with most medications, the risks associated with fetal drug exposure need to be weighed against the risks of uncontrolled maternal disease. The goal for treating women taking antiepileptic medications is to maintain the lowest effective dose, with monotherapy being preferred to polytherapy. For women who require polytherapy for seizure control, including the fewest medications at the lowest effective doses is recommended.

One of the explanations for increased frequency of seizures during pregnancy is a subtherapeutic antiepileptic medication level in the blood. Because of the physiologic changes that occur during pregnancy that affect the volume of distribution and metabolism of medications, monitoring of antiepileptic medication levels in the blood is recommended. For example, levels of levetiracetam have been shown to be as low as 40% of baseline concentrations during pregnancy. Levels should be checked periodically with appropriate adjustment of medication dosage in conjunction with the patient's antiepileptic medication prescriber. Serum concentrations will return to baseline levels postpartum, necessitating gradual dose reductions to avoid excessively high serum levels.

Folic acid intake is encouraged in all pregnant women to reduce the risks of major fetal anomalies, particularly of the brain and spine. Increased folate supplementation also may be needed in women who are taking enzyme-inducing antiepileptic medications that reduce serum folate levels, because these antiepileptic medications increase the risk of a fetus developing a neural tube defect. These tend to be the first-generation antiepileptic medications, particularly carbamazepine, phenytoin, phenobarbital, and primidone. Valproic acid also may interfere with folate metabolism. However, it is unclear whether increased folic acid intake reduces the risk of fetal anomalies, and an optimal dose has not been established.

Epilepsy Foundation. Epilepsy and pregnancy. Epilepsy Foundation; 2014. Accessed March 21, 2022. https://www.epilepsy.com/living-epilepsy/epilepsy-and/women/epilepsy-and-pregnancy

Hessler A, Dolbeck K. Seizures. Clin Update Womens Health Care 2021;XX(1):1–26.

Neural tube defects. Practice Bulletin No. 187. American College of Obstetricians and Gynecologists. Obstet Gynecol 2017;130:e279–90. doi: 10.1097/AOG.0000000000002412 https://journals.lww.com/greenjournal/Fulltext/2017/12000/Practice_Bulletin_No__187__Neural_Tube_Defects.41.aspx

Sazgar M. Treatment of women with epilepsy. Continuum (Minneap Minn) 2019;25:408–30. doi: 10.1212/CON.0000000000000713 https://journals.lww.com/continuum/Abstract/2019/04000/Treatment_of_Women_With_Epilepsy.9.aspx

Stephen LJ, Harden C, Tomson T, Brodie MJ. Management of epilepsy in women. Lancet Neurol 2019;18:481–91. doi: 10.1016/S1474-4422(18)30495-2 https://www.thelancet.com/journals/laneur/article/PIIS1474-4422(18)30495-2/fulltext

The North American AED (Antiepileptic Drug) Pregnancy Registry. Accessed March 21, 2022. https://www.aedpregnancyregistry.org/

Tomson T, Battino D, Bonizzoni E, Craig J, Lindhout D, Perucca E, et al. Comparative risk of major congenital malformations with eight different antiepileptic drugs: a prospective cohort study of the EURAP registry. EURAP Study Group. Lancet Neurol 2018;17:530–8. doi: 10.1016/S1474-4422(18)30107-8 https://www.thelancet.com/journals/laneur/article/PIIS1474-4422(18)30107-8/fulltext.

Veroniki AA, Cogo E, Rios P, Straus SE, Finkelstein Y, Kealey R, et al. Comparative safety of anti-epileptic drugs during pregnancy: a systematic review and network meta-analysis of congenital malformations and prenatal outcomes. BMC Med 2017;15:95–1. doi: 10.1186/s12916-017-0845-1 https://bmcmedicine.biomedcentral.com/articles/10.1186/s12916-017-0845-1

100 Adnexal mass in pregnancy

A 33-year-old gravida 2, para 1, presents at 15 1/7 weeks of gestation for follow-up imaging of a right adnexal mass incidentally noted on ultrasonographic evaluation at 8 weeks of gestation. The right adnexa was visualized (Fig. 100-1). The most likely diagnosis is

(A) endometrioma
(B) hydrosalpinx
* (C) mature cystic teratoma
(D) serous cystadenoma
(E) theca lutein cyst

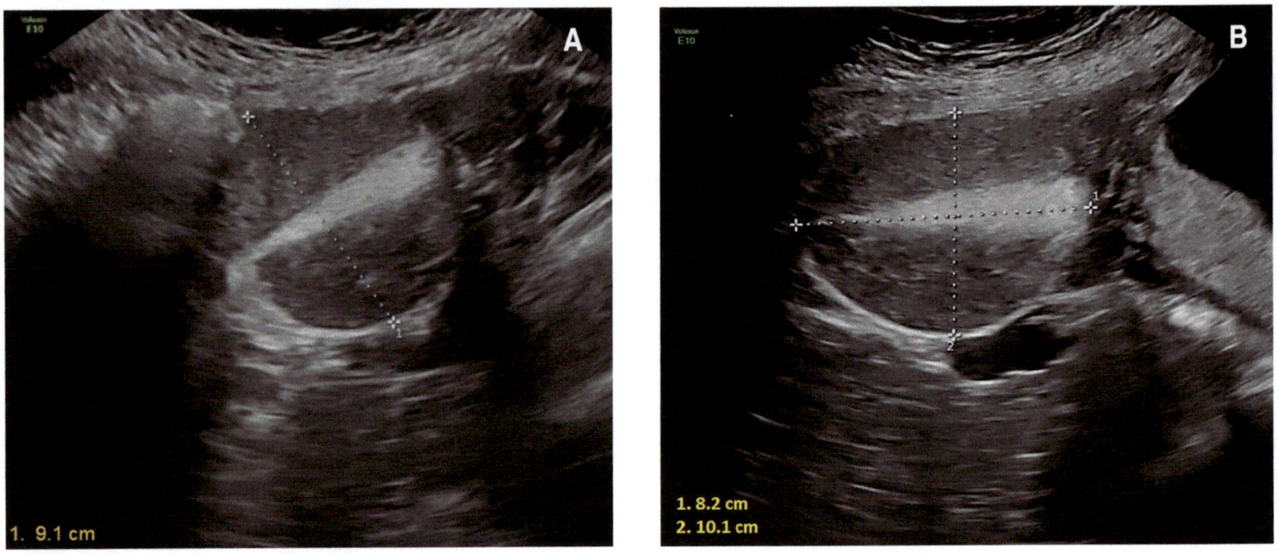

FIGURE 100-1. A and B. Ultrasonographic images of patient's right adnexa showing measurements in two orthogonal planes.

The evaluation of the adnexa is a now a standard component of first-trimester ultrasonography, and as a result, the diagnosis of adnexal masses in pregnancy has increased. Adnexal masses include masses of the ovary, fallopian tube, or surrounding structures. The reported incidence of adnexal masses in pregnancy ranges from 0.05% to 3.2% of live births with approximately 17% being malignant. Most of these masses are incidentally identified and are benign.

Nearly 70% of adnexal cysts detected in the first trimester resolve spontaneously. However, some masses may result in complications that require further management, either because they cause symptoms, or they are concerning for malignancy. Persistent masses are more likely to be associated with adverse clinical outcomes. These include masses that are greater than 5 cm and are multicystic or complex in appearance; however, a large proportion of these masses also resolve during pregnancy. Therefore, clinicians should recognize the various types of adnexal masses that may be visualized during the ultrasound evaluation to develop a differential diagnosis and guide management decisions.

Although many women with adnexal masses are asymptomatic, an adnexal mass can predispose the ovary to torsion. Torsion is more frequent in pregnant than nonpregnant women. It is estimated to occur in up to 7% of adnexal masses during pregnancy and is considered a surgical emergency. When the adnexa twists around its vascular pedicle on the long axis, it results in venous and lymphatic obstruction, which can lead to stasis, venous congestion, hemorrhage, and necrosis. Ultrasound imaging may show a congested, edematous ovary, and if torsion is complete, there often is an absence of blood flow. Torsion is more common with masses greater than 5 cm in size and commonly occurs with cystic teratomas. Symptoms include sudden onset of severe abdominal pain, nausea, and vomiting. The pain is often intermittent. Most ovarian torsions occur before 20 weeks of gestation.

Ultrasonographic evaluation of the adnexa is important and often includes transabdominal and transvaginal examination. A transvaginal approach allows improved imaging of the pelvis. Color Doppler also can be implemented to assess vascular flow. Ultrasonographic features associated with an increased risk of malignancy include size greater than 10 cm, solid or complex appearance, multilocular cysts, excrescences or papillary projections, irregular borders, increased vascularity, and ascites. Depending upon the ultrasonographic findings and differential diagnosis, management may include observation, further imaging, or a surgical procedure.

The most common adnexal masses found in pregnancy are functional cysts, including corpus luteum and follicular cysts and mature cystic teratomas. Corpus luteum cysts are fluid-filled cysts with smooth, thick walls and the classic ultrasonographic finding of a ring of vascularity around the cyst on color Doppler (termed the "ring of fire"). They range in size from approximately 2.5 to 6 cm. These progesterone-producing cysts typically begin to regress after 8 weeks of gestation and often resolve in the second trimester. The ultrasonographic appearance may become more complex if bleeding occurs within the cysts. A hemorrhagic cyst can display multiple fine strands of fibrin within the cyst. Over time, the cyst can appear to have debris and an organized clot within it.

Mature cystic teratomas, often called dermoid cysts, are the most common benign germ cell tumor in premenopausal women, and this is the correct diagnosis for the described patient. Mature cystic teratomas tend to have a classic ultrasonographic appearance. As seen in the figures, they usually are heterogenous, well-circumscribed masses containing echogenic material that may appear to be in layers. Calcifications (teeth) or punctate and linear echogenic foci (hair) may be seen. They often have a peripherally placed hyperechoic solid-appearing area composed of sebum, bones, and hair. They are persistent and are the most common adnexal mass associated with ovarian torsion in pregnancy.

Endometriomas, often called chocolate cysts, are a manifestation of endometriosis seen in women of reproductive age. Although endometriomas can have a variable appearance, the classic appearance in a premenopausal woman is a unilocular thick-walled cyst with diffuse homogeneous, ground-glass appearance. There is no internal flow with color Doppler. Tiny echogenic wall foci can distinguish an endometrioma from a hemorrhagic cyst. During pregnancy, the appearance of an endometrioma can change secondary to decidualization, resulting in solid vascular projections into the cyst cavity. This is a rare occurrence but can mimic ovarian carcinoma.

Hydrosalpinx refers to a fluid-filled dilatation of the fallopian tube secondary to an occlusion at the distal end. Ultrasonographically, it appears as a tubular-shaped cystic structure separate from the ipsilateral ovary. Indentations on the opposite sides of the wall (often called the waist sign) are a strong predictor of a hydrosalpinx and, in combination with a tubular cystic mass, are pathognomonic for hydrosalpinx. Incomplete septa from the fallopian tube walls folding on themselves also may be visualized.

The mass in the current figure is not consistent with a serous cystadenoma, which is the most frequent ovarian epithelial neoplasm. The ultrasonographic appearance usually is a smooth, thin-walled, unilocular, anechoic cyst that can be quite large (10 cm on average). There may be fine septations, and there is no flow on color Doppler.

Theca lutein cysts can develop in response to significant elevations of β-human chorionic gonadotropin resulting in hyperplasia of the theca and granulosa cells. They may be associated with gestational trophoblastic disease (complete molar pregnancy) and are less commonly associated with multiple gestations, ovulation induction, fetal hydrops, or hyperthyroidism. They often are bilateral and involve ovarian enlargement with multiple thin-walled cysts of fairly uniform size, usually 2–3 cm.

Other potential adnexal masses that may be encountered during pregnancy include paraovarian cysts, leiomyomas, fibromas, and ovarian malignancies.

Canavan TP. Sonographic tips for evaluation of adnexal masses in pregnancy. Clin Obstet Gynecol 2017;60:575–85. doi: 10.1097/GRF.0000000000000302 https://journals.lww.com/clinicalobgyn/Abstract/2017/09000/Sonographic_Tips_for_Evaluation_of_Adnexal_Masses.16.aspx

Evaluation and management of adnexal masses. Practice Bulletin No. 174. American College of Obstetricians and Gynecologists. Obstet Gynecol 2016;128:e210–26. doi: 10.1097/AOG.0000000000001768 https://journals.lww.com/greenjournal/Fulltext/2016/11000/Practice_Bulletin_No__174__Evaluation_and.52.aspx

Goh W, Bohrer J, Zalud I. Management of the adnexal mass in pregnancy. Curr Opin Obstet Gynecol 2014;26:49–53. doi: 10.1097/GCO.0000000000000048 https://journals.lww.com/co-obgyn/Abstract/2014/04000/Management_of_the_adnexal_mass_in_pregnancy.2.aspx

Khati NJ, Kim T, Riess J. Imaging of benign adnexal disease. Radiol Clin North Am 2020;58:257–73. doi: 10.1016/j.rcl.2019.10.009 https://www.radiologic.theclinics.com/article/S0033-8389(19)30148-4/fulltext

McMinn E, Schwartz N. Adnexal masses in pregnancy. Clin Obstet Gynecol 2020;63:392–404. doi: 10.1097/GRF.0000000000000528 https://journals.lww.com/clinicalobgyn/Abstract/2020/06000/Adnexal_Masses_in_Pregnancy.18.aspx

101 Thromboprophylaxis

A 38-year-old gravida 1 has been prescribed low-molecular-weight heparin daily during her pregnancy because her mother experienced a deep vein thrombosis during pregnancy, and she and her mother are heterozygous for factor V Leiden mutation. She is scheduled for induction of labor at 39 weeks of gestation and desires an epidural for pain management during labor. The most appropriate timing for discontinuation of this patient's anticoagulation before epidural placement is

(A) 6 hours
* (B) 12 hours
(C) 24 hours
(D) 48 hours

Venous thromboembolism (VTE), which encompasses both deep vein thrombosis and pulmonary embolism, is a leading cause of maternal morbidity and mortality in the United States. Evidence suggests that the incidence of VTE in pregnancy is increasing. When vaginal delivery hospitalizations were evaluated from 2006 to 2012, there was a significant increase in VTE incidence (from 15.6 to 29.8 per 100,000 deliveries). Therefore, it is likely that the number of women receiving anticoagulation during pregnancy will continue to increase.

Pregnancy is a known risk factor for VTE because of the associated physiologic and anatomic changes. Risk factors that further increase the risk of VTE in pregnancy include increasing age, prolonged immobilization, obesity, inherited thrombophilia, previous VTE, and cesarean birth. When a woman undergoes a cesarean birth, the risk of VTE is increased fourfold compared with vaginal delivery. This increased risk continues postpartum, particularly during the first 6 weeks after delivery.

Pharmacologic thromboprophylaxis is an intervention to consider in women at risk of developing a VTE during pregnancy. Anticoagulation regimens include either low-molecular-weight heparin or unfractionated heparin, and dosing regimens range from prophylactic to intermediate to adjusted-dose (therapeutic). Appendix G gives anticoagulation regimen definitions. Low-molecular-weight heparin generally is the anticoagulant of choice during pregnancy because of its ease of administration, better safety and bioavailability profiles, and more predictable dosing when compared with unfractionated heparin. Benefits include fewer bleeding complications and a lower incidence of heparin-induced thrombocytopenia in pregnant women receiving low-molecular-weight heparin compared with unfractionated heparin. Although protamine sulfate results in a full reversal of unfractionated heparin and only a 60–80% reversal of low-molecular-weight heparin, little is known about its use in pregnancy to facilitate the provision of neuraxial anesthesia.

Neuraxial blockade is an important modality for pain management in the obstetric patient and provides superior pain relief in addition to decreasing circulating catecholamines. For the woman who undergoes a cesarean birth, neuraxial anesthesia affords both maternal and fetal benefits when compared with general anesthesia. However, when women are on anticoagulation, considerations must be made to minimize potential risks associated with administration of neuraxial anesthesia, namely spinal epidural hematoma. Available data are very limited but suggest that this risk is quite low (1:200,000–1:250,000). One systematic review did not identify any cases of spinal epidural hematoma in obstetric patients who were receiving unfractionated heparin or low-molecular-weight heparin for thromboprophylaxis.

The Society for Obstetric Anesthesia and Perinatology has developed a consensus statement on the anesthetic management of pregnant and postpartum women receiving anticoagulation. Specific guidelines for timing of neuraxial administration and removal of catheters in women on anticoagulants have been established, and they differ in their recommendations for dosing regimen and agent (Appendix G). In addition to recommended timing of the last dose of anticoagulant, there is also a difference between low-molecular-weight heparin and unfractionated heparin regarding the recommendation to assess coagulation status before administration of a neuraxial blockade. With low-molecular-weight heparin, obtaining coagulation laboratory values is not considered necessary; however, with unfractionated heparin laboratory evaluation is recommended for prophylactic and therapeutic dosing regimens because of the larger variability in response to unfractionated heparin.

Consequently, advanced delivery planning in women on anticoagulation is recommended to optimize pregnancy outcomes. Because labor may occur before the scheduled date, patients should be educated to hold their anticoagulation dose if they suspect they are in labor or they experience leaking of fluid or vaginal bleeding.

In the current scenario, the patient is heterozygous for factor V Leiden, a low-risk thrombophilia, and has a first-degree relative who has had a VTE, and she qualifies for taking prophylactic low-molecular-weight heparin during her pregnancy and for 6 weeks postpartum. For delivery planning, she should discontinue her heparin the day before her planned induction of labor so at least 12 hours elapse before she receives epidural anesthesia. Anticoagulation should be resumed after delivery with the dosing regimen being equal to or greater than the antepartum treatment. Although the optimal time to resume anticoagulation after delivery has not been established, the general recommendation is to restart no sooner than 4–6 hours after vaginal delivery and 6–12 hours after cesarean birth. Additionally, when regional anesthesia has been administered, guidelines have been established regarding timing of catheter removal and resumption of anticoagulation based on the dosage regimen (Table 101-1).

When therapeutic dosing of low-molecular-weight heparin is prescribed during pregnancy, neuraxial blockade should not be administered until 24 hours after the last dose. There are no current scenarios in which discontinuing anticoagulation 48 hours before epidural placement is required.

When postpartum anticoagulation is planned, it is important to remember to place pneumatic compression devices until the patient is ambulatory and anticoagulation is restarted.

TABLE 101-1. Timing of Neuraxial Anesthesia in Relation to Pharmacologic Anticoagulation

DOSAGE REGIMEN	INTRAPARTUM, ELECTIVE PROCEDURE	INTRAPARTUM, URGENT/ EMERGENT PROCEDURE	POSTPARTUM
UFH prophylaxis (7,500 units SC twice daily or 10,000 units SC twice daily)	Hold dose for 12 h and assess coagulation status before administering neuraxial anesthesia.	Hold dose for 12 h and assess coagulation status before administering neuraxial anesthesia. However, in urgent cases with greater competing risks from general anesthesia, placement of neuraxial anesthesia may be appropriate.	Wait at least 1 h after neuraxial blockade and catheter removal before restarting heparin.
UFH adjusted-dose (greater than 10,000 units per dose or less than 20,000 units per day)	Hold dose for 24 h and assess coagulation status before administering neuraxial blockade.	If at least 24 h since last dose and aPTT within normal limits or undetectable anti-Xa, likely low risk of neuraxial blockade.	Wait at least 1 h after neuraxial blockade or catheter removal before restarting heparin.
Low-dose LMWH prophylaxis	Wait 12 h after last dose before neuraxial blockade.	Insufficient data to make a recommendation for placement of neuraxial blockade less than 12 h from last dose of LMWH. In high-risk situations in which intervention is needed, risks of general anesthesia may outweigh risks of spinal epidural hematoma.	Wait at least 12 h after neuraxial blockade and at least 4 h after catheter removal to restart LMWH prophylaxis.
LMWH intermediate-dose or adjusted-dose	Wait 24 h after last dose before neuraxial blockade.	If less than 24 h, insufficient evidence to recommend proceeding with neuraxial blockade.	Consider waiting at least 24 h after neuraxial blockade *and* at least 4 h after catheter removal to restart LMWH anticoagulation.

Abbreviations: aPTT, activated partial thromboplastin clotting time; LMWH, low-molecular-weight heparin; SC, subcutaneously; UFH, unfractionated heparin.

Data from Leffert L, Butwick A, Carvalho B, Arendt K, Bates SM, Friedman A, et al. The Society for Obstetric Anesthesia and Perinatology consensus statement on the anesthetic management of pregnant and postpartum women receiving thromboprophylaxis or higher dose anticoagulants. SOAP VTE Taskforce. Anesth Analg 2018;126:928–44. doi: 10.1213/ANE.0000000000002530 https://journals.lww.com/anesthesia-analgesia/Fulltext/2018/03000/The_Society_for_Obstetric_Anesthesia_and.33.aspx

Horlocker TT, Vandermeulen E, Kopp SL, Gogarten W, Leffert LR, Benzon HT. Regional anesthesia in the patient receiving antithrombotic or thrombolytic therapy: American Society of Regional Anesthesia and Pain Medicine Evidence-Based guidelines (Fourth Edition) [published erratum appears in Reg Anesth Pain Med 2018;43:566]. Reg Anesth Pain Med 2018;43:263–309. doi: 10.1097/AAP.0000000000000763 https://rapm.bmj.com/content/43/3/263.long

Inherited thrombophilias in pregnancy. ACOG Practice Bulletin No. 197. American College of Obstetricians and Gynecologists [published erratum appears in Obstet Gynecol 2018;132:1069]. Obstet Gynecol 2018;132:e18–34. doi: 10.1097/AOG.0000000000002703 https://journals.lww.com/greenjournal/Fulltext/2018/07000/ACOG_Practice_Bulletin_No__197__Inherited.55.aspx

Leffert L, Butwick A, Carvalho B, Arendt K, Bates SM, Friedman A, et al. The Society for Obstetric Anesthesia and Perinatology consensus statement on the anesthetic management of pregnant and postpartum women receiving thromboprophylaxis or higher dose anticoagulants. SOAP VTE Taskforce. Anesth Analg 2018;126:928–44. doi: 10.1213/ANE.0000000000002530 https://journals.lww.com/anesthesia-analgesia/Fulltext/2018/03000/The_Society_for_Obstetric_Anesthesia_and.33.aspx

Thromboembolism in pregnancy. ACOG Practice Bulletin No. 196. American College of Obstetricians and Gynecologists [published erratum appears in Obstet Gynecol 2018;132:1068]. Obstet Gynecol 2018;132:e1–17. doi: 10.1097/AOG.0000000000002706 https://journals.lww.com/greenjournal/Fulltext/2018/07000/ACOG_Practice_Bulletin_No__196__Thromboembolism_in.54.aspx

102 Vaginal birth after cesarean

A 38-year-old gravida 3, para 1, with a previous cesarean birth at 38 weeks of gestation presents to labor and delivery with a report of leaking fluid. She reports that her first cesarean birth was performed for breech presentation at term. Ruptured membranes are confirmed. The cervix is 4-cm dilated, 50% effaced, with fetal station at −2. Fetal heart rate tracing shows a baseline of 135 beats per minute, moderate variability, the presence of accelerations, and the absence of decelerations. She had planned to deliver at a hospital 30 miles away. With regard to delivery planning, the most appropriate next step is to

* (A) offer a trial of labor
(B) perform immediate repeat cesarean birth
(C) perform ultrasonographic evaluation of the lower uterine segment
(D) transfer the patient to her primary obstetrician

Cesarean birth is one of the most commonly performed abdominal surgeries in the United States, with rates increasing since the 1970s. Cesarean birth carries increased risks to the patient compared with vaginal birth, including increased risk of hemorrhage, infection, and venous thromboembolism. In a subsequent pregnancy, vaginal birth may decrease these risks compared with cesarean birth.

Risks of labor after cesarean include uterine rupture, need for emergent cesarean birth, hemorrhage, infection, and surgical injury. These risks are increased with labor after cesarean compared with elective repeat cesarean birth; however, labor after cesarean carries a decreased risk of maternal death. Neonatal risks increase with labor after cesarean, most of which are related to uterine rupture and the need for emergent cesarean birth. Successful vaginal birth after cesarean carries lower maternal risks than elective repeat cesarean birth.

The likelihood of successful vaginal birth after cesarean depends on several factors: the number of previous cesareans, indication for previous cesarean, the need for labor induction versus spontaneous labor, age, body mass index, and gestational age. Candidates for trial of labor after cesarean (TOLAC) include patients who have had one or two previous cesareans with low transverse uterine incisions. Those with a history of classical or T incision generally are not considered candidates for TOLAC because of an increased risk of uterine rupture.

In the setting of unknown uterine scar, data suggest that overall risk of uterine rupture is not significantly increased. In the absence of concern for previous classical uterine incision, these patients may be offered TOLAC. History that would raise suspicion for a previous classical incision would include cesarean for extremely preterm delivery. A vertical skin incision performed at the time of a term cesarean birth does not correlate with a vertical uterine incision and should not preclude offering a TOLAC. In the clinical scenario presented above, a low transverse uterine incision is most likely in the setting of term breech delivery. Although ultrasonographic evaluation of the lower uterine segment may provide information about the thickness of the previous uterine scar and may help predict the risk of uterine rupture, there is no recommendation for its routine use. Transfer of this patient would be a violation of the Emergency Medical Treatment and Labor Act given the ruptured membranes and likely early labor.

Cunningham FG, Leveno KJ, Bloom SL, Dashe JS, Hoffman BL, Casey BM, et al. Williams obstetrics. 25th ed. McGraw-Hill Education; 2018.

Prelabor rupture of membranes: ACOG Practice Bulletin No. 217. American College of Obstetricians and Gynecologists. Obstet Gynecol 2020;135:e80–97. doi: 10.1097/AOG.0000000000003700 https://journals.lww.com/greenjournal/Fulltext/2020/03000/Prelabor_Rupture_of_Membranes__ACOG_Practice.47.aspx

Vaginal birth after cesarean delivery. ACOG Practice Bulletin No. 205. American College of Obstetricians and Gynecologists. Obstet Gynecol 2019;133:e110–27. doi: 10.1097/AOG.0000000000003078 https://journals.lww.com/greenjournal/Fulltext/2019/02000/ACOG_Practice_Bulletin_No__205__Vaginal_Birth.40.aspx

103 Nausea and vomiting of pregnancy

A 39-year-old primigravida at 14 weeks of gestation presents to the emergency department with intractable nausea and vomiting. This is her third presentation for nausea and vomiting. The patient reports that she has self-treated with marijuana. She has been treated with doxylamine, pyridoxine, and ondansetron with no improvement in her symptoms. She mentions that the only thing that seems to be helping is frequent hot showers. On presentation, she is afebrile, her blood pressure is 100/62 mm Hg, and her heart rate is 110 beats per minute. Her weight is decreased to 65 kg from 76 kg before pregnancy. She is hospitalized for intravenous hydration and optimization of antiemetic therapy. The best next step to resolve her nausea and vomiting is

* (A) cessation of marijuana use
(B) methylprednisolone taper
(C) metoclopramide
(D) psychotherapy

Nausea and vomiting are among the most common complications of pregnancy, affecting between 50% and 80% of pregnant women. Hyperemesis gravidarum, or extreme nausea and vomiting of pregnancy, affects 0.3–3% of pregnancies. *Hyperemesis gravidarum* is defined as 1) persistent vomiting in pregnancy not related to other causes, accompanied by 2) a measure of acute starvation, typically ketonuria, and 3) weight loss of at least 5% of prepregnancy weight. Hyperemesis gravidarum is associated with an increased incidence of small-for-gestational-age newborns, can result in severe complications leading to hospitalization, and can significantly affect the quality of life of the pregnant woman.

When a pregnant patient presents with nausea and vomiting, the effect on quality of life can be evaluated using standardized assessment tools. One such tool is the Pregnancy Unique Quantification of Emesis/Nausea Index (PUQE) that assesses the severity of symptoms (Table 103-1). This tool has been validated in multiple populations and may help assess the severity of symptoms in the first trimester and guide early treatment of nausea and vomiting to prevent progression to hyperemesis gravidarum.

In addition to quantitatively evaluating symptoms, obstetrician–gynecologists should take a careful history and rule out other potential causes of nausea and vomiting. A history of nausea and vomiting that predates pregnancy likely has other underlying causes, for example, inflammatory bowel syndrome, gastroparesis, pancreatitis, or cholelithiasis. Additionally, nausea and vomiting that start after 9–10 weeks of gestation are unlikely to be related to pregnancy. If symptoms are accompanied by abdominal pain, tenderness, fever, headache, or an abnormal neurologic examination, they are likely to have causes beyond pregnancy. Similarly, if a goiter is present, thyroid disease may be a cause. Although psychiatric causes should be considered in patients with nausea and vomiting

TABLE 103-1. Modified Pregnancy-Unique Quantification of Emesis and Nausea

Circle the answer that best suits your situation from the beginning of your pregnancy.

1. ON AVERAGE IN A DAY, FOR HOW LONG DO YOU FEEL NAUSEATED OR SICK TO YOUR STOMACH?				
Not at all (1)	1 h or less (2)	2–3 h (3)	4–6 h (4)	More than 6 h (5)
2. ON AVERAGE IN A DAY, HOW MANY TIMES DO YOU VOMIT OR THROW UP?				
7 or more times (5)	5–6 times (4)	3–4 times (3)	1–2 times (2)	I did not throw up (1)
3. ON AVERAGE IN A DAY, HOW MANY TIMES DO YOU HAVE RETCHING OR DRY HEAVES WITHOUT BRINGING ANYTHING UP?				
None (1)	1–2 times (2)	3–4 times (3)	5–6 times (4)	7 or more times (5)
Total score (sum of replies to 1, 2, and 3): mild NVP, 6 or less; moderate NVP, 7–12; severe NVP, 13 or more.				

Abbreviation: NVP, nausea and vomiting of pregnancy.

Reprinted from Lacasse A, Rey E, Ferreira E, Morin C, Bérard A. Validity of a modified Pregnancy-Unique Quantification of Emesis and Nausea (PUQE) scoring index to assess severity of nausea and vomiting of pregnancy. Am J Obstet Gynecol 2008;198:71.e1–7. doi: 10.1016/j.ajog.2007.05.051 https://www.ajog.org/article/S0002-9378(07)00716-8/fulltext

of pregnancy, recent literature has illustrated that conversion disorder, abnormal stress response, and other psychologic disorders are not typical causes and are not more common among patients with hyperemesis gravidarum. Finally, it is important to evaluate substance use as an underlying cause of nausea and vomiting in pregnancy.

Cannabis, or marijuana, has antiemetic qualities and is used to treat nausea related to chemotherapy. At least 3–5% of pregnant women self-report marijuana use during pregnancy, and a recent study showed that women with hyperemesis gravidarum were more likely to report marijuana use during gestation. Additionally, marijuana is legalized for medicinal use in many states, and severe or intractable nausea is a condition for use in most of these states. Marijuana was shown to be similar to ondansetron and superior to prochlorperazine in the treatment of nausea related to chemotherapy. However, there is no clear evidence of benefit for marijuana use for hyperemesis gravidarum.

Recreational marijuana use is legal in some states, and many states have legalized medical marijuana. Both are illegal under federal law. Despite federal restrictions, select state legalization has contributed to the false perception that marijuana is safe in pregnancy. Recent studies have shown that 20–65% of women believe there is no risk of harm from smoking marijuana as often as twice a week. In fact, marijuana crosses the placenta and may have adverse consequences for the fetus and pregnancy. It is somewhat difficult to separate the effects of marijuana use from other potential confounding exposures to tobacco, alcohol, or other drugs. However, evidence from recent meta-analyses has illustrated an increased risk of low birth weight and fetal growth restriction. There also may be an association with increased risk of stillbirth. Concurrent marijuana and tobacco use may increase preterm birth rates. Additionally, medical marijuana is not regulated, and there are no standardizations of dose and formulation. For these reasons, pregnant women or women contemplating pregnancy should be encouraged to stop using medical marijuana and use therapies with more evidence of safety in pregnancy.

Importantly, despite its antiemetic qualities, cannabis can cause users to experience a syndrome associated with cyclic nausea, vomiting, and abdominal pain known as *cannabinoid hyperemesis syndrome*. This syndrome, which was first described in 2004, is a paradoxical vomiting syndrome that occurs episodically in those who use marijuana more than once a week. Classically, the symptoms are relieved by hot showers or baths; compulsive bathing is specific and pathognomonic for the diagnosis of cannabinoid hyperemesis syndrome. There are many hypotheses regarding etiology, the most common being that cannabinoid stimulation of vascular receptors causes splanchnic vasodilation and mesenteric congestion. Exposure to hot water redistributes blood flow to the skin and could explain symptom relief. Additional symptoms may include agitation, diaphoresis, tachycardia, hypotension, and weight loss.

There have been several cases of cannabinoid hyperemesis syndrome reported in pregnancy. Often, pregnant patients experiencing these symptoms undergo a workup and treatment for hyperemesis gravidarum, sometimes resulting in extensive laboratory and imaging studies. The usual treatments for nausea and vomiting in pregnancy, including vitamin B_6, doxylamine, ondansetron, promethazine, metoclopramide, and corticosteroids, do not help, and symptoms will generally last 24–48 hours at a time. The syndrome is likely to recur if marijuana is used again. For the described patient, methylprednisolone taper, psychotherapy, and total parenteral nutrition are unlikely to help; recognition of cannabinoid hyperemesis syndrome and cessation of marijuana use are the best approach to relieve symptoms. Given the increasing use of marijuana for recreational and medical purposes and the increasing number of U.S. states with legalization of both types of marijuana, obstetricians should consider cannabinoid hyperemesis syndrome in the evaluation and treatment of nausea and vomiting of pregnancy.

Alaniz VI, Liss J, Metz TD, Stickrath E. Cannabinoid hyperemesis syndrome: a cause of refractory nausea and vomiting in pregnancy. Obstet Gynecol 2015;125:1484–6. doi: 10.1097/AOG.0000000000000595 https://journals.lww.com/greenjournal/Fulltext/2015/06000/Cannabinoid_Hyperemesis_Syndrome__A_Cause_of.30.aspx

Chocron Y, Zuber JP, Vaucher J. Cannabinoid hyperemesis syndrome. BMJ 2019;366:l4336. doi: 10.1136/bmj.l4336 https://www.bmj.com/content/366/bmj.l4336.long

Marijuana use during pregnancy and lactation. Committee Opinion No. 722. American College of Obstetricians and Gynecologists. Obstet Gynecol 2017;130:e205–9. doi: 10.1097/AOG.0000000000002354 https://journals.lww.com/greenjournal/Fulltext/2017/10000/Committee_Opinion_No__722__Marijuana_Use_During.59.aspx

Metz TD, Borgelt LM. Marijuana use in pregnancy and while breastfeeding. Obstet Gynecol 2018;132:1198–210. doi: 10.1097/AOG.0000000000002878 https://journals.lww.com/greenjournal/Fulltext/2018/11000/Marijuana_Use_in_Pregnancy_and_While_Breastfeeding.17.aspx

Nausea and vomiting of pregnancy. ACOG Practice Bulletin No. 189. American College of Obstetricians and Gynecologists. Obstet Gynecol 2018;131:e15–30. doi: 10.1097/AOG.0000000000002456 https://journals.lww.com/greenjournal/Fulltext/2018/01000/ACOG_Practice_Bulletin_No__189__Nausea_And.39.aspx

Roberson EK, Patrick WK, Hurwitz EL. Marijuana use and maternal experiences of severe nausea during pregnancy in Hawai'i. Hawaii J Med Public Health 2014;73:283–7. https://www.ncbi.nlm.nih.gov/pmc/articles/PMC4174692/

104 Penicillin allergy

A 27-year-old gravida 1, para 0, will be undergoing primary cesarean birth for breech presentation following an unsuccessful external cephalic version. She reports that she is allergic to penicillin and states that her allergic reaction was a rash after treatment with amoxicillin as a child. Rectovaginal culture at 37 weeks of gestation is positive for group B streptococcus (GBS), which is sensitive to ampicillin, clindamycin, and erythromycin. The most appropriate antibiotic surgical prophylaxis for this patient is

(A) ampicillin and sulbactam
(B) azithromycin
* (C) cefazolin
(D) clindamycin and gentamicin
(E) vancomycin

In patients undergoing cesarean birth, prophylactic antibiotics are recommended to reduce surgical site infection. First-generation cephalosporins, usually cefazolin, are used most commonly for prophylaxis in patients without allergy. Second-generation cephalosporins also provide adequate coverage but are significantly more expensive. Cefazolin provides adequate coverage of appropriate skin flora, has good bactericidal activity, and rapidly reaches appropriate levels in tissue, making it a good choice for antibiotic prophylaxis.

Up to 25% of patients report a penicillin allergy, but documentation of allergies is inconsistent. A true hypersensitivity reaction to penicillin exists in 1 in 2,500 to 1 in 25,000 women. In patients reporting allergy, 90–99% do not have a true hypersensitivity reaction. Severe reactions include anaphylaxis, angioedema, and urticaria. Many patients will report adverse effects such as nausea and vomiting as allergy. Less than 10% of patients who report a penicillin allergy will have a reaction to cephalosporin. Skin testing can provide specific information about the actual allergy, but this has generally not been performed in pregnancy because of the risk of anaphylaxis to the fetus. More recent data suggest that skin testing in pregnancy is safe and should be considered. In a recent study, anaphylaxis occurred in only 4% of pregnant patients undergoing penicillin allergy testing, and no one suffered any significant adverse effects.

In patients who have a penicillin allergy, it is important to determine whether the reaction is a true allergy, hypersensitivity, or simply an adverse effect. Those who are at high risk of anaphylaxis (they have a history of anaphylaxis, angioedema, or urticaria) should receive an alternative to cefazolin at the time of cesarean birth. The usual antibiotic choice in this setting is clindamycin plus an aminoglycoside, such as gentamicin. In patients who have a mild reaction to penicillin, including rash, cephalosporins can be used. In one large study, patients who received alternative preoperative antibiotics because of penicillin allergy had a significantly increased risk of surgical site infection—although this finding was not specific to cesarean birth.

In the clinical scenario above, the patient should receive cefazolin because it provides the best coverage and her risk of anaphylaxis is low. Similarly, were this patient in labor and in need of GBS prophylaxis, cefazolin would be the appropriate antibiotic choice. Ampicillin and sulbactam provide adequate coverage for surgical prophylaxis but are more expensive than cefazolin, and they would not be the preferred option for this patient. In a patient already being treated for intra-amniotic infection, continuing ampicillin and sulbactam is appropriate and provides adequate coverage with the addition of azithromycin. Patients should only be treated with clindamycin for GBS if they have a high risk of cephalosporin allergy and have a culture showing that GBS is sensitive to clindamycin and erythromycin. Clindamycin with gentamicin is an appropriate surgical prophylaxis choice for patients with true penicillin allergy with risk of anaphylaxis. Azithromycin often is added for surgical prophylaxis for unscheduled cesarean birth in laboring and ruptured patients but is not sufficient for monotherapy. Vancomycin is appropriate for use in patients with methicillin-resistant *Staphylococcus aureus* colonization; however, it also is not sufficient for monotherapy and would be combined with cefazolin or another β-lactam antibiotic.

Blumenthal KG, Ryan EE, Li Y, Lee H, Kuhlen JL, Shenoy ES. The impact of a reported penicillin allergy on surgical site infection risk. Clin Infect Dis 2018;66:329–36. doi: 10.1093/cid/cix794 https://academic.oup.com/cid/article/66/3/329/4372047

Desravines N, Waldron J, Venkatesh KK, Kwan M, Boggess KA. Outpatient penicillin allergy testing in pregnant women who report an allergy. Obstet Gynecol 2021;137:56–61. doi: 10.1097/AOG.0000000000004213 https://journals.lww.com/greenjournal/Fulltext/2021/01000/Outpatient_Penicillin_Allergy_Testing_in_Pregnant.8.aspx

Shenoy ES, Macy E, Rowe T, Blumenthal KG. Evaluation and management of penicillin allergy: a review. JAMA 2019;321:188–99. doi: 10.1001/jama.2018.19283 https://jamanetwork.com/journals/jama/fullarticle/2720732

Use of prophylactic antibiotics in labor and delivery. ACOG Practice Bulletin No. 199. American College of Obstetricians and Gynecologists [published erratum appears in Obstet Gynecol 2019;134:883–884]. Obstet Gynecol 2018;132:e103-19. doi: 10.1097/AOG.0000000000002833 https://journals.lww.com/greenjournal/Fulltext/2018/09000/ACOG_Practice_Bulletin_No__199__Use_of.67.aspx

105 Disseminated intravascular coagulation

A 34-year-old gravida 3, para 2, presents at 36 weeks of gestation for her third cesarean birth. Her pregnancy is complicated by placenta previa. Placenta accreta is suspected at the time of delivery, requiring immediate hysterectomy, which is complicated by adhesive disease and heavy intraoperative bleeding. Massive transfusion protocol is initiated. Total quantitative blood loss is 6,350 mL. She is intubated and transferred to the intensive care unit for monitoring. Her temperature is 37.1 °C (98.8 °F), her blood pressure is 122/70 mm Hg, and she is ventilated with pressure support only. She is sedated, but otherwise her physical examination is normal. Telemetry shows peaked T-waves and wide QRS interval (Fig. 105-1). The most likely massive transfusion complication is

* (A) electrolyte derangement
(B) febrile hemolytic reaction
(C) transfusion-associated circulatory overload (TACO)
(D) transfusion-related acute lung injury (TRALI)

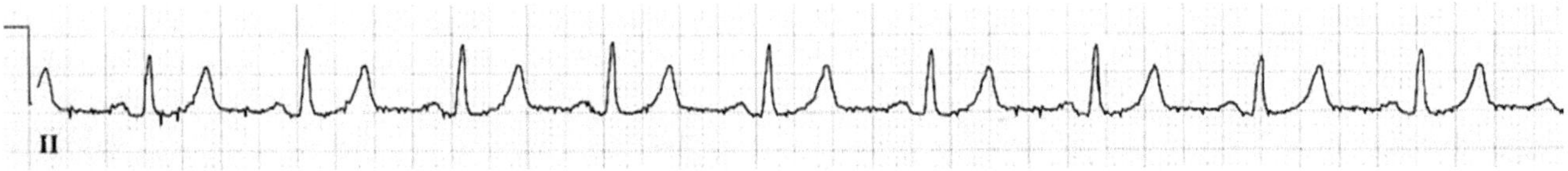

FIGURE 105-1. Postoperative electrocardiogram. (Image courtesy of Baystate Medical Center Division of Nephrology.)

Postpartum hemorrhage is a cumulative blood loss of 1,000 mL or greater in the first 24 hours after vaginal or cesarean birth. Primary postpartum hemorrhage occurs within this 24-hour period and causes include uterine atony, lacerations, retained placenta, coagulopathy, uterine inversion, and placenta accreta. Placenta accreta can lead to particularly high blood loss when undiagnosed before delivery, as is the case with this patient.

Massive transfusion usually will require a transfusion of 10 or more units of packed red blood cells within 24 hours, or 4 units within 1 hour, with an ongoing need for more blood. The recommended transfusion ratio is 1:1:1 for packed red blood cells, fresh frozen plasma, and platelets, but this comes largely from trauma literature, and experience in obstetric cohorts is predominantly retrospective. Studies in civilian trauma units and combat hospitals have shown that component replacement rarely is necessary with acute replacement of 5–10 units of packed red blood cells. Evaluation of platelets, clotting studies, and fibrinogen concentration are reasonable to guide treatment. Platelets should be maintained above 50×10^9/L. A fibrinogen concentration below 150 mg/dL or a prolonged prothrombin time should prompt replacement therapy with plasma. Thromboelastography and rotational thromboelastography are point-of-care tests that can assess coagulation status in the patient. They indicate time to clot formation, clot strength, and fibrinolysis. These data may be used to refine blood product usage according to which portion of the coagulation cascade is affected but should be reserved for trained personnel to avoid misinterpretation and incorrect blood product replacement.

Lifesaving blood transfusion does come with risks, particularly when using large volumes during a massive transfusion protocol. Packed red blood cells contain high levels of potassium and citrate and can lead to hyperkalemia and citrate toxicity with hypocalcemia. Electrolytes should be closely monitored during any massive transfusion, with corrective therapy in the setting of abnormal and critical values, although there are no guidelines to suggest how often serum testing should occur, and obstetricians should refer to their local protocols. This patient received a massive transfusion and has electrocardiogram changes suggestive of hyperkalemia, represented by the peaked T-waves and wide QRS interval. A large volume or rapid infusion of red blood cells are the highest risk situations that can lead to hyperkalemia, and in some cases life-threatening levels. A unit of packed red blood cells may contain on average 27 mEq/L potassium, but the concentration tends to increase as the unit ages and potassium exits the intracellular red blood cell space. Surgical stress, shock, metabolic acidosis, hyperglycemia, hypocalcemia, and hypothermia all increase the risk of hyperkalemia after transfusion.

Immediate treatment of hyperkalemia includes intravenous insulin and nebulized β-2 agonist. Hypocalcemia also can complicate massive transfusion and has a linear concentration-dependent relationship with mortality. In a series of 71 patients who received a massive transfusion protocol, 59% had periods of severe hypocalcemia with an ionized calcium less than or equal to 1.0 mmol/L. The rate of hypocalcemia ranged from 22% for those receiving 4 units of packed red blood cells to

83% if the patient received more than 13 units. Intravenous calcium gluconate is the treatment for hypocalcemia.

Transfusion febrile nonhemolytic reactions occur in 0.8 per 1,000 units transfused. Acute hemolytic transfusion reaction occurs in 0.19 per 1,000 units transfused and is characterized by fever, hypotension, tachycardia, dyspnea, and chest or back pain. The patient also may report severe anxiety and flushing. Preventable errors, such as mislabeling specimens, are the most common cause of these reactions. This patient does not exhibit symptoms of an acute hemolytic reaction.

Transfusion-related acute lung injury occurs in 0.1 per 1,000 units transfused and, like an acute hemolytic reaction, can present with severe dyspnea. However, it also will be associated with a noncardiogenic pulmonary edema and hypoxia that usually develop within 6 hours of transfusion. Transfusion-related acute lung injury is the most common cause of transfusion-related mortality. This patient has normal vital signs and is only on pressure support ventilation.

In the setting of pulmonary edema, increasing ventilation requirements would be expected, making TRALI an unlikely diagnosis. This condition appears very similar to acute respiratory distress syndrome with normal cardiac evaluation. This is in contrast to TACO, which can lead to left heart failure and pulmonary edema with elevated brain natriuretic peptides due to the positive fluid balance. Transfusion-related acute lung injury and TACO should be considered within the differential diagnosis for any patient who experiences respiratory distress after a massive transfusion.

Cunningham FG, Leveno KJ, Bloom SL, Dashe JS, Hoffman BL, Casey BM, et al. Williams obstetrics. 25th ed. McGraw-Hill Education; 2018.

Hall C, Nagengast AK, Knapp C, Behrens B, Dewey EN, Goodman A, et al. Massive transfusions and severe hypocalcemia: an opportunity for monitoring and supplementation guidelines. Transfusion 2021;61(suppl 1):S188–94. doi: 10.1111/trf.16496 https://onlinelibrary.wiley.com/doi/10.1111/trf.16496

Postpartum hemorrhage. Practice Bulletin No. 183. American College of Obstetricians and Gynecologists. Obstet Gynecol 2017;130:e168–86. doi: 10.1097/AOG.0000000000002351 https://journals.lww.com/greenjournal/Fulltext/2017/10000/Practice_Bulletin_No__183__Postpartum_Hemorrhage.56.aspx

Quantitative blood loss in obstetric hemorrhage. ACOG Committee Opinion No. 794. American College of Obstetricians and Gynecologists. Obstet Gynecol 2019;134:e150–6. doi: 10.1097/AOG.0000000000003564 https://journals.lww.com/greenjournal/Fulltext/2019/12000/Quantitative_Blood_Loss_in_Obstetric_Hemorrhage_.40.aspx

Smith HM, Farrow SJ, Ackerman JD, Stubbs JR, Sprung J. Cardiac arrests associated with hyperkalemia during red blood cell transfusion: a case series. Anesth Analg 2008;106:1062–9, table of contents. doi: 10.1213/ane.0b013e318164f03d https://journals.lww.com/anesthesia-analgesia/Fulltext/2008/04000/Cardiac_Arrests_Associated_with_Hyperkalemia.6.aspx

106 Breastfeeding challenges

A 42-year-old gravida 2, para 2, presents for her routine 6-week postpartum visit. On breast examination, you palpate a 4-cm mass in the upper outer quadrant of her right breast. She reports that it has been present for about 1 month. It is nontender and is not erythematous. She has not had any fevers or chills. The best next step is to

(A) apply warm compresses and massage the area
* (B) obtain breast ultrasonography
(C) perform an incision and drainage
(D) prescribe dicloxacillin
(E) reevaluate the breast in 4 weeks

It is common for lactating women to experience breast pain and tenderness or notice breast lumps. Often these lumps are secondary to a plugged milk duct, engorgement, or mastitis—all of which are treatable. However, some breast lumps are persistent and, in rare cases, may be an indication of a malignancy. The differential diagnosis of a palpable mass in a lactating woman includes galactocele, fibroadenoma, lactating adenoma, mastitis or abscess, and pregnancy-associated breast cancer.

Breast cancer is the most common invasive cancer diagnosed during pregnancy. Pregnancy-associated breast cancer refers to the diagnosis of cancer during pregnancy, throughout the first year postpartum, or during lactation. Although pregnancy confers a decreased risk of breast cancer in the long term, there may be a transient increase in risk during pregnancy and lactation. The rate of pregnancy-associated breast cancer, which accounts for around 3% of all breast cancer diagnoses, is increasing, in part because of delayed childbearing. Diagnosis often is delayed in pregnant or lactating women, leading to a worse prognosis.

A palpable mass is the most common presentation of pregnancy-associated breast cancer. Other less common signs and symptoms include pain, nipple discharge, diffuse breast enlargement, and milk rejection by the infant. Breast examinations and imaging are more challenging during pregnancy and lactation secondary to physiological and structural breast changes. These changes may conceal a breast mass. This may lead to delayed diagnosis, which is one reason why women with pregnancy-associated breast cancer often present with more advanced disease when compared with age-matched nonpregnant women. There also is evidence to suggest that pregnancy-associated breast cancer may be biologically more aggressive than age-matched non-pregnancy-associated breast cancer.

If there is no evidence of mastitis or another common cause for a palpable mass with breastfeeding, such as a plugged duct, further evaluation is needed to avoid a delay in diagnosis. In pregnant and lactating women, breast ultrasonography is the first-line imaging choice for a palpable breast mass. These women often are younger with dense breast tissue, which reduces the sensitivity of mammography. In addition to defining benign etiologies, such as simple cysts or galactoceles, ultrasonography has the highest sensitivity for diagnosing pregnancy-associated breast cancer.

If further evaluation is needed, mammography or digital breast tomosynthesis may be performed. Mammography is not contraindicated during pregnancy or lactation. The fetal radiation dose from a four-view mammogram is negligible. Magnetic resonance imaging is not recommended as an initial screening modality in pregnant or lactating women. This is primarily because of the limited safety data on gadolinium during pregnancy and lactation. Biopsy is recommended if there are suspicious imaging findings. More than 80% of breast biopsies during pregnancy and lactation are benign.

In the described scenario, a lactating woman with a persistent, palpable breast mass requires further evaluation with ultrasound imaging. Other management options at this point, including warm compresses and reevaluation in 4 weeks, will only delay a diagnosis, which could worsen prognosis. Warm compresses often are recommended when a plugged milk duct is suspected. An incision and drainage would not be indicated because she has no signs of an infection or abscess. Also, imaging should be done before performing such a procedure. Prescribing dicloxacillin would be appropriate if the diagnosis were mastitis, which is not consistent with her clinical presentation.

All pregnant and lactating women with a persistent palpable mass should undergo ultrasound imaging followed by further evaluation and possible biopsy if suspicious findings result to avoid a delay in diagnosis. Additionally, if a pregnant woman is in the age range when breast cancer screening is recommended, it is important to offer routine breast cancer screening during pregnancy and lactation, particularly if their individual risk is increased. Although guidelines vary regarding when to initiate screening, the American College of Obstetricians and Gynecologists recommends that average-risk women be offered screening mammography beginning at age 40 years. If they have not initiated screening in their 40s, they should begin screening mammography by no later than 50 years.

Berens P, Brodribb W. ABM clinical protocol #20: engorgement, revised 2016. Breastfeed Med 2016;11:159–63. doi: 10.1089/bfm.2016.29008.pjb https://www.liebertpub.com/doi/10.1089/bfm.2016.29008.pjb

Breastfeeding challenges. ACOG Committee Opinion No. 820. American College of Obstetricians and Gynecologists. Obstet Gynecol 2021;137:e42–53. doi: 10.1097/AOG.0000000000004253 https://journals.lww.com/greenjournal/Fulltext/2021/02000/Breastfeeding_Challenges__ACOG_Committee_Opinion,.46.aspx

diFlorio-Alexander RM, Slanetz PJ, Moy L, Baron P, Didwania AD, Heller SL, et al. ACR Appropriateness Criteria® breast imaging of pregnant and lactating women. Expert Panel on Breast Imaging. J Am Coll Radiol 2018;15:S263–75. doi: 10.1016/j.jacr.2018.09.013 https://www.jacr.org/article/S1546-1440(18)31155-4/fulltext

Johnson HM, Lewis TC, Mitchell KB. Breast cancer screening during lactation: ensuring optimal surveillance for breastfeeding women. Obstet Gynecol 2020;135:194–8. doi: 10.1097/AOG.0000000000003600 https://journals.lww.com/greenjournal/Fulltext/2020/01000/Breast_Cancer_Screening_During_Lactation__Ensuring.25.aspx

Optimizing support for breastfeeding as part of obstetric practice. ACOG Committee Opinion No. 756. American College of Obstetricians and Gynecologists. Obstet Gynecol 2018;132:e187–96. doi: 10.1097/AOG.0000000000002890 https://journals.lww.com/greenjournal/Fulltext/2018/10000/ACOG_Committee_Opinion_No__756__Optimizing_Support.62.aspx

107 Cell-free DNA microdeletion detection

A 38-year-old patient with a normal body mass index (BMI) presents for a prenatal visit and genetic testing. She and her partner have an unremarkable genetic history in their families. She decided to have cell-free DNA (cfDNA) screening with a microdeletion panel. The results indicate that the fetus has a high risk of 22q11 deletion syndrome. The most likely cause of a false-positive screening test for this condition in this patient is

(A) advanced maternal age
(B) BMI
(C) family history
* (D) low disease incidence
(E) low fetal fraction

When screening tests for fetal indication are offered, patients should be counseled on test performance, particularly on positive and negative predictive values, because these are arguably the most important factors for the individual patient when interpreting their results. Sensitivity of a screening test is the probability of correctly identifying the presence of a condition among a population known to have the condition, and specificity is the probability of a test to correctly identify patients who do not have the condition among a population known to be negative for the condition. The positive predictive value is the probability of correctly identifying all patients who have the condition out of all patients tested. A negative predictive value is the probability that the screening test will correctly identify all patients without the condition among all patients tested. These terms can be represented mathematically with the aid of a common 2 × 2 table (Fig. 107-1).

The availability of cfDNA technology to obstetric patients has rapidly evolved, and advances have led commercial platforms to offer screening for single-gene disorders to the general obstetric population. Single-gene disorder screening has been marketed in the setting of advanced paternal age, and microdeletion screening (eg, 22q11.2 deletion syndrome) has been marketed to the general obstetric population, but the accuracy of these tests and the positive and negative predictive values for single-gene disorders and microdeletions in the general population are not known. Cri-du-chat syndrome (5pter), DiGeorge syndrome (22q11.2 deletion syndrome), and Prader–Willi and Angelman syndromes (15q11.2-q13.1) are some of the disorders for which testing is available with commercially marketed cfDNA tests. However, the positive predictive values varied widely in laboratory studies and were as low as 0% in some studies, depending on the disorder. Table 107-1 reflects the range in positive predictive values for commonly offered single-gene and microdeletion screening tests. Even in fetuses with ultrasonographic findings suspicious for 22q11.2 deletion syndrome, the positive predictive value ranges from 34% to 67%. At an incidence of 1 in 2,000 to 1 in 6,000 live births, there is a high likelihood that a high-risk result for 22q11.2 deletion syndrome is a false-positive in the general population.

Although certain single-gene disorders do increase with paternal age, advanced maternal age is associated with increasing risk of aneuploidy, not microdeletions and single-gene disorders. The quantity of fetal DNA in maternal blood is known as the *fetal fraction*. There are several things that can affect fetal fraction, including gestational age, BMI, aneuploidy, and multiple gestation. The described patient has a normal BMI, and her fetal fraction is unlikely to be affected by this parameter. Nor would a low fetal fraction increase the risk of a false-positive result for microdeletion.

In the setting of low fetal fraction, a risk result would not be reported for microdeletions. Because this patient reports no history consistent with 22q11.2 deletion syndrome (or conditions that would be associated with an undiagnosed case) in herself or her family, it is unlikely this test result represents a true-positive result. Cell-free DNA testing for 22q11.2 syndrome should not be performed in the setting of maternal diagnosis for this disorder nor for screening in the general obstetric population.

		Patient condition status	
		Positive	Negative
Screening test result	Positive	True positive (TP)	False positive (FP)
	Negative	False negative (FN)	True negative (TN)

Sensitivity = [TP/(TP+FN)] × 100

Specificity = [TN/(TN+FP)] × 100

Positive predictive value (PPV) = [TP/(TP+FP)] × 100

Negative predictive value (NPV) = [TN/(FN+TN)] × 100

FIGURE 107-1. Test sensitivity, specificity, and predictive value. (Modified from Trevethan R. Sensitivity, specificity, and predictive values: foundations, pliabilities, and pitfalls in research and practice. Front Public Health 2017;5:307. doi: 10.3389/fpubh.2017.00307 https://www.frontiersin.org/articles/10.3389/fpubh.2017.00307/full)

TABLE 107-1. Positive Predictive Value for Microdeletion Disorders Available Through Cell-Free DNA Testing

MICRODELETION	POSITIVE PREDICTIVE VALUE RANGE (UNSELECTED POPULATION)
22q11.2 deletion (DiGeorge syndrome)	18–29%
5pter (Cri-du-chat syndrome)	0–17%
15q11.2-q13.1 (Prader–Willi and Angelman syndromes)	0–100%

Modified from Petersen AK, Cheung SW, Smith JL, Bi W, Ward PA, Peacock S, et al. Positive predictive value estimates for cell-free noninvasive prenatal screening from data of a large referral genetic diagnostic laboratory. Am J Obstet Gynecol 2017;217:691.e1–6. doi: 10.1016/j.ajog.2017.10.005 https://www.ajog.org/article/S0002-9378(17)31187-0/fulltext.

American College of Obstetricians and Gynecologists. Cell-free DNA to screen for single-gene disorders. Practice Advisory. ACOG; 2019. Accessed March 17, 2022. https://www.acog.org/clinical/clinical-guidance/practice-advisory/articles/2019/02/cell-free-dna-to-screen-for-single-gene-disorders

Gross SJ, Stosic M, McDonald-McGinn DM, Bassett AS, Norvez A, Dhamankar R, et al. Clinical experience with single-nucleotide polymorphism-based non-invasive prenatal screening for 22q11.2 deletion syndrome. Ultrasound Obstet Gynecol 2016;47:177–83. doi: 10.1002/uog.15754 https://obgyn.onlinelibrary.wiley.com/doi/10.1002/uog.15754

Petersen AK, Cheung SW, Smith JL, Bi W, Ward PA, Peacock S, et al. Positive predictive value estimates for cell-free noninvasive prenatal screening from data of a large referral genetic diagnostic laboratory. Am J Obstet Gynecol 2017;217:691.e1–6. doi: 10.1016/j.ajog.2017.10.005 https://www.ajog.org/article/S0002-9378(17)31187-0/fulltext

Screening for fetal chromosomal abnormalities: ACOG Practice Bulletin No. 226. American College of Obstetricians and Gynecologists. Obstet Gynecol 2020;136:e48–69. doi: 10.1097/AOG.0000000000004084 https://journals.lww.com/greenjournal/Fulltext/2020/10000/Screening_for_Fetal_Chromosomal_Abnormalities_.44.aspx

Society for Maternal–Fetal Medicine. Twenty things physicians and patients should question. Choosing Wisely. ABIM Foundation; 2021. Accessed March 17, 2022. https://www.choosingwisely.org/societies/society-for-maternal-fetal-medicine/

Trevethan R. Sensitivity, specificity, and predictive values: foundations, pliabilities, and pitfalls in research and practice. Front Public Health 2017;5:307. doi: 10.3389/fpubh.2017.00307 https://www.frontiersin.org/articles/10.3389/fpubh.2017.00307/full

108–112 Genetic carrier screening

Match the genetic disorder (108–112) to the appropriate patient pedigree (A–C):

(A) Pedigree A

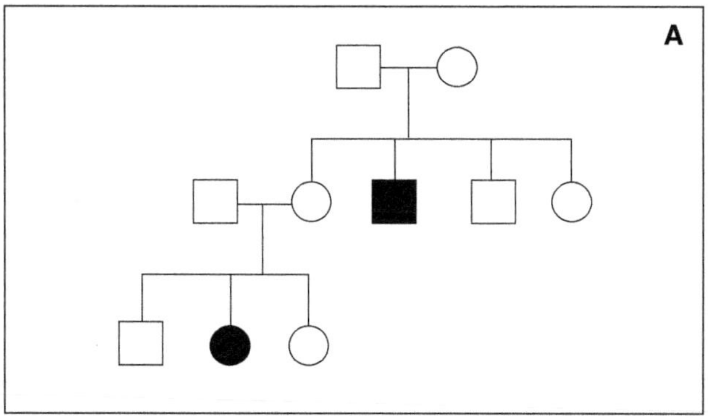

(B) Pedigree B

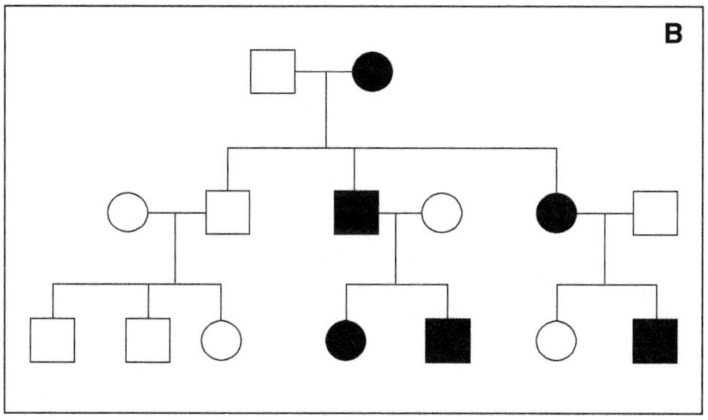

(C) Pedigree C

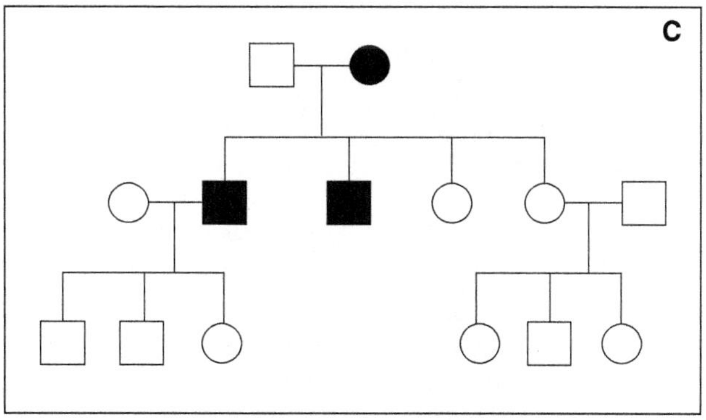

108. A. Spinal muscular atrophy

109. C. Hemophilia A

110. A. Cystic fibrosis (CF)

111. B. Neurofibromatosis

112. B. Marfan syndrome

Genetic carrier screening should be offered to every pregnant woman, preferably before pregnancy. Carrier screening should be performed only once in an individual's lifetime as long as the result is maintained in the patient's record. If a patient is a carrier for an autosomal recessive (AR) condition, the reproductive partner also should be tested. If both partners are carriers of a genetic condition, genetic counseling should be offered and options for advanced reproductive technologies should be discussed. If both partners are found to be carriers after pregnancy is established, prenatal diagnosis options should be discussed. The genetic counseling visit should include obtaining relevant family history and screening for consanguinity. According to the American College of Obstetricians and Gynecologists, screening for spinal muscular atrophy and CF should be offered to all women considering pregnancy. Both of these conditions are inherited through an AR pattern of inheritance.

Genetic conditions are categorized by their mode of inheritance. Mendelian or single-gene disorders are inherited as AR, autosomal dominant (AD), codominant, or X-linked. Genes come in pairs, and with AD disorders, the presence of one abnormal copy will result in the disease. The gene that causes an AD condition or trait has a 50% chance of being passed to offspring with each pregnancy. Autosomal dominant disorders can affect offspring of either sex, meaning affected males can have affected male children. Autosomal dominant conditions often appear in every generation, as illustrated in Pedigree B. The birth of affected children from unaffected parents may be due to incomplete penetrance, variable expressivity, or *de novo* mutations.

Autosomal recessive diseases, such as CF and spinal muscular atrophy, occur when both copies of the gene are inherited (Pedigree A) (Fig. 108–112-1). Individuals with only one copy of the gene are called *carriers* or described as heterozygotes. Depending on the disease state, the clinical degree of disease or implication of carrier state varies. When an affected child is identified with an AR condition, both parents are obligate carriers, and thus the parents would have a 25% chance of having an affected child with each pregnancy. There also is a 66% chance that an unaffected sibling of that couple is a carrier of the AR gene. Review of the family history or pedigree of an AR condition is characterized by affected males and females, and the trait usually skips generations.

With some diseases, the pattern of inheritance can appear non-Mendelian. For example, affected individuals have a single copy of the AR gene but exhibit disease characteristics, or individuals with an AD disease have different degrees of severity (Fig. 108–112-2). Although it is possible that the second copy of an AR gene is not identified (because of the presence of an intron or variant type), it also is possible that the clinical condition has varying penetrance and expressivity. Diseases with varying penetrance and expressivity often are still inherited through Mendelian pattern, but identification in the family history can be challenging. The phenotype refers to the clinical manifestation of the disease and is determined by several factors. Disease penetrance indicates whether the abnormal gene is expressed. When a dominant gene produces the same recognizable phenotypic expression in everyone who carries it, it is said to have complete penetrance. One example

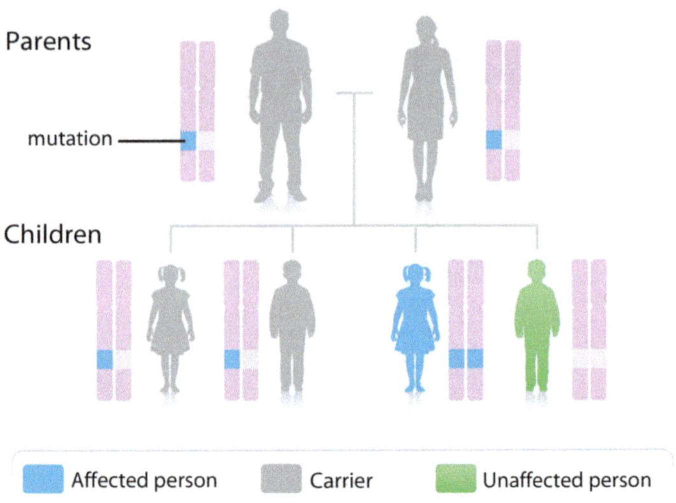

FIGURE 108-112-1. Autosomal recessive.

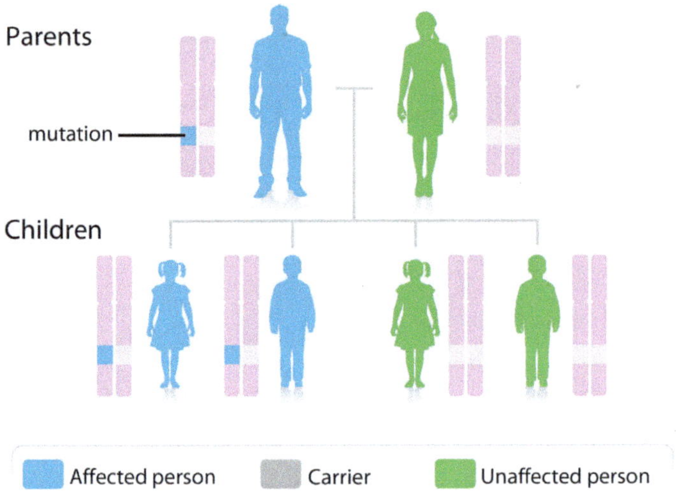

FIGURE 108-112-2. Autosomal dominant.

of a condition with incomplete penetrance is DiGeorge syndrome. The degree to which a penetrant gene is expressed—ie, the range of phenotypic features or the number of organ systems affected—is called *expressivity.* If individuals who carry the affected gene do not have the same phenotypes, the gene is said to have *variable expressivity*. An example of a disease with variable expressivity is neurofibromatosis, in which some individuals have skin manifestations, but others have central nervous system tumors.

Examples of AR conditions from this question include CF and spinal muscular atrophy. Cystic fibrosis is caused by a mutation in one gene (cystic fibrosis transmembrane conductance regulator [*CFTR*]) located on chromosome 7. Numerous mutations that lead to CF disease have been identified (more than 1,700 to date). Carrier frequency ranges from 1/24 to approximately 1/60 (see Table 108–112-1). Cystic fibrosis is a progressive multisystem disease that primarily affects pulmonary, pancreatic, and gastrointestinal systems, does not cause intellectual disability, and can increase the risk of primary infertility. If a woman is a carrier of CF mutation and her partner is unavailable for testing, genetic counseling and baseline population risk estimates should be shared with the patient to provide information regarding the risk of an affected child. If both partners are CF carriers, genetic counseling is recommended and diagnostic testing or assisted reproductive technologies with preimplantation genetic diagnosis for monogenic disorders may be desired.

Spinal muscular atrophy is another example of an AR condition. The disorder is caused by mutation in the *SMN1* gene and leads to progressive degeneration of spinal cord motor neurons, resulting in weakness and muscle atrophy. Carrier frequencies in most populations are estimated at 1 in 40 to 1 in 60, but frequency appears to be lower in Hispanic women (see Table 108–112-2).

Examples of AD conditions in this question (Pedigree B) include neurofibromatosis and Marfan syndrome. Neurofibromatosis is an example of an AD condition with variable expressivity. Recall expressivity is the degree to which a penetrant gene is expressed, meaning it has a wide range of phenotypic features. Pathogenic variations in the *NF1* gene, located on chromosome 17q11.2, result in loss of production or reduced function of the proteins. Using molecular screening, the rate of pathogenic variants for neurofibromatosis is estimated at less than 100%. The penetrance of neurofibromatosis is complete.

Marfan syndrome is an example of an AD condition involving the fibrillin 1 (*FBN1*) gene, and over 1,800 mutations have been identified. A smaller fraction of Marfan syndrome is related to mutations in TGF-beta receptor (*TGFBR2*). Both mutations are inherited in an AD pattern and variable expressivity is widely noted.

X-linked diseases (Pedigree C) most often are recessive and primarily affect men, given that they have a single copy of the X chromosome (Fig. 108–112-3). Examples of X-linked conditions and diseases include color blindness, hemophilia A, and Duchenne muscular dystrophy. Women who carry the X-linked recessive gene often are unaffected unless they have a skewed X inactivation or carry two copies of the abnormal gene. When a woman carries a gene causing an X-linked recessive trait or disease, she has a 50% chance of passing on the gene with each pregnancy and, therefore, each of her sons will have a 50% chance of being affected and each of her daughters will have a 50% chance of being a carrier. When the man has an X-linked disease, none of his sons will be affected but all daughters will be carriers. The pedigree of an X-linked recessive condition demonstrates greater prevalence of affected males than females and no male-to-male transmission is seen. If a woman has the condition (is affected), then all sons will be affected.

TABLE 108-112-1. Cystic Fibrosis Detection and Carrier Rates Before and After Testing

REPORTED RACIAL OR ETHNIC GROUP	DETECTION RATE (%)*	INDIVIDUAL CARRIER RISK BEFORE TESTING	APPROXIMATE INDIVIDUAL CARRIER RISK AFTER NEGATIVE TEST RESULT†
Ashkenazi Jewish	94	1/24	1/380
Non-Hispanic White	88	1/25	1/200
Hispanic White	72	1/58	1/200
Black	64	1/61	1/170
Asian American	49	1/94	1/180

*Detection rate data based on use of a 23-mutation panel.

†Bayesian statistics used to calculate approximate carrier risk after a negative test result.

Modified from the American College of Medical Genetics. Technical standards and guidelines for CFTR mutation testing. In: Standards and guidelines for clinical genetics laboratories. ACMG; 2011. Accessed February 25, 2022. https://www.acmg.net//docs/CFTR_Mutation_Testing_2011.pdf.

TABLE 108-112-2. Spinal Muscular Atrophy Carrier Risk Based on Ethnicity and Residual Risk Assuming Negative Test Results

REPORTED RACIAL OR ETHNIC GROUP	CARRIER DETECTION RATE (%)	CARRIER RISK BY ETHNICITY	RESIDUAL RISK 2 COPIES *SMN1*	RESIDUAL RISK 3 COPIES *SMN1*
Non-Hispanic White	95	1:35	1:632	1: 3,500
Ashkenazi Jewish	90	1:41	1:350	1: 4,000
Asian	93	1:53	1:628	1: 5,000
Black	71	1:66	1:121	1: 3,000
Hispanic	91	1:117	1:1,061	1: 11,000

Modified from Carrier screening for genetic conditions. Committee Opinion No. 691. American College of Obstetricians and Gynecologists. Obstet Gynecol 2017;129:e41–55. doi: 10.1097/AOG.0000000000001952. https://journals.lww.com/greenjournal/Fulltext/2017/03000/Committee_Opinion_No__691__Carrier_Screening_for.48.aspx.

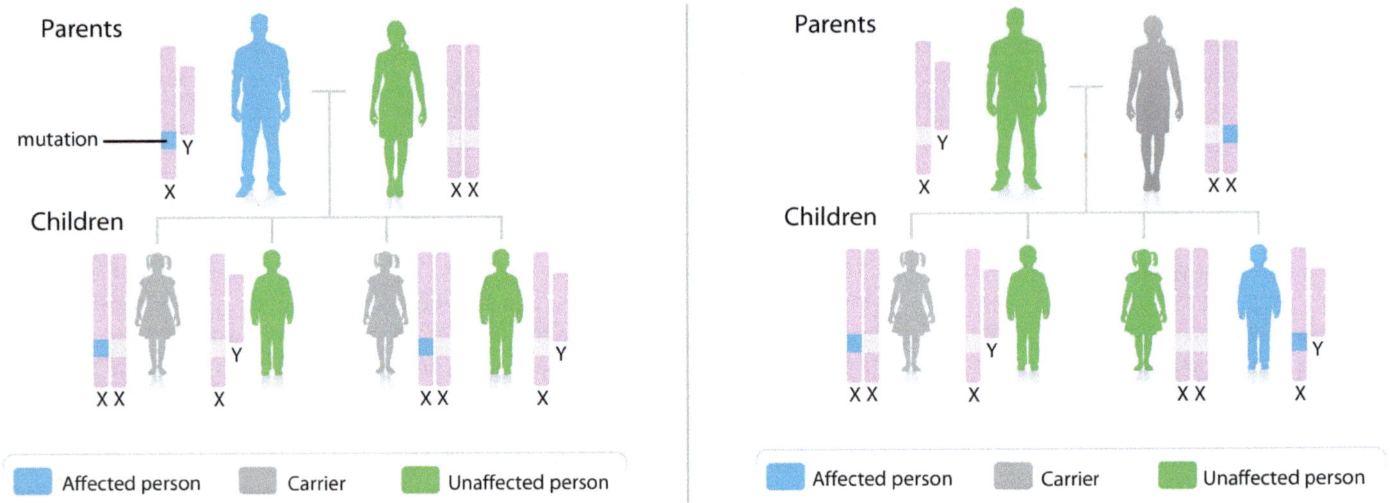

FIGURE 108-112-3. X-linked recessive.

Hemophilia A is an example of an X-linked recessive disease and typically refers to factor VIII deficiency caused by variation in the *F8* gene. In most cases, hemophilia is then characterized as mild, moderate, or severe depending on the percent of factor activity that is normal. Males are affected with disease because they have a single copy of the X chromosome that has the defective gene. Affected males can transmit only the affected trait to their daughters who are obligate carriers. Females are most often asymptomatic carriers but because of X inactivation can have bleeding problems similar to affected males. Female carriers have a 50% chance to transmit the abnormal X chromosome, making one half of their sons affected and one half of their daughters carriers.

The term *codominant* is used when the genes in each gene pair are expressed in the phenotype. The best example of this is blood type (type AB blood). A pedigree reflecting codominant conditions was not offered in this discussion.

American College of Medical Genetics. Technical standards and guidelines for CFTR mutation testing. In: Standards and guidelines for clinical genetics laboratories. ACMG; 2011. Accessed February 25, 2022. https://www.acmg.net//docs/CFTR_Mutation_Testing_2011.pdf

Carrier screening for genetic conditions. Committee Opinion No. 691. American College of Obstetricians and Gynecologists. Obstet Gynecol 2017;129:e41–55. doi: 10.1097/AOG.0000000000001952 https://journals.lww.com/greenjournal/Fulltext/2017/03000/Committee_Opinion_No__691__Carrier_Screening_for.48.aspx

Carrier screening in the age of genomic medicine. Committee Opinion No. 690. American College of Obstetricians and Gynecologists. Obstet Gynecol 2017;129:e35–40. doi: 10.1097/AOG.0000000000001951 https://journals.lww.com/greenjournal/Fulltext/2017/03000/Committee_Opinion_No__690__Carrier_Screening_in.47.aspx

Ferreira JC, Schreiber-Agus N, Carter SM, Klugman S, Gregg AR, Gross SJ. Carrier testing for Ashkenazi Jewish disorders in the prenatal setting: navigating the genetic maze. Am J Obstet Gynecol 2014;211:197–204. doi: 10.1016/j.ajog.2014.02.001 https://www.ajog.org/article/S0002-9378(14)00117-3/fulltext

Modern genetics in obstetrics and gynecology. ACOG Technology Assessment in Obstetrics and Gynecology No. 14. American College of Obstetricians and Gynecologists. Obstet Gynecol 2018;132:e143–68. doi: 10.1097/AOG.0000000000002831

113–115 Headache in pregnancy

For each clinical scenario (113–115), choose the best next step (A–D).

(A) Administer caffeine
(B) Order computed tomography (CT) imaging
(C) Order magnetic resonance arteriogram and venogram
(D) Place a blood patch

113. B. A 45-year-old at 38 weeks of gestation presents with acute onset of blurry vision, an unsteady gait, and a diffuse, severe headache. She has no history of headaches. Her blood pressure is 100/60 mm Hg, papilledema is noted on fundoscopic examination, and laboratory results are normal.

114. C. A 31-year-old who is 2 weeks postpartum presents with a new, sudden, painful headache that woke her from sleep this morning. The headache did not respond to acetaminophen or ibuprofen. Her blood pressure was 165/100 mm Hg on admission. Liver function and platelets are normal, and a protein/creatinine ratio is 1.0. The next morning, the headache returns despite use of magnesium sulfate, antihypertensives, and analgesics. Magnetic resonance imaging reveals no pathology.

115. A. A 20-year-old on postpartum day 1 has a frontal headache that is worse when she is sitting or standing but resolves when she lies supine. Her labor was uncomplicated, with use of epidural analgesia.

Headaches affect approximately 50% of the population worldwide and 25–30% of pregnant individuals. Headaches are divided into two groups: primary and secondary. Examples of a primary headache include migraine, tension, and cluster headaches. Primary headaches account for approximately 90% of headaches in the first trimester and 50–75% of headaches postpartum. In contrast, a secondary headache is a symptom of another process (Box 113–115-1). Secondary headaches occur more commonly starting in the second trimester through the postpartum period.

Physicians should suspect a secondary headache when a patient reports no prior history of headaches and has associated neurologic findings and hypertension. Other significant findings in the patient's history can include cancer, head trauma, a change in a prepregnancy headache pattern, a thunderclap or severe headache, age greater than 50 years, or a headache related to activity or position. A history and physical examination with vital signs, screening neurologic examination, and neck examination will help clarify the cause of a secondary headache.

In Scenario 113, the patient's presentation is concerning for a stroke in pregnancy, specifically a cerebral venous thrombosis, which accounts for less than 1% of all strokes. The headache is present in up to 90% of patients with a cerebral venous thrombosis and most often is diffuse, progressive, and severe. It can

BOX 113-115-1

Causes of Secondary Headaches in Pregnancy and Postpartum

- Cerebrovascular disorders: aneurysmal subarachnoid hemorrhage, acute ischemic or hemorrhagic stroke, CVT, cervical artery dissection, and RVCS
- Preeclampsia/eclampsia
- PRES
- Postdural puncture headache
- Pneumocephalus
- Brain tumor
- RVCS
- Idiopathic intracranial hypertension
- Chiari malformation
- Third ventricle colloid cyst

Abbreviations: CVT, cerebral venous thrombosis; PRES, posterior reversible encephalopathy syndrome; RVCS, reversible cerebral vasoconstriction syndrome.

Data from O'Neal MA. Headaches complicating pregnancy and the postpartum period. Pract Neurol 2017;17:191–202. doi: 10.1136/practneurol-2016-001589 https://pn.bmj.com/content/17/3/191.long *and* Robbins MS. Headache in pregnancy. Continuum (Minneap Minn) 2018;24:1092–107. doi: 10.1212/CON.0000000000000642 https://journals.lww.com/continuum/Abstract/2018/08000/Headache_in_Pregnancy.10.aspx

be unilateral, thunderclap, and worse when supine. Neurologic findings, including seizures (seen in up to 40% of individuals) and visual field or focal neurologic deficits, can be present. Nausea, vomiting, and papilledema are secondary to the intracranial hypertension. Medical conditions associated with an increased risk of cerebral venous thrombosis include diabetes mellitus, gestational diabetes, migraine, or obesity. In the described patient, the best next step is an emergent CT. Magnetic resonance imaging and laboratory evaluation for nonpregnancy-related causes may be considered after the initial CT imaging.

The patient described in Scenario 114 has a postpartum headache that is isolated or relapsing, and often is described as a thunderclap headache. The clinical characteristics and timing of the headache are significant and help to distinguish between posterior reversible encephalopathy syndrome and reversible cerebral vasoconstriction syndrome (Table 113–115-1). Focal neurologic findings are seen with both. Reversible cerebral vasoconstriction syndrome is more common postpartum. Posterior reversible encephalopathy syndrome is more common antepartum. Preeclampsia, posterior reversible encephalopathy syndrome, and reversible cerebral vasoconstriction syndrome share common features of hypertension and the possibility of seizures. Reversible cerebral vasoconstriction syndrome can present with a single or relapsing thunderclap headache, whereas in posterior reversible encephalopathy syndrome there may be vision loss.

In Scenario 114, an initial magnetic resonance imaging study did not reveal any intracranial lesions as the cause of the neurologic deficits. The best next step in the treatment of this patient would be to evaluate for arterial narrowing on magnetic resonance angiogram, which supports a diagnosis of reversible cerebral vasoconstriction syndrome. If vasogenic edema is evident on the study, then the diagnosis would be posterior reversible encephalopathy syndrome. Reversible cerebral vasoconstriction syndrome and posterior reversible encephalopathy syndrome are believed to begin with endothelial dysfunction that leads to expansion of the vasculature with rupture and surrounding edema.

The postdural puncture headache described in Scenario 115 occurs after the use of regional anesthesia. The pathognomonic findings for a postdural puncture headache include onset within 48 hours of regional anesthesia, a frontal headache preventing sitting or standing, and resolution in the supine position. Conservative treatment starts with fluids and caffeine and is, therefore, the best next step in Scenario 115. If the headache does not resolve, evaluation for a blood patch is indicated.

TABLE 113–115-1. Symptoms and Timing of Cerebral Venous Thrombosis, Reversible Cerebral Vasoconstriction Syndrome, and Posterior Reversible Encephalopathy Syndrome

CAUSE	HEADACHE CHARACTERISTICS	ADDITIONAL FINDINGS	TIMING
CVT	Variable Most often diffuse, progressive, severe Can be unilateral, sudden, migraine like, or mild	Nausea and vomiting Papilledema Seizure Visual field defects Focal neurologic deficits	Highest incidence in early postpartum period (fivefold greater than first trimester)
RCVS	Severe (thunderclap) Diffuse Single or relapsing over 1–2 wk Triggered by exertion or Valsalva	Focal neurologic deficit Sometimes seizures Hypertension	Postpartum more than antepartum usually within the first week after birth
PRES	Insidious onset Occipital Bilateral Dull No prodrome Progresses over 48 h Present in two-thirds of patients	Impaired conscious Focal neurologic deficits Seizures Vision loss Hypertensive encephalopathy	Antepartum more than postpartum
Preeclampsia or eclampsia	Progressive bilateral pulsing Temporal, frontal, occipital, diffuse Worse with physical activity	Visual changes	Antepartum and postpartum

Abbreviations: CVT, cerebral venous thrombosis; PRES, posterior reversible encephalopathy syndrome; RVCS, reversible cerebral vasoconstriction syndrome.

Data from Robbins MS. Headache in pregnancy. Continuum (Minneap Minn) 2018;24:1092–107. doi: 10.1212/CON.0000000000000642 https://journals.lww.com/continuum/Abstract/2018/08000/Headache_in_Pregnancy.10.aspx *and* Negro A, Delaruelle Z, Ivanova TA, Khan S, Ornello R, Raffaelli B, et al. Headache and pregnancy: a systematic review. European Headache Federation School of Advanced Studies (EHF-SAS). J Headache Pain 2017;18:106–0. doi: 10.1186/s10194-017-0816-0 https://thejournalofheadacheandpain.biomedcentral.com/articles/10.1186/s10194-017-0816-0

Burch R. Epidemiology and treatment of menstrual migraine and migraine during pregnancy and lactation: a narrative review. Headache 2020;60:200–16. doi: 10.1111/head.13665 https://headachejournal.onlinelibrary.wiley.com/doi/10.1111/head.13665

Ferro JM, Aguiar de Sousa D. Cerebral venous thrombosis: an update. Curr Neurol Neurosci Rep 2019;19:74–x. doi: 10.1007/s11910-019-0988-x https://link.springer.com/article/10.1007%2Fs11910-019-0988-x

Jones A, Cometa MA, Euliano T, Lopez BM. Postpartum headache-unmasking the zebra among the horses: a case report. A A Pract 2020;14:e01340. doi: 10.1213/XAA.0000000000001340 https://journals.lww.com/aacr/Abstract/2020/11000/Postpartum_Headache_Unmasking_the_Zebra_Among_the.6.aspx

Karjalainen L, Tikkanen M, Rantanen K, Aarnio K, Korhonen A, Saaros A, et al. Stroke in pregnancy and puerperium: validated incidence trends with risk factor analysis in Finland 1987–2016. Neurology 2021;96:e2564–75. doi: 10.1212/WNL.0000000000011990 https://n.neurology.org/content/96/21/e2564.long

Lucas S. Migraine and other headache disorders. Clin Update Womens Health Care 2019;XVIII(4):1–55. https://www.acog.org/-/media/project/acog/acogorg/clinical/files/clinical-updates/2019/07/migraine-and-other-headache-disorders.pdf

Negro A, Delaruelle Z, Ivanova TA, Khan S, Ornello R, Raffaelli B, et al. Headache and pregnancy: a systematic review. European Headache Federation School of Advanced Studies (EHF-SAS). J Headache Pain 2017;18:106–0. doi: 10.1186/s10194-017-0816-0 https://thejournalofheadacheandpain.biomedcentral.com/articles/10.1186/s10194-017-0816-0

O'Neal MA. Headaches complicating pregnancy and the postpartum period. Pract Neurol 2017;17:191–202. doi: 10.1136/practneurol-2016-001589 https://pn.bmj.com/content/17/3/191.long

Robbins MS. Headache in pregnancy. Continuum (Minneap Minn) 2018;24:1092–107. doi: 10.1212/CON.0000000000000642 https://journals.lww.com/continuum/Abstract/2018/08000/Headache_in_Pregnancy.10.aspx

116–119 Contraception in a breastfeeding patient

For each clinical scenario (116–119), choose the optimal contraceptive method (A–E).

(A) Copper intrauterine device (IUD)
(B) Etonogestrel implant
(C) Levonorgestrel IUD
(D) Oral estrogen and progestogen combination pills
(E) Progestin-only pills

116. A. A 23-year-old gravida 3, para 2, is admitted for a repeat cesarean birth. She is planning on breastfeeding and requests the longest-lasting reversible contraceptive option.

117. E. A 38-year-old gravida 2, para 2, presents for a 4-week postpartum visit and requests contraception. They are a current smoker, and they are breastfeeding. They decline inserting anything in their body or any injections for contraception.

118. D. A 28-year-old gravida 3, para 3, presents 3 months after giving birth. She is breastfeeding. She reports worsening acne and would like a contraceptive method to reduce this.

119. B. A 29-year-old gravida 2, para 2, on postpartum day 1 requests long-acting reversible contraception before her discharge from the hospital.

The medical indications and contraindications for methods of contraception are the same for immediately postpartum and non-postpartum individuals with one distinction: the increased risk of thromboembolism postpartum. The thromboembolic risk is highest immediately postpartum and is 60-fold higher compared with the risk of a thromboembolic event for a nonpregnant individual. This risk persists through the first 6 weeks after delivery and starts to decrease 21 days after birth. Births occurring less than 18 months after a previous birth are considered short-interval or rapid-repeat pregnancies. Rapid-repeat pregnancies are associated with preterm births, small-for-gestational-age newborns, increased neonatal intensive care unit admissions, gestational diabetes mellitus, obesity, placental abruption, and uterine rupture after cesarean birth. The American College of Obstetricians and Gynecologists recommends IUD placement within 10 minutes of placental delivery in vaginal and cesarean births as an effective way to reduce short-interval and unintended pregnancies.

Postpartum contraception is protective against short-interval birth. Options for contraception can be organized based on effectiveness with permanent sterilization (vasectomy, tubal ligation, bilateral salpingectomy) and long-acting reversible contraception methods (IUD, subdermal contraceptive implant) being the most effective and the most likely to be continued. User-dependent hormone contraception methods (combined hormone contraception, combined patch, combined ring, progestin-only pills, or injection) are comparatively less effective. Fertility awareness and withdrawal, and barrier methods, such as female condom, male condom, diaphragm, and the cervical cup, have the widest range of pregnancy rates when comparing perfect use to typical use.

Intrauterine devices placed within 10 minutes of delivery of the placenta have an expulsion rate of 10–27%. The rate increases in the few days after delivery and then decreases at 2 weeks after delivery because the involution of the uterus mostly is complete. The risk of perforation when placing an IUD is 0.1%. Intrauterine devices have the lowest failure rate compared with other reversible methods of contraception. Hormone-containing IUDs are approved for up to 3–7 years of use. The copper IUD is approved for up to 10 years of use and has evidence for 12 years of use. The patient in Scenario 116 requests the longest-acting reversible method of contraception, which is the copper IUD. Contraindications to IUD placement at the time of birth are postpartum hemorrhage, chorioamnionitis, and sepsis. There is no increased risk of thrombosis or effect on breastfeeding with postpartum IUD use.

The patient in Scenario 117 declines having anything placed inside them, thus eliminating the contraceptive implant or IUD. They smoke and are over the age of age 35 years, which increases the risk of a thromboembolic event when using combined hormone contraception regardless of postpartum status. Progestin-only pills may be used in individuals who smoke over age 35. There is no difference in breastfeeding continuation or incidence of supplementation with formula when initiating progestin-only contraception within the first 6 weeks after delivery. This makes a progestin-only pill the recommended option for the patient in Scenario 117. The progestin-only injection of depot medroxyprogesterone acetate (DMPA) would be another option for this patient if they had been open to an injection. Reported continuation rates at 3 and 12 months are 75.7% and 66.7%, respectively, in adolescents. There were no consistent differences reported between users of the DMPA injection when compared with nonhormonal methods of contraception with respect to the continuation of breastfeeding over time.

Approximately 3 weeks postpartum, 41% of women will experience some breastfeeding difficulties, irrespective of hormone-containing contraceptive use. There is no change in the quantity of ingested milk, the number of daily feedings, or infant growth parameters for combined hormone-containing contraception, the etonogestrel implant, the copper IUD, and the levonorgestrel IUD. Furthermore, when breastfeeding women who initiated any type of hormone-containing contraception were compared with breastfeeding women who did not, the incidence of concerns related to milk supply were the same (hazard ratio, 1.18; 95% CI, 0.94–1.47). The patient in Scenario 3 is more than 42 days postpartum, she is breastfeeding, and she is experiencing acne. Combined hormone-containing contraception has been shown to decrease acne by increasing sex hormone binding globulin, reducing testosterone. A combined hormonal pill is the recommended option for the patient in Scenario 118.

The recommended option for the patient in Scenario 119 is the etonogestrel implant. The patient delivered the placenta more than 10 minutes ago. The risk of expulsion of an IUD is increased when placed more than 10 minutes and less than 28 days postpartum and, therefore, is not recommended. Studies of the etonogestrel implant in adolescents revealed a trend toward increased breastfeeding rates when placed immediately after delivery. The removal rates with the implant are similar in postpartum women and nonpregnant women.

Bryant AG, Bauer AE, Muddana A, Wouk K, Chetwynd E, Yourkavitch J, et al. The Lactational Effects of Contraceptive Hormones: an Evaluation (LECHE) study. Contraception 2019;100:48–53. doi: 10.1016/j.contraception.2019.03.040 https://www.contraceptionjournal.org/article/S0010-7824(19)30103-9/fulltext

Jackson E, Glasier A. Return of ovulation and menses in postpartum nonlactating women: a systematic review. Obstet Gynecol 2011;117:657–62. doi: 10.1097/AOG.0b013e31820ce18c https://journals.lww.com/greenjournal/Fulltext/2011/03000/Return_of_Ovulation_and_Menses_in_Postpartum.20.aspx

Lacy MM, McMurtry Baird S, Scott TA, Barker B, Zite NB. Statewide quality improvement initiative to implement immediate postpartum long-acting reversible contraception. Am J Obstet Gynecol 2020;222: S910e1–8. doi: 10.1016/j.ajog.2019.11.1272 https://www.ajog.org/article/S0002-9378(19)32693-6/fulltext

Optimizing postpartum care. ACOG Committee Opinion No. 736. American College of Obstetricians and Gynecologists. Obstet Gynecol 2018;131:e140–50. doi: 10.1097/AOG.0000000000002633 https://journals.lww.com/greenjournal/Fulltext/2018/05000/ACOG_Committee_Opinion_No__736__Optimizing.42.aspx

Stanton TA, Blumenthal PD. Postpartum hormonal contraception in breastfeeding women. Curr Opin Obstet Gynecol 2019;31:441–6. doi: 10.1097/GCO.0000000000000571 https://journals.lww.com/co-obgyn/Abstract/2019/12000/Postpartum_hormonal_contraception_in_breastfeeding.12.aspx

Taub RL, Jensen JT. Advances in contraception: new options for postpartum women. Expert Opin Pharmacother 2017;18:677–88. doi: 10.1080/14656566.2017.1316370 https://www.tandfonline.com/doi/abs/10.1080/14656566.2017.1316370

120–124 Teratogenic drugs

For each ultrasound finding (120–124), choose the most likely maternal condition(s) (A–E) that contributed to the increased risk of congenital malformation(s).

(A) Generalized seizure disorder
(B) Severe refractory bipolar disorder
(C) Autoimmune hepatitis with recent liver transplant
(D) Mechanical heart valve
(E) Chronic hypertension and insulin-requiring diabetes mellitus

120. A. Spina bifida, craniofacial and cardiovascular anomalies

121. B. Ebstein anomaly, polyhydramnios, diabetes insipidus

122. D. Absent nasal bone, limb hypoplasia with stippled epiphyses, ventral midline dysplasia

123. E. Oligohydramnios, fetal lung hypoplasia, skeletal malformations

124. C. Cleft lip and ear, and eye abnormalities

The patient in Scenario 120, who was treated for generalized seizures, has epilepsy and might have been on an older-generation medication, such as valproic acid, with resultant fetal ultrasound findings of spina bifida, craniofacial, and cardiovascular abnormalities. The treatment of generalized tonic-clonic seizures may be accomplished with a variety of antiepileptic medications. These medications include newer-generation antiepileptics as well as older medications and can be prescribed as monotherapy or polytherapy. As a group, monotherapy and use of newer-generation antiepileptic medications are associated with decreased risk of congenital anomaly when compared with the older-generation medications. Of the older antiepileptic medications, valproic acid carries increased risk of preterm birth, poor neurodevelopmental outcomes, and structural anomalies such as neural tube defects, fetal cardiac malformations, and craniofacial abnormalities (cleft lip or palate and craniosynostosis). The risk of fetal cardiac malformation among women on valproic acid can have odds ratios as high as 6–10 when used in combination with phenytoin or phenobarbital. In comparison, the risk of fetal cardiac malformation with levetiracetam or lamotrigine has odds ratio of less than 1 when used in monotherapy.

Following a shared decision-making model, a patient continued on valproic acid during pregnancy should have supplemental folic acid. Detailed fetal ultrasound examination at 18–22 weeks of gestation is recommended to screen for anomalies, including neural tube defects and cardiovascular and craniofacial abnormalities. Women taking antiepileptic medications have a higher risk of miscarriage and teratogenicity compared with those not taking antiepileptic medications (specific rates are described in Table 120–124-1). Another benefit of newer-generation antiepileptic medications is that they can be used to treat maternal mood disorders when clinically indicated in addition to epilepsy.

TABLE 120-124-1. Antiepileptic Drugs and Congenital Anomaly Risks

MEDICATION AS MONOTHERAPY	ODDS RATIO FOR MAJOR CONGENITAL MALFORMATION (95% CI)
Ethosuximide	3.04 (1.23–7.07)
Valproate	2.93 (2.36–3.69)
Topiramate	1.90 (1.17–2.97)
Phenobarbital	1.83 (1.35–2.47)
Phenytoin	1.67 (1.3–2.17)
Carbamazepine	1.37 (1.1–1.71)
Gabapentin	1.00 (0.47–1.89)
Levetiracetam	0.72 (0.43–1.16)
Lamotrigine	0.96 (0.72–1.25)

Adapted from Veroniki AA, Cogo E, Rios P, Straus SE, Finkelstein Y, Kealey R, et al. Comparative safety of anti-epileptic drugs during pregnancy: a systematic review and network meta-analysis of congenital malformations and prenatal outcomes. BMC Med 2017;15:95-1. doi: 10.1186/s12916-017-0845-1 https://bmcmedicine.biomedcentral.com/articles/10.1186/s12916-017-0845-1

The patient in Scenario 121 has a history of refractory bipolar disorder, which indicates a lack of response to first-line medications such as newer generation mood stabilizers. During pregnancy, women with bipolar disorder are at risk of relapse and recurrence of mood cycling as well as increased adverse obstetric outcomes. The intent of pharmacotherapy maintenance in bipolar disorder is to delay and prevent recurrence of new mood episodes, reduce the risk of suicide, and improve psychosocial functioning. In such a situation, lithium is considered one of the most effective maintenance medications and has been widely used. Lithium use during pregnancy carries an increased risk of fetal heart defects and congenital anomalies, in particular Ebstein anomaly.

Pregnancy is not an absolute contraindication to lithium therapy, and women who are stable on lithium or those who experienced poor control with other treatments can consider use of lithium at the lowest effective dose, with shared decision making taking place. In the later weeks of gestation, ongoing lithium exposure has been associated with polyhydramnios, preterm delivery, neonatal cardiac arrhythmias, hypoglycemia, diabetes insipidus, and reversible thyroid function changes. The symptoms of lithium toxicity in the neonate may include lethargy and poor suck reflexes that may last as long as 7 days after delivery. For patients considering pregnancy, a discussion of risks and benefits and a trial of medications with less teratogenic risk may be considered by their psychiatrist.

Physiologic changes of pregnancy may affect metabolism and distribution of lithium, and close monitoring of the medication concentration is recommended during pregnancy and postpartum. The decision to continue or discontinue lithium therapy during pregnancy should balance the maternal risk of bipolar exacerbation with the risks of lithium use in pregnancy. A shared decision-making model is recommended as well as input from a psychiatrist or mental health professional.

The patient in Scenario 122 has a history of mechanical heart valve replacement and is likely on warfarin, which is a vitamin K antagonist. Women of reproductive age typically are recommended to receive bioprosthetic valve replacements when allowable given the significant risk associated with therapeutic anticoagulation. Women of reproductive potential who have mechanical prosthetic valves pose a unique challenge, because no anticoagulation regimen is completely safe or has been proved to prevent thromboembolism. Each anticoagulation option has drawbacks, whether risk of bleeding, increased risk of thromboembolism, or both.

Vitamin K antagonist therapy is the safest anticoagulant option for the woman but carries the risks of fetal spontaneous miscarriage, embryopathy, and intracranial bleeding secondary to the medication crossing the placenta. A woman receiving warfarin is recommended to have an international normalized ratio of 2.5–3.5 throughout pregnancy; however, in decision making with a cardiologist, different international normalized ratios may be tolerated with use in mechanical valves at higher or lower flow locations in the heart (mitral versus aortic). The risks associated with warfarin use during pregnancy include nasal hypoplasia, stippled epiphysis, and a higher incidence of fetal intraventricular hemorrhage, particularly with operative vaginal delivery. The risk of spontaneous pregnancy loss or warfarin embryopathy is estimated between 0.6% and 6% depending on the dose of warfarin used. Low-molecular-weight heparin does not cross the placenta and, therefore, does not carry fetal risks of bleeding. However, there is a higher risk of maternal valve thrombosis, thromboembolism, and death with use of injectable anticoagulants. These risks may be related more to inadequate dosing, failed monitoring, or subtherapeutic anti-Xa levels rather than a failure of the medication's effectiveness.

The patient in Scenario 123 has chronic hypertension and insulin-dependent diabetes. She likely is taking an angiotensin receptor inhibitor, and her risk of oligohydramnios, fetal lung hypoplasia, and skeletal malformations is increased. For women with chronic hypertension during pregnancy, one of the first evaluations (other than length and severity of her disease) is review of her antihypertensive medication(s). The medication classes with the highest risk of congenital anomalies include angiotensin-receptor blockers and angiotensin-converting enzyme inhibitors. These medications, which are active against renin-dependent vasoconstriction, often are the first-line medication choice in nonpregnant patients with hypertension and diabetes or hypertension and renal disease, coronary ischemia, heart failure, or pulmonary edema.

Angiotensin receptor blockers and angiotensin-converting enzyme inhibitors are teratogenic, and exposure in the first trimester should be avoided when possible. The risks of exposure of these medications to the fetus include fetal renal dysgenesis and calvarial hypoplasia, and prolonged use is associated with increased risk of fetal growth restriction. When angiotensin-converting enzyme inhibitor therapy is considered throughout pregnancy, consultation with a maternal–fetal medicine subspecialist is advised. Medications often used for pregnant women with chronic hypertension include calcium channel blockers and β-blockers because these medications have proved safe and effective.

The patient in Scenario 124 has a recent history of a solid organ transplant, and based on the anomalies listed, she is likely on mycophenolate. Most experts agree that pregnancy should be avoided in the first year after a solid organ transplant because of increased risks of organ rejection, allograft failure caused by changes in the metabolism of medications, and physiologic changes in renal function during pregnancy affecting medication pharmacokinetics. Mycophenolate can be used after a transplant or in reproductive-aged women as maintenance therapy for rheumatologic conditions such as lupus nephritis. Mycophenolate inhibits purine biosynthesis, and similar to methotrexate, it is teratogenic and increases the risk of pregnancy loss. Mycophenolate has been associated with increased risk of cleft lip and palate, micrognathia, microtia, and auditory canal abnormalities.

The use of mycophenolate is contraindicated in pregnancy. Furthermore, if a woman who is more than 1 year post transplant elects to pursue pregnancy, modifications to her immunosuppressive regimen should be discussed with her transplant care team and maternal–fetal medicine subspecialists. If she and her medical team elect to discontinue mycophenolate, expert opinion suggests that pregnancy should be delayed for 6 weeks. Other antirejection medications that may be used during pregnancy, depending on selection with the transplant team, with more favorable side effect profiles include the following: tacrolimus or cyclosporine, azathioprine, and low-dose prednisone.

Chronic hypertension in pregnancy. ACOG Practice Bulletin No. 203. American College of Obstetricians and Gynecologists. Obstet Gynecol 2019;133:e26–50. doi: 10.1097/AOG.0000000000003020 https://journals.lww.com/greenjournal/Fulltext/2019/01000/ACOG_Practice_Bulletin_No__203__Chronic.50.aspx

Coscia LA, Armenti DP, King RW, Sifontis NM, Constantinescu S, Moritz MJ. Update on the teratogenicity of maternal mycophenolate mofetil. J Pediatr Genet 2015;4:42–55. doi: 10.1055/s-0035-1556743 https://www.ncbi.nlm.nih.gov/pmc/articles/PMC4944211/

Fornaro M, Maritan E, Ferranti R, Zaninotto L, Miola A, Anastasia A, et al. Lithium exposure during pregnancy and the postpartum period: a systematic review and meta-analysis of safety and efficacy outcomes. Am J Psychiatry 2020;177:76–92. doi: 10.1176/appi.ajp.2019.19030228 https://ajp.psychiatryonline.org/doi/10.1176/appi.ajp.2019.19030228

Gynecologic management of adolescents and young women with cardiac conditions. ACOG Committee Opinion No. 813. American College of Obstetricians and Gynecologists. Obstet Gynecol 2020;136:e90–9. doi: 10.1097/AOG.0000000000004133 https://journals.lww.com/greenjournal/Fulltext/2020/11000/Gynecologic_Considerations_for_Adolescents_and.48.aspx

Immune modulating therapies in pregnancy and lactation. ACOG Committee Opinion No. 776. American College of Obstetricians and Gynecologists. Obstet Gynecol 2019;133:e287–95. doi: 10.1097/AOG.0000000000003176 https://journals.lww.com/greenjournal/Fulltext/2019/04000/ACOG_Committee_Opinion_No__776__Immune_Modulating.61.aspx

Nanna M, Stergiopoulos K. Pregnancy complicated by valvular heart disease: an update. J Am Heart Assoc 2014;3:e000712. doi: 10.1161/JAHA.113.000712 https://www.ahajournals.org/doi/10.1161/JAHA.113.000712

Use of psychiatric medications during pregnancy and lactation. ACOG Practice Bulletin No. 92. American College of Obstetricians and Gynecologists. Obstet Gynecol 2008;111:1001–20. doi: 10.1097/AOG.0b013e31816fd910 https://journals.lww.com/greenjournal/Citation/2008/04000/ACOG_Practice_Bulletin_No__92__Use_of_Psychiatric.39.aspx

Veroniki AA, Cogo E, Rios P, Straus SE, Finkelstein Y, Kealey R, et al. Comparative safety of anti-epileptic drugs during pregnancy: a systematic review and network meta-analysis of congenital malformations and prenatal outcomes. BMC Med 2017;15:95–1. doi: 10.1186/s12916-017-0845-1 https://bmcmedicine.biomedcentral.com/articles/10.1186/s12916-017-0845-1

125–128 Operative vaginal delivery

For each of the following clinical scenarios (125–128), select the most appropriate type of forceps (A–D) to assist in a vaginal delivery.

(A) Tucker-McLane forceps
(B) Simpson-Luikart forceps
(C) Piper forceps
(D) Kielland forceps

125. B. A nulliparous patient at term with a prolonged second stage of labor.

126. D. A nulliparous patient at term in labor with nonreassuring tracing and a left occiput transverse presentation.

127. A. A multiparous patient at term with maternal cardiac disease necessitating a passive second stage of labor.

128. C. A multiparous patient at term with diamniotic-dichorionic twins. The second twin is delivered by breech extraction, and additional assistance is needed with the aftercoming head.

The rate of operative vaginal delivery in the United States has decreased over the past few decades. The decrease in operative vaginal delivery rates coincides with increasing rates of cesarean birth. However, operative vaginal delivery can expedite a safe vaginal birth when maternal or fetal indications are present. Furthermore, operative vaginal delivery is beneficial for the parturient because it avoids the risks of cesarean birth, including higher rates of acute blood loss anemia, infection, prolonged healing, increased costs, and long-term issues associated with higher-order cesarean birth and subsequent placenta accreta spectrum. For a fetus with signs of decreased tolerance of labor, successful operative vaginal delivery can shorten intrapartum stressors and expedite effective delivery.

Operative vaginal delivery remains an important part of obstetric care and can be accomplished either with forceps or a vacuum extractor. Various types of forceps and vacuum extractors have been developed for this purpose. Potential indications for operative vaginal delivery include 1) prolonged second stage of labor, 2) suspicion of immediate or potential fetal compromise, or 3) shortening of the second stage of labor for maternal benefit.

Operative vaginal deliveries are classified by the station of the presenting part at instrument application and degree of rotation necessary for delivery (Table 125–128-1). The criteria for types of forceps deliveries (low versus outlet forceps) also are listed in this table. Figure 125–128-1 depicts the pelvis divided into four planes that represent the station of the presenting fetal part as it relates to operative vaginal delivery. A midforceps application would be used when the presenting fetal part is located between the middle of the inner border of the pubic symphysis and the junction of the second and third sacral vertebrae. Low forceps would be required when the presenting fetal part is at the smallest obstetric plane in the pelvis, composed of the lower, inner border of the symphysis pubis and the sacrococcygeal joint, and is surrounded laterally by the ischial spines. Finally, the pelvic outlet is quadrilateral in shape and bounded by the sacrococcygeal joint, ischial tuberosities laterally, and the inferior border of the symphysis pubis and often is the station for outlet operative vaginal delivery.

The prerequisites for operative vaginal delivery are listed in Table 125–128-2. Before considering assisted vaginal delivery, the obstetrician should assess the adequacy of the maternal pelvis, the estimated fetal weight, station, and position, as well as the adequacy of anesthesia. Operative delivery is contraindicated in the absence of a fully dilated cervix, lack of engagement in the pelvis, or inability to determine position of the vertex fetus.

Forceps and vacuum extractors are acceptable for operative vaginal delivery. The choice is determined by obstetrician preference and experience as well as clinical indications. Vacuum extraction is believed to be easier to learn and may be used when asynclitism prevents successful forceps articulation and placement. Forceps provide a more secure application and can be used to accomplish completion of a passive second stage of labor and to perform operative vaginal delivery at less than 34 weeks of gestation. A forceps-assisted vaginal delivery has a higher risk of vaginal, cervical, and soft tissue lacerations and hematoma formation, with a stronger association of third-degree and fourth-degree maternal perineal lacerations (20% risk

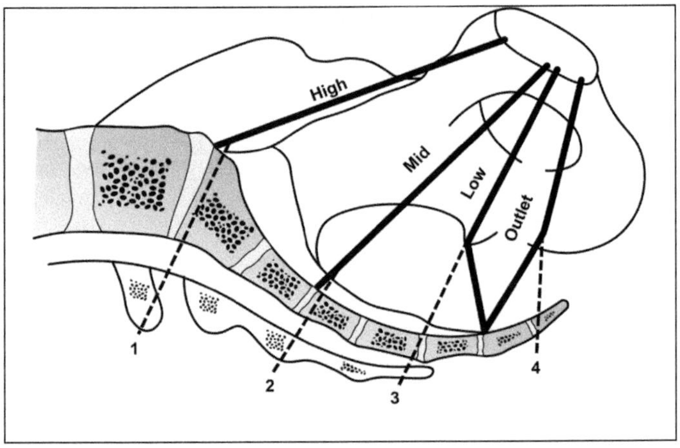

FIGURE 125-128-1. The four major planes of the pelvis. Reprinted from American College of Obstetricians and Gynecologists. Dennen's forceps deliveries. 4th ed. American College of Obstetricians and Gynecologists; 2001.

TABLE 125-128-1. Criteria for Types of Forceps Deliveries

OUTLET FORCEPS	LOW FORCEPS	MIDFORCEPS
Fetal scalp is visible at the introitus without separating the labia.	Leading point of the fetal skull is at station +2 or more and not on the pelvic floor.	Station is above +2 cm but head is engaged.
Fetal head is at or on the perineum.	Without rotation: Rotation is 45 degrees or less (right or left occiput anterior to occiput anterior or right or left occiput posterior to occiput posterior).	
Fetal skull has reached the pelvic floor	With rotation: Rotation is greater than 45 degrees.	
Sagittal suture is in an anterior posterior diameter or right or left occiput anterior or posterior position. (Rotation does not exceed 45 degrees.)		

Adapted from Operative vaginal birth. ACOG Practice Bulletin No. 219. American College of Obstetricians and Gynecologists. Obstet Gynecol 2020;135:e149–59. doi: 10.1097/AOG.0000000000003764 https://journals.lww.com/greenjournal/Fulltext/2020/04000/Operative_Vaginal_Birth__ACOG_Practice_Bulletin,.57.aspx

Modified and adapted by ACOG from Royal Australian and New Zealand College of Obstetricians and Gynaecologists. Instrumental vaginal birth (C-Obs 16). RANZCOG; 2020. Accessed February 11, 2022. https://ranzcog.edu.au/RANZCOG_SITE/media/RANZCOG-MEDIA/Women%27s%20Health/Statement%20and%20guidelines/Clinical-Obstetrics/Instrumental-vaginal-birth-(C-Obs-16)-Review-March-2020.pdf?ext=.pdf

TABLE 125-128-2. Prerequisites for Operative Vaginal Delivery (As easy to remember as A, B, Cs)

A	**Adequate** anesthesia, **Adequate** Pelvis
B	Maternal **Bladder** emptied
C	**Cephalic** presentation with known position of the fetal head
D	**Dilation** of cervix is complete/fully **Dilated** and membranes ruptured
E	**Engagement** of the fetal head
F	In**FORMED** patient of risks and benefits, and she desires to proceed
G	**Gameplan:** Willingness to halt attempted vaginal delivery if appears unsuccessful and can offer cesarean

Data from Operative vaginal birth. ACOG Practice Bulletin No. 219. American College of Obstetricians and Gynecologists. Obstet Gynecol 2020;135:e149–59. doi: 10.1097/AOG.0000000000003764 https://journals.lww.com/greenjournal/Fulltext/2020/04000/Operative_Vaginal_Birth__ACOG_Practice_Bulletin,.57.aspx.

of third- or fourth-degree lacerations during forceps-assisted vaginal delivery compared to 2% with spontaneous birth). Forceps-assisted vaginal delivery has a slight increased risk over vacuum-assisted vaginal delivery of transient facial forceps marks, bruising, lacerations, and facial nerve injuries. Less commonly, forceps-assisted vaginal delivery carries a risk of skull fracture and intracranial hemorrhage in the case of falx or tentorial laceration, but these rarely have been reported.

Vacuum-assisted vaginal delivery is reportedly less associated with maternal genital tract trauma (10% risk of third- or fourth-degree lacerations) but is discouraged at less than 34 weeks of gestation. When compared with cesarean birth, vacuum-assisted vaginal delivery carries a higher risk of cephalohematoma, scalp laceration, fracture, and brachial plexus injury, but not central neurologic complications. If used with torsion and traction by the vacuum cup, vacuum-assisted vaginal delivery rarely can cause severe intracranial hemorrhage (epidural, subdural, intraparenchymal, subarachnoid), intraventricular hemorrhage, and subgaleal hemorrhage in the neonate. The risk of these complications remains low, and large database studies to establish complication rates are ongoing. In summary, operative vaginal delivery increases the overall risk of hematomas, urethral injury, and extension of an episiotomy, with the degree or frequency of complication being inversely related to operative experience. Operative vaginal delivery is contraindicated if the fetal presenting part is not engaged, the position is unknown, or the fetus is suspected to have a bone demineralization condition, such as osteogenesis imperfecta, or a bleeding disorder, such as alloimmune thrombocytopenia, hemophilia, or von Willebrand disease.

Although reported rates of neonatal complications remain relatively low, the weight of available evidence appears to be against routine use of sequential instruments at operative vaginal delivery (progressing from vacuum extractor to forceps or vice versa). Midforceps- and rotational forceps-assisted deliveries are appropriate in select circumstances and with significant operator experience. Kielland forceps can be used for rotation with good outcomes, resulting in a reduction in cesarean births. In patients with occiput posterior position with arrest of descent in the second stage of labor, there may be a benefit to attempting rotation either with forceps or manual rotation.

In Scenario 125, the nulliparous patient with a prolonged second stage of labor would be best assisted by Simpson–Luikart forceps (Fig. 125–128-2). The Simpson–Luikart forceps have blades that assist the molded head well and have parallel, separated shanks and a long tapering cephalic curve. The fetal head is likely to have significant molding; therefore, the Simpson–Luikart forceps are the appropriate choice.

In Scenario 126, the patient has a left occiput transverse presentation. Both manual and instrumental rotation are options. The most commonly used forceps for rotations are Kielland forceps (Fig. 125–128-3). Kielland forceps have a slightly backward pelvic curve with blades shaped for the cephalic curves, with overlapping shanks and a longer distance between the heels of the blades and the intersection point on the shank. The sliding lock can correct for asynclitism. Kielland forceps may be applied using the inverse or

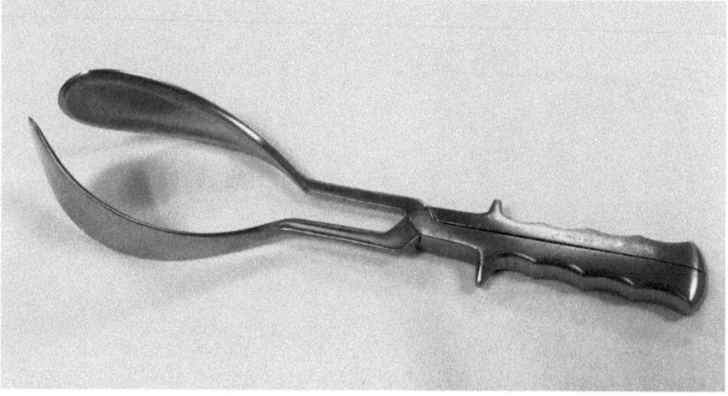

FIGURE 125-128-2. Simpson–Luikart forceps. The running obstetrician. 2015. Accessed April 21, 2022. http://www.runningobstetrician.com/obstetrics

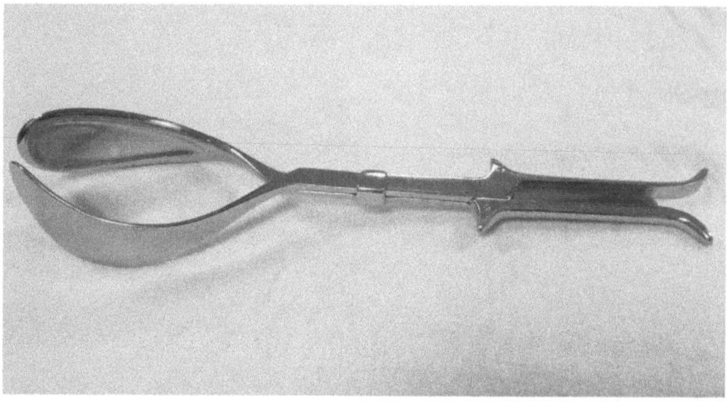

FIGURE 125-128-3. Kielland forceps. The running obstetrician. 2015. Accessed April 21, 2022. http://www.runningobstetrician.com/obstetrics

classical method versus a wandering method of application. Following drainage of the maternal bladder, the anterior blade is always placed first, and with left occiput transverse, that would mean the right blade is placed first. The classical placement involves inverting the forceps to introduce it near the fetal ear, with the inner surface of the blade's cephalic curve facing ventrally. The blade is then rotated on its own long axis away from the occiput and toward the midline. The wandering method of application is when the operator applies the anterior blade by gliding or wandering the blade around the face to the anterior ear. Once the anterior blade is placed, the posterior blade is placed, the forceps articulated, and the rotation is completed. Rotational forceps are highly effective in accomplishing vaginal delivery, but in less experienced hands they pose an increased risk of maternal soft tissue trauma. Delivery is not accomplished with Kielland forceps. They are instead used for rotation only. Following the rotational maneuver, they are removed and either maternal effort or another instrument may be used to effect delivery.

In Scenario 127, Tucker–McLane forceps, or another pair of Elliott-type forceps, should be used in this multiparous patient needing a passive second stage of labor. The Tucker–McLane forceps (Fig. 125–128-4) have narrower, overlapping shanks and a rounder cephalic curve in the blades accommodating the less molded fetal head typical in multiparous patients. Elliot forceps have similar accommodations for round, unmolded heads.

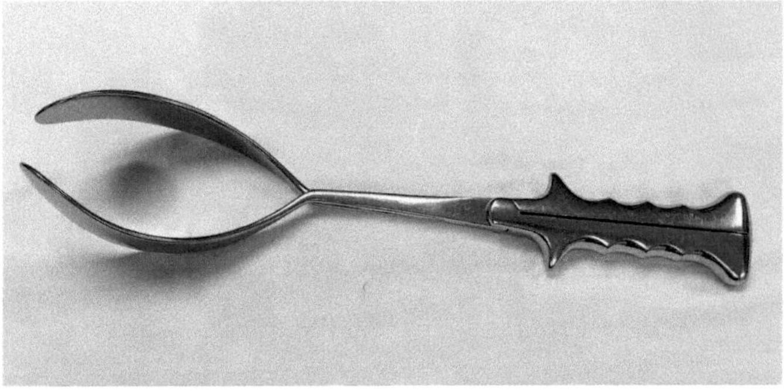

FIGURE 125-128-4. Tucker-McClane forceps. The running obstetrician. 2015. Accessed April 21, 2022. http://www.runningobstetrician.com/obstetrics

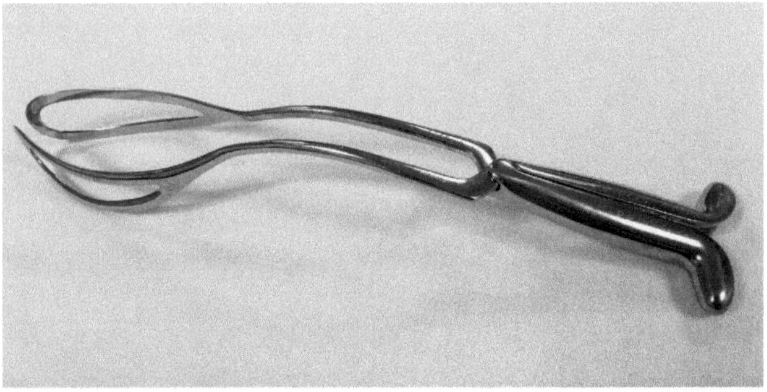

FIGURE 125-128-5. Piper forceps. The running obstetrician. 2015. Accessed April 21, 2022. http://www.runningobstetrician.com/obstetrics

In Scenario 128, the breech fetus should be delivered with Piper forceps only (Fig. 125–128-5). Piper forceps are designed for the aftercoming fetal head and have a pelvic curve rather than a cephalic curve. They also have longer shanks and are designed to accommodate a longer distance between the operator and the blades, giving more spring to the Piper forceps and reducing compression on the fetal head. Piper forceps should be applied after the shoulders and arms have been delivered and the head is in the maternal pelvis with the fetal chin oriented posteriorly. An assistant is critical when using Piper forceps because they help hold the neonate while the operator is applying the Piper forceps. Piper forceps should be placed with the operator in a kneeling or low sitting position in front of the patient. Use of Piper forceps to deliver the fetal head often helps create head flexion, reducing the presenting diameter and accomplishing delivery of the head through the maternal pelvis. This is different than head entrapment, in which the head is stuck in the maternal cervix, and Piper forceps should not be used in such a scenario.

Hale RW. Dennen's forceps deliveries. 4th ed. American College of Obstetricians and Gynecologists; 2001.

Morosky C. The running obstetrician. Accessed February 11, 2022. https://www.runningobstetrician.com/meet-the-founder

Operative vaginal birth. ACOG Practice Bulletin No. 219. American College of Obstetricians and Gynecologists. Obstet Gynecol 2020;135:e149–59. doi: 10.1097/AOG.0000000000003764 https://journals.lww.com/greenjournal/Fulltext/2020/04000/Operative_Vaginal_Birth__ACOG_Practice_Bulletin,.57.aspx

129–133 Thrombocytopenia in pregnancy

Match each clinical scenario (129–133) with the most likely diagnosis (A–E).

(A) Acute fatty liver of pregnancy
(B) Gestational thrombocytopenia
(C) Immune thrombocytopenia (ITP)
(D) Preeclampsia with severe features
(E) Thrombotic thrombocytopenic purpura (TTP)

129. C. A nulliparous patient presents at 7 weeks of gestation. She has no significant medical history. Her platelet count is 35,000/mm³.

130. A. A nulliparous patient at 32 weeks of gestation presents with nausea and abdominal pain. Examination reveals a blood pressure of 150/100 mm Hg and evidence of jaundice. Laboratory test results include an ammonia level of 60 micromoles/L and platelet count of 68,000/mm³.

131. B. A multiparous patient at 30 weeks of gestation has a routine third-trimester platelet count of 105,000/mm³ and normal blood pressure.

132. E. A nulliparous patient at 18 weeks of gestation presents with headache, abdominal pain, fever, and decreased fetal movement. On examination, she is noted to have petechiae and a fetal death. Laboratory testing reveals a hematocrit of 24%, platelet count of 10,000/mm³, and proteinuria.

133. D. A nulliparous patient at 34 weeks of gestation presents with a headache and epigastric pain. On examination, she is found to have new-onset hypertension. Laboratory testing reveals an aspartate aminotransferase of 220 IU/L, alanine aminotransferase of 250 IU/L, and a platelet count of 98,000/mm³.

A variety of causes of thrombocytopenia are encountered in pregnancy. *Thrombocytopenia* is defined as a platelet count of less than 150,000/mm³ and is managed based on the clinical status, degree, and etiology of the thrombocytopenia. Some variation in platelet counts exists during pregnancy, with a trend toward lower averages seen during the third trimester, but otherwise platelet counts usually are not significantly altered by pregnancy. The differential diagnosis can be divided by conditions that either increase platelet destruction or decrease platelet production as noted in Table 129–133-1. Increased destruction is more commonly noted in pregnancy and can entail immunologic activation, platelet consumption from bleeding, or abnormal platelet activation. Decreased production of platelets is associated with marrow disorders or nutritional deficiencies rather than thrombocytopenia.

The patient in Scenario 129 has ITP, which includes processes that lead to impaired platelet production and T cell-mediated destruction. Because there are no hallmark signs or true diagnostic tests, it is diagnosed by exclusion of other etiologies. Primary ITP is diagnosed based on the absence of triggering causes or other associated conditions and can be divided into three categories: 1) newly diagnosed (up to 3 months since diagnosis), 2) persistent (3–12 months since diagnosis), and 3) chronic (12 months or longer since diagnosis). Adults with ITP eventually achieve a stable and safe platelet count but may require multiple therapies and management of bleeding complications before stability.

Both onset and exacerbations of ITP occur at a higher incidence during pregnancy than in the general adult population. Women with ITP have normally functioning platelets, and the management goal is to minimize the risk of bleeding for the woman and the fetus during pregnancy and delivery—not to maintain normal platelet ranges. During pregnancy, treatment should be initiated for symptomatic bleeding, with the exception of the time around delivery. As delivery approaches (approximately 35–37 weeks of gestation), the obstetrician–gynecologist may opt for medical therapies, such as intravenous immunoglobulin or corticosteroid courses, or both, sufficient to improve maternal platelet counts to enable regional anesthesia or other indicated procedures. These therapies have not been shown to decrease risk of neonatal thrombocytopenia. Because maternal immunoglobulin G antiplatelet antibodies can cross the placenta, the newborn also is at risk of thrombocytopenia, and procedures associated with increased bleeding risk to the fetus should be avoided during labor. The occurrence of severe fetal or neonatal thrombocytopenia (platelet count less than 50,000/mm³ is low) is not correlated with maternal platelet level.

The patient in Scenario 130 has acute fatty liver of pregnancy, a rare and life-threatening hepatobiliary condition unique to pregnancy, in particular during the third trimester. Acute fatty liver of pregnancy occurs more frequently in nulliparous patients, those with multiple gestations, and when the fetus is male. Although the pathogenesis is not well understood, it appears to be related to defective mitochondrial fatty acid oxidation in the woman and the affected fetus, which results in accumulation of fatty acids deposited in the maternal liver. Presenting features include nausea and vomiting, epigastric pain, malaise, and jaundice.

Given the overlap of signs and symptoms with HELLP (hemolysis, elevated liver enzymes, and low platelet count) syndrome and other hypertensive disorders, a set of criteria for diagnosis have been established known as the Swansea Criteria (Table 129–133-2). The diagnosis of acute fatty liver of pregnancy requires six of the criteria listed without other identifying causes. Hyperbilirubinemia, coagulopathy, and hepatic encephalopathy are poor prognostic signs. Around 10% of women will have concordant disseminated intravascular coagulopathy, which has major complications, including liver, renal, and respiratory failure; encephalitis; pancreatitis; and death.

A multidisciplinary care team is necessary to manage acute fatty liver of pregnancy. The priority is delivery of the fetus, regardless of gestational age, because delivery initiates resolution of the disease. Following delivery, supportive care often is required to stabilize the patient until her liver recovers. After diagnosis, the affected woman and her neonate should be tested for the genetic disorder mitochondrial fatty acid oxidation,

TABLE 129-133-1. Thrombocytopenia in Pregnancy

HYPERTENSIVE DISORDERS	IMMUNE THROMBOCYTOPENIA		ASSOCIATION WITH SYSTEMIC CONDITIONS	OTHER
	PRIMARY ITP	SECONDARY ITP		
Preeclampsia HELLP syndrome	Immune Thrombocytopenia	Antiphospholipid antibody syndrome Systemic lupus erythematosus Infectious (HIV, hepatitis C, cytomegalovirus, *Helicobacter pylori*) Drug-induced (heparins, antimicrobials, anticonvulsants, analgesics)	Disseminated intravascular coagulation Thrombotic thrombocytopenia/ hemolytic uremic syndrome Bone marrow disorders Nutritional deficiencies Splenic sequestration	Congenital thrombocytopenia Gestational thrombocytopenia

Adapted from Thrombocytopenia in pregnancy. ACOG Practice Bulletin No. 207. American College of Obstetricians and Gynecologists. Obstet Gynecol 2019;133:e181–93. doi: 10.1097/AOG.0000000000003100 https://journals.lww.com/greenjournal/Fulltext/2019/03000/ACOG_Practice_Bulletin_No__207__Thrombocytopenia.43.aspx.

TABLE 129-133-2. Swansea Criteria for Acute Fatty Liver of Pregnancy*

SYMPTOMS AND SIGNS	LABORATORY ABNORMALITIES	OTHER ABNORMALITIES
Vomiting	Bilirubin level greater than 14 micromoles/L (0.8 mg/dL)	Ascites or hyperechogenic liver on ultrasound
Abdominal pain	Hypoglycemia (low blood glucose level of less than 4 mmol/L [72 mg/dL])	Microvesicular steatosis on liver biopsy
Polydipsia or polyuria	Leukocyte count: greater than 11×10^9/L (11,000 per microliter)	
Encephalopathy	Increased uric acid level; greater than 5.7 mg/dL or 340 micromoles/L (5.7 mg/dL)	
	Increased ammonia level: greater than 47 micromoles/L (66 micrograms/dL)	
	Increased aminotransferase levels (alanine aminotransferase or aspartate aminotransferase level: greater than 42 U/L)	
	Renal impairment (creatinine level: greater than 150 micromoles/L [1.7 mg/dL])	
	Coagulopathy (prothrombin time greater than 14 s [prothrombin time international normalized ratio of 1.2] or activated thromboplastin time greater than 34 s)	

*In the absence of an alternative cause, six or more of these criteria should be present to establish a diagnosis of acute fatty liver of pregnancy.

Reprinted from Vierling JM, Stribling RJ. Liver disease: reproductive considerations. Clin Update Womens Health Care 2017;XVI(1):1–42. https://www.acog.org/clinical/journals-and-publications/clinical-updates/2017/01/liver-disease-reproductive-considerations.

most commonly long-chain 3-hydroxyacyl-coenzyme A dehydrogenase deficiency.

The patient in Scenario 131 has gestational thrombocytopenia, which often is noted incidentally on third-trimester laboratory studies. Gestational thrombocytopenia occurs in approximately 5–10% of pregnant women and can be notable for platelet counts that are low but typically stay above 75,000/mm^3. The key characteristics of gestational thrombocytopenia are

- Onset typically is in the mid-second to third trimester but can occur anytime during pregnancy.
- The patient is asymptomatic with no history of bleeding.
- The patient has no history of thrombocytopenia outside of pregnancy.
- There is a low incidence of fetal and neonatal thrombocytopenia.
- No other identifiable cause for thrombocytopenia is present.
- Thrombocytopenia resolves postpartum, within 12 months after delivery.

The diagnosis of gestational thrombocytopenia is one of exclusion, and no specific treatment is needed or recommended. Pregnancies complicated by gestational thrombocytopenia usually are not at increased risk of maternal bleeding or fetal complications. Although no evidence currently guides the frequency of platelet evaluation or additional testing, many women are offered serial platelet counts leading up to delivery. If platelet counts trend below 100,000/mm^3, corticosteroid therapy can be considered to accomplish regional anesthetic at delivery. A repeat platelet count should be obtained 1–3 months postpartum to evaluate for resolution.

The patient in Scenario 132 has TTP, an acute, rare, and life-threatening disorder caused by a deficiency of ADAMTS13, von Willebrand factor cleaving protease, or both. Although data are sparse, the initial presentation and diagnosis of TTP are not uncommon during pregnancy given TTP's prevalence in women and presentation in adults in their 30s or 40s. Furthermore, at least one half of all acute episodes of TTP occur in women of childbearing age, with pregnancy often being the initial, and sometimes only, precipitating event leading to diagnosis. The initial presentation of TTP typically appears similar to preeclampsia with severe features, but earlier in gestation, during the mid-second or early-third trimester.

Women with TTP may demonstrate severe thrombocytopenia during pregnancy (usually with platelet counts less than 50,000/mm^3), hemolysis on peripheral blood smear, temporary neurologic symptoms, and acute kidney injury, and may have a fetal death. Diagnosis and treatment before 20 weeks of gestation are associated with the best outcomes. Treatment of TTP during pregnancy depends on the presence or absence of ADAMTS13 antibody and often requires serial plasmapheresis to effect remission with or without the addition of immunosuppressive therapies. Risk of TTP relapse in subsequent pregnancies is as high as 50%.

The patient in Scenario 133 most likely has preeclampsia with severe features, specifically HELLP syndrome. Hypertensive disorders in pregnancy are the cause of up to 20% of cases of maternal thrombocytopenia. Of women with preeclampsia, only around 10% will have HELLP syndrome. The diagnosis of HELLP syndrome can be made when microangiopathic hemolytic anemia and elevated liver function test results are found in association with hypertension and thrombocytopenia with a platelet count of less than 100,000/mm^3. The cause of decreasing platelet counts is uncertain but appears to be associated with increased platelet consumption and platelet activation. Unlike other causes of thrombocytopenia, platelet function can be impaired. Hemolysis, elevated liver enzymes, and low platelet count syndrome is associated with preterm birth and fetal growth restriction, conditions that are thought to be independent of low platelets and more associated with preeclampsia.

The treatment for HELLP syndrome is delivery, usually in conjunction with the administration of magnesium sulfate to prevent seizures. Expectant management and delay of delivery for antenatal corticosteroids are based on strict selection criteria and are best accomplished in a tertiary care center. The route of delivery should be determined by routine obstetric indications. Platelet transfusions should be considered when a platelet count is less than 50,000/mm^3 and cesarean birth is indicated or if disseminated intravascular coagulation is suspected.

Gestational hypertension and preeclampsia. ACOG Practice Bulletin No. 222. American College of Obstetricians and Gynecologists. Obstet Gynecol 2020;135:e237–60. doi: 10.1097/AOG.0000000000003891 https://journals.lww.com/greenjournal/Fulltext/2020/06000/Gestational_Hypertension_and_Preeclampsia__ACOG.46.aspx

Kaufman RM, Djulbegovic B, Gernsheimer T, Kleinman S, Tinmouth AT, Capocelli KE, et al. Platelet transfusion: a clinical practice guideline from the AABB. Ann Intern Med 2015;162:205–13. doi: 10.7326/M14-1589 https://www.acpjournals.org/doi/full/10.7326/M14-1589

Provan D, Stasi R, Newland AC, Blanchette VS, Bolton-Maggs P, Bussel JB, et al. International consensus report on the investigation and management of primary immune thrombocytopenia. Blood 2010;115:168–86. doi: 10.1182/blood-2009-06-225565 https://ashpublications.org/blood/article/115/2/168/26966/International-consensus-report-on-the

Scully M, Thomas M, Underwood M, Watson H, Langley K, Camilleri RS, et al. Thrombotic thrombocytopenic purpura and pregnancy: presentation, management, and subsequent pregnancy outcomes. Collaborators of the UK TTP Registry. Blood 2014;124:211–9. doi: 10.1182/blood-2014-02-553131 https://ashpublications.org/blood/article/124/2/211/32922/Thrombotic-thrombocytopenic-purpura-and-pregnancy

Thrombocytopenia in pregnancy. ACOG Practice Bulletin No. 207. American College of Obstetricians and Gynecologists. Obstet Gynecol 2019;133:e181–93. doi: 10.1097/AOG.0000000000003100 https://journals.lww.com/greenjournal/Fulltext/2019/03000/ACOG_Practice_Bulletin_No__207__Thrombocytopenia.43.aspx

Vierling JM, Stribling RJ. Liver disease: reproductive considerations. Clin Update Womens Health Care 2017;XVI(1):1–42. https://www.acog.org/clinical/journals-and-publications/clinical-updates/2017/01/liver-disease-reproductive-considerations

134–138 Preterm birth prevention

For each clinical scenario (134–138), choose the most appropriate next step for preterm birth prevention (A–C).

(A) Cerclage
(B) Cervical length screening
(C) Expectant management

134. A. A 23-year-old gravida 2, para 1, presents for fetal anatomy ultrasonography at 19 weeks of gestation. She has no history of preterm birth. Her cervical length on examination is 4 mm, and the cervix is dilated 5 mm.

135. B. A 33-year-old gravida 2, para 1, presents for fetal anatomy ultrasonography at 19 weeks of gestation. She has a history of spontaneous preterm delivery at 30 weeks of gestation. Her cervical length is 26 mm, and the cervix is closed on examination.

136. A. A 28-year-old gravida 2, para 1, presents for initiation of prenatal care at 12 weeks of gestation. She has a history of asymptomatic cervical dilation, requiring cerclage placement at 20 weeks in her last pregnancy.

137. A. A 30-year-old gravida 2, para 1, presents for transvaginal ultrasonography at 16 weeks of gestation because of a history of spontaneous preterm birth at 28 weeks of gestation. Her cervical length is 20 mm, and the cervix is closed on examination.

138. C. A 25-year-old gravida 3, para 2, presents for her anatomy ultrasonography at 19 weeks of gestation. She has no history of preterm birth. Her cervical length is 29 mm, and the cervix is closed on examination.

Cervical insufficiency is a term used to describe the inability of the cervix to maintain pregnancy without any evidence of uterine contractions or labor. The pathophysiology is poorly understood. Risk factors include surgical procedures or trauma to the cervix (eg, conization, loop electrosurgical excision procedures, and lacerations), müllerian anomalies, and collagen or elastin deficiencies. The diagnosis is challenging because of the lack of diagnostic criteria and objective findings. Criteria that raise suspicion for the diagnosis are painless cervical dilation after 14 and typically before 24 weeks of gestation; absence of contractions or labor; and absence of other identifiable causes, such as bleeding (abruption), infection, or membrane rupture.

A cerclage may be indicated by obstetric history, ultrasonographic examination, or physical examination of the cervix. The American College of Obstetricians and Gynecologists' indications are outlined in Box 134–138-1. In a systematic review of pregnant women with singletons who underwent cerclage placement because of history, ultrasound indication, or physical examination indication, women with cerclage were less likely to have preterm births before 37, 34 (average relative risk, 0.77; 95% CI, 0.66–0.89), and 28 weeks of gestation.

BOX 134–138-1

Indications for Cervical Cerclage in Women With Singleton Pregnancies

History
- History of one or more second-trimester pregnancy losses related to painless cervical dilation and in the absence of labor or abruptio placentae
- Prior cerclage due to painless cervical dilation in the second trimester

Physical examination
- Painless cervical dilation in the second trimester

Ultrasonographic finding with a history of prior preterm birth
- Current singleton pregnancy, prior spontaneous preterm birth at less than 34 weeks of gestation, and short cervical length (less than 25 mm) before 24 weeks of gestation

Reprinted from Cerclage for the management of cervical insufficiency. Practice Bulletin No. 142. American College of Obstetricians and Gynecologists. Obstet Gynecol 2014;123:372–9. doi: 10.1097/01.AOG.0000443276.68274.cc https://journals.lww.com/greenjournal/Fulltext/2014/02000/Practice_Bulletin_No__142__Cerclage_for_the.33.aspx.

Ultrasonographic assessment of cervical length has been shown to be the best predictor of preterm birth. The definition of a *short cervix* varies, ranging from 20 to 30 mm. The risk of spontaneous preterm birth is inversely proportional to cervical length. The risk of extreme preterm birth (less than 28 weeks of gestation) is highest for women with a cervical length of less than 15 mm.

The patient described in Scenario 134 has a short, dilated cervix and meets criteria for an examination-indicated cerclage. The majority of published data examining the effects of physical examination-indicated cerclage are from observational studies. These studies suggest that cerclage is beneficial because it improves neonatal survival rates and prolongs pregnancy by approximately 1 month.

For women with a prior spontaneous preterm birth who either do not have a clear history of cervical insufficiency or who prefer the monitoring of cervical length in lieu of outright cerclage placement, cervical length screening typically is performed every 1–2 weeks from 16 to 24 weeks of gestation. In a woman with a prior spontaneous preterm birth, a *short cervix* is defined as less than 25 mm. In these women, a cerclage may be offered and could be beneficial. The patient described in Scenario 135 does not have a cervical length less than 25 mm and, therefore, does not need a cerclage. The Society for Maternal-Fetal Medicine recommends repeat cervical length every 1–4 weeks for women with a prior spontaneous preterm birth and a cervical length of 26–29 mm (borderline short cervix). Screening should start around 16 0/7 weeks and continue until 24 0/7 weeks of gestation or until a cerclage is placed, whichever comes first.

The patient described in Scenario 136 has a history consistent with cervical insufficiency and underwent cerclage placement during her previous pregnancy. She meets criteria for a history-indicated cerclage. Cerclage placement compared with no cerclage has been shown to decrease the risk of preterm delivery before 33 weeks of gestation (83 [13%] compared with 110 [17%], P=.03) in this setting.

The patient described in Scenario 137 has a history of spontaneous preterm birth and a short cervix (less than 25 mm), and she meets criteria to offer cerclage placement. The patient described in Scenario 138 has no history of preterm birth and has a normal cervical length (greater than 25 mm). No intervention is indicated, and expectant management is recommended.

Alfirevic Z, Stampalija T, Medley N. Cervical stitch (cerclage) for preventing preterm birth in singleton pregnancy. Cochrane Database of Systematic Reviews 2017, Issue 6. Art. No.: CD008991. doi: 10.1002/14651858.CD008991.pub3 http://dx.doi.org/10.1002/14651858.CD008991.pub3

Cerclage for the management of cervical insufficiency. Practice Bulletin No. 142. American College of Obstetricians and Gynecologists. Obstet Gynecol 2014;123:372–9. doi: 10.1097/01.AOG.0000443276.68274.cc https://journals.lww.com/greenjournal/Fulltext/2014/02000/Practice_Bulletin_No__142__Cerclage_for_the.33.aspx

McIntosh J, Feltovich H, Berghella V, Manuck T. The role of routine cervical length screening in selected high- and low-risk women for preterm birth prevention. Society for Maternal–Fetal Medicine (SMFM). Am J Obstet Gynecol 2016;215:B2–7. doi: 10.1016/j.ajog.2016.04.027 https://www.ajog.org/article/S0002-9378(16)30112-0/fulltext

Society for Maternal–Fetal Medicine. SMFM preterm birth toolkit. SMFM; 2016. Accessed February 28, 2022. https://www.smfm.org/publications/231-smfm-preterm-birth-toolkit

Suhag A, Berghella V. Cervical cerclage. Clin Obstet Gynecol 2014;57:557–67. doi: 10.1097/GRF.0000000000000044 https://journals.lww.com/clinicalobgyn/Abstract/2014/09000/Cervical_Cerclage.16.aspx

139–143 Group B streptococci

For each clinical scenario (139–143), choose the recommended intrapartum group B streptococcus (GBS) prophylaxis strategy (A–E).

(A) Cefazolin
(B) Clindamycin
(C) Penicillin
(D) Prophylaxis not indicated
(E) Vancomycin

139. C. A 26-year-old gravida 2, para 1, presents in spontaneous labor at 38 weeks of gestation. Current GBS status is unknown, but she was a GBS carrier in her prior pregnancy. She has no allergies to medications.

140. A. A 30-year-old gravida 3, para 2, presents for scheduled induction of labor at 39 weeks of gestation. Earlier in the pregnancy, she had a urine culture positive for GBS at 10^2 colony-forming units/mL. She has a history of a mild rash after taking penicillin as a young child.

141. D. A 39-year-old gravida 1, para 0, at 37 weeks of gestation is being induced for chronic hypertension. Her amniotic membranes have been ruptured for 24 hours, she is 3-cm dilated, and she is continuing to labor. A GBS screening culture was negative at 36 weeks of gestation. She has no allergies to medications.

142. E. A 20-year-old gravida 1, para 0, presents in spontaneous preterm labor at 37 weeks of gestation. Her intrapartum nucleic acid amplification test (NAAT) GBS screening was negative. Amniotic membranes have been ruptured greater than 18 hours, and on cervical examination she is 6-cm dilated. She has a history of hives with penicillin.

143. C. A 33-year-old gravida 2, para 1, is in spontaneous preterm labor at 36 weeks of gestation. A GBS culture was negative at 28 weeks of gestation when she was admitted for a prior episode of preterm labor. She has no allergies to medications.

Group B streptococcus (also known as *Streptococcus agalactiae*) is the leading cause of infection in the newborn. *Early-onset GBS disease* is defined as infection occurring within the first week of life. In the 1970s, the reported case-fatality ratios for invasive GBS were as high as 50%. In the 1980s, studies emerged showing that intravenous antibiotics given to the woman during labor could effectively prevent invasive disease in the newborn. With the use of intrapartum prophylaxis, the risk of early-onset GBS disease from intrapartum exposure is very low. Today, a woman who tests positive for GBS colonization and receives antibiotics during labor has a 1 in 4,000 chance of having a newborn with GBS disease, whereas a woman who tests positive for GBS colonization and does not receive antibiotics during labor has a 1 in 200 chance of having a newborn with GBS disease.

A rectovaginal GBS culture should be obtained in all pregnant women at 36 0/7 to 37 6/7 weeks of gestation (unless delivery is anticipated before then) to allow for the 5-week window of valid culture results, given that women will most likely deliver before 41 weeks of gestation. The indications for intrapartum prophylaxis are shown in Table 139–143-1. Intravenous penicillin is the antimicrobial of choice for intrapartum prophylaxis because GBS is exquisitely sensitive to penicillins. First-generation cephalosporins (ie, cefazolin) also are acceptable for women reporting a low-risk penicillin allergy (such as a nonurticarial maculopapular rash or pruritus without rash).

For women with a high-risk penicillin allergy (immunoglobulin E mediated, anaphylaxis), clindamycin is recommended if susceptibility has been demonstrated. Penicillin allergy testing is another option in women who report an allergy. Most patients who report penicillin allergy are actually penicillin tolerant. Testing can confirm the presence or absence of true allergy, allowing for use of penicillin both intrapartum and for future health indications if they arise. In the event a high-risk allergy is confirmed or suspected, and clindamycin susceptibility is unknown or resistant, women should receive intravenous vancomycin.

Women who have unknown GBS culture results but report a history of GBS colonization in a previous pregnancy, as with the patient in Scenario 139, have an increased risk of early-onset GBS disease in the newborn. The American College of

TABLE 139-143-1. Indications for Intrapartum GBS Prophylaxis to Prevent Neonatal Group B Streptococcal Early-Onset Disease

INTRAPARTUM GBS PROPHYLAXIS INDICATED	INTRAPARTUM GBS PROPHYLAXIS NOT INDICATED
Maternal history • Previous neonate with invasive GBS disease	• Colonization with GBS during a previous pregnancy (unless colonization status in current pregnancy is unknown at onset of labor at term)
Current pregnancy • Positive GBS culture obtained at 36 0/7 wk of gestation or more during current pregnancy (unless a cesarean birth is performed before onset of labor for a woman with intact amniotic membranes) • GBS bacteriuria during any trimester of the current pregnancy	• Negative vaginal–rectal GBS culture obtained at 36 0/7 wk of gestation or more during the current pregnancy • Cesarean birth performed before onset of labor on a woman with intact amniotic membranes, regardless of GBS colonization status or gestational age
Intrapartum • Unknown GBS status at the onset of labor (culture not done or results unknown) and any of the following: — Birth at less than 37 0/7 wk of gestation — Amniotic membrane rupture 18 h or more — Intrapartum temperature 38.0 °C (100.4 °F) or higher* — Intrapartum NAAT result positive for GBS — Intrapartum NAAT result negative but risk factors develop (ie, less than 37 0/7 wk of gestation, amniotic membrane rupture 18 h or more, or maternal temperature 38.0 °C [100.4 °F] or higher) — Known GBS positive status in a previous pregnancy	• Negative vaginal–rectal GBS culture obtained at 36 0/7 wk of gestation or more during the current pregnancy, regardless of intrapartum risk factors • Unknown GBS status at onset of labor, NAAT result negative and no intrapartum risk factors present (ie, less than 37 0/7 wk of gestation, amniotic membrane rupture 18 h or more, or maternal temperature 38 °C [100.4 °F] or higher)

Abbreviations: GBS, group B streptococcus; NAAT, nucleic acid amplification test.

*If intra-amniotic infection is suspected, broad-spectrum antibiotic therapy that includes an agent known to be active against GBS should replace GBS prophylaxis.

Reprinted from Prevention of group B streptococcal early-onset disease in newborns. ACOG Committee Opinion No. 797. American College of Obstetricians and Gynecologists [published erratum appears in Obstet Gynecol 2020;135:978–9]. Obstet Gynecol 2020;135:e51–72. doi: 10.1097/AOG.0000000000003668 https://journals.lww.com/greenjournal/Fulltext/2020/02000/Prevention_of_Group_B_Streptococcal_Early_Onset.43.aspx.

Modified from Verani JR, McGee L, Schra SJ. Prevention of perinatal group B streptococcal disease—revised guidelines from CDC, 2010. Division of Bacterial Diseases, National Center for Immunization and Respiratory Diseases, Centers for Disease Control and Prevention CDC). MMWR Recomm Rep 2010;59:1–36.

Obstetricians and Gynecologists considers women with a history of GBS to be candidates for GBS prophylaxis in the setting of unknown GBS status.

Women who have had a positive culture result at any point in the pregnancy, including rectovaginal or urine culture, should receive intrapartum prophylaxis regardless of when the culture was obtained. The patient in Scenario 140 had a positive urine culture and, therefore, should receive prophylaxis. With a low-risk penicillin allergy, a first-generation cephalosporin could be used. Approximately 80% of patients with immunoglobulin E-mediated penicillin allergy lose their sensitivity after 10 years.

In the setting of a negative culture result within the past 5 weeks, as with the patient in clinical Scenario 141, GBS prophylaxis is not indicated. However, if the GBS culture result was unknown, and the patient were preterm or had prolonged ruptured membranes (greater than 18 hours), prophylaxis would be indicated.

The patient described in Scenario 142 had negative intrapartum GBS screening NAAT, but now has a risk factor given that she has had ruptured membranes for 18 hours. Nucleic acid amplification-based testing can be used at the time of presentation for labor, but the 1- to 2-hour turnaround time does not allow for the full enrichment broth incubation step that is required to maximize results. Thus, the sensitivity is diminished, and the failure rate of NAAT-based testing is up to 7–10%. Given that this patient has developed additional risk factors, she should receive prophylaxis, and because of her high-risk allergy to penicillin, she should receive vancomycin.

The patient described in Scenario 143 had a negative GBS culture more than 5 weeks ago. Additionally, she is at risk of preterm delivery. Therefore, she should receive intrapartum prophylaxis and penicillin is appropriate.

American Society for Microbiology. Guidelines for the detection and identification of group B streptococcus. ASM; 2021. Accessed March 1, 2022. https://asm.org/Guideline/Guidelines-for-the-Detection-and-Identification-of

Centers for Disease Control and Prevention. Preventing group B strep disease in newborns. Accessed February 28, 2022. https://www.cdc.gov/groupbstrep/about/prevention.html

Prevention of group B streptococcal early-onset disease in newborns. ACOG Committee Opinion No. 797. American College of Obstetricians and Gynecologists [published erratum appears in Obstet Gynecol 2020;135:978–9]. Obstet Gynecol 2020;135:e51–72. doi: 10.1097/AOG.0000000000003668 https://journals.lww.com/greenjournal/Fulltext/2020/02000/Prevention_of_Group_B_Streptococcal_Early_Onset.43.aspx

144–147 Abnormal ultrasound findings

For each ultrasound image (Figs. 144–147) choose the likely diagnosis (A–F).

(A) Ascites
(B) Bowel obstruction
(C) Echogenic bowel
(D) Gastroschisis
(E) Hydronephrosis
(F) Omphalocele

144. F

145. D

146. E

147. A

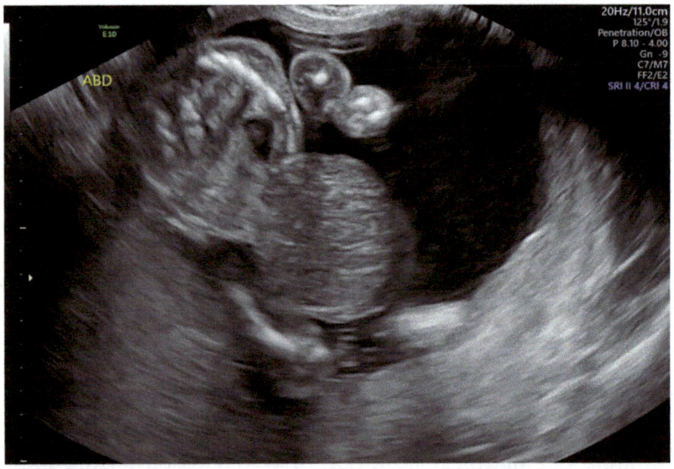

FIGURE 144. Fetal ultrasonography.

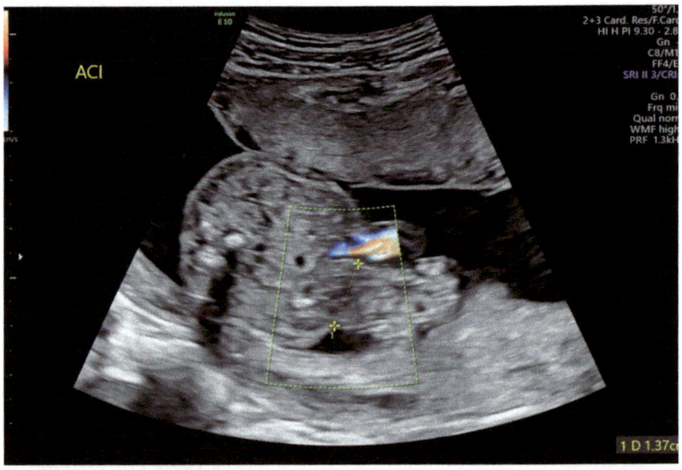

FIGURE 145. Fetal ultrasonography.

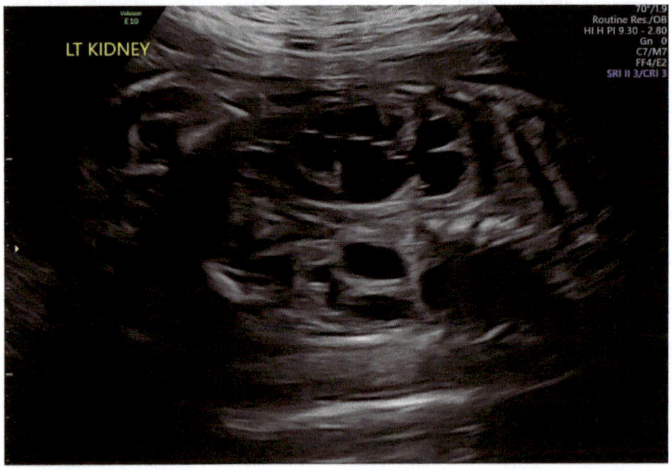

FIGURE 146. Fetal ultrasonography.

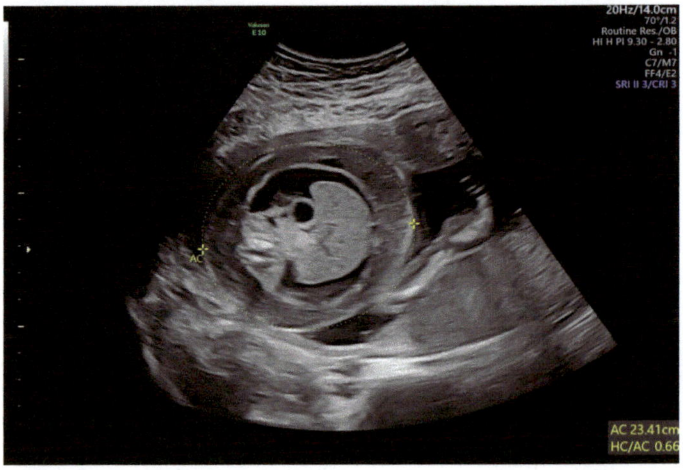

FIGURE 147. Fetal ultrasonography.

Obstetric ultrasonography is an important component of prenatal care in the United States. Ultrasound examinations in pregnancy are performed with transabdominal, transvaginal, and less commonly, transperineal approaches. The American College of Obstetricians and Gynecologists (ACOG), American College of Radiology, American Institute of Ultrasound in Medicine, *Eunice Kennedy Shriver* National Institute of Child Health and Human Development, Society for Maternal-Fetal Medicine, and Society of Radiologists in Ultrasound have adopted uniform terminology for the performance of ultrasonography in the second trimester and the third trimester: *standard*, *limited*, and *specialized*. A standard obstetric ultrasound examination includes assessment of fetal presentation and number, amniotic fluid, cardiac activity, placental position, fetal biometry, and an anatomic survey. A limited examination is performed to investigate a specific question, such as confirming fetal viability with cardiac activity, evaluating amniotic fluid volume, or assessing the fetal presentation. A specialized examination also is referred to as detailed or targeted and is performed to assess for fetal anomalies when there is an increased risk in that patient, or if an abnormality is suspected based on limited or standard ultrasonographic examination.

Many obstetricians perform and interpret ultrasonographic examinations, and ACOG recommends that obstetricians receive specific training in obstetric ultrasonography and be familiar with the anatomy, physiology, and pathophysiology of the pelvis, pregnant uterus, and fetus. Physicians are responsible for the quality and accuracy of ultrasound examinations performed in their names, the documentation of examinations, and quality control and safety of the ultrasonography, environment, and procedures performed.

The fetal gastrointestinal tract can be imaged starting in the late first trimester with visualization of the fetal stomach and the abdominal wall. The ventral abdominal wall defects most commonly seen are omphalocele and gastroschisis. Omphaloceles involve the umbilicus, often contain the liver, and are covered by a membrane. This diagnosis is associated with aneuploidy, other anomalies, fetal growth restriction, and a higher risk of fetal death. Gastroschisis involves free loops of bowel (without liver) herniated to the right of the umbilical cord insertion site, and are less commonly associated with aneuploidy or other anomalies. The fetus in Figure 144 has an omphalocele with a midline defect that is likely covered by a membrane with no free loops of bowel. The fetus in Figure 145 has gastroschisis with a midline defect next to the umbilical cord and free loops of extruded bowel.

The small intestine is sometimes noted to have an increased echogenicity; this finding is generally referred to as echogenic bowel. Although there are no standard criteria for this diagnosis, it typically is diagnosed when the fetal bowel is at least as echogenic as bone with imaging performed with reduced gain, and without harmonics to reduce the risk of overdiagnosis. It is thought to be caused by abnormal bowel contents (such as meconium or blood) or edema of the bowel wall. Echogenic bowel is associated with an increased risk of trisomy 21, fetal cystic fibrosis, or congenital infection, and a higher risk of complications, such as fetal growth restriction and stillbirth.

Bowel obstruction may occur in utero with duodenal or jejunoileal obstruction. Ultrasonographic findings with fetal bowel obstruction include dilated loops of bowel, polyhydramnios, a dilated stomach, and echogenic bowel. Duodenal atresia has a well-known ultrasonographic "double bubble sign" showing a dilated duodenum just beyond the fetal stomach. Fetal bowel obstruction may be caused by vascular disruption leading to ischemic necrosis of bowel (most common in jejunoileal obstruction), bowel atresia, or extrinsic constriction. Duodenal atresia is strongly associated with fetal trisomy 21.

Fetal ascites is characterized by excess intraperitoneal fluid in the fetal abdomen. It may be caused by leakage of bowel or bladder contents, a ruptured ovarian cyst, and other etiologies, and often is associated with hydrops fetalis. Hydrops fetalis consists of two or more of the following findings: ascites, skin edema, pleural effusion, pericaridal effusion, polyhydramnios, and placental thickening. Approximately 10% of the thousands of possible etiologies of hydrops fetalis are caused by immune hydrops secondary to fetal anemia from maternal red blood cell alloimmunization. The diagnosis of nonimmune hydrops encompasses the remainder of cases, and some common causes include fetal cardiac abnormalities (such as arrythmia or congenital heart defect), chromosomal abnormalities (such as monosomy X), and hematologic abnormalities (eg, α-thalassemia). The exact mechanism causing hydrops fetalis is not always known but may be secondary to decreased lymphatic return or lymphatic vessel dysplasia, increased interstitial fluid, or an inflammatory reaction leading to increased capillary permeability. When hydrops fetalis is diagnosed, a detailed evaluation can identify the underlying cause. The fetus in Figure 147 has ascites and skin edema, which indicate hydrops fetalis.

Normal renal function is established in a fetus by the ninth week of gestation. The fetal bladder can be seen after 9 weeks of gestation, and the kidneys at 11–12 weeks of gestation. Assessment of the fetal urinary tract includes the amniotic fluid volume in addition to the kidneys and bladder. After 14 weeks of gestation, approximately two-thirds of the amnitoic fluid is produced by fetal urination, and one-third from pulmonary fluid.

Abnormalities of the fetal kidneys compose approximately 20% of all major fetal anomalies. Dilation of the fetal kidneys is one of the most common renal abnormalities, which is diagnosed by an increase in fluid in the anteroposterior diameter of the renal pelvis. This is commonly referred to as urinary tract dilation (formerly referred to as pyelectasis or pelviectasis). Urinary tract dilation is diagnosed when the anteroposterior diameter of the kidney is greater than 4 mm at less than 28 weeks of gestation or greater than 7 mm after 28 weeks of gestation. *Hydronephrosis* is a similiar term and includes significant calyceal dilation in addition to dilation of the renal pelvis. The fetus in Figure 146 has severe bilateral urinary tract dilation, or hydronephrosis. Hydronephrosis may be caused by transient dilation, vesicoureteral reflux, ureteropelvic junction obstruction, or ureterovesical junction obstruction. Lower urinary tract obstruction causes an enlarged fetal bladder and enlarged ureters and increased fluid in the renal pelvis. This can be caused by abnormalities in urethral valves, urethra, and other less common syndromes.

Mendez-Figueroa H, Chauhan SP. Evaluation of hydrops fetalis. In: Norton ME, Scoutt LM, Feldstein VA, editors. Callen's ultrasonography in obstetrics and gynecology. 6th ed. Elsevier; 2017. p. 633–52.

Nadel A. Ultrasound evaluation of the fetal gastrointestinal tract and abdominal wall. In: Norton ME, Scoutt LM, Feldstein VA, editors. Callen's ultrasonography in obstetrics and gynecology. 6th ed. Elsevier; 2017. p. 460–502.

Odibo AO, Dicke JM. Fetal genitourinary tract. In: Norton ME, Scoutt LM, Feldstein VA, editors. Callen's ultrasonography in obstetrics and gynecology. 6th ed. Elsevier; 2017. p. 503–38.

Ultrasound in pregnancy. Practice Bulletin No. 175. American College of Obstetricians and Gynecologists. Obstet Gynecol 2016;128:e241–56. doi: 10.1097/AOG.0000000000001815 https://journals.lww.com/greenjournal/Fulltext/2016/12000/Practice_Bulletin_No__175__Ultrasound_in_Pregnancy.53.aspx

148–151 Labor dystocia and indications for cesarean birth

For each clinical scenario (148–151), choose the best diagnosis (A–E).

(A) Arrest of dilation
(B) Protracted dilation
(C) Arrest of descent
(D) Unsuccessful induction
(E) Normal labor

148. D. A gravida 2, para 0, at term presented with prelabor rupture of membranes 24 hours ago. She has received oxytocin for 18 hours with no cervical change.

149. A. A gravida 2, para 1, at term presented in latent labor and progressed to a cervical dilation of 7 cm. Her cervix has remained unchanged for the past 6 hours despite oxytocin administration and ruptured membranes.

150. C. A gravida 1, para 0, at term presented in spontaneous labor, received an epidural, and progressed to complete dilation. After 4 hours of pushing, the fetal head remains at +2 station.

151. E. A gravida 1, para 0, at term presented in spontaneous latent labor 14 hours ago. Membranes remain intact, and cervical dilation has progressed from 2 cm on admission to 5 cm.

Labor dystocia is defined as an abnormality in the labor progress. These abnormalities may be due to insufficient expulsive effort of the uterus or maternal pushing efforts, fetal size or pelvic anatomy, or both. To reduce the incidence of primary cesarean birth, it is important to have standard definitions of labor dysfunction (Table 148–151-1).

The patient in scenario 148 has been on Pitocin with ruptured membranes for 18 hours without progress and, therefore, meets the criteria for unsuccessful induction. At this point, continued attempts at induction may lead to complications, such as intra-amniotic infection or hemorrhage, with a low chance of success.

Labor is categorized into latent and active phases. Previously, the *active phase* was defined as beginning at 4-cm cervical dilation. More current data suggest that 6 cm should be used as the threshold for active labor, because the rate of cervical change between 4 and 6 cm is slower than previously thought. Therefore, a diagnosis of active-phase arrest should not be made until the patient has achieved 6-cm cervical dilation. Cesarean birth for active-phase arrest should be performed only in the setting of 6-cm dilation with ruptured membranes, and no progressive cervical dilation with 4 hours of adequate uterine activity or 6 hours of oxytocin administration. The patient in Scenario 149 meets the criteria for arrest of dilation.

Similarly, the definition of protracted labor has changed over time. Previously, *protracted dilation* was defined as less than 1.2-cm dilation per hour in the active phase. Data from the Consortium on Safe Labor indicate that slower rates are still within the normal range and that rates as low as 0.5 cm per hour can be seen in nulliparous women.

Current recommendations for cesarean birth for arrest of descent are intended to decrease cesarean birth rates while minimizing adverse maternal and fetal outcomes. Recommendations from the Consortium on Safe Labor are to allow a second stage of at least 2 hours for multiparous patients and 3 hours for nulliparous patients. These are minimums, and longer durations can be reasonable if fetal status remains reassuring. The patient in Scenario 150 meets the criteria for arrest of descent.

It was previously thought that women undergoing induction of labor had a higher rate of cesarean birth than those with spontaneous labor. However, current data suggest that when induction is compared with expectant management, rates of cesarean birth are the same or lower in the setting of labor induction. Cesarean birth for failed induction should be reserved for cases in which the patient has had ruptured membranes for at least 12–18 hours with oxytocin administration. Allowing a latent phase of 24 hours or longer will further

TABLE 148-151-1. Recommendations for the Safe Prevention of Primary Cesarean Birth

RECOMMENDATIONS	GRADE OF RECOMMENDATIONS
FIRST STAGE OF LABOR	
A prolonged latent phase (eg, greater than 20 h in nulliparous women and greater than 14 h in multiparous women) should not be an indication for cesarean birth.	1B Strong recommendation, moderate-quality evidence
Slow but progressive labor in the first stage of labor should not be an indication for cesarean birth.	1B Strong recommendation, moderate-quality evidence
Cervical dilation of 6 cm should be considered the threshold for the active phase of most women in labor. Thus, before 6 cm of dilation is achieved, standards of active phase progress should not be applied.	1B Strong recommendation, moderate-quality evidence
Cesarean birth for active phase arrest in the first stage of labor should be reserved for women at or beyond 6 cm of dilation with ruptured membranes who fail to progress despite 4 h of adequate uterine activity, or at least 6 h of oxytocin administration with inadequate uterine activity and no cervical change.	1B Strong recommendation, moderate-quality evidence
SECOND STAGE OF LABOR	
A specific absolute maximum length of time spent in the second stage of labor beyond which all women should undergo operative delivery has not been identified.	1C Strong recommendation, low-quality evidence
Before diagnosing arrest of labor in the second stage, if the maternal and fetal conditions permit, allow for the following: • At least 2 h of pushing in multiparous women (1B) • At least 3 h of pushing in nulliparous women (1B) Longer durations may be appropriate on an individualized basis (eg, with the use of epidural analgesia or with fetal malposition) as long as progress is being documented. (1B)	1B Strong recommendation, moderate-quality evidence
Operative vaginal delivery in the second stage of labor by experienced and well-trained physicians should be considered a safe, acceptable alternative to cesarean birth. Training in, and ongoing maintenance of, practical skills related to operative vaginal delivery should be encouraged.	1B Strong recommendation, moderate-quality evidence
Manual rotation of the fetal occiput in the setting of fetal malposition in the second stage of labor is a reasonable intervention to consider before moving to operative vaginal delivery or cesarean birth. In order to safely prevent cesarean birth in the setting of malposition, it is important to assess the fetal position in the second stage of labor, particularly in the setting of abnormal fetal descent.	1B Strong recommendation, moderate-quality evidence
FETAL HEART RATE MONITORING	
Amnioinfusion for repetitive variable fetal heart rate decelerations may safely reduce the rate of cesarean birth.	1A Strong recommendation, high-quality evidence
Scalp stimulation can be used as a means of assessing fetal acid–base status when abnormal or indeterminate (formerly, nonreassuring) fetal heart patterns (eg, minimal variability) are present and is a safe alternative to cesarean birth in this setting.	1C Strong recommendation, low-quality evidence
INDUCTION OF LABOR	
Before 41 0/7 wk of gestation, induction of labor generally should be performed based on maternal and fetal medical indications. Inductions at 41 0/7 wk of gestation and beyond should be performed to reduce the risk of cesarean birth and the risk of perinatal morbidity and mortality.	1A Strong recommendation, high-quality evidence
Cervical ripening methods should be used when labor is induced in women with an unfavorable cervix.	1B Strong recommendation, moderate-quality evidence
If the maternal and fetal status allow, cesarean birth for failed induction of labor in the latent phase can be avoided by allowing longer durations of the latent phase (up to 24 h or longer) and requiring that oxytocin be administered for at least 12–18 h after membrane rupture before deeming the induction a failure.	1B Strong recommendation, moderate-quality evidence

(continued)

Table 148–151-1 *(continued)*

FETAL MALPRESENTATION	
Fetal presentation should be assessed and documented beginning at 36 0/7 wk of gestation to allow for external cephalic version to be offered.	1C Strong recommendation, low-quality evidence
SUSPECTED FETAL MACROSOMIA	
Cesarean birth to avoid potential birth trauma should be limited to estimated fetal weights of at least 5,000 g in women without diabetes and at least 4,500 g in women with diabetes. The prevalence of birth weight of 5,000 g or more is rare, and patients should be counseled that estimates of fetal weight, particularly late in gestation, are imprecise.	2C Weak recommendation, low-quality evidence
EXCESSIVE MATERNAL WEIGHT GAIN	
Women should be counseled about the IOM maternal weight guidelines in an attempt to avoid excessive weight gain.	1B Strong recommendation, moderate-quality evidence
TWIN GESTATIONS	
Perinatal outcomes for twin gestations in which the first twin is in cephalic presentation are not improved by cesarean birth. Thus, women with either cephalic/cephalic-presenting twins or cephalic/noncephalic presenting twins should be counseled to attempt vaginal delivery.	1B Strong recommendation, moderate-quality evidence
OTHER	
Individuals, organizations, and governing bodies should work to ensure that research is conducted to provide a better knowledge base to guide decisions regarding cesarean birth and to encourage policy changes that safely lower the rate of primary cesarean delivery.	1C Strong recommendation, low-quality evidence

Abbreviation: IOM, Institute of Medicine.

Reprinted from Safe prevention of the primary cesarean delivery. Obstetric Care Consensus No. 1. American College of Obstetricians and Gynecologists. Obstet Gynecol 2014;123:693–711. doi: 10.1097/01.AOG.0000444441.04111.1d https://journals.lww.com/greenjournal/Fulltext/2014/03000/Obstetric_Care_Consensus_No__1__Safe_Prevention_of.41.aspx

decrease the need for cesarean birth. The patient in Scenario 148 meets the criteria for unsuccessful induction.

In the primigravida in Scenario 151, cervical change in the latent phase is occurring at an appropriate rate, and she is having normal labor; therefore, expectant management is appropriate in this patient.

Cunningham FG, Leveno KJ, Bloom SL, Dashe JS, Hoffman BL, Casey BM, et al. Williams obstetrics. 25th ed. McGraw-Hill Education; 2018.

Safe prevention of the primary cesarean delivery. Obstetric Care Consensus No. 1. American College of Obstetricians and Gynecologists. Obstet Gynecol 2014;123:693–711. doi: 10.1097/01.AOG.0000444441.04111.1d https://journals.lww.com/greenjournal/Fulltext/2014/03000/Obstetric_Care_Consensus_No__1__Safe_Prevention_of.41.aspx

152–156 Hepatitis B testing

For each hepatitis B virus testing result (152–156), choose the most likely status (A–E).

(A) Acutely infected
(B) Chronically infected
(C) Immune because of hepatitis B vaccination
(D) Immune because of natural infection
(E) Susceptible to infection

152. E.

HBsAg	Negative
IgG anti-HBc	Negative
IgG anti-HBs	Negative

153. B.

HBsAg	Positive
IgG anti-HBc	Positive
IgM anti-HBc	Negative
IgG anti-HBs	Negative

154. A.

HBsAg	Positive
IgG anti-HBc	Positive
IgM anti-HBc	Positive
IgG anti-HBs	Negative

155. D.

HBsAg	Negative
IgG anti-HBc	Positive
IgG anti-HBs	Positive

156. C.

HBsAg	Negative
IgG anti-HBc	Negative
IgG anti-HBs	Positive

Testing for infectious diseases is a routine part of prenatal care in the United States. Pregnancy permits access to health care for many women who would not otherwise receive medical screening and intervention. Additionally, certain infectious diseases can affect maternal and neonatal outcomes in pregnancy. The goal of routine obstetric screening is to identify at-risk pregnancies and take action to prevent or minimize risks. There are effective, if not curative, therapies for human immunodeficiency virus (HIV), herpes simplex virus, syphilis, chlamydia, gonorrhea, and tuberculosis. Obstetric and pediatric interventions can help reduce the vertical transmission of HIV, herpes simplex virus, hepatitis B virus, hepatitis C virus, and chlamydia. Routine prenatal care should include screening for HIV, syphilis, hepatitis B virus, and chlamydia.

Recommendations from the Centers for Disease Control and Prevention (CDC) and the U.S. Preventive Services Task Force were published in 2020 regarding routine screening for hepatitis C virus. The CDC recommends that all pregnant patients be screened for hepatitis C in every pregnancy unless the population prevalence is less than 0.1%. The U.S. Preventive Services Task Force recommends universal screening of pregnant adults and recommends that consideration be given to screening pregnant adolescents. Screening is conducted with a serum evaluation for anti-hepatitis C virus antibodies.

Hepatitis B virus screening is performed in all women during each pregnancy, even in women who have been previously vaccinated. Repeat screening in the third trimester should be considered in patients with more than one sexual partner in the preceding 6 months, those with sexually transmitted infections since the last hepatitis B screening, recent or current intravenous drug use, or in patients with an active sexual partner who is hepatitis B surface antigen positive. Hepatitis B virus has three antigens: 1) the surface antigen (HBsAg), which is expressed on the viral surface and actively circulates in the serum during infection; 2) the core antigen (HbcAg), which is only found in the hepatocyte; and 3) the e antigen (HbeAg), which is indicative of a high viral load with active virus replication.

Screening in pregnancy is conducted with evaluation of HbsAg. The presence of the HbsAg is indicative of active infection. Patients with HbsAg who have immunoglobulin G (IgG) and immunoglobulin M (IgM) have an acute infection. The IgM anti-HBc generally clears within 6 months of the initial infection; therefore, a chronically infected patient will have persistent HbsAg but only anti-HBc (IgG) antibodies. Although not routinely evaluated, individuals with immunity to hepatitis B virus will test negative for HbsAg, because there is no active infection, but will have antibodies. Those with anti-HBc and anti-HBs antibodies are immune after a previous natural infection because only natural infection will elicit core antibodies. A patient immune from previous vaccination will demonstrate only anti-HBs antibodies.

The patient in Scenario 152 has no demonstrated antigens or antibodies, is susceptible to infection, and is a candidate for vaccination. The patient in Scenario 153 has an active infection because HbsAg is present. The IgG anti-HBc is positive, but the IgM anti-HBc is negative, indicating a chronic infection. The patient in Scenario 154 also has an active infection based on the HbsAg positivity, but the presence of IgM anti-HBc indicates an acute infection. The patient in Scenario 155 has immunity to hepatitis B based on the presence of IgG anti-HBs, but the immunity is derived from a past infection because IgG anti-HBc are also present. Finally, the patient in Scenario 156 has immunity to hepatitis B with the presence of IgG anti-HBs, but this immunity was derived from vaccination because there are no IgG anti-HBc.

American Academy of Pediatrics, American College of Obstetricians, and Gynecologists. Guidelines for perinatal care. 8th ed. AAP, ACOG; 2017.

American College of Obstetricians and Gynecologists. Routine hepatitis C virus screening in pregnant individuals. Practice Advisory. ACOG; 2021. Accessed March 3, 2022. https://www.acog.org/clinical/clinical-guidance/practice-advisory/articles/2021/05/routine-hepatitis-c-virus-screening-in-pregnant-individuals

Prenatal and perinatal human immunodeficiency virus testing. ACOG Committee Opinion No. 752. American College of Obstetricians and Gynecologists. Obstet Gynecol 2018;132:e138–42. doi: 10.1097/AOG.0000000000002825 https://journals.lww.com/greenjournal/Fulltext/2018/09000/ACOG_Committee_Opinion_No__752__Prenatal_and.70.aspx

Viral hepatitis in pregnancy. ACOG Practice Bulletin No. 86. American College of Obstetricians and Gynecologists. Obstet Gynecol 2007;110:941–56. doi: 10.1097/01.AOG.0000263930.28382.2a https://journals.lww.com/greenjournal/Citation/2007/10000/ACOG_Practice_Bulletin_No__86__Viral_Hepatitis_in.50.aspx

157–161 Maternal levels of care

For each clinical scenario 157–161, choose the minimum level of maternal care necessary given the resources anticipated (A–E).

(A) Birth center
(B) Level I
(C) Level II
(D) Level III
(E) Level IV

157. B. Uncomplicated diamniotic–dichorionic twin pregnancy at term

158. D. Anterior placenta with three previous cesarean births and ultrasound findings suspicious for a placenta accreta

159. E. Severe maternal pulmonary hypertension

160. C. Placenta previa and no previous uterine surgery

161. A. Uncomplicated antenatal course and a singleton vertex fetus in labor at 41 weeks of gestation

In the United States, maternal mortality and severe maternal morbidity have increased significantly over the last several decades. Based on data shared by maternal mortality review committees, as many as 60% of pregnancy-related deaths from 2013 to 2017 were potentially preventable. Most births in the United States occur in accredited birth centers and hospitals that offer basic and specialty maternity care, and many of these are in rural or underserved communities. The development and implementation of regionalized maternal care is critical to improving pregnancy outcomes.

Designation of maternal levels of care is an effort to improve perinatal morbidity and mortality. The guidelines help to ensure patients are cared for in facilities with adequate expertise and resources to address their medical complexity. To be effective, higher-level hospitals must facilitate patient transfer from lower-level hospitals. Outreach education is an excellent way to create a network capable of providing care for women with various medical needs across a diverse geographic area.

Data demonstrate that regionalized perinatal care provides advantages for high-risk neonates. Outcomes are better when patients with complicated conditions are treated in high-volume hospitals. Maternal mortality is decreased in areas with a larger concentration of maternal–fetal medicine subspecialists. These findings suggest a correlation between expertise and resources at delivering hospitals and outcomes for women giving birth in these facilities. Designated levels of maternal care provide direction regarding the optimal location for low-risk and high-risk care for pregnant women.

Although nomenclature about maternal care facilities has varied, the most recent consensus of the American College of Obstetricians and Gynecologists and the Society for Maternal-Fetal Medicine divide maternal care facilities into five categories (Appendix D). The first category is birth centers, and hospitals with obstetric units are identified as Levels I to IV. Birth centers are expected to provide perinatal care for low-risk, singleton, and cephalic pregnancies in a home-like environment. Each birth center should have an established relationship with local hospitals where patients can be transferred when more acute care is necessary. Regulations for birth centers vary by state.

Level I hospital facilities can provide care to women with low-risk pregnancies anticipating uncomplicated births. Emergency cesarean birth services are available, as are routine obstetric support services (eg, access to ultrasonography and anesthesia services). These facilities also are capable of stabilizing and transferring high-risk patients to another facility with an appropriate level of maternal care when needed. Level II facilities provide specialty care, including management of high-risk pregnancies in carefully selected patients. At these facilities, nurses are trained to provide more acute perinatal care, and maternal–fetal medicine consultation is readily available. Medical and surgical consultation and 24-hour, 7-day-a-week anesthesia services are available at Level II facilities.

Subspecialty care, including the comprehensive management of severe maternal and fetal complications, is available at Level III facilities. Nurses are trained to care for women with complicated and less common maternal illnesses and obstetric and fetal complications. In addition, the full range of imaging, laboratory, and consultant services are required for the care of patients with high-risk pregnancies.

In addition to the services offered at levels of care I to III, Level IV facilities have the resources and experience necessary to care for the most complex and critically ill pregnant women throughout the antepartum, intrapartum, and postpartum periods. Level IV facilities require on-site consultants in maternal–fetal medicine, as well as medical, surgical, and subspecialty consultants, to be available at all times.

Although specific outcomes data are not available, concentrating women with high-risk conditions in high-level facilities allows the physicians and staff to maintain skills and develop further expertise in the treatment of patients with complex pregnancies. Outreach education disseminates educational materials and best practices to local obstetrician–gynecologists, thus advancing the local skills and knowledge base at lower-level hospitals. Successful implementation of levels of care requires coordinated specialized services, continuing education, facilitation of transport of patients to facilities with appropriate levels of care, and data collection to assess the effect on maternal outcomes.

Levels of care should be guided by local and state regulations, national accreditation and professional organization guidelines, and identified need. Because available services and needs vary by region, one must consider how best to use this level-of-care system without creating harmful barriers to care. Travel distance, availability of a subspecialist, and third-party payer issues are examples of challenges to effective implementation that must be addressed as part of this effort. Finally, maternal and neonatal levels of care would not necessarily coincide at a given facility. The needs of the woman and fetus must be incorporated into the determination of the appropriate facilities to care for women and their newborns before, during, and after delivery.

In Scenario 157, given a twin pregnancy without other complications, a Level I center is appropriate. In Scenario 158 with antepartum concern for placenta accreta, a Level III center is optimal, given the possible need for cesarean hysterectomy and the resources anticipated for that procedure. In Scenario 159, with severe maternal pulmonary hypertension, a Level IV center with on-site pulmonary and cardiac medicine and intensive care unit specialists who routinely coordinate care with on-site maternal–fetal medicine specialists is most appropriate. In Scenario 160, given a placenta previa without previous uterine surgery, a Level II center, with obstetrician–gynecologists or maternal–fetal medicine subspecialists providing delivery services and available at all times, is best. For the patient in Scenario 161, with an uncomplicated medical and antenatal course, anticipating an uncomplicated birth in a birth center is appropriate. Appendix D, although not comprehensive, outlines the capabilities and professionals available at various levels of maternal care.

American Academy of Pediatrics, American College of Obstetricians and Gynecologists. Guidelines for perinatal care. 8th ed. AAP, ACOG; 2017.

Centers for Disease Control and Prevention. Pregnancy mortality surveillance system. CDC; 2020. Accessed February 24, 2022. https://www.cdc.gov/reproductivehealth/maternal-mortality/pregnancy-mortality-surveillance-system.htm?CDC_AA_refVal=https%3A%2F%2Fwww.cdc.gov%2Freproductivehealth%2Fmaternalinfanthealth%2Fpregnancy-mortality-surveillance-system.html

Levels of maternal care. Obstetric Care Consensus No. 9. American College of Obstetricians and Gynecologists [published erratum appears in Obstet Gynecol 2019;134:883]. Obstet Gynecol 2019;134:e41–55. doi: 10.1097/AOG.0000000000003383 https://journals.lww.com/greenjournal/pages/articleviewer.aspx?year=2019&issue=08000&article=00044&type=Fulltext

Petersen EE, Davis NL, Goodman D, Cox S, Mayes N, Johnston E, et al. Vital signs: pregnancy-related deaths, United States, 2011–2015, and strategies for prevention, 13 states, 2013–2017. MMWR Morb Mortal Wkly Rep 2019;68:423–9. doi: 10.15585/mmwr.mm6818e1 https://www.cdc.gov/mmwr/volumes/68/wr/mm6818e1.htm?s_cid=mm6818e1_w

162–166 Apgar score

For each term neonate (162–166), choose the correct Apgar score (A–E).

(A) 4
(B) 5
(C) 6
(D) 7
(E) 8

162. E. A neonate, precipitously delivered, has blue feet and hands. The heart rate is 95 beats per minute. The neonate is crying, with active movement and good respiratory effort.

163. A. A neonate, delivered by forceps, is pale and has a weak cry. The heart rate is 90 beats per minute. The neonate grimaces with weak flexion.

164. D. A neonate, delivered by breech extraction (twin B), has blue feet and hands. The heart rate has increased to 110 beats per minute. When stimulated, the infant grimaces, with some flexion, and has begun crying loudly.

165. B. A neonate was delivered by cesarean birth after an unsuccessful vacuum delivery. The infant is pale and demonstrates a weak cry. The heart rate is 105 beats per minute. There is some flexion and a grimace to stimulation.

166. C. A neonate who was delivered by cesarean birth for breech is acrocyanotic, and the heart rate is 110 beats per minute. The infant grimaces and has weak flexion. The infant demonstrates a weak cry.

Dr. Virginia Apgar devised a scoring system in 1952 intended to rapidly assess a neonate's clinical status. The Apgar score measures color, heart rate, reflexes, muscle tone, and respiration. The neonate is scored from 0 to 2 in each of these categories (Fig. 162–166-1), and the sum of the score can range from 0 to 10. Apgar scores are not used to determine the need for initial resuscitation but are useful to gauge a neonate's response to resuscitation—resuscitation should be initiated before assigning the 1-minute Apgar score.

Apgar scores typically are assessed at 1 and 5 minutes, but for neonates with a 5-minute score totaling fewer than 7 points, 10-, 15-, and 20-minute scores also are calculated. Umbilical artery cord gases may provide more information in neonates with a 5-minute Apgar score below 6 points, when available. Cord gas, pH, Pco_2, and Po_2 are stable from a clamped section of the umbilical cord for up to 90 minutes, whereas base excess and lactate should be interpreted with caution after 20 minutes. For neonates with a score of 0 points for at least 10 minutes, neonatal resuscitation guidelines deem that cessation of resuscitative efforts may be appropriate.

The Apgar score is affected by maternal sedation, congenital malformations, gestational age, and interobserver variability. It should not be used to predict adverse neurologic outcome. Although 5- and 10-minute Apgar scores of fewer than 5 points are associated with an increased risk of cerebral palsy, the risk of developing cerebral palsy in these neonates is low. In the setting of neonatal encephalopathy, 5-minute Apgar scores greater than 6 points suggest that peripartum hypoxia is not the etiology of the encephalopathy.

The neonate in Scenario 162 is assigned 1 point for color, 1 point for heart rate, and 2 points each for reflex irritability, muscle tone, and respiration, for a total of 8 points. The neonate in Scenario 163 is assigned no points for color and 1 point each for heart rate, reflex irritability, muscle tone, and respiration, for a total of 4 points. The neonate in Scenario 164 is assigned 1 point for color, 2 points each for heart rate and respiration, and 1 point each for reflex irritability and muscle tone, for a total of 7. The neonate in Scenario 165 is assigned no points for color, 2 points for heart rate, and 1 point each for reflex irritability, muscle tone, and respiration, for a total of 5 points. The neonate is Scenario 166 is assigned 1 point for color, 2 points for heart rate, and 1 point each for reflex irritability, muscle tone, and respiration, for a total of 6 points.

Apgar Score

Gestational age ________________wk

Sign	0	1	2	1 min	5 min	10 min	15 min	20 min
Color	Blue or Pale	Acrocyanotic	Completely Pink					
Heart rate	Absent	Less than 100 min	Greater than 100 min					
Reflex irritability	No Response	Grimace	Cry or Active Withdrawal					
Muscle tone	Limp	Some Flexion	Active Motion					
Respiration	Absent	Weak Cry; Hypoventilation	Good, Crying					
			Total					

Comments

Resuscitation

Minutes	1	5	10	15	20
Oxygen					
PPV/NCPAP					
ETT					
Chest Compressions					
Epinephrine					

FIGURE 162-166-1. Expanded Apgar score form. Abbreviations: ETT, endotracheal tube; PPV/NCPAP, positive-pressure ventilation/nasal continuous positive airway pressure. Record the score in the appropriate place at specific time intervals. The additional resuscitative measures (if appropriate) are recorded at the same time that the score is reported using a check mark in the appropriate box. Use the comment box to list other factors including maternal medications and/or the response to resuscitation between the recorded times of scoring. (Reprinted from The Apgar score. Committee Opinion No. 644. American College of Obstetricians and Gynecologists. Obstet Gynecol 2015;126:e52–5. doi: 10.1097/AOG.0000000000001108 https://journals.lww.com/greenjournal/Fulltext/2015/10000/Committee_Opinion_No__644__The_Apgar_Score.54.aspx)

American Academy of Pediatrics, American Heart Association. Textbook of neonatal resuscitation. 8th ed. AAP; 2021.

American College of Obstetricians and Gynecologists, American Academy of Pediatrics. Neonatal encephalopathy and neurologic outcome. 2nd ed. ACOG; AAP; 2014. https://www.acog.org/clinical/clinical-guidance/task-force-report/articles/2014/neonatal-encephalopathy-and-neurologic-outcome

167–171 Intrapartum electronic fetal monitoring

For each clinical scenario (167–171), choose the most appropriate *Eunice Kennedy Shriver* National Institute of Child Health and Human Development (NICHD) fetal heart rate tracing classification or fetal testing interpretation (A–E).

(A) Category I
(B) Category II
(C) Category III
(D) Nonreactive nonstress test (NST)
(E) Reactive NST

167. D. A 38-year-old gravida 3, para 2, at 35 weeks of gestation with hypertension and gestational diabetes mellitus presents for scheduled prenatal testing (Fig. 167–171-1).

168. A. A 17-year-old gravida 1, para 0, in triage with abdominal pain at 37 weeks of gestation is having regular uterine contractions. Her cervix is 6-cm dilated and fully effaced (Fig. 167–171-2).

169. E. A 28-year-old gravida 1, para 0, at 36 weeks of gestation and with type 1 diabetes mellitus presents for an office visit with scheduled fetal testing (Fig. 167–171-3).

170. C. A 30-year-old gravida 2, para 1, at 36 weeks of gestation presents to triage for evaluation after a low-speed motor vehicle collision. She is contracting painfully every 1–2 minutes (Fig. 167–171-4).

171. B. A 23-year-old gravida 3, para 0, is admitted in early labor with spontaneously ruptured membranes (Fig. 167–171-5).

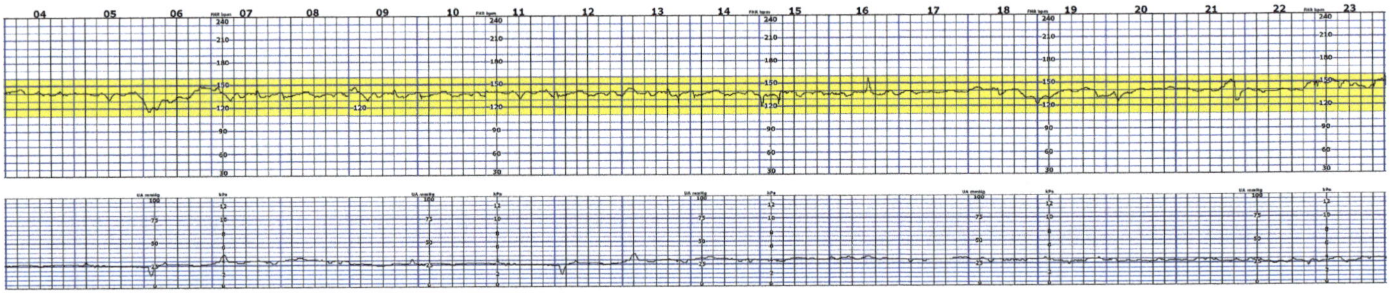

FIGURE 167-171-1. Patient's fetal heart rate tracing. (Image courtesy of James Woods, MD, and periFACTS OB/GYN Academy.)

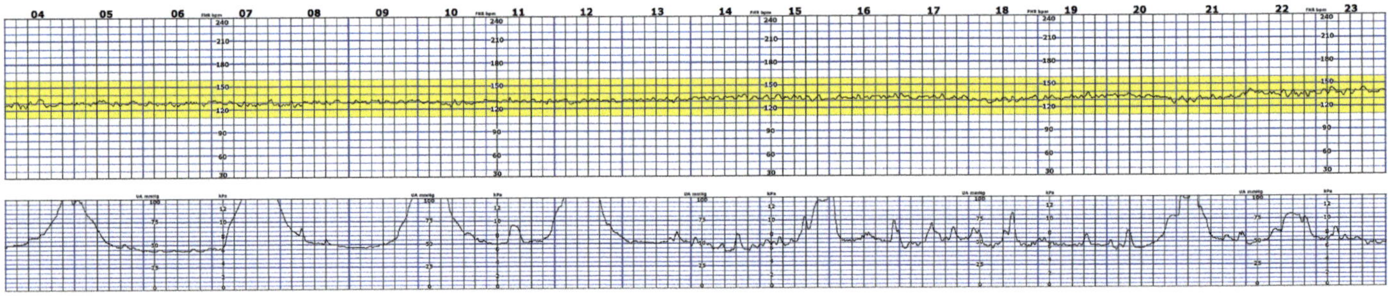

FIGURE 167-171-2. Patient's fetal heart rate tracing. (Image courtesy of James Woods, MD, and periFACTS OB/GYN Academy.)

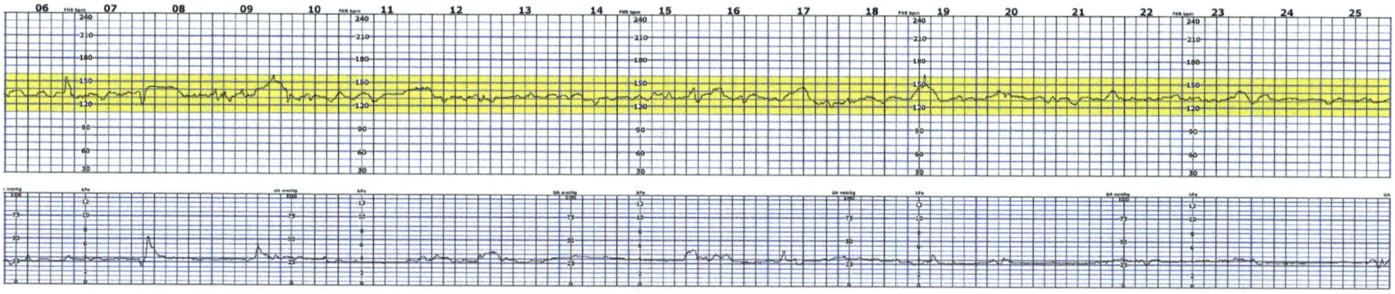

FIGURE 167-171-3. Patient's fetal heart rate tracing. (Image courtesy of James Woods, MD, and periFACTS OB/GYN Academy.)

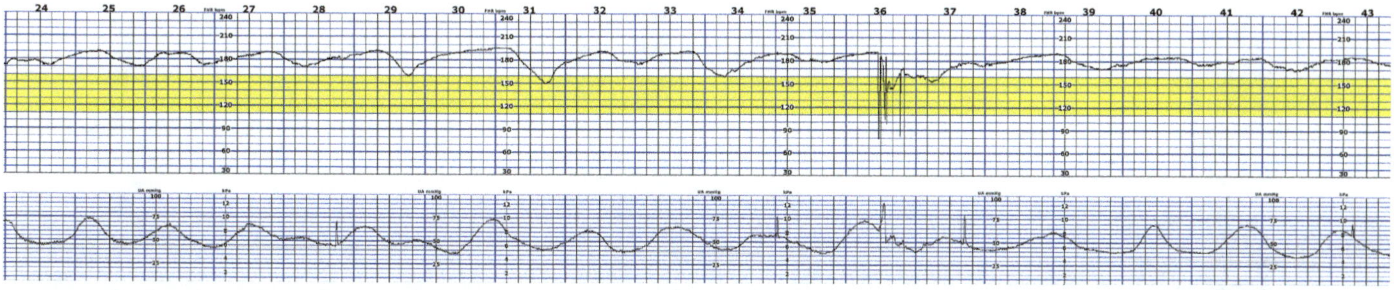

FIGURE 167-171-4. Patient's fetal heart rate tracing. (Image courtesy of James Woods, MD, and periFACTS OB/GYN Academy.)

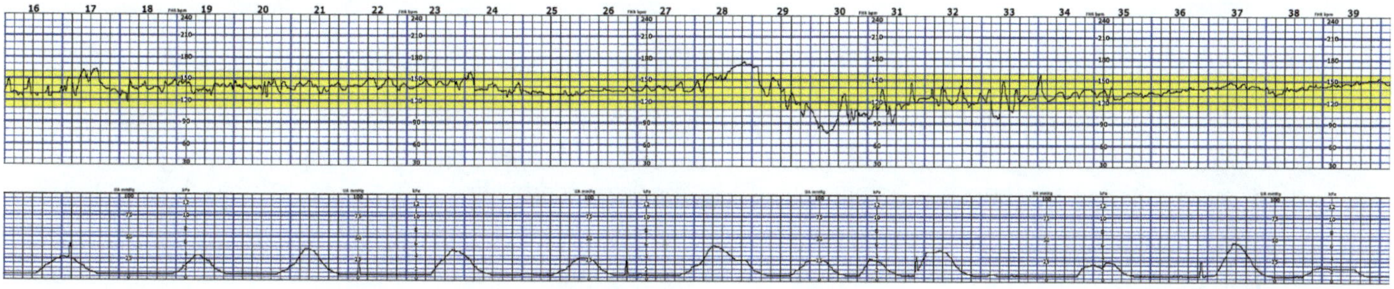

FIGURE 167-171-5. Patient's fetal heart rate tracing. (Image courtesy of James Woods, MD, and periFACTS OB/GYN Academy.)

Electronic fetal monitoring (EFM) is used widely throughout the United States for laboring patients. Although the intent of EFM at its inception was to reduce the incidence of cerebral palsy and fetal death, reliable evidence shows that its use is associated with an increase in operative vaginal delivery and cesarean birth for abnormal tracings or acidosis. The use of EFM has not been shown to reduce perinatal mortality or cerebral palsy but has reduced the risk of neonatal seizures, according to a meta-analysis of randomized clinical trials that compare EFM with intermittent auscultation of the fetal heart rate. The positive predictive value of the EFM in predicting cases of cerebral palsy is 0.14% (ie, only 1–2 out of 1,000 fetuses with non-reassuring tracings will in fact develop cerebral palsy). Given the current understanding that 70% of cases of cerebral palsy occur before the onset of labor and that only 4% of encephalopathy cases are directly attributable to intrapartum events, it is unreasonable to expect EFM to reduce the rate of cerebral palsy significantly.

A task force from the American College of Obstetricians and Gynecologists and the Society for Maternal-Fetal Medicine reaffirmed the use of electronic fetal heart rate monitoring in 2008. This task force created a three-tiered system for the interpretation and nomenclature of intrapartum fetal heart rate tracings to reduce the variety of terminology at that time for the description and reporting of intrapartum tracings and to update the understanding of interpretation with evidence-based guidelines. This system was developed for the intrapartum interpretation and reporting of EFM and is not used for patients who are not in labor. Appendix H shows a summary of the three-tiered interpretation and terminology.

An NST is conducted by monitoring the fetal heart rate for 20 minutes. A reactive NST features at least two accelerations of the fetal heart rate peaking 15 beats per minute (bpm) above the baseline during a minimum of 15 seconds. Extending the duration of the NST to 40 minutes is acceptable if accelerations are not observed, and vibroacoustic stimulation is permissible. Some modification to interpretation of the NST has been provided for fetuses at earlier gestational ages. Accelerations consisting of a fetal heart rate elevation of 10 bpm over a minimum of 10 seconds are considered sufficient for pregnancies between 24 and 32 weeks of gestation. The negative predictive value for stillbirth after a reactive NST is 99.8% (ie, a stillbirth rate of 1.9 per 1,000 gestations).

In Scenario 167, the fetal heart rate is 140 bpm with moderate variability and variable decelerations. There are not at least two accelerations lasting at least 15 seconds with a peak at least

15 bpm above baseline. This is a nonreactive NST. Because this patient is not in labor, the category system is not applicable.

In Scenario 168, the fetal heart rate is 130 bpm with moderate variability. There are no accelerations or decelerations. Because the patient is in labor, the most appropriate description of this tracing is a Category I fetal heart rate pattern.

In Scenario 169, the fetal heart rate is 130 bpm with moderate variability. There are more than two accelerations lasting at least 15 seconds with a peak at least 15 bpm above baseline. Given that this is a scenario without labor, this is best described as a reactive NST.

In Scenario 170, the fetal heart rate is 180–190 bpm, with absent variability and recurrent late decelerations. This is a Category III fetal heart rate pattern and is concerning for a placental abruption.

In Scenario 171, the fetal heart rate is 140 bpm with moderate variability and a variable deceleration. Given that the patient is in early labor, this is a Category II fetal heart rate pattern.

Intrapartum fetal heart rate monitoring: nomenclature, interpretation, and general management principles. ACOG Practice Bulletin No. 106. American College of Obstetricians and Gynecologists. Obstet Gynecol 2009;114:192–202. doi: 10.1097/AOG.0b013e3181aef106 https://journals.lww.com/greenjournal/Citation/2009/07000/ACOG_Practice_Bulletin_No__106__Intrapartum_Fetal.51.aspx

Management of intrapartum fetal heart rate tracings. Practice Bulletin No. 116. American College of Obstetricians and Gynecologists. Obstet Gynecol 2010;116:1232–40. doi: 10.1097/AOG.0b013e3182004fa9 https://journals.lww.com/greenjournal/Citation/2010/11000/Practice_Bulletin_No__116__Management_of.53.aspx

Timmins AE, Clark SL. How to approach intrapartum category II tracings. Obstet Gynecol Clin North Am 2015;42:363–75. doi: 10.1016/j.ogc.2015.01.013 https://www.obgyn.theclinics.com/article/S0889-8545(15)00027-3/fulltext

172–175 Preterm prelabor rupture of membranes

A 33-year-old gravida 3, para 2, is admitted at 34 weeks of gestation with preterm prelabor rupture of membranes (PPROM). Both of her previous births were vaginal deliveries. The biophysical profile is 10/10. The patient is not experiencing contractions or vaginal bleeding. She is afebrile, and there is no uterine tenderness. She expresses concern regarding neonatal intensive care unit admission. Continued expectant management until 37 weeks could have the following effect (A–C) on the listed morbidities (172–175).

(A) Increased
(B) Decreased
(C) Unchanged

172. A. Maternal hemorrhage

173. B. Neonatal respiratory distress

174. C. Neonatal sepsis

175. A. Maternal infection

Preterm prelabor rupture of membranes is defined as rupture of membranes before 37 weeks of completed gestation. Preterm prelabor rupture of membranes complicates approximately 2–3% of all pregnancies in the United States and accounts for a significant portion of preterm births.

Management decisions depend on gestational age and evaluation of the relative risks of delivery versus the risks of expectant management (eg, infection, placental abruption, umbilical cord accident, and stillbirth) when pregnancy is allowed to progress to a later gestational age. These include risks to the woman and fetus.

In the setting of PPROM, birth occurs within 1 week of membrane rupture in more than 50% of patients. Intra-amniotic infection occurs in 15–35% of women, and postpartum infection occurs in approximately 15–25% of women. Placental abruption is less common, occurring in 2–5% of pregnancies.

The most important risks to the fetus after PPROM are the complications of prematurity. These include respiratory distress, sepsis, intraventricular hemorrhage, and necrotizing enterocolitis. In addition, PPROM has been associated with an increased risk of neurodevelopmental impairment and neonatal white matter damage. There is no clear evidence that immediate delivery after presentation with PPROM will prevent these complications. A large cohort study published in 2017 suggested that prolonged latency duration, when adjusted for gestational age, does not worsen neonatal prognosis in terms of survival, survival without morbidity, and early-onset sepsis. In the setting of PPROM, delivery is indicated when intra-amniotic infection is diagnosed, if there is a significant placental abruption, or if the fetal heart rate tracing is non-reassuring.

A meta-analysis of 12 randomized control trials published in 2017 concluded there was evidence to guide clinical practice toward expectant management versus immediate delivery in the setting of PPROM. Although there were no differences in neonatal sepsis between women who gave birth immediately compared with those who chose expectant management, immediate delivery carried a higher risk to neonates for respiratory distress, the need for ventilation, neonatal mortality, neonatal intensive care unit admission, and the likelihood of cesarean birth.

Many centers have recommended immediate delivery for all women if PPROM occurs between 34 and 37 weeks of gestation. A large randomized trial published in 2018 evaluated immediate delivery versus expectant management in patients with PPROM between 34 and 37 weeks of gestation and found some benefits associated with expectant management. There was no significant difference in the primary outcome (neonatal sepsis) or the secondary outcome (composite neonatal morbidity); however, neonates who were delivered immediately had increased rates of respiratory distress and mechanical ventilation, as well as increased hospitalization durations. With expectant management there was an increased risk of adverse maternal outcomes, including hemorrhage and infection.

In the setting of PPROM, hospitalized observation is optimal to allow careful monitoring for signs or symptoms of infection, labor, or placental abruption. Care should be individualized, and patients should be thoroughly counseled with an emphasis on shared decision making.

In the scenario above, expectant management is a reasonable option. The patient should be counseled about the potential increased risks of maternal infection and hemorrhage and the decreased risk of neonatal respiratory distress syndrome.

Lorthe E, Ancel PY, Torchin H, Kaminski M, Langer B, Subtil D, et al. Impact of latency duration on the prognosis of preterm infants after preterm premature rupture of membranes at 24 to 32 weeks' gestation: a national population-based cohort study. J Pediatr 2017;182:47–52.e2. doi: 10.1016/j.jpeds.2016.11.074 https://www.jpeds.com/article/S0022-3476(16)31382-8/fulltext

Medically indicated late-preterm and early-term deliveries. ACOG Committee Opinion No. 831. American College of Obstetricians and Gynecologists. Obstet Gynecol 2021;138:e35–9. doi: 10.1097/AOG.0000000000004447 https://journals.lww.com/greenjournal/Fulltext/2021/07000/Medically_Indicated_Late_Preterm_and_Early_Term.38.aspx

Prelabor rupture of membranes. ACOG Practice Bulletin No. 217. American College of Obstetricians and Gynecologists. Obstet Gynecol 2020;135:e80–97. doi: 10.1097/AOG.0000000000003700 https://journals.lww.com/greenjournal/Fulltext/2020/03000/Prelabor_Rupture_of_Membranes__ACOG_Practice.47.aspx

Quist-Nelson J, de Ruigh AA, Seidler AL, van der Ham DP, Willekes C, Berghella V, et al. Immediate delivery compared with expectant management in late preterm prelabor rupture of membranes: an individual participant data meta-analysis. Preterm Premature Rupture of Membranes Meta-analysis (PPROMM) Collaboration. Obstet Gynecol 2018;131:269–79. doi: 10.1097/AOG.0000000000002447 https://journals.lww.com/greenjournal/Fulltext/2018/02000/Immediate_Delivery_Compared_With_Expectant.11.aspx

176–179 COVID-19 pandemic population health effects

For each of the following diagnoses (176–179), choose whether the diagnosis prevalence decreased, increased, or was unchanged (A–C) during the first year of the COVID-19 pandemic.

(A) Decreased
(B) Increased
(C) Unchanged

176. A. Influenza

177. B. Opioid overdose

178. C. Stillbirth

179. B. Postpartum depression

The global COVID-19 pandemic was declared in March 2020, and population-level infection control measures were instituted soon after. Distancing between people, face coverings, and increased hand washing were recommended to reduce the spread of severe acute respiratory syndrome coronavirus 2 (SARS-CoV-2), the causative agent of COVID-19. In the United States, local and state governments instituted lockdowns and business closures, varying in degree based on locality. Social isolation increased with these stay-at-home orders, and these individual measures may be associated with unintended effects on the obstetric population.

Because the infection control methods were intended to reduce transmission of a respiratory virus, it remains highly likely that this was the cause of the reduction in the number of cases of influenza during the 2020 influenza season. Following initiation of the above recommendations, the percentage of respiratory specimens positive for influenza fell from approximately 20% to 1–2% over the course of the pandemic. Australia also instituted similar guidelines to reduce the spread of COVID-19 and saw similar decreases in influenza rates.

Lockdown and stay-at-home orders increased the social isolation experienced by many people. Visit rates for mental health conditions, suicide attempts, and drug and opioid overdoses were higher from March through October 2020 compared with the same time period in 2019. This increase in social isolation also was found in postpartum women, who experienced a higher degree of postpartum depression and anxiety as reflected in change in scores on the Edinburgh Postpartum Depression Scale during the pandemic. This effect was not limited to the United States. Patients studied in China and Italy experienced the increased risk of perinatal depression and anxiety, and depressive rates were positively associated with the numbers of new infections and deaths per day being reported. Thoughts of self-harm also increased during the pandemic, and this was compounded by health care systems that were burdened with the ongoing pandemic and potentially had fewer resources to treat these women.

Willingness to seek in-person care also may have decreased during the pandemic, with fewer pregnant women seeking early care for potential complications because of fear of contracting SARS-CoV-2, and fewer women attending prenatal visits in-person or undergoing assessments for antenatal surveillance. Modeling of the indirect effects of the pandemic has estimated a reduction in antepartum and postpartum care of 18% and 52%, respectively. The effects of the pandemic on prenatal care and access were seen in low-resource countries as well, where misinformation and fears about contracting the virus led to a significant number of patients foregoing any prenatal care at all. The result of these decreased visits may have contributed to the initial reports of increased stillbirth rates during the COVID-19 pandemic. However, as more data became available through broader administrative datasets, the risk of stillbirth in the general population was unchanged in the first year after the pandemic in the U.S. (0.58% pre-pandemic and 0.64% in the first post-pandemic year). Stillbirth rates did increase for patients infected with COVID-19. In the pre-Delta variant period, the risk of stillbirth was 0.98% for COVID-19-affected pregnancies (adjusted risk, 1.47), further increasing to 2.7% during the Delta wave (adjusted risk ratio, 4.04). The highest risk appears to be among patients with chronic hypertension, multiple gestation, placental abruption, maternal cardiac event, sepsis, shock, acute respiratory distress syndrome, mechanical ventilation, or intensive care unit admission.

The direct effects of COVID-19 infection on pregnancy are becoming clearer as the pandemic continues and more pregnant women are infected. Pregnant individuals are expected to have the same rate of an asymptomatic or mild infection of COVID-19 compared with nonpregnant patients. However, pregnant women with severe disease are at a high risk of admission to the intensive care unit, mechanical ventilation, stillbirth, and maternal death. One of the most common obstetric complications from having COVID-19 is preterm birth, but it appears to be iatrogenic among patients with moderate to severe disease. The rate of cesarean birth is also higher in these patients, although the reason is unclear from systematic reviews. Cesarean birth is not recommended for the indication of COVID-19 but may be due to more aggressive management early in the pandemic or iatrogenic preterm deliveries for patients with respiratory failure. Possible associations with complications, such as fetal growth restriction and preeclampsia, are less clear.

A prospective study found pregnant patients with severe COVID-19 may present with a preeclampsia-like syndrome with abnormal ratios of soluble fms-like tyrosine kinase 1 to placental growth factor (sFLT/PIGF) and uterine artery Doppler, which may explain some of the overlap in symptoms. Fortunately, vertical transmission seems rare, and the pathophysiology of transmission remains unclear at the time of publication. Breast milk is not suspected to cause neonatal infection, and maternal antibodies have been found in breast milk samples of infected women. Reduction in neonatal transmission should be done through masking and meticulous handwashing.

DeSisto CL, Wallace B, Simeone RM, Polen K, Ko JY, Meaney-Delman D, et al. Risk for stillbirth among women with and without COVID-19 at delivery hospitalization—United States, March 2020–September 2021. MMWR Morb Mortal Wkly Rep 2021;70:1640–5. doi: 10.15585/mmwr.mm7047e1 https://www.cdc.gov/mmwr/volumes/70/wr/mm7047e1.htm

Holland KM, Jones C, Vivolo-Kantor AM, Idaikkadar N, Zwald M, Hoots B, et al. Trends in US emergency department visits for mental health, overdose, and violence outcomes before and during the COVID-19 pandemic. JAMA Psychiatry 2021;78:372–9. doi: 10.1001/jamapsychiatry.2020.4402 https://jamanetwork.com/journals/jamapsychiatry/fullarticle/2775991

Khalil A, von Dadelszen P, Draycott T, Ugwumadu A, O'Brien P, Magee L. Change in the incidence of stillbirth and preterm delivery during the COVID-19 pandemic. JAMA 2020;324:705–6. doi: 10.1001/jama.2020.12746 https://jamanetwork.com/journals/jama/fullarticle/2768389

Kotlar B, Gerson E, Petrillo S, Langer A, Tiemeier H. The impact of the COVID-19 pandemic on maternal and perinatal health: a scoping review. Reprod Health 2021;18:10–6. doi: 10.1186/s12978-021-01070-6 https://reproductive-health-journal.biomedcentral.com/articles/10.1186/s12978-021-01070-6

Olsen SJ, Azziz-Baumgartner E, Budd AP, Brammer L, Sullivan S, Pineda RF, et al. Decreased influenza activity during the COVID-19 pandemic—United States, Australia, Chile, and South Africa, 2020. MMWR Morb Mortal Wkly Rep 2020;69:1305–9. doi: 10.15585/mmwr.mm6937a6 https://www.cdc.gov/mmwr/volumes/69/wr/mm6937a6.htm?s_cid=mm6937a6_w

Perzow SED, Hennessey EP, Hoffman MC, Grote NK, Davis EP, Hankin BL. Mental health of pregnant and postpartum women in response to the COVID-19 pandemic. J Affect Disord Rep 2021;4:100123. doi: 10.1016/j.jadr.2021.100123 https://www.ncbi.nlm.nih.gov/pmc/articles/PMC7904453/

180–184 Preeclampsia and its imitators

For each of the following clinical scenarios (180–184), choose the most likely diagnosis (A–E).

(A) Acute fatty liver of pregnancy
(B) COVID-19
(C) HELLP (hemolysis, elevated liver enzymes, and low platelet count) syndrome
(D) Preeclampsia with severe features
(E) Systemic lupus erythematosus (SLE) flare

180. C. A primigravida presents for a routine prenatal visit at 41 weeks of gestation. She has noticed increased fatigue and severe headache over the past 2 days. On physical examination, she has bilateral lower-extremity pitting edema and clonus. Her blood pressure is 160/105 mm Hg. Laboratory studies show a white blood cell count of 10.4×10^9/L, platelet count of 52,000/mm^3, hemoglobin of 9.6 mg/dL, creatinine of 1.0 mg/dL, serum alanine aminotransferase of 88 units/L, lactate dehydrogenase of 722 units/L, and total urine protein–creatinine ratio of 0.25.

181. B. A patient at 29 weeks of gestation presents to the emergency department with malaise for 3 days, headache, and cough. She is lethargic and has difficulty breathing. Vital signs are a temperature of 38.4 °C (101.1 °F), blood pressure of 130/90 mm Hg, pulse of 130 beats per minute, and respiratory rate of 24 breaths per minute. Her pulse oximetry is 92% on room air. Chest X-ray shows bilateral opacities. Laboratory studies show a white blood cell count of 12.0×10^9/L, platelet count of 110,000/mm^3, hemoglobin of 8.2 mg/dL, creatinine of 1.2 mg/dL, and serum alanine aminotransferase of 62 units/L.

182. A. A multigravida at 37 weeks of gestation presents with malaise, nausea, and decreased fetal movement for 24 hours. She appears ill. Her temperature is normal, blood pressure is 140/80 mm Hg, and pulse is 114 bpm. She has right upper quadrant pain with scleral icterus. Laboratory studies show a white blood cell count of 14.3×10^9/L, platelet count of 120,000/mm^3, creatinine of 1.3 mg/dL, glucose of 49 mg/dL, and serum alanine aminotransferase of 450 units/L. The urine protein–creatinine ratio is 0.32. Fetal cardiac activity is absent on ultrasonography.

183. D. A primigravida at 29 weeks of gestation presents with an unrelenting headache and difficulty breathing. Her temperature is 36.8 °C (98.2 °F), blood pressure is 180/110 mm Hg, respiratory rate is 23 breaths per minute, and pulse oximetry is 95% on room air. She has bilateral crackles on her pulmonary examination. Laboratory studies show a white blood cell count of 12.4×10^9/L, platelet count of 95,000/mm^3, hemoglobin of 13.2 mg/dL, creatinine of 1.1 mg/dL, serum alanine aminotransferase of 24 units/L, lactate dehydrogenase of 450 units/L, and urine protein–creatinine ratio of 0.5. Chest X-ray shows pulmonary edema with bilateral pleural effusions.

184. E. A 23-year-old gravida 4, para 0, at 21 weeks of gestation presents with severe headache and confusion. Her temperature is 37.0 °C (98.6 °F), and blood pressure is 150/94 mm Hg. On physical examination, there is lower-extremity pitting edema to the hips. Computed tomography of the head is negative for thrombus or mass. Laboratory studies show white blood cell count of 4.5×10^9/L, platelets count of 87,000/mm^3, hemoglobin of 11.4 mg/dL, creatinine of 1.9 mg/dL, serum aspartate aminotransferase of 30 units/L, and urine protein–creatinine ratio of 4.6. Urinalysis shows 4+ protein, erythrocytes 6/HPF, and granular and hyaline casts. Serial laboratory tests and symptoms are stable over 24 hours.

The incidence of preeclampsia is approximately 2–8% worldwide, but other disease processes can mimic the presentation of preeclampsia in several clinical scenarios. Full consideration of laboratory values, vital signs, and clinical presentation will allow for an accurate diagnosis and appropriate treatment.

Patient 180 is a primigravida and is in late-term pregnancy, which increases the risk of hypertensive disease of pregnancy (Table 180–184-1). She has severe-range blood pressure exhibited by systolic blood pressure greater than 160 mm Hg (the diastolic blood pressure is in the mild range at less than 110 mm Hg). She has lower-extremity edema and clonus, but these are not considered part of the diagnostic criteria for preeclampsia with severe features, although her headache is. Laboratory values are notable for hemolysis (low hemoglobin and lactate dehydrogenase greater than 600 units/L), low platelet count (less than 100,000/mm^3), and elevated liver enzymes that are twice the upper limit of normal. Proteinuria is not required to meet diagnostic criteria for HELLP (hemolysis, elevated liver enzymes, and low platelet count) syndrome. This patient meets the full diagnostic criteria for HELLP syndrome, although hemolysis may not always be present and may be considered partial HELLP syndrome. Treatment includes delivery, with cesarean birth reserved for typical obstetric indications, seizure prophylaxis with magnesium sulfate infusion, and antihypertensives within 30 minutes of sustained severe-range blood pressure (greater than 160/110 mm Hg). Hemolysis, elevated liver enzymes, and low platelet count syndrome may have an atypical presentation, with up to 15% of cases without associated proteinuria or hypertension.

Patient 181 presents with fever, cough, and respiratory distress more consistent with an infectious process than with preeclampsia. Although she has a mild thrombocytopenia and mildly elevated blood pressure, her chest X-ray is consistent with pneumonia. Fever is not expected in preeclampsia with severe features. This patient's symptoms are most consistent with COVID-19 pneumonia. The approach to treatment for COVID-19 pneumonia in pregnancy is the same as in the nonobstetric population.

Patient 182 has symptoms suspicious for liver involvement given her malaise, vomiting, and jaundice. She has mild-range

TABLE 180-184-1. Differential Diagnosis of Hypertensive Disease in Pregnancy

	GESTATIONAL HTN/ PREECLAMPSIA WITHOUT SEVERE FEATURES	PREECLAMPSIA WITH SEVERE FEATURES	HELLP SYNDROME	ACUTE FATTY LIVER OF PREGNANCY	COVID-19	SLE FLARE
Gestational age at onset (weeks)	Greater than 20	Greater than 20	Greater than 20	Greater than 20	Any	Any
Symptoms	Asymptomatic	Headache, visual changes, abdominal pain, pulmonary edema, oliguria, seizures with eclampsia	Asymptomatic or headache, visual changes, abdominal pain, pulmonary edema, oliguria	Malaise, lethargy, jaundice, headache, abdominal pain, nausea/ vomiting, agitation, confusion	Cough, fever, sore throat, difficulty breathing, vomiting, diarrhea, headache	Headache, joint pain, rash
Blood pressure	↑	↑↑/↑↑↑	↑/↑↑↑	↑	↓/↑	Normal/↑
Fever	No	No	No	Possible	Yes	No
Platelets	Normal	Normal/↓↓	↓↓	Normal/↓	Normal/↓↓	Normal/↓↓
Liver enzymes	Normal	Normal/↑↑	↑↑	↑↑↑	↑↑	Normal/↑↑
LDH	Normal	Normal/↑↑	↑↑	Normal/↑↑		Normal/↑↑
Bilirubin	Normal	Normal/↑↑	Normal/↑↑	↑↑		Normal
Glucose	Normal	Normal	Normal	↓↓	Normal	Normal
Ammonia	Normal	Normal	Normal	↑	Normal	Normal
Proteinuria	Normal (GHTN)/↑↑ (preeclampsia without severe features)	Normal (if other symptoms present)/↑↑↑	Normal/↑↑↑	Normal/↑↑	Normal	Normal/↑↑↑ (also hematuria)
Pulmonary edema	No	Possible	Possible	No	Usually no, ground-glass opacities in pneumonia	Possible

Abbreviations: HELLP, hemolysis, elevated liver enzymes, low platelet count; HTN, hypertension; LDH, lactate dehydrogenase; SLE, systemic lupus erythematosus.

blood pressure with elevated creatinine, liver enzymes, and proteinuria that would suggest preeclampsia with severe features. However, this diagnosis is not consistent with hypoglycemia. This makes the most likely diagnosis acute fatty liver of pregnancy. An elevated ammonia level would also be consistent with this diagnosis. Acute fatty liver of pregnancy and HELLP syndrome have overlapping clinical presentation and laboratory findings, but the jaundice and hypoglycemia make acute fatty liver of pregnancy the more appropriate diagnosis, present in 70% and 90% of cases, respectively. Acute fatty liver of pregnancy is a rare, but potentially life-threatening, disease for the patient and fetus.

Patient 183 presents with severe features of preeclampsia (headache, severe range blood pressures, and thrombocytopenia). She does not have hemolysis or transaminitis, which would have given her a diagnosis of HELLP syndrome. Although she also has respiratory symptoms, chest X-ray findings are not consistent with pneumonia, but rather pulmonary edema, also a severe feature of preeclampsia.

Patient 184 is a gravida 4 without any live births who presents just after 20 weeks of gestation with hypertension. She has no history of chronic hypertension, and because she is beyond 20 weeks of gestation, another cause should be sought. Her headache and elevated creatinine could be suggestive of preeclampsia with severe features, but her joint pain and confusion are not consistent with this diagnosis, and preeclampsia at 21 weeks of gestation is rare. In this scenario, the fact that she has hyaline casts in her urine with stable laboratory values over a course of observation makes her presentation suspicious for SLE flare. Consideration should also be given to evaluation for antiphospholipid syndrome given her history of recurrent pregnancy loss.

Systemic lupus erythematosus may have its initial presentation in pregnancy, and it is important to discern the difference between an SLE flare and preeclampsia with severe features because the management is not the same. A new diagnosis of lupus or recurrent SLE flare can be treated with immune modulators or corticosteroids, and laboratory findings will usually improve with treatment. Complement levels may be useful if baseline levels are known, because they can decrease during an active SLE flare. However, they may be mildly reduced in preeclampsia as well, and should be considered an adjunctive, but not necessarily diagnostic, test in the evaluation of the patient. Conversely, complement levels are likely most helpful in their negative predictive value, as normal complement levels rule out an acute lupus flare. There is no one laboratory test that can differentiate SLE from preeclampsia because both diseases can exist concurrently and have similar laboratory derangements. The clinical context is important in these cases, and often a short period of observation, with or without treatment with corticosteroids, may clarify the diagnosis.

Gestational hypertension and preeclampsia. ACOG Practice Bulletin No. 222. American College of Obstetricians and Gynecologists. Obstet Gynecol 2020;135:e237–60. doi: 10.1097/AOG.0000000000003891 https://journals.lww.com/greenjournal/Fulltext/2020/06000/Gestational_Hypertension_and_Preeclampsia__ACOG.46.aspx

Halscott T, Vaught J. Society for Maternal–Fetal Medicine management considerations for pregnant patients with COVID-19. SMFM COVID-19 Task Force. 2021. https://s3.amazonaws.com/cdn.smfm.org/media/2734/SMFM_COVID_Management_of_COVID_pos_preg_patients_2-2-21_(final).pdf

Loscalzo J, Fauci AS, Kasper DL, Hauser S, Longo D, Jameson JL. Harrison's principles of internal medicine. 21st ed. McGraw-Hill Companies; 2022.

Resnik R, Lockwood CJ, Moore TR, Greene ME, Copel JA, Silver RM, editors. Creasy and Resnik's maternal–fetal medicine: principles and practice. 8th ed. Elsevier; 2018.

Vigil-de Gracia P, Montufar-Rueda C. Acute fatty liver of pregnancy: diagnosis, treatment, and outcome based on 35 consecutive cases. J Matern Fetal Neonatal Med 2011;24:1143–6. doi: 10.3109/14767058.2010.531325 https://www.tandfonline.com/doi/abs/10.3109/14767058.2010.531325

185–188 Ultrasonographic findings of common aneuploidy

For each second-trimester fetal ultrasound finding (185–188), choose the most likely abnormal fetal karyotype (A–D).

(A) 69,XXY
(B) 45,X
(C) 47,XY (+21)
(D) 47,XX (+18)

185. B. Cystic hygroma

186. A. Large cystic placenta

187. D. Omphalocele

188. C. Thickened nuchal fold

Second-trimester ultrasonography is an important component of screening for fetal chromosomal abnormalities. Ultrasonography can identify structural abnormalities that may be associated with an abnormal karyotype. All pregnant women should be offered screening for chromosomal abnormalities, including second-trimester ultrasonography.

Cystic hygroma, an enlarged hypoechoic space extending along the length of the fetal back with clearly visible septations, is thought to result from abnormal fetal lymphatic drainage. Cystic hygromas may be seen in the first or second trimester and are associated with a high rate of fetal aneuploidy (50–70%). In the first trimester, cystic hygroma is equally likely to be associated with 45,X and trisomy 21; however, when cystic hygromas are diagnosed in aneuploid fetuses in the second trimester, nearly 75% have Turner syndrome (45,X). Cystic hygroma generally is not associated with triploidy (69,XXY) or trisomy 18.

There are three different presentations of Turner syndrome: 1) first-trimester abortion (98%), 2) second-trimester hydrops fetalis resulting in fetal death, and 3) a fetus with cystic hygroma. Ultrasound findings associated with Turner syndrome include renal anomalies; cardiac anomalies, including coarctation of the aorta and hypoplastic left heart; and short femur. In the scenario above of a cystic hygroma on second-trimester ultrasound, 45,X (Turner syndrome) is the most likely karyotype.

Triploidy (69,XXY), a complete extra set of chromosomes, occurs in approximately 1–3% of fertilizations, most of which are spontaneous abortions. It is estimated that only 3% of triploid pregnancies survive to being recognized pregnancies, and triploidy generally is believed to be lethal.

Triploidy occurs from fertilization of 1) one oocyte by two sperm (dispermy), 2) one oocyte by diploid sperm (diandry), or 3) diploid oocyte by one sperm (digyny). Two distinct phenotypes of triploid fetuses have been described, and they differ based on the parental origin of the extra set of chromosomes. Type I triploidy of paternal origin (dispermy or diandry) results in a normally grown fetus with a normal head size and a large, cystic placenta (69,XXY). In general, normal placental thickness is approximately 1 mm per week of gestational age; greater than 4-cm thick always is considered abnormal. This type of triploidy also is known as a partial molar pregnancy. Type II triploidy, which is of maternal origin (dygyny), usually presents as a growth-restricted fetus with a large head and a normal-appearing but small placenta. Multiple additional anomalies, including craniofacial abnormalities, syndactyly, cardiac defects, abnormal genitalia, and brain anomalies, also may be found. Triploidy is not commonly associated with cystic hygroma, omphalocele, or thickened nuchal fold; therefore, large cystic placenta is most likely associated with the 69,XXY karyotype (triploidy).

Omphalocele is a midline, membrane-covered abdominal wall defect in which bowel, liver, or both, herniate into the base of the umbilical cord. Umbilical vessels typically insert into the membrane and can be seen coursing through the omphalocele sac. Omphaloceles with defects greater than 5 cm often contain the liver or other abdominopelvic organs. Smaller defects usually contain only the small bowel. Omphalocele is strongly associated with structural and chromosomal abnormalities with rates ranging from 15% to 45%, depending on the study. The most associated aneuploidy is trisomy 18. Although about 20% of fetuses with trisomy 18 have omphalocele, 62–78% of aneuploid fetuses with omphalocele have trisomy 18. Aneuploidy and other syndromes occur more commonly in fetuses with smaller omphaloceles without liver herniation. Although fetuses with larger, liver-containing omphaloceles may be at lower risk of chromosomal abnormalities or syndrome, they are at risk of significant morbidity and mortality because of the omphalocele itself. Omphalocele rarely is associated with trisomy 21, triploidy, or Turner syndrome. Therefore, for the second-trimester ultrasound finding of omphalocele, the most likely karyotype is 47,XY (+18) (trisomy 18).

Multiple soft markers have been described to improve ultrasonographic detection of trisomy 21 in high-risk women. Nuchal fold thickness of 6 mm or greater is considered a strong predictive marker for trisomy 21, with a likelihood ratio of 49. The nuchal fold is measured in a standard posterior fossa view of the fetal head. The distance is measured between calipers placed at the outer edge of the occipital bone and the outer skin edge. As with nuchal translucency, the risk of fetal aneuploidy increases with increasing nuchal fold. Thickened nuchal fold also may be associated with cardiac abnormalities. Triploidy, trisomy 18, and Turner syndrome generally are not associated with thickened nuchal fold. Therefore, in the case of second-trimester ultrasonography with thickened nuchal fold, the most likely karyotype is 47,XY (+21) (trisomy 21).

When structural anomalies or soft sonographic markers are identified on second-trimester ultrasonography, the risk of chromosomal abnormality associated with each finding should be considered within the complete clinical context. The patient should be counseled regarding the risk of aneuploidy associated with the finding, and diagnostic testing with amniocentesis or screening testing with cell-free DNA or quad screen should be offered. Patients may also be offered genetic counseling and maternal–fetal medicine consultation. This is recommended if more than one marker is identified, or if screening or diagnostic testing is abnormal.

Aagaard-Tillery KM, Malone FD, Nyberg DA, Porter TF, Cuckle HS, Fuchs K et al. Role of second-trimester genetic sonography after Down syndrome screening. Obstet Gynecol 2009;114:1189–96. doi: 10.1097/AOG.0b013e3181c15064 https://journals.lww.com/greenjournal/Fulltext/2009/12000/Role_of_Second_Trimester_Genetic_Sonography_After.6.aspx

Afshar Y, Platt LD. Turner syndrome (monosomy X). In: Copel JA, D'Alton ME, Feltovich H, Gratacós E, Krakow D, Odibo AO, et al, editors. Obstetric imaging: fetal diagnosis and care. 2nd ed. Elsevier; 2018. p. 613–7.

Gainer JA. Triploidy. In: Copel JA, D'Alton ME, Feltovich H, Gratacós E, Krakow D, Odido AO, et al, editors. Obstetric imaging: fetal diagnosis and care. 2nd ed. Elsevier; 2018. p. 598–602.

Marshall J, Salemi JL, Tanner JP, Ramakrishnan R, Feldkamp ML, Marengo LK, et al. Prevalence, correlates, and outcomes of omphalocele in the United States, 1995–2005. National Birth Defects Prevention Network. Obstet Gynecol 2015;126:284–93. doi: 10.1097/AOG.0000000000000920 https://journals.lww.com/greenjournal/pages/articleviewer.aspx?year=2015&issue=08000&article=00010&type=Fulltext

Screening for fetal chromosomal abnormalities: ACOG Practice Bulletin No. 226. American College of Obstetricians and Gynecologists. Obstet Gynecol 2020;136:e48–69. doi: 10.1097/AOG.0000000000004084 https://journals.lww.com/greenjournal/Fulltext/2020/10000/Screening_for_Fetal_Chromosomal_Abnormalities_.44.aspx

189–192 Antepartum fetal surveillance

For each clinical scenario (189–192), choose the most appropriate timing of antepartum fetal surveillance with nonstress test or biophysical profile (A–D).

(A) No ongoing surveillance
(B) Once weekly
(C) Twice weekly
(D) Once weekly plus once-weekly umbilical artery Doppler assessment

189. A. A 26-year-old gravida 1 at 34 weeks of gestation was found to have a maximum vertical pocket of amniotic fluid of 8.5 cm and amniotic fluid index of 26 cm on ultrasonographic evaluation. She has had an otherwise uncomplicated pregnancy.

190. D. A 29-year-old gravida 1 at 33 weeks of gestation underwent ultrasonographic evaluation for the finding of a fundal height of 29 cm. The estimated fetal weight was at the 12th percentile, and the abdominal circumference was at the 5th percentile.

191. B. A 36-year-old gravida 2, para 1, is at 33 weeks of gestation and has a history of chronic hypertension. She has no other pregnancy complications and her blood pressure has been well controlled on labetalol.

192. C. A 23-year-old gravida 2, para 1, at 31 weeks of gestation has been diagnosed with preeclampsia without severe features. An ultrasonographic evaluation of the fetus showed an estimated fetal weight of 1,650 grams (33rd percentile).

The goal of antenatal fetal surveillance is to reduce the risk of stillbirth. It attempts to differentiate a fetus at risk of hypoxic injury or death from a normally oxygenated fetus so timely delivery can be performed. A potential consequence of antenatal surveillance is that the reduction in the risk of stillbirth may result in iatrogenic prematurity, which carries its own risks. There is a lack of data supporting the effectiveness of this additional surveillance on improving perinatal outcomes because the outcome—stillbirth—remains rare. Therefore, it is difficult to provide evidence-based, specific guidelines for all maternal and fetal indications that may be associated with an increased stillbirth risk. The American College of Obstetricians and Gynecologists has developed guidance regarding antenatal surveillance, including when to start and how frequently to test (Table 189–192-1). These recommendations are based on expert opinion and data from observational studies.

Although these guidelines exist, shared decision making continues to be an important component of developing a surveillance plan, and an individualized approach may be necessary. Available testing options include nonstress tests, biophysical profiles, modified biophysical profiles, and the contraction stress test. There are advantages and disadvantages of each modality, and the choice of test depends on the gestational age, need for other evaluations, and available resources.

For most patients, initiating testing at 32 weeks of gestation is considered appropriate. However, certain clinical situations may necessitate earlier testing. Earlier testing should be performed only at a gestational age when delivery for perinatal benefit would be considered. On the other hand, there are clinical scenarios in which initiating testing later than 32 weeks of gestation is recommended, such as uncomplicated gestations with dichorionic–diamniotic twins, pregnancies complicated

TABLE 189-192-1. Factors Associated With an Increased Risk of Stillbirth and Suggested Strategies for Antenatal Fetal Surveillance After Viability

FACTOR	SUGGESTED GESTATIONAL AGE TO BEGIN ANTENATAL FETAL SURVEILLANCE	SUGGESTED FREQUENCY OF ANTENATAL FETAL SURVEILLANCE
FETAL		
Growth restriction[1]		
UAD: normal or with elevated impedance to flow in umbilical artery with diastolic flow present; with normal AFI and no other concurrent maternal or fetal conditions	At diagnosis[2]	Once or twice weekly
UAD: AEDV or concurrent conditions (oligohydramnios, maternal comorbidity [eg, preeclampsia, chronic hypertension])	At diagnosis[2]	Twice weekly[3] or consider inpatient management
UAD: REDV	At diagnosis[2]	Inpatient management[3]
Multiple gestation		
Twins, uncomplicated dichorionic	36 0/7 weeks	Weekly
Twins, dichorionic, complicated by maternal or fetal disorders, such as fetal growth restriction	At diagnosis[2]	Individualized
Twins, uncomplicated monochorionic-diamniotic	32 0/7 weeks[4]	Weekly
Twins, complicated monochorionic-diamniotic (ie, TTTS)	Individualized	Individualized
Twins, monoamniotic	Individualized	Individualized
Triplets and higher order multiples	Individualized	Individualized
Decreased fetal movement	At diagnosis[3]	Once[5]
Fetal anomalies and aneuploidy	Individualized	Individualized
MATERNAL		
Hypertension, chronic		
Controlled with medications	32 0/7 weeks	Weekly
Poorly controlled or with associated medical conditions	At diagnosis[2]	Individualized
Gestational hypertension/preeclampsia		
Without severe features	At diagnosis[2,3]	Twice weekly
With severe features	At diagnosis[2,3]	Daily

(continued)

Table 189–192-1 *(continued)*

Diabetes		
Gestational, controlled on medications without other comorbidities	32 0/7 weeks	Once or twice weekly
Gestational, poorly controlled	32 0/7 weeks	Twice weekly
Pregestational	32 0/7 weeks[6]	Twice weekly
Systemic lupus erythematosus		
Uncomplicated	By 32 0/7 weeks	Weekly
Complicated[7]	At diagnosis[2]	Individualized
Antiphospholipid syndrome	By 32 0/7 weeks[8]	Twice weekly
Sickle cell disease		
Uncomplicated	32 0/7 weeks	Once or twice weekly
Complicated[9]	At diagnosis[2]	Individualized
Hemoglobinopathies other than Hb SS disease	Individualized	Individualized
Renal disease (Cr greater than 1.4 mg/dL)	32 0/7 weeks	Once or twice weekly
Thyroid disorders, poorly controlled	Individualized	Individualized
In vitro fertilization	36 0/7 weeks	Weekly
Substance use		
Alcohol, 5 or more drinks per week	36 0/7 weeks	Weekly
Polysubstance use	Individualized	Individualized
Prepregnancy BMI		
Prepregnancy BMI 35.0–39.9 kg/m^2	37 0/7 weeks	Weekly
Prepregnancy BMI 40 kg/m^2 or above	34 0/7 weeks	Weekly
Maternal age older than 35 years	Individualized[10]	Individualized
OBSTETRIC		
Previous stillbirth		
At or after 32 0/7 weeks	32 0/7 weeks[11]	Once or twice weekly
Before 32 0/7 weeks of gestation	Individualized	Individualized
History of other adverse pregnancy outcomes in immediately preceding pregnancy		
Previous fetal growth restriction requiring preterm delivery	32 0/7 weeks	Weekly
Previous preeclampsia requiring preterm delivery	32 0/7 weeks	Weekly
Cholestasis	At diagnosis[2]	Once or twice weekly
Late term	41 0/7 weeks	Once or twice weekly
Abnormal serum markers[12]		
PAPP-A less than or equal to the fifth percentile (0.4 MoM)	36 0/7 weeks	Weekly
Second-trimester Inhibin A equal to or greater than 2.0 MoM	36 0/7 weeks	Weekly
PLACENTAL		
Chronic placental abruption[13]	At diagnosis[2]	Once or twice weekly
Vasa previa	Individualized	Individualized
Velamentous cord insertion	36 0/7 weeks	Weekly
Single umbilical artery	36 0/7 weeks	Weekly

(continued)

Table 189–192-1 *(continued)*

Isolated oligohydramnios (single deepest vertical pocket less than 2 cm)	At diagnosis[2,3]	Once or twice weekly
Polyhydramnios, moderate to severe (deepest vertical pocket equal to or greater than 12 cm or AFI equal to or greater than 30 cm)	32 0/7–34 0/7 weeks[14]	Once or twice weekly

Abbreviations: AEDV, absent end-diastolic velocity; AFI, amniotic fluid index; BMI, body mass index; Cr, creatinine; MoM, multiples of the median; PAPP-A, pregnancy-associated plasma protein A; REDV, reversed end-diastolic flow; TTTS, twin-to-twin transfusion syndrome; UAD, umbilical artery Doppler.

The guidance offered in this table should be construed only as suggestions, not mandates. Ultimately, individualization about if and when to offer antenatal fetal surveillance is advised.

[1]Estimated fetal weight or abdominal circumference less than the 10th percentile.

[2]Or at a gestational age when delivery would be considered because of abnormal test results.

[3]If not delivered.

[4]In addition to routine surveillance for twin–twin transfusion syndrome and other monochorionic twin complications.

[5]Repeat if decreased fetal movement recurs.

[6]Or earlier for poor glycemic control or end-organ damage.

[7]Such as active lupus nephritis, recent lupus flare, antiphospholipid antibodies with prior fetal loss, anti-RO/SSA or anti-La/SSB antibodies, or thrombosis.

[8]Individualize, take into consideration obstetric history, number of positive antibodies, and current pregnancy complications.

[9]Such as maternal hypertension, vaso-occlusive crisis, placental insufficiency, fetal growth restriction.

[10]Based on cumulative risk when present with other factors.

[11]Or starting 1–2 weeks before the gestational age of the previous stillbirth.

[12]If serum screening for aneuploidy is performed, the results may be considered in determining whether antenatal fetal surveillance should be performed.

[13]In individuals who are candidates for outpatient management.

[14]Or at diagnosis if diagnosed after 32 0/7–34 0/7 weeks.

Reprinted from Indications for outpatient antenatal fetal surveillance. ACOG Committee Opinion No. 828. American College of Obstetricians and Gynecologists. Obstet Gynecol 2021;137:e177–97. doi: 10.1097/AOG.0000000000004407 https://journals.lww.com/greenjournal/Fulltext/2021/06000/Indications_for_Outpatient_Antenatal_Fetal.42.aspx

by obesity, pregnancies achieved by in vitro fertilization, and several other indications (Table 189–192-1).

The ideal frequency of fetal surveillance has not been determined. Weekly testing often is suggested; however, individualization is encouraged because there are high-risk clinical situations in which more frequent testing (twice weekly or more often) may be beneficial.

In Scenario 189, polyhydramnios is noted on ultrasonography. Polyhydramnios can be classified, based on deepest maximum vertical pocket, as mild (8–11 cm), moderate (12–15 cm), or severe (16 cm or greater). Because polyhydramnios has been associated with an increased risk of stillbirth, antenatal fetal surveillance typically is recommended for those with moderate to severe polyhydramnios, but not mild polyhydramnios, as is seen in this scenario. Therefore, no additional surveillance is indicated. Follow-up fluid assessment can be considered to ensure there is no progression to moderate or severe polyhydramnios. *Oligohydramnios*, defined as a deepest vertical pocket less than 2 cm, also is associated with an increased risk of stillbirth (14 in 1,000) because it often is a consequence of placental insufficiency. Antenatal fetal surveillance is recommended once or twice weekly on diagnosis of oligohydramnios if delivery for perinatal benefit is an option.

In Scenario 190, the fetus has a diagnosis of growth restriction. *Fetal growth restriction* is defined as an estimated fetal weight or abdominal circumference that is less than the 10th percentile for gestational age. This patient meets criteria because the abdominal circumference measures at the 5th percentile. Once fetal growth restriction is diagnosed, umbilical artery Doppler velocimetry is recommended in addition to standard fetal surveillance with nonstress tests or biophysical profiles. Umbilical artery Doppler assesses resistance to flow in the fetoplacental vascular system. An abnormal result suggests placental insufficiency and is an important measure of fetal well-being. The use of umbilical artery Doppler in fetuses with fetal growth restriction has been shown to reduce the risk of perinatal death. For this patient, once-weekly nonstress test or biophysical profile and once-weekly umbilical artery Doppler assessment are recommended.

In Scenario 191, risk factors include advanced maternal age and chronic hypertension that is well controlled on medications. Hypertensive disorders of pregnancy require additional surveillance during pregnancy. Women with chronic hypertension are at increased risk of stillbirth. The risk varies with the degree of hypertension and other comorbidities. If diagnosed with superimposed preeclampsia, the risk is increased more than fourfold. With chronic hypertension currently well controlled on medications, once-weekly antenatal surveillance is recommended starting at 32 weeks of gestation. If other complications occur, such as fetal growth restriction, more frequent testing should be considered.

In Scenario 192, the diagnosis is preeclampsia without severe features or other complicating factors, such as fetal growth restriction. With preeclampsia or gestational hypertension, fetal surveillance is recommended to start at the time of diagnosis or at a gestational age that delivery would be considered for perinatal benefit. Twice-weekly surveillance is recommended until delivery. If the patient's status changes and she meets criteria for severe features, then daily surveillance is recommended.

Antepartum fetal surveillance. ACOG Practice Bulletin No. 229. American College of Obstetricians and Gynecologists. Obstet Gynecol 2021;137:e116–27. doi: 10.1097/AOG.0000000000004410 https://journals.lww.com/greenjournal/Fulltext/2021/06000/Antepartum_Fetal_Surveillance__ACOG_Practice.37.aspx

Fetal growth restriction. ACOG Practice Bulletin No.227. American College of Obstetricians and Gynecologists. Obstet Gynecol 2021;137:e16–28. doi: 10.1097/AOG.0000000000004251 https://journals.lww.com/greenjournal/pages/articleviewer.aspx?year=2021&issue=02000&article=00043&type=Fulltext

Gestational diabetes mellitus. ACOG Practice Bulletin No. 190. American College of Obstetricians and Gynecologists. Obstet Gynecol 2018;131:e49–64. doi: 10.1097/AOG.0000000000002501 https://journals.lww.com/greenjournal/Fulltext/2018/02000/ACOG_Practice_Bulletin_No__190__Gestational.37.aspx

Indications for outpatient antenatal fetal surveillance. ACOG Committee Opinion No. 828. American College of Obstetricians and Gynecologists. Obstet Gynecol 2021;137:e177–97. doi: 10.1097/AOG.0000000000004407 https://journals.lww.com/greenjournal/Fulltext/2021/06000/Indications_for_Outpatient_Antenatal_Fetal.42.aspx

Martins JG. Society for Maternal–Fetal Medicine Consult Series #52: Diagnosis and management of fetal growth restriction (Replaces Clinical Guideline Number 3, April 2012). Am J Obstet Gynecol 2020;223:B2–17. doi: 10.1016/j.ajog.2020.05.010 https://www.ajog.org/article/S0002-9378(20)30535-4/fulltext

Pregestational diabetes mellitus. ACOG Practice Bulletin No. 201. American College of Obstetricians and Gynecologists. Obstet Gynecol 2018;132:e228–48. doi: 10.1097/AOG.0000000000002960 https://journals.lww.com/greenjournal/Fulltext/2018/12000/ACOG_Practice_Bulletin_No__201__Pregestational.48.aspx

193–196 Health disparities and health equity in obstetrics

For each scenario of racial and ethnic disparity in obstetrics (193–196), choose the underlying cause (A–D).

(A) Health inequity
(B) Implicit bias
(C) Social determinants of health
(D) Structural racism

193. D. The lack of diversity among physicians perpetuates a system of decreased quality of care for marginalized populations.

194. B. Seventy-three percent of a group of medical students falsely believe that there are biological differences in pain among people of different races.

195. C. Lack of transportation is associated with fewer prenatal visits and increased rate of preeclampsia.

196. A. Racial and ethnic minorities tend to receive lower quality of health care than nonminorities, even when controlling for access factors, such as insurance status and income.

Racial and ethnic disparities in obstetric care and outcomes are prevalent in the United States. The National Institutes of Health defines *disparities* as racial- or ethnic-based differences in the overall rate of disease incidence, prevalence, morbidity, and mortality when populations are compared with the general population. Reducing these disparities in health and health care should be a top priority for all health care professionals. The root causes of these disparities must be understood to address them.

Structural racism is an important contributor to racial disparity. Structural racism is defined as the "totality of ways in which societies foster racial discrimination through mutually reinforcing systems of housing, education, employment, earnings, benefits, media, health care, and criminal justice." Put another way, the Aspen Institute defines structural racism as "a system in which public policies, institutional practices, cultural representations, and other norms work in various, often reinforcing ways to perpetuate racial group inequity."

One example of structural racism is the systematic implementation of racial residential segregation. Unfair lending practices and housing discrimination have led to the racial segregation of neighborhoods, and this segregation has been linked to poor health outcomes. Minority neighborhoods have higher rates of tobacco advertisements and less access to affordable, healthy food, and this has contributed to increased obesity and preterm birth.

Another example of structural racism is the lack of diversity among health care professionals. This lack of diversity exists at every level, from medical school admissions to obstetrics and gynecology residency programs as well as among practicing obstetrician–gynecologists. Studies have consistently demonstrated that when the physician is the same race as the patient, patient trust and outcomes, including infant mortality, are improved. Although the other answers also may involve structural racism, the systemic factors that result in a lack of diversity in health care professionals are the best examples of structural racism. Structural racism must be dismantled to decrease racial disparity.

Implicit bias is defined by the Kirwan Institute for the Study of Race and Ethnicity as "the attitudes or stereotypes that affect our understanding, actions and decisions in an unconscious manner." A major cause of racial disparity is the implicit biases health care professionals may have about groups that may lead to differential treatment. Most health care professionals carry these implicit biases, and this negatively affects patient–physician interactions, delivery of care, and health outcomes.

A well-studied example is the false belief, held by some health care professionals, that there are biological differences in pain. A recent study showed that 73% of medical students endorsed at least one false belief about biological differences in pain by race. This implicit bias has led to well-documented differences in pain management by race: Black patients are less likely to have adequate treatment of pain and less likely to receive epidural analgesia. The other answer choices do not involve obstetricians' unconscious perceptions or attitudes.

Social determinants of health are defined by the U.S. Department of Health and Human Services as the "conditions in the environments where people are born, live, learn, work, play, and worship that affect a wide range of health and quality of life outcomes and risks." Social determinants of health can include economic status, education access and quality, immigration status, neighborhoods, access to transportation, and availability of familial support systems.

Patient access to transportation is an important social determinant of health. Numerous studies have illustrated that patients' ability to access transportation is correlated to their ability to attend prenatal care appointments and can affect obstetric outcomes, including preeclampsia and preterm birth. Although other factors may contribute to disparities in access to prenatal care and increased preeclampsia, the transportation concern mentioned in this answer choice is a social determinant of health.

Health inequity refers to differences in health outcomes and their risk factors between groups that occur systematically and are avoidable and unfair or unjust. It is important to distinguish inequity from inequality. Although the terms are sometime used interchangeably, "inequality" implies the unequal distribution of resources or treatment, regardless of need or outcomes. Striving for equity focuses on reaching more equal outcomes and recognizes that traditionally disadvantaged populations may need more support or resources to achieve the same health outcomes. The distinction between equity and equality is important because even if equal resources are allotted, inequity will continue to exist. Even when factors such as insurance status and income are equal, racial and ethnic minorities tend to receive lower quality health care and experience reduced access compared with nonminorities. Of the answer choices, this is the best example of health inequity.

Gillispie-Bell V. The contrast of color: why the black community continues to suffer health disparities. Obstet Gynecol 2021;137:220–4. doi: 10.1097/AOG.0000000000004226 https://journals.lww.com/greenjournal/Fulltext/2021/02000/The_Contrast_of_Color__Why_the_Black_Community.4.aspx

Johnson JD, Louis JM. Does race or ethnicity play a role in the origin, pathophysiology, and outcomes of preeclampsia? An expert review of the literature. Am J Obstet Gynecol 2022;226:S876–85. doi: 10.1016/j.ajog.2020.07.038 https://www.ajog.org/article/S0002-9378(20)30769-9/fulltext

Kirwan Institute. Kirwan Institute for the Study of Race and Ethnicity. Ohio State University; 2012. Accessed March 23, 2022. https://kirwaninstitute.osu.edu/article/understanding-implicit-bias

Racial and ethnic disparities in obstetrics and gynecology. ACOG Committee Opinion No. 649. American College of Obstetricians and Gynecologists. Obstet Gynecol 2015;126:e130–4. doi: 10.1097/AOG.0000000000001213 https://journals.lww.com/greenjournal/Fulltext/2015/12000/Committee_Opinion_No__649__Racial_and_Ethnic.57.aspx

197–200 Informed consent and shared decision making

A 28-year-old primigravida at 16 weeks of gestation with a history of Marfan syndrome undergoes maternal echocardiogram and is found to have an aortic root that is dilated to 52 mm. She is considered World Health Organization Class IV with extremely high risk of maternal morbidity or mortality, and pregnancy is contraindicated. For this patient scenario, match the possible next steps in 197–200 to the ethical principles they represent (A–D).

(A) Autonomy
(B) Beneficence
(C) Conscientious refusal
(D) Fiduciary responsibility

197. A. Provide continued pregnancy care according to her wishes after informed consent.

198. B. Advise the patient that you recommend termination of pregnancy and perform the procedure after informed consent.

199. C. Decline to perform pregnancy termination because you are morally opposed to pregnancy termination.

200. D. Refer the patient to a different physician because you are morally opposed to pregnancy termination.

Informed consent is one of the most important tenets of care and treatment for the pregnant woman. Several important ethical principles underlie the process of informed consent. It is important for the obstetrician to understand these principles to achieve informed consent and determine how to proceed when the patient does not consent to what the obstetrician believes to be in the best interest of the patient and fetus.

The goal of informed consent is to give the patient adequate, accurate, and understandable information that can help the patient and physician use shared decision making to reach a treatment plan. To obtain informed consent, the physician should first assess the patient's ability to understand the relevant treatment information and the implications of alternatives to treatment. In doing so, the physician may evaluate a patient's decision-making capacity and her ability to understand the consequences of declining treatment. Relevant information should be presented in an accurate and sensitive manner. The physician can give this information in the way that the patient prefers to receive information: written, verbal, or both. The obstetrician should describe the diagnosis or differential diagnosis, the nature and purpose of the interventions, treatment alternatives, and the risks, burdens, and expected benefits of all options, including declining treatment. Documentation of informed consent and the decision of the patient or their surrogate should be clearly outlined in the medical record, including placing a copy of a signed written consent in the record.

The four pillars of principle-based medical ethics are autonomy, beneficence, nonmaleficence, and justice. *Autonomy*, which literally means self-rule, is the patient's right to determine their own treatment plan. Respect for autonomy provides the strong foundation for informed consent, in which a patient who is adequately informed and has capacity freely agrees to treatment or nontreatment. Adults are presumed to have capacity, and an adult patient with capacity can decline treatment, including in labor and delivery and when declining treatment might affect the patient's or fetus's health and survival. If there is doubt about the patient's decision-making capacity, consultation with experts in psychiatry, ethics, and the law can be obtained in the interest of respecting the patient's autonomy. For patients who either temporarily or permanently lose decision-making capacity, autonomy is best respected by adhering to advanced directives, if they are available. If they are not available, a surrogate decision maker who is either legally designated by the patient or the next of kin can provide a "substituted judgment" that reflects the patient's autonomy. Autonomy often is considered the "first among equals" of the pillars of medical ethics, and when actions taken based on ethical principles conflict, respect for patient autonomy often prevails. In Scenario 197, if the patient desires continued pregnancy care after informed consent, you should provide it out of respect for the patient's autonomy.

The next important principles are beneficence and nonmaleficence. *Beneficence*, which is the act of producing good, is the ethical principle that obligates a person to promote the well-being of others. It requires the physician to act in a way that benefits the patient. *Nonmaleficence* is the ethical obligation to avoid causing harm or injury. In medicine, nonmaleficence is best described by the maxim *primum non nocere*, or "first, do no harm." These principles are usually considered part of the same principle because they are interrelated and part of almost every treatment decision a physician makes. Beneficence, nonmaleficence, or both, can conflict with the obligation to respect autonomy when the patient desires care that may, in the physician's view, not be in the patient's best interest or have the potential to cause harm. In this case, the physician must work with the patient through shared decision making to reach a solution, which ideally fulfills all three principles. These principles can be complicated during pregnancy, when that which benefits or does not cause harm to the patient may have the opposite effect on the fetus. When this occurs, the obstetrician's primary responsibility is the pregnant woman.

It may be helpful to consider that the obstetrician has an obligation of beneficence and nonmaleficence to the pregnant patient, and a motivation of beneficence toward the fetus. Usually, these two converge and actions benefit both the patient and fetus. However, when benefit for the patient and the fetus conflict, the patient and the patient's autonomy take priority. In Scenario 198, beneficence and the mother's health would lead you to counsel the patient you recommend pregnancy termination for her health and perform the procedure after informed consent.

Justice is one of the more complex ethical principles supporting informed consent. Justice requires that the pregnant patient be offered what is due to them and that medical resources be allocated appropriately in the broader community. Justice also requires that patients be treated similarly regardless of race and ethnicity or payor status. For the obstetrician, the principle of justice applies when determining clinic hours, prioritizing operating room times, and determining order or timing of various patients' discharge from the hospital. As part of informed consent, justice requires that all treatment options that are appropriate be discussed with a patient regardless of their insurance status or ability to pay.

Conscientious refusal is an important ethical principle that can come into play as the physician attempts to obtain informed consent and respect patient's autonomy. This refers to the physician's own autonomy and their right to refuse to provide a patient with care to which the physician objects. Generally, the principle of conscientious refusal is limited to when the physician declines to provide the patient with care that is considered standard or potentially beneficial to the patient. Conscientious refusals that undermine the patient's access to care can conflict with the patient's autonomy, beneficence, nonmaleficence, and justice and must be approached with caution. There are limitations to conscientious refusal. In Scenario 199, a physician may decline to perform termination based on conscientious refusal if they are morally opposed to termination.

The physician has a *fiduciary responsibility* to the patient. This fiduciary responsibility obliges the physician to act in good faith to promote the patient's health. The physician is obligated, in the setting of conscientious refusal, to provide the patient with alternatives to achieve the care that they desire, particularly if that care is considered standard of care. When the patient's wishes conflict with the physician's personal belief systems, the physician should respect this fiduciary responsibility. In the setting of conscientious refusal, the physician is obligated to provide the patient with accurate and unbiased medical information as part of informed consent. The physician must make appropriate referrals to provide the patient with the full range of medical options. In Scenario 200, if a physician is morally opposed to pregnancy termination, they have a fiduciary responsibility to refer the patient to a different physician.

For the case in question, the aortic root dilation in the setting of Marfan syndrome and the associated high potential for severe maternal morbidity or even mortality due to abdominal aortic aneurysm make pregnancy contraindicated. In this case, the best interests of the woman and the fetus diverge. Informed consent is critical. After the physician assesses the patient's decision-making capacity and presents all relevant information and options, the patient faces a difficult decision. Advising the patient to terminate and performing the pregnancy termination fulfill the obligation of beneficence to the patient. In this case, beneficence and nonmaleficence to the patient supersede these obligations to the fetus.

If the patient desires pregnancy termination, and the physician feels performing termination would violate their conscience or moral code, the physician can use conscientious refusal and decline to perform the procedure. In this case, the physician should fulfill their fiduciary responsibility to the patient by referring the patient to a physician who is willing to perform pregnancy termination if that is the patient's wish. After informed consent, if the patient desires to continue the pregnancy despite understanding that it places her at substantial risk, the principle of autonomy prevails and should be respected. In this case, the physician should document the informed consent and continue to provide the patient pregnancy care.

Ethical decision making in obstetrics and gynecology, ACOG Committee Opinion No. 390. American College of Obstetrics and Gynecology. Obstet Gynecol 2007;110:1479–87. doi: 10.1097/01.AOG.0000291573.09193.36 https://journals.lww.com/greenjournal/Citation/2007/12000/ACOG_Committee_Opinion_No__390__Ethical_Decision.53.aspx

Informed consent and shared decision making in obstetrics and gynecology. ACOG Committee Opinion No. 819. American College of Obstetricians. Obstet Gynecol 2021;137:e34–41. doi: 10.1097/AOG.0000000000004247 https://journals.lww.com/greenjournal/Fulltext/2021/02000/Informed_Consent_and_Shared_Decision_Making_in.45.aspx

Refusal of medically recommended treatment during pregnancy. Committee Opinion No. 664. American College of Obstetricians and Gynecologists. Obstet Gynecol 2016;127:e175–82. doi: 10.1097/AOG.0000000000001485 https://journals.lww.com/greenjournal/Fulltext/2016/06000/Committee_Opinion_No__664__Refusal_of_Medically.45.aspx

Regitz-Zagrosek V, Blomstrom Lundqvist C, Borghi C, Cifkova R, Ferreira R, Foidart JM, et al. ESC guidelines on the management of cardiovascular diseases during pregnancy: the task force on the management of cardiovascular diseases during pregnancy of the European Society of Cardiology (ESC). ESC Committee for Practice Guidelines. Eur Heart J 2011;32:3147–97. doi: 10.1093/eurheartj/ehr218 https://academic.oup.com/eurheartj/article/32/24/3147/462571

The limits of conscientious refusal in reproductive medicine. ACOG Committee Opinion No. 385. American College of Obstetricians and Gynecologists. Obstet Gynecol 2007;110:1203–8. doi: 10.1097/01.AOG.0000291561.48203.27 https://journals.lww.com/greenjournal/Citation/2007/11000/ACOG_Committee_Opinion_No__385__The_Limits_of.50.aspx

201–204 Anticoagulation

For each clinical scenario (201–204), choose the most appropriate anticoagulation recommendation (A–C).

(A) Prophylactic anticoagulation
(B) Surveillance without coagulation
(C) Therapeutic (adjusted dose) anticoagulation

201. B. A 35-year-old gravida 4, para 2, presents at 12 1/7 weeks of gestation with a body mass index (BMI) of 42 experienced a deep vein thrombosis (DVT) 3 years ago after knee surgery. She was prescribed and completed 3 months of anticoagulation therapy. Testing was negative for factor V Leiden, prothrombin gene mutation, and deficiencies in antithrombin, Protein S, and Protein C.

202. C. A 38-year-old gravida 2, para 1, at 8 2/7 weeks of gestation has a history of two previous DVTs, one after a long airplane flight, and the second after foot surgery. Testing reveals that she is heterozygous for factor V Leiden and the prothrombin G20210A mutation. Testing for deficiencies in antithrombin, Protein S, and Protein C was negative. After her second DVT, she was started on rivaroxaban, an anti-Xa inhibitor.

203. A. A 21-year-old gravida 1 with a BMI of 31 underwent an uncomplicated cesarean birth. She is heterozygous for the factor V Leiden mutation. She has no personal history of a venous thromboembolism (VTE). Her mother experienced a DVT at age 45.

204. B. A 25-year-old gravida 1 underwent a full-term vaginal delivery. She smokes one-half pack of cigarettes daily, and her BMI is 24. She has no personal history of VTE. Her maternal aunt was diagnosed with a pulmonary embolism after a surgical procedure at age 54 years.

Venous thromboembolism is a leading cause of maternal morbidity and mortality worldwide and in the United States. Approximately 75–80% of venous thromboemboli in pregnancy are deep vein thrombi and 20–25% are pulmonary emboli, with about one half occurring during pregnancy and one half in the postpartum period. Pregnancy is associated with physiologic and anatomic changes that increase the risk of VTE, such as hypercoagulability, venous stasis, decreased venous outflow, compression of the inferior vena cava and pelvic veins by the uterus, and decreased mobility. Women with inherited thrombophilias (Box 201–204-1) are at additional risk of VTE in pregnancy, as are those with a personal or family history of VTE. Patients at increased risk of VTE should be administered anticoagulation during pregnancy and postpartum. Acquired risk factors include triggering events, such as recent surgery, prolonged immobilization, pregnancy, trauma, and presence of an indwelling venous catheter. Other acquired risk factors include medical diseases, such as antiphospholipid syndrome, malignancy, and myeloproliferative disorders, and having two or more episodes of VTE in the past.

BOX 201-204-1

Inherited Thrombophilia Categories

Low Risk
- Factor V Leiden heterozygotes
- Prothrombin G20210A mutation heterozygotes
- Protein C and S deficiencies

High Risk
- Antithrombin deficiency
- Compound heterozygotes for prothrombin G20210A mutation and factor V Leiden
- Homozygotes for prothrombin G20210A mutation and factor V Leiden

An antepartum and postpartum anticoagulation regimen should be considered for each woman based on her level of risk. If anticoagulation is chosen over surveillance, low-molecular-weight heparin usually is the anticoagulant of choice given its safety and ease of dosing. A prophylactic dose typically is given once daily, and for treatment of active VTE or prevention in the highest risk women, it is administered as a weight-based, therapeutic dose. Women receiving anticoagulation with low-molecular-weight heparin may be switched to unfractionated heparin, which has a shorter half-life, in anticipation of birth. For women on prophylactic unfractionated heparin or low-molecular-weight heparin, anticoagulants should be held at least 12 hours before regional anesthesia placement and delivery. For women on therapeutic doses of unfractionated heparin or low-molecular-weight heparin, anticoagulants should be held at least 24 hours. Additionally, coagulation status should be evaluated before administering regional anesthesia to women on unfractionated heparin. In general, anticoagulation is resumed

4–6 hours after vaginal delivery and 6–12 hours after cesarean birth (Appendix G). If pharmacologic management is recommended during pregnancy, it typically is continued for at least 6 weeks postpartum. Although the risk of VTE is likely increased up to 12 weeks postpartum, the risk is especially increased during the first 6 weeks.

In Scenario 201, surveillance without anticoagulation is recommended. This patient has not been diagnosed with an inherited thrombophilia. Although she experienced a DVT 3 years ago, it was after knee surgery, which is considered a provoked VTE associated with a transient risk factor. Risk of recurrent DVT is considered significantly lower in women with a single previous VTE associated with a transient risk factor not related to pregnancy or hormone use, compared with women who have experienced a previous unprovoked or pregnancy- or hormone-related VTE. Therefore, clinical vigilance is favored in the antepartum period. If she undergoes a cesarean birth, postpartum prophylactic anticoagulation could be considered because she would now have an additional risk factor for VTE (cesarean birth).

In Scenario 202, therapeutic anticoagulation is recommended. This patient has a history of two prior DVTs, both provoked, and she is a compound heterozygote for factor V Leiden and prothrombin gene mutation, which is considered a high-risk thrombophilia. Because of this combination of history and thrombophilia, she previously had been started on long-term anticoagulation (rivaroxaban) by her hematologist. When a woman who is on long-term anticoagulation becomes pregnant, the recommendation is to continue anticoagulation (therapeutic or adjusted-dose) during the pregnancy. She must be transitioned to low-molecular-weight heparin upon confirmation of a viable pregnancy because rivaroxaban is not recommended in pregnancy.

The patient in Scenario 203 should have prophylactic anticoagulation. She has a low-risk thrombophilia and no history of VTE; therefore, she does not meet criteria for antepartum anticoagulation. However, she has additional risk factors, including a BMI over 30, cesarean birth, and a first-degree relative with a previous DVT. Because of these factors, her risk of VTE postpartum is increased and prophylactic anticoagulation should be considered.

For the patient in Scenario 204, surveillance without anticoagulation is recommended. Although she has a family history of VTE, it did not occur in a first-degree relative, and she does not have additional risk factors that would warrant postpartum anticoagulation.

Bates SM, Rajasekhar A, Middeldorp S, McLintock C, Rodger MA, James AH, et al. American Society of Hematology 2018 guidelines for management of venous thromboembolism: venous thromboembolism in the context of pregnancy. Blood Adv 2018;2:3317–59. doi: 10.1182/bloodadvances.2018024802 https://ashpublications.org/bloodadvances/article/2/22/3317/16094/American-Society-of-Hematology-2018-guidelines-for

Lamont MC, McDermott C, Thomson AJ, Greer IA. United Kingdom recommendations for obstetric venous thromboembolism prophylaxis: evidence and rationale. Semin Perinatol 2019;43:222–8. doi: 10.1053/j.semperi.2019.03.008 https://www.sciencedirect.com/science/article/abs/pii/S0146000519300333

Resnik R, Lockwood CJ, Moore TR, Greene ME, Copel JA, Silver RM, editors. Creasy and Resnik's maternal–fetal medicine: principles and practice. 8th ed. Elsevier; 2018.

Thromboembolism in pregnancy. ACOG Practice Bulletin No. 196. American College of Obstetricians and Gynecologists [published erratum appears in Obstet Gynecol 2018;132:1068]. Obstet Gynecol 2018;132:e1–17. doi: 10.1097/AOG.0000000000002706 https://journals.lww.com/greenjournal/Fulltext/2018/07000/ACOG_Practice_Bulletin_No__196__Thromboembolism_in.54.aspx

205–208 Intimate partner violence

For each clinical scenario (205–208), choose the type of intimate partner violence (A–D).

(A) Physical violence
(B) Psychologic aggression
(C) Reproductive coercion
(D) Sexual violence

205. A. A pregnant patient presents after falling down the stairs. With questioning, she reveals she was shoved by her partner.

206. D. A pregnant patient reports that her partner shares suggestive photographs of her on social media without her consent or knowledge.

207. B. A patient informs you that her partner repeatedly threatens to hurt her children.

208. C. A patient has an unplanned pregnancy, and she reports that her partner threatens to hurt her if she seeks pregnancy termination.

Intimate partner violence, or any form of physical or psychologic abuse that occurs between people in a relationship, is a pervasive problem that affects women of every socioeconomic background, race, ethnicity, educational background, and sexual orientation. Although the true incidence is hard to determine because of underreporting, intimate partner violence is most prevalent among women of reproductive age. It is estimated that more than one in three women has experienced intimate partner violence in their lifetime and that intimate partner violence may occur in 20–30% of pregnant patients.

The term *intimate partner violence*, as defined by the Centers for Disease Control and Prevention, refers to physical violence, sexual violence, stalking, or psychologic harm by a current or previous partner or spouse. It is a public health problem. Because victims of intimate partner violence are more likely to seek health care while pregnant, obstetricians have an important opportunity and responsibility to screen for intimate partner violence.

Physicians must understand the various types of intimate partner violence to recognize them among patients. An intimate partner is a person with whom a patient has an ongoing close and personal relationship. Intimacy between partners may be characterized by emotional connectedness, regular contact, physical contact, sexual behavior, and familiarity and involvement in each other's lives. Intimate partners may identify as couples or may not, can include individuals of the same or opposite sex, and can include spouses, boyfriends or girlfriends, dating partners, or sexual partners. If the individuals do not have an ongoing relationship but have a history of a relationship, they are considered intimate partners.

Physical violence occurs when a person hurts or attempts to hurt a partner using physical force. This can include throwing objects, beating, threatening with a weapon, using a weapon, kicking, biting, slapping, hitting, strangling, choking, pulling hair, punching, and use of restraints. Physical violence also includes coercing other people to commit any of the above acts. Physical violence can be recognized in patients with acute injuries to the head, face, breasts, abdomen, or genitalia. Patients also may present with less overt signs, including reports of abdominal pain or symptoms, palpitations, chronic pelvic pain, urinary frequency or urgency, and recurrent vaginal symptoms. These symptoms may be the direct result of physical abuse or may represent somatization due to internalized stress. In Scenario 205, a pregnant patient who presents after being shoved down the stairs by her partner is experiencing physical violence.

Sexual violence is defined as a sexual act attempted or committed by another person without voluntary consent or against someone who cannot consent or cannot refuse the sexual act. A partner may be unable to consent because of their age, disability, being incapacitated by voluntary or involuntary use of drugs or alcohol, or being asleep or unconscious. Similarly, a person may be unable to refuse if they are under threat of or experiencing physical violence, pressure, or misuse of authority. Sexual violence includes completed or attempted forced penetration or forcing the victim to penetrate a perpetrator or someone else. It includes any form of unwanted sexual contact or noncontact unwanted sexual experience. Sexual violence can also include nonphysically forced sexual contact that occurs after verbal pressure or intimidation. Some acts of noncontact unwanted sexual violence may occur without the victim's knowledge, including unwanted filming or taking or disseminating photographs of a sexual nature of the victim. In Scenario 206, the patient whose partner is sharing illicit photographs of her on social media without her consent or knowledge is experiencing sexual violence.

Psychologic aggression includes the use of verbal and nonverbal communication with the intent to exert control over a person and harm them mentally or emotionally. This may not include physical violence and may not be perceived as aggression because it can be covert in nature. Examples of psychological aggression include name-calling, humiliation, degradation, and threats of physical violence through words or gestures. It also can involve coercive control by limiting access to transportation, money, friends, family, and communication. Psychologic aggression is an essential component of intimate partner violence because it may often precede physical or sexual violence. The effect of psychologic aggression can be just as significant as that of physical violence on a partner, although its presence may be harder to identify. The patient in Scenario 207 whose partner is repeatedly threatening harm to her children is experiencing psychologic aggression.

Reproductive coercion involves behaviors that a partner uses to maintain power and control over their partner's reproductive health. Reproductive coercion includes explicit attempts to impregnate a partner against their will by birth control sabotage, including replacing birth control, removing birth control, forced non-condom use, or destroying condoms. Reproductive coercion includes pregnancy coercion, which involves threats or acts of violence if a person does not comply with their partner's wishes regarding continuation or termination of a pregnancy. This may result in a partner being forced to proceed with pregnancy termination or being forced to carry a pregnancy and also may include injuring a partner in such a way that she may have a miscarriage. Approximately 20% of women with a history of abuse seeking care in family planning clinics have experienced pregnancy coercion or birth control sabotage. The patient in Scenario 208 who has an unplanned pregnancy and is being threatened by her partner if she seeks pregnancy termination is experiencing reproductive coercion.

Intimate partner violence is common and has many consequences. Intimate partner violence may result in physical or psychologic injury and even homicide. In pregnancy, it is associated with poor gestational weight gain, preterm birth, stillbirth, abruption, and low birth weight. Violence can escalate during pregnancy or the postpartum period, and homicide remains a leading cause of maternal mortality, with most attacks perpetrated by current or former intimate partners. There is a large societal cost to intimate partner violence with loss of financial stability of families, increased homelessness of women and children who leave violent relationships, and direct costs of medical care as well as lost productivity from paid work.

Health care professionals play an important role in stopping the cycle of intimate partner violence by screening and offering support and referral for patients. The U.S. Department of Health and Human Services and the National Academy of Medicine (formerly the Institute of Medicine) recommend that intimate partner violence screening be a core part of women's health visits. Because of the unique opportunity for repeated follow-up that occurs during pregnancy, obstetricians should screen for intimate partner violence at the first prenatal visit, at least once per trimester, and at the postpartum visit. Additionally, obstetricians should be well-informed regarding signs of human trafficking, including patients with signs of abuse or neglect that may be accompanied by an individual who does not let the patient speak for themselves, refuses to allow for privacy, or insists on interpreting for them in place of a professional.

Patient self-administered or computerized screenings are just as effective as clinician interview in terms of disclosure rates. Patients should be screened in a private and safe setting and not in front of family, friends, or caregivers. They should be questioned using nonstigmatizing language, avoiding terms such as "rape," "abuse," and "battered." Patients should be reassured that screening is done universally and confidentially. Screening should be incorporated into medical history by integrating questions into all intake forms so that patients are screened whether or not abuse is suspected. Office staff should regularly receive training about intimate partner violence and screening. Examples of screening questions are given in Box 205–208-1.

If a patient discloses that they are involved in intimate partner violence, the physician should evaluate the immediate safety of the patient and her children and assist in formulating a safety plan. The patient can be offered community resources and appropriate referrals.

Physicians should assess the patient's readiness for assistance and be careful to avoid forcing the patient to accept assistance. Violence and aggression may increase if the partner suspects that the patient is seeking assistance. Cellphone call logs and internet usage may be monitored by abusers. Physicians can help by offering a private phone and giving patients access to the National Domestic Violence hotline (Box 205–208-2). Additionally, physicians should accurately document the clinical interaction, including pictures and descriptions as needed, for the medical record so that it could be used as evidence for future legal proceedings.

BOX 205-208-1

Sample Intimate Partner Violence Screening Questions

Patients should be screened for intimate partner violence during new patient visits, annual examinations, initial prenatal visits, each trimester of pregnancy, and the postpartum checkup in a private manner.

Framing Statement

"We're asking all of our patients about safe and healthy relationships because it can have such a large impact on your health."*

Confidentiality

"Before we get started, I want you to know that everything here is confidential, meaning that I won't talk to anyone else about what is said unless you tell me that... [insert the laws in your state about what is necessary to disclose]."*

Sample Questions

"Has your current partner ever threatened you or made you feel afraid?"

"Has your partner ever hit, choked, or physically hurt you?"

"Has your partner ever forced you to do something sexually that you did not want to do, or refused your request to use condoms?"*

"Does your partner support your decision about when or if you want to become pregnant?"*

"Has your partner ever tampered with your birth control or tried to get you pregnant when you didn't want to be?"*

*Data from Chamberlain L, Levenson R. Reproductive health and partner violence guidelines: an integrated response to intimate partner violence and reproductive coercion. Family Violence Prevention Fund; 2010. Accessed March 25, 2022. http://www.futureswithoutviolence.org/userfiles/file/HealthCare/Repro_Guide.pdf

BOX 205-208-2

Resources

Domestic Shelters, https://www.domesticshelters.org/
Futures Without Violence, www.futureswithoutviolence.org
National Coalition Against Domestic Violence, https://ncadv.org
National Domestic Violence Hotline, 1-800-799-SAFE (7233), https://www.thehotline.org/
Safe Alliance, https://www.safealliance.org/

Centers for Disease Control and Prevention. Violence prevention. CDC; 2021. Accessed March 25, 2022. https://www.cdc.gov/violenceprevention/intimatepartnerviolence/index.html

Chamberlain L, Levenson R. Reproductive health and partner violence guidelines: an integrated response to intimate partner violence and reproductive coercion. Family Violence Prevention Fund; 2010. Accessed March 25, 2022. http://www.futureswithoutviolence.org/userfiles/file/HealthCare/Repro_Guide.pdf

Chisholm CA, Bullock L, Ferguson JE II. Intimate partner violence and pregnancy: epidemiology and impact. Am J Obstet Gynecol 2017;217:1414. doi: 10.1016/j.ajog.2017.05.042 https://www.ajog.org/article/S0002-9378(17)30659-2/fulltext

Intimate partner violence. ACOG Committee Opinion No. 518. American College of Obstetricians and Gynecologists. Obstet Gynecol 2012;119:412–7. doi: 10.1097/AOG.0b013e318249ff74 https://journals.lww.com/greenjournal/Citation/2012/02000/Committee_Opinion_No__518__Intimate_Partner.51.aspx

Miller E, Decker MR, McCauley HL, Tancredi DJ, Levenson RR, Waldman J, et al. Pregnancy coercion, intimate partner violence and unintended pregnancy. Contraception 2010;81:316–22. doi: 10.1016/j.contraception.2009.12.004 https://www.contraceptionjournal.org/article/S0010-7824(09)00522-8/fulltext

209–213 Vaccines in pregnancy

For each vaccine (209–213), choose the appropriate recommendation for administration during pregnancy (A–C).

(A) Contraindicated during pregnancy
(B) Indicated during every pregnancy
(C) May be given during pregnancy in indicated persons

209. C. Hepatitis A

210. B. Tetanus toxoid, reduced diphtheria toxoid, and acellular pertussis (Tdap)

211. A. Varicella

212. A. Measles–mumps–rubella

213. B. Inactivated influenza

Pregnancy represents an opportunity for patients, clinicians, and health systems to address the preventive care needs of women and children. It often allows access to medical care and coverage of services that patients do not have when they are not pregnant or postpartum.

Vaccination is vital to the well-being of the woman and child, but also to population health. The obstetrician should inquire about vaccination status for every patient during pregnancy and provide the appropriate immunizations or direct the patient to facilities that can administer the vaccines. There is no evidence of maternal harm or fetal compromise with the administration of inactivated virus vaccines, bacterial vaccines, and toxoid vaccines. Only activated virus vaccines are contraindicated in pregnant patients.

An inactivated, age-appropriate influenza vaccine is recommended for every woman who is or will be pregnant during the influenza season, which generally extends from September through May. The vaccine can be given in any trimester and should be given as early in the season as possible. Influenza infection during pregnancy has higher rates of morbidity and mortality versus infection in nonpregnant women, including higher rates of pneumonia, hospitalization, and intensive care unit admission. Influenza during pregnancy also increases fetal morbidity and mortality, with higher rates of congenital anomalies, spontaneous abortions, preterm delivery, and low birth weight.

For patients with egg allergies manifesting as hives or lesser symptoms, any age-appropriate inactivated influenza virus vaccination may be administered. For those with more severe egg allergies, including those who have demonstrated angioedema, respiratory distress, or required epinephrine administration, any age-appropriate inactivated influenza virus vaccination may still be given, but should be done under direct medical observation with personnel trained to recognize an allergic reaction and equipped to manage it. The only contraindication to an influenza vaccination is a previous severe allergic reaction to the vaccine not related to an egg allergy.

The Tdap vaccine also is recommended in every pregnancy for all patients. Pertussis infection has the greatest morbidity and mortality in infants less than 3 months of age, but the neonatal vaccination series cannot start until 6 weeks of age at the earliest. The method known as *cocooning* refers to vaccinating all persons around the infant who are not previously vaccinated and is recommended at least 2 weeks before contact with the newborn. Cocooning has not been demonstrated as an effective strategy for reducing disease transmission. In addition, all pregnant patients should receive the Tdap vaccine between 27 and 36 weeks of gestation to trigger a maternal antibody response with passive transfer to the fetus. From data thus far, administration of the Tdap vaccine earlier in the window may have more effective passive immunity in the neonate based on cord blood titers. For pregnant patients who require the vaccination earlier in pregnancy, such as for an injury, there is no need to repeat it in the 27- to 36-weeks-of-gestation window, as long as it was a Tdap and not just a tetanus booster.

Vaccinations that are recommended for certain pregnant populations (Appendix F) include the pneumococcal, meningococcal, hepatitis A, and hepatitis B vaccines. The 23-valent pneumococcal polysaccharide vaccine is recommended in reproductive-aged women with heart or lung disease, diabetes mellitus, or sickle cell disease, whereas the 13-valent pneumococcal vaccine is recommended for reproductive-aged women with immunocompromise, such as human immunodeficiency virus (HIV) or asplenia. The 13-valent pneumococcal vaccine should be deferred in pregnancy unless the patient is at increased risk of pneumococcal disease.

The quadrivalent conjugate meningococcal vaccine is recommended for all adolescents 11–18 years of age, for women with HIV, patients with complement component deficiency and those with anatomic asplenia or functional asplenia, such as sickle cell disease, and in patients exposed to meningococcal outbreaks. The meningococcal serogroup B vaccine generally is deferred in pregnancy unless the patient is at increased risk of acquiring a meningococcal B infection.

The hepatitis A vaccine should be offered to pregnant women not previously vaccinated who have chronic liver disease, clotting disorders, or substance use disorder. It also should be offered to those who are traveling to endemic locations and those who work with nonhuman primates. Similarly, the hepatitis B vaccine should be offered to pregnant patients not previously vaccinated who have chronic liver disease, HIV, current or recent intravenous drug use, or a history of sexually transmitted infection, in patients with more than one previous sexual partner in the last 6 months, and in patients with household contacts or sexual partners who are hepatitis B surface antigen positive.

Live-attenuated virus vaccines are relatively contraindicated during pregnancy depending on the indication. These include live-attenuated virus influenza vaccines, the measles–mumps–rubella vaccine, and the varicella vaccine. Although they are contraindicated during pregnancy, there is no scientific evidence that inadvertent administration has led to congenital rubella or congenital varicella with the respective vaccines. The human papillomavirus vaccine also should be deferred during pregnancy, although no adverse events have been linked to inadvertent administration to pregnant patients. The measles–mumps–rubella, varicella, and human papillomavirus vaccines can be safely given in the postpartum period, including to lactating mothers when indicated.

The Ebola, rabies, and yellow fever vaccines also are live-attenuated vaccines. Pregnant patients for whom there is an anticipated exposure risk of these diseases, which have considerable morbidity and mortality, should be individually counseled, and the risks versus benefits of vaccination during pregnancy should be discussed.

Vaccination against severe acute respiratory syndrome coronavirus 2 (SARS-CoV-2), the causative agent of coronavirus disease COVID-19 is an evolving topic. The American College of Obstetricians and Gynecologists recommends that all eligible persons aged 12 years and older, including pregnant and lactating individuals, receive a COVID-19 vaccine or vaccine series. No specific vaccination is preferred in pregnancy. Neither pregnancy nor breastfeeding should preclude a patient from receiving a COVID-19 vaccination should they desire the immunization. Clinicians should remain up to date on the developments with the COVID-19 vaccines and be prepared to counsel pregnant patients who are considering the immunization. Neither consultation with a clinician nor a pregnancy test should be required before receiving this vaccine.

American College of Obstetricians and Gynecologists. COVID-19 vaccination considerations for obstetric–gynecologic care. Practice Advisory. ACOG; 2020. Accessed March 3, 2022. https://www.acog.org/clinical/clinical-guidance/practice-advisory/articles/2020/12/covid-19-vaccination-considerations-for-obstetric-gynecologic-care

Influenza vaccination during pregnancy. ACOG Committee Opinion No. 732. American College of Obstetricians and Gynecologists. Obstet Gynecol 2018;131:e109–14. doi: 10.1097/AOG.0000000000002588 https://journals.lww.com/greenjournal/Fulltext/2018/04000/ACOG_Committee_Opinion_No__732__Influenza.45.aspx

Maternal immunization. ACOG Committee Opinion No. 741. American College of Obstetricians and Gynecologists. Obstet Gynecol 2018;131:e214–7. doi: 10.1097/AOG.0000000000002662 https://journals.lww.com/greenjournal/Fulltext/2018/06000/Maternal_Immunization__ACOG_Committee_Opinion,.60.aspx

Update on immunization and pregnancy: tetanus, diphtheria, and pertussis vaccination. Committee Opinion No. 718. American College of Obstetricians and Gynecologists. Obstet Gynecol 2017;130:e153–7. doi: 10.1097/AOG.0000000000002301 https://journals.lww.com/greenjournal/Fulltext/2017/09000/Committee_Opinion_No__718__Update_on_Immunization.49.aspx

214–218 Electronic fetal heart rate monitoring

For each clinical scenario (214–218), choose the best next management option.

(A) Amnioinfusion
(B) Cesarean birth
(C) Decrease of oxytocin
(D) Expectant management
(E) Operative vaginal delivery

214. C. A 24-year-old gravida 1, para 0, is undergoing induction of labor with oxytocin at 41 weeks of gestation. Vaginal examination reveals the cervix to be 6 cm, 100% effaced, soft and anterior, with the fetal vertex at +2 station (Fig. 214–218-1).

215. D. A 22-year-old gravida 2, para 0, is admitted at 37 weeks of gestation with prelabor rupture of membranes. Oxytocin is initiated. Vaginal examination reveals the cervix to be 4-cm dilated, 80% effaced, soft and anterior, with the fetal vertex at 0 station (Fig. 214–218-2).

216. B. A 31-year-old gravida 3, para 2, has a history of two previous cesarean births and elects to undergo a trial of labor. She is admitted at 41 weeks of gestation with ruptured membranes. Oxytocin is initiated. She receives epidural anesthesia. Several hours later, she reports increased lower abdominal pain. Vaginal examination reveals the cervix to be 7-cm dilated with the fetal vertex at −4 station and significant vaginal bleeding (Fig. 214–218-3).

217. A. A 38-year-old gravida 4, para 3, is admitted for spontaneous rupture of membranes at 39 weeks of gestation. She is admitted for expectant management. Several hours later, her cervix is 5-cm dilated, 50% effaced, and −2 station (Fig. 214–218-4).

218. E. A 37-year-old gravida 7, para 6, presents to labor and delivery in active labor at 36 weeks of gestation. She has a history of cesarean birth at 32 weeks of gestation for her second child and has since had four vaginal deliveries. She requires oxytocin augmentation after placement of an epidural. Vaginal examination reveals the cervix to be 10-cm dilated and fully effaced, with the fetal vertex at +3 station in the occiput anterior position (Fig. 214–218-5).

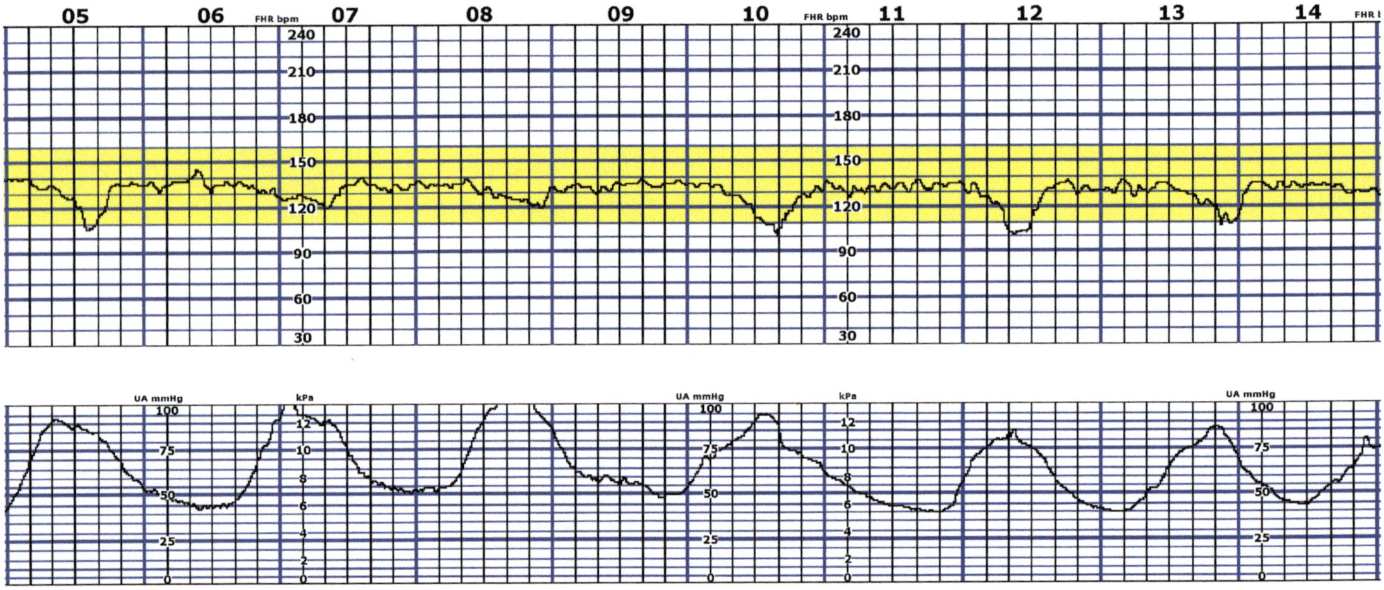

FIGURE 214-218-1. Fetal heart tracing in patient 214. (Image courtesy of James Woods, MD, and periFacts OB/GYN Academy.)

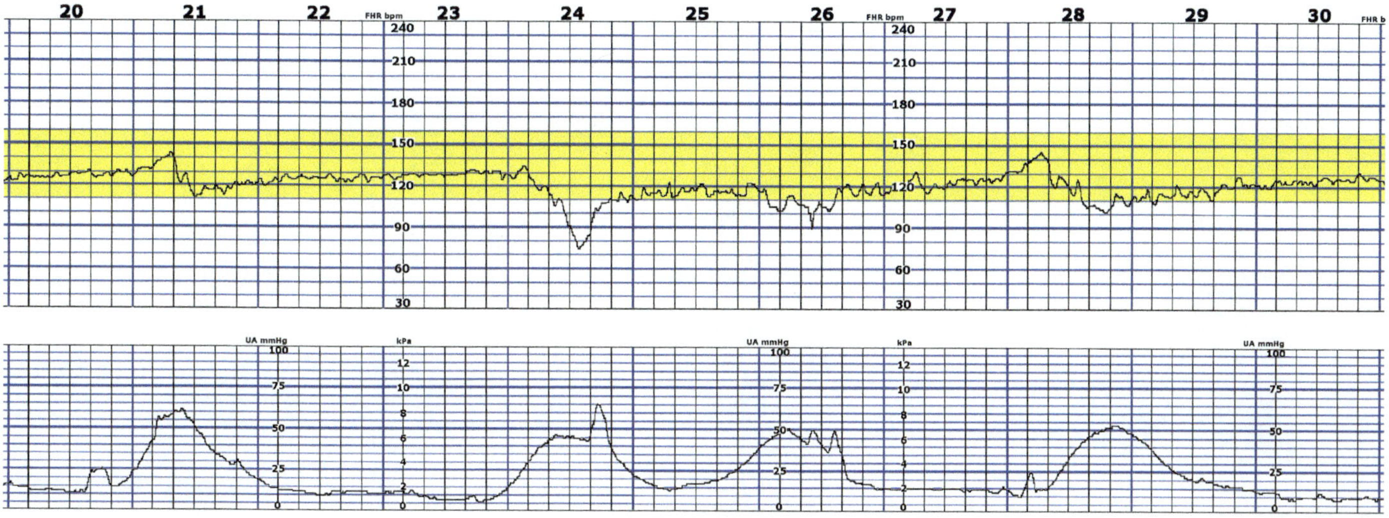

FIGURE 214-218-2. Fetal heart tracing in patient 215. (Image courtesy of James Woods, MD, and periFacts OB/GYN Academy.)

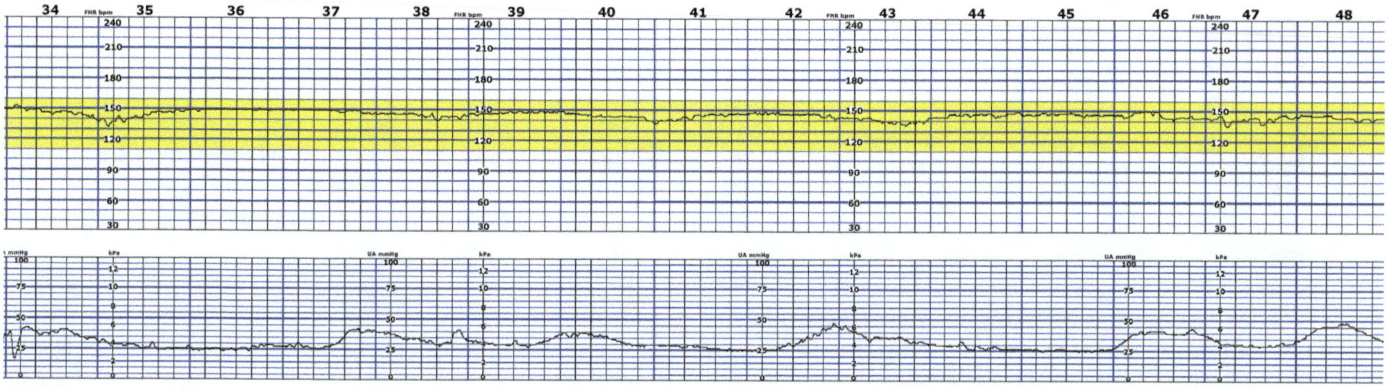

FIGURE 214-218-3. Fetal heart tracing in patient 216. (Image courtesy of James Woods, MD, and periFacts OB/GYN Academy.)

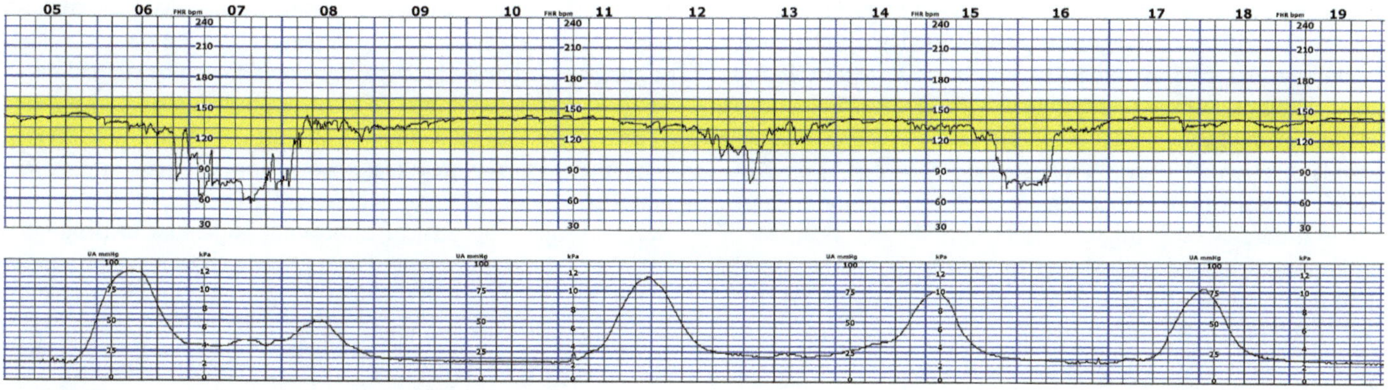

FIGURE 214-218-4. Fetal heart tracing in patient 217.

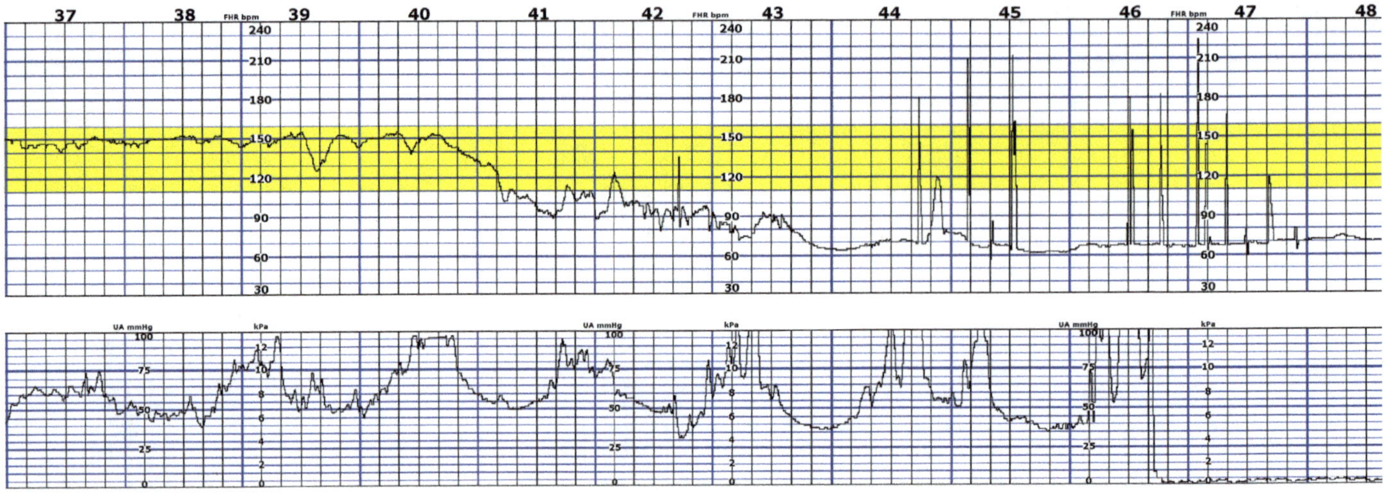

FIGURE 214-218-5. Fetal heart tracing in patient 218. (Image courtesy of James Woods, MD, and periFacts OB/GYN Academy.)

Since the inception of electronic fetal monitoring, significant intra-observer and interobserver variations in interpretation have existed. The subjective nature of fetal heart rate interpretation and assessment has led to inconsistent management plans by practitioners. In recent years, there have been increased efforts to standardize the nomenclature, interpretation, and management of the intrapartum fetal heart rate monitoring. In 2008, the American College of Obstetricians and Gynecologists, the *Eunice Kennedy Shriver* National Institute of Child Health and Human Development, and the Society for Maternal-Fetal Medicine updated approaches to the interpretation and nomenclature of electronic fetal monitoring, resulting in the development of a three-tiered classification system to assist practitioners in their decision-making process (Appendix H).

The vast majority of fetal heart tracings in labor are appropriately identified as Category II. One of the largest challenges in intrapartum care is the management of Category II fetal heart tracings. An article published in 2013, "Intrapartum Management of Category II Fetal Heart Rate Tracings: Towards Standardization of Care," proposed an algorithm (Fig. 214–218-6) to assist in the management of these common tracings. When used clinically, this algorithm (and the clarifications of definitions listed in Appendix H) may help clinicians comply with the standard of care based on the best available evidence and a widely recognized approach.

In Scenario 214, the patient has tachysystole, with more than five contractions in 10 minutes. The fetal baseline is in the normal range, between 130 and 140 beats per minute (bpm), with moderate variability and recurrent variable decelerations. This is a Category II tracing (recurrent variable decelerations with moderate variability). The oxytocin dose should be reduced.

In Scenario 215, the patient is having contractions every 2–3 minutes. The fetal heart rate baseline is 140 bpm, with moderate variability. There is a variable deceleration with one contraction. This is a Category II tracing (variable deceleration with moderate variability). Expectant management is the appropriate choice.

In Scenario 216, the patient's uterine contractions are occurring every 2–5 minutes. The fetal heart rate shows tachycardia at about 170 bpm. There are recurrent late decelerations with minimal variability. In the context of the patient's symptoms and physical examination (vaginal bleeding and loss of station), uterine rupture should be suspected. Emergent cesarean birth should be performed.

In Scenario 217, the patient is having contractions every 2–3 minutes. The fetal heart rate is 135 bpm, with moderate variability and recurrent variable decelerations. This is a Category II tracing (recurrent variable decelerations with moderate variability). Variable decelerations are associated with umbilical cord compression and are not necessarily temporally related to uterine contractions. Management of these decelerations is largely dependent on the patient's labor status, frequency of decelerations, and other potential signs of fetal intolerance of labor. In many circumstances, observation is an appropriate management option; however, the described patient requires more than observation at this point in her care because of the depth and repetitive nature of the variable decelerations. The goal of improving persistent or prolonged variable decelerations should be relieving the possible umbilical cord compression. Although there is limited evidence that demonstrates improvement in short-term and long-term neonatal outcomes, maternal repositioning and amnioinfusion are considered options as initial interventions. Amnioinfusion has been shown to decrease the frequency of variable decelerations and ultimately the incidence of cesarean births secondary to fetal intolerance of labor. Amnioinfusion would be the most appropriate option for the treatment of this patient.

In Scenario 218, the patient is having contractions every 2 minutes. The fetal heart rate is 135 bpm, with moderate variability. Progressive fetal bradycardia develops. This is a Category III tracing. Given the patient's examination, operative vaginal delivery would be most expeditious.

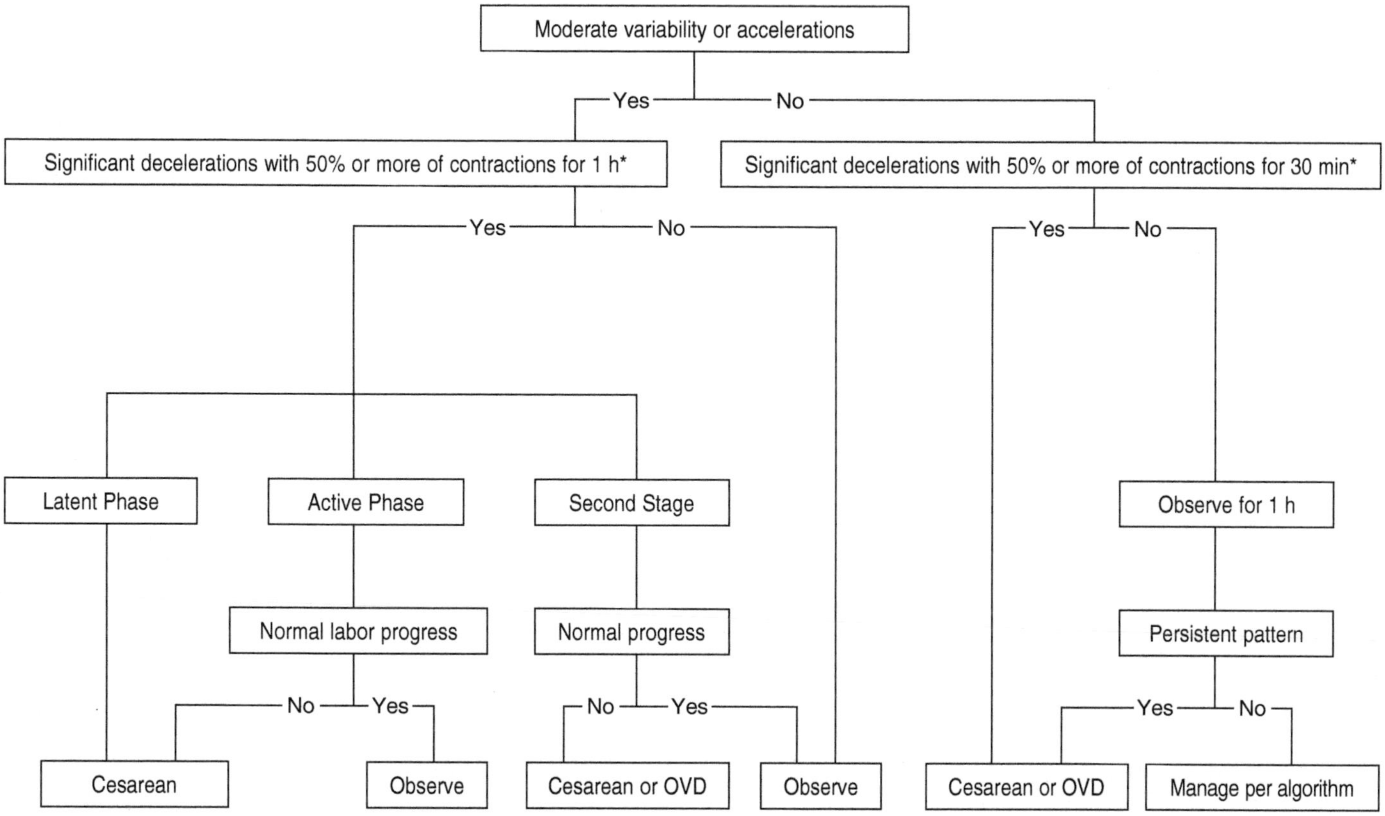

FIGURE 214-218-6. Algorithm for management of Category II fetal heart rate tracings. *That have not resolved with appropriate conservative corrective measures, which may include supplemental oxygen, maternal position changes, intravenous fluid administration, correction of hypotension, reduction or discontinuation of uterine stimulation, administration of uterine relaxant, amnioinfusion, and/or changes in second stage breathing and pushing techniques. (Reprinted from Clark SL, Nageotte MP, Garite TJ, Freeman RK, Miller DA, Simpson KR, et al. Intrapartum management of category II fetal heart rate tracings: towards standardization of care. Am J Obstet Gynecol 2013;209:89–97. doi: 10.1016/j.ajog.2013.04.030 https://www.ajog.org/article/S0002-9378(13)00405-5/fulltext)

Clark SL, Nageotte MP, Garite TJ, Freeman RK, Miller DA, Simpson KR, et al. Intrapartum management of category II fetal heart rate tracings: towards standardization of care. Am J Obstet Gynecol 2013;209:89–97. doi: 10.1016/j.ajog.2013.04.030 https://www.ajog.org/article/S0002-9378(13)00405-5/fulltext

Intrapartum fetal heart rate monitoring: nomenclature, interpretation, and general management principles. ACOG Practice Bulletin No. 106. American College of Obstetricians and Gynecologists. Obstet Gynecol 2009;114:192–202. doi: 10.1097/AOG.0b013e3181aef106 https://journals.lww.com/greenjournal/Citation/2009/07000/ACOG_Practice_Bulletin_No__106__Intrapartum_Fetal.51.aspx

Management of intrapartum fetal heart rate tracings. Practice Bulletin No. 116. American College of Obstetricians and Gynecologists. Obstet Gynecol 2010;116:1232–40. doi: 10.1097/AOG.0b013e3182004fa9 https://journals.lww.com/greenjournal/Citation/2010/11000/Practice_Bulletin_No__116__Management_of.53.aspx

Timmins AE, Clark SL. How to approach intrapartum category II tracings. Obstet Gynecol Clin North Am 2015;42:363–75. doi: 10.1016/j.ogc.2015.01.013 https://www.obgyn.theclinics.com/article/S0889-8545(15)00027-3/fulltext

Appendix A

Normal Values for Laboratory Tests*

ANALYTE	CONVENTIONAL UNITS
Alanine aminotransferase (ALT), serum	10–28 units/L
Alkaline phosphatase, serum	30–120 units/L
Pregnancy	30–229 units/L
Amniotic fluid index	5–25 cm
Amylase	
Serum	20–96 units/L
Pregnancy	15–81 units/L
Aspartate aminotransferase (AST), serum	10–59 units/L
Bicarbonate	
Arterial blood	21–27 mEq/L
Serum	23–28 mEq/L
Pregnancy	18–26 mEq/L
Bilirubin	
Birth to 1 d	1.0–6.0 mg/dL
1–2 d	6.0–7.5 mg/dL
2–5 d	4.0–13.5 mg/dL
5 d to death	0.2–1.2 mg/dL
Blood gases	
Base deficit (calculated)	Less than 3 mEq/L
Base excess, blood	-2 to +3 mEq/L
Arterial and capillary	
Oxygen saturation (So_2)	95% or greater
Pao_2	75–100 mm Hg or greater
$Paco_2$	32–53 mm Hg
Venous	
Pvo_2	30–40 mm Hg
$Pvco_2$	41–51 mm Hg
pH	
Arterial	7.35–7.45
Venous	7.31–7.41
CA 125, serum	Less than 35 units/mL
Calcium, ionized, serum	4.64–5.28 mg/dL
Chloride, serum and plasma (Hep)	98–107 mEq/L
Cholesterol, serum	
Total	
Desirable	Less than 200 mg/dL
Borderline high	200–239 mg/dL
High	240 mg/dL or more
Pregnancy	141–339 mg/dL
High-density lipoprotein (HDL)	40 mg/dL or greater
Pregnancy	40–87 mg/dL
Low-density lipoprotein (LDL)	
Desirable	Less than 100 mg/dL
Borderline high	130–159 mg/dL
High	Greater than 160 mg/dL
Pregnancy	60–224 mg/dL
Triglycerides, serum, fasting	
Desirable	Less than 100 mg/dL
Borderline high	150–199 mg/dL
High	200–499 mg/dL
Pregnancy	40–453 mg/dL
Cortisol, plasma	
8 AM	5–23 micrograms/dL
4 PM	3–16 micrograms/dL
10 PM	Less than 50% of 8 AM value
Pregnancy	7–50 micrograms/dL

(continued)

*Values listed are specific for adults or women, if relevant, unless otherwise differentiated. This table is provided as a reference for normal laboratory values. Note that each laboratory has its own normal values. When treating patients, readers also should refer to the normal values determined by their laboratory.

Normal Values for Laboratory Tests (continued)

ANALYTE	CONVENTIONAL UNITS
Creatinine, serum	0.6–1.1 mg/dL
Pregnancy	0.4–0.8 mg/dL
Dehydroepiandrosterone sulfate, serum or plasma	
Premenopausal	12–379 micrograms/mL
Postmenopausal	30–260 micrograms/mL
Pregnancy	30–611 micrograms/mL
Erythrocyte	
Count	4.2–5.4 × 10^9/L
Sedimentation rate	
Westergren method	0–20 mm/h
Pregnancy	4–70 mm/h
Erythrocyte measures	
Mean corpuscular hemoglobin	27–31 pg
Mean corpuscular hemoglobin concentration	33–37 g/dL
Mean corpuscular volume	81–99 mm^3
Red cell distribution width	10% ± 1.5%
Estradiol-17β	
Follicular phase	10–180 pg/mL
Mid-cycle peak	100–300 pg/mL
Luteal phase	40–200 pg/mL
Postmenopausal	Less than 10 pg/mL
Child	0.8–56 pg/mL
Pregnancy	188–7,192 pg/mL
Ferritin, serum	10–120 micrograms/L
Fibrinogen, plasma	200–400 mg/dL
Pregnancy	250–650 mg/dL
Follicle-stimulating hormone	
Follicular phase	2–9 mIU/mL
Mid-cycle	4–22 mIU/mL
Premenopause	2.8–17.2 mIU/mL
Postmenopause	Greater than 30 mIU/mL
Child	
Tanner stages	1/2 0.5–8.0 mIU/mL
Tanner stages	3–5 1–12 mIU/mL
Glucose	
Fasting, blood	65–95 mg/dL
2-h postprandial	Less than 120 mg/dL
Random, blood	65–110 mg/dL
Serum	65–95 mg/dL
Hematocrit	37–47%
Pregnancy	32–40%
Hemoglobin	12–16 g/dL
Newborn	17.0–23.0 g/dL
Child (varies with age)	11.2–16.5 g/dL
Fetal, percentage	Less than 2% of total hemoglobin
Pregnancy	9.5–15 g/dL
Hemoglobin A_{1c} (nondiabetic)	4.2–5.7
β-Human chorionic gonadotropin	0–5 mIU/mL
Pregnant	Greater than 5 mIU/mL
Postmenopausal	Less than 7.0 mIU/L
17α-Hydroxyprogesterone	
Child	32–63 ng/dL
Follicular phase	Less than 80 ng/dL
Luteal phase	Less than 285 ng/dL
Postmenopausal	Less than 51 ng/dL
Pregnancy	8–340 ng/dL
25-Hydroxyvitamin D	30–60 ng/mL
Iron, serum	50–70 micrograms/dL
Binding capacity, total	254–425 micrograms/dL

(continued)

Normal Values for Laboratory Tests (continued)

ANALYTE	CONVENTIONAL UNITS
Lactate dehydrogenase, serum	
Newborn	290–775 U/L
Neonate	545–2,000 U/L
Infant	180–430 U/L
Child	110–190 U/L
Adult	100–190 U/L
Older than 60 years	110–210 U/L
Pregnancy	80–520 U/L
Leukocytes	
Total	4.5–11 × 10^9/L
Pregnancy	5.5–15 × 10^9/L
Differential counts	
Basophils	0–1%
Eosinophils	0–3%
Lymphocytes	30–45%
Monocytes	0–6%
Band neutrophils	0–5%
Segmented neutrophils	50–70%
Lipase	
60 years or younger	10–140 units/L
Older than 60 years	18–180 units/L
Luteinizing hormone	
Follicular phase	1–12 mIU/mL
Midcycle peak	9–80 mIU/mL
Postmenopause	Greater than 30 mIU/mL
Child	
Tanner stages 1–3	Less than 9 mIU/mL
Tanner stages 4, 5	1–15 mIU/mL
Magnesium	
Adult	1.6–2.6 mg/dL
Child	1.7–2.1 mg/dL
Newborn	1.5–2.2 mg/dL
Partial thromboplastin time, activated	Less than 39 s
Pregnancy	Less than 35 s
Phosphate, inorganic serum	2.7–4.5 mg/dL
Platelet count	150,000–450,000 per microliter
Potassium	3.5–5.0 mEq/L
Progesterone	
Premenarchal	0.1–0.3 ng/dL
Follicular phase	0.1–0.7 ng/dL
Luteal phase	2–25 ng/dL
First trimester	11–44 ng/mL
Second trimester	25–83 ng/mL
Third trimester	58–214 ng/mL
Prolactin	2.5–19 ng/mL
Pregnant	80–400 ng/mL
Prothrombin time–international normalized ratio	
Birth to 6 mo	1.0–1.6
6 mo to adult	0.9–1.2
Pulmonary function	
Peak expiratory flow rate	400–700 L/min
Forced expiratory volume	3.5–5 L (varies by height and age)
Forced vital capacity	3.5–5 L (varies by height and age)
Reticulocyte count	0.5–1.5%
Semen analysis	
Count	Greater than 20 million/mL
Motility, total	40–81%
Morphology	4% normal forms and greater
Sodium, serum	135–145 mEq/L

(continued)

Normal Values for Laboratory Tests (continued)

ANALYTE	CONVENTIONAL UNITS
Testosterone, female	
Total	17–70 ng/dL
Pregnant	3–4 × normal
Postmenopause	8–35 ng/dL
Thyroid-stimulating hormone	0.5–5 mIU/mL
Thyroxine, serum (T_4)	
Free	0.8–1.8 ng/dL
Total	15–12 micrograms/dL
Triiodothyronine, serum (T_3)	
Total	80–180 ng/dL
Reverse	10–24 ng/dL
Free	0.2–0.5 ng/dL
Urea nitrogen, blood	
Adult	8–20 mg/dL
Pregnancy	3–12 mg/dL
Uric acid, serum	2.5–6.2 mg/dL
Child	2.0–5.5 mg/dL
Urinalysis	
Epithelial cells	0–3 HPF
Erythrocytes	0–3 HPF
Leukocytes	0–4 HPF
Protein (albumin)	
Qualitative	None detected
Quantitative	10–100 mg/24 h
Pregnancy	Less than 300 mg/24 h
Urine-specific gravity	
Normal hydration and volume	1.005–1.030
Concentrated	1.025–1.035
Diluted	1.001–1.010

Appendix B [34 and 92]

TABLE B-1. Bishop Scoring System

	FACTOR				
SCORE	**DILATION (CM)**	**POSITION OF CERVIX**	**EFFACEMENT (%)**	**STATION***	**CERVICAL CONSISTENCY**
0	Closed	Posterior	0–30	–3	Firm
1	1–2	Midposition	40–50	–2	Medium
2	3–4	Anterior	60–70	–1, 0	Soft
3	5–6	—	80	+1, +2	—

*Station reflects a –3 to +3 scale.

Modified from Bishop EH. Pelvic scoring for elective induction. Obstet Gynecol 1964;24:266–8. https://journals.lww.com/greenjournal/pages/articleviewer.aspx

Appendix C [38, 81, 86]

BOX C-1

Preeclampsia With Severe Features

- Systolic blood pressure of 160 mm Hg or more, or diastolic blood pressure of 110 mm Hg or more on two occasions at least 4 h apart (unless antihypertensive therapy is initiated before this time)
- Thrombocytopenia (platelet count less than 100×10^9/L)
- Impaired liver function that is not accounted for by alternative diagnoses and as indicated by abnormally elevated blood concentrations of liver enzymes (to more than twice the upper limit normal concentrations), or by severe persistent right upper quadrant or epigastric pain unresponsive to medica tions
- Renal insufficiency (serum creatinine concentration more than 1.1 mg/dL or a doubling of the serum creatinine concentration in the absence of other renal disease)
- Pulmonary edema
- New-onset headache unresponsive to medication and not accounted for by alternative diagnoses
- Visual disturbances

Reprinted from Gestational hypertension and preeclampsia. ACOG Practice Bulletin No. 222. American College of Obstetricians and Gynecologists. Obstet Gynecol 2020;135:e237–60. doi: 10.1097/AOG.0000000000003891 https://journals.lww.com/greenjournal/Fulltext/2020/06000/Gestational_Hypertension_and_Preeclampsia__ACOG.46.aspx

Appendix D [43 and 157-161]

TABLE D-1. Levels of Maternal Care: Definitions, Capabilities, and Health Care Professionals*

ACCREDITED BIRTH CENTER	
Definition	Care for low-risk women with uncomplicated singleton term vertex pregnancies who are expected to have an uncomplicated birth
Capabilities and health care professionals	· Refer to birthcenters.org for American Association of Birth Centers' Standards for Birth Centers.
LEVEL I (BASIC CARE)	
Definition	Care of low- to moderate-risk pregnancies with ability to detect, stabilize, and initiate management of unanticipated maternal–fetal or neonatal problems that occur during the antepartum, intrapartum, or postpartum period until the patient can be transferred to a facility at which specialty maternal care is available
Capabilities	· Capability and equipment to provide low-risk and appropriate moderate-risk maternal care and a readiness at all times to initiate emergency procedures to meet unexpected needs of women and newborns within the center. This includes – ability to begin emergency cesarean delivery within a time interval that best incorporates maternal and fetal risks and benefits. – limited obstetric ultrasonography with interpretation readily available at all times.† – support services readily available at all times,† including laboratory testing and blood bank. – capability to implement patient safety bundles‡ for common causes of preventable maternal morbidity, such as management of maternal venous thromboembolism, obstetric hemorrhage, and maternal severe hypertension in pregnancy.§ – ability at all times† to initiate massive transfusion protocol, with process to obtain more blood and component therapy as needed. · Stabilization and the ability to facilitate transport to a higher-level hospital when necessary. This includes – risk identification and determination of conditions necessitating consultation, referral, and transfer. – a mechanism and procedure for transfer/transport to a higher-level hospital available at all times.† – a reliable, accurate, and comprehensive communication system between participating hospitals, hospital personnel, and transport teams. · Ability, in collaboration with higher-level facility partners, to initiate and sustain education and quality improvement programs to maximize patient safety.
Health care professionals	· Every birth attended by at least one qualified birthing professional (midwife,‖ family physician, or ob-gyn) and an appropriately trained and qualified RN with level-appropriate competencies as demonstrated by nursing competency documentation. · Physician with privileges to perform emergency cesarean delivery readily available at all times.† · Primary maternal care professionals, including midwives,‖ family physicians, or ob-gyns readily available at all times.† · Appropriately trained and qualified RNs with level-appropriate competencies as demonstrated by nursing competency documentation readily available at all times.† · Nursing leadership has level-appropriate formal training and experience in maternal care. · Anesthesia professionals, such as anesthesiologists, nurse anesthetists, or anesthesiologist assistants working with an anesthesiologist,¶ for labor analgesia and surgical anesthesia readily available at all times.†

(continued)

Table D-1 *(continued)*

LEVEL II (SPECIALTY CARE)	
Definition	Level I facility plus care of appropriate moderate- to high-risk antepartum, intrapartum, or postpartum conditions
Capabilities	Level I facility capabilities plus • Computed tomography scan, magnetic resonance imaging, nonobstetric ultrasound imaging, and maternal echocardiography with interpretation readily available daily (at all times not required). • Standard obstetric ultrasound imaging with interpretation readily available at all times.†
Health care professionals	Level I facility health care professionals plus • Ob-gyn readily available at all times.† – Based upon available resources and facility determination of the most appropriate staffing, it may be acceptable for a family physician with obstetric fellowship training or equivalent training and skills in obstetrics, and with surgical skill and privileges to perform cesarean delivery to meet the criteria for being readily available at all times. • Physician obstetric leadership is a board-certified# ob-gyn with experience in obstetric care. – Based upon available resources and facility determination of the most appropriate staffing, it may be acceptable for such leader to be board certified in another specialty with privileges and expertise in obstetric care including with surgical skill and privileges to perform cesarean delivery. • An MFM readily available at all times† for consultation onsite, by phone, or by telemedicine, as needed. • Anesthesiologist readily available at all times.† • Internal or family medicine physicians and general surgeons readily available at all times† for obstetric patients.
LEVEL III (SUBSPECIALTY CARE)	
Definition	Level II facility plus care of more complex maternal medical conditions, obstetric complications, and fetal conditions
Capabilities	Level II facility capabilities plus • In-house availability of all blood components. • Computed tomography scan, magnetic resonance imaging, maternal echocardiography, and nonobstetric ultrasound imaging services and interpretation readily available at all times.† • Specialized obstetric ultrasound and fetal assessment, including Doppler studies, with interpretation readily available at all times.† • Basic interventional radiology (capable of performing uterine artery embolization) readily available at all times.† • Appropriate equipment and personnel physically present at all times** onsite to ventilate and monitor women in labor and delivery until they can be safely transferred to the ICU. • Onsite medical and surgical ICUs that accept pregnant women and women in the postpartum period. The ICUs have adult critical care professionals physically present at all times.** An MFM is readily available at all times† to actively communicate or consult for all obstetric patients in the ICU. • Documented mechanism to facilitate and accept maternal transfers/transports. • Provide outreach education and patient transfer feedback to level I and II designated facilities to address maternal care quality issues. • Provide perinatal system leadership if acting as a regional center (for example, in areas where level IV facilities are not available) (see Level IV).

(continued)

Table D-1 (*continued*)

Health care professionals	Level II health care professionals plus • Nursing leaders and adequate number of RNs who have special training and experience in the management of women with complex and critical maternal illnesses and obstetric complications • Board-certified# ob-gyn physically present** at all times • An MFM with inpatient privileges readily available at all times,† either onsite, by phone, or by telemedicine. Timing of need to be onsite is directed by urgency of clinical situation. However, MFM must be able to be onsite to provide direct care within 24 h. • Director of maternal–fetal medicine service is a board-certified MFM. • Director of obstetric service is a board-certified ob-gyn or MFM. • Board-certified anesthesiologist# physically present** at all times. • Director of obstetric anesthesia services is board-certified anesthesiologist with obstetric anesthesia fellowship training or experience in obstetric anesthesia. • Full complement of subspecialists, such as subspecialists in critical care, general surgery, infectious disease, hematology, cardiology, nephrology, neurology, gastroenterology, internal medicine, behavioral health, and neonatology, readily available for inpatient consultation at all times.†
LEVEL IV (REGIONAL PERINATAL HEALTH CARE CENTERS)	
Definition	Level III facility plus on-site medical and surgical care of the most complex maternal conditions and critically ill pregnant women and fetuses throughout antepartum, intrapartum, and postpartum care
Capabilities	Level III facility capabilities plus • On-site medical and surgical care of complex maternal conditions with the availability of critical care unit or ICU beds. • On-site ICU care for obstetric patients with primary or co-management by maternal–fetal medicine team. Co-management includes at least daily rounds by an MFM with interaction with the ICU team and other subspecialists with daily documentation. In some settings, the ICU is in an adjoining or connected building, which is acceptable as long as maternal–fetal medicine care is as noted above. If the woman must be transported by ambulance to the ICU, this is not considered onsite. • Perinatal system leadership, including facilitation of collaboration with facilities in the region, analysis and review of system perinatal outcome and quality data, provision of outreach education and assistance with quality improvement as needed.
Health care professionals	Level III health care professionals plus • Maternal–fetal medicine care team with expertise to manage highly complex, critically ill, or unstable maternal patients. A board-certified MFM attending with full inpatient privileges is readily available at all times† for consultation and management. This includes co-management of ICU-admitted obstetric patients. • Nursing Service Line leadership with advanced degree and national certification. • Continuous availability of adequate numbers of RNs who have experience in the care of women with complex medical illnesses and obstetric complications with close collaboration between critical care nurses and obstetric nurses with expertise in caring for critically ill women. • Board-certified anesthesiologist with obstetric anesthesia fellowship training or experience in obstetric anesthesia physically present at all times.** • At least one of the following adult subspecialties readily available at all times for consultation and treatment as needed onsite: neurosurgery, cardiac surgery, or transplant. If the facility does not have all three subspecialties available, there should be a process in place to transfer women to a facility that can provide the needed service.

(*continued*)

Table D-1 (*continued*)

Abbreviations: CMs, certified midwives; CNMs, certified nurse-midwives; ICU, intensive care unit; MFM, maternal-fetal medicine subspecialists; ob-gyns, obstetrician-gynecologists; RNs, registered nurses.

*These guidelines are limited to maternal needs. Consideration of fetal or neonatal needs and the appropriate level of care should occur following existing guidelines. In fact, levels of maternal care and levels of neonatal care may not match within facilities. Additionally, these are guidelines, and local issues will affect systems of implementation for regionalized maternal care, perinatal care, or both.

†Readily available at all times: the specific person should be available 24 hours a day, 7 days a week for consultation and assistance, and able to be physically present onsite within a time frame that incorporates maternal and fetal or neonatal risks and benefits with the provision of care. Further defining this time frame should be individualized by facilities and regions, with input from their obstetric care professionals. If referring to the availability of a service, the service should be available 24 hours a day, 7 days a week, unless otherwise specified.

‡Available at https://safehealthcareforeverywoman.org/patient-safety-bundles.

§See also Emergent therapy for acute-onset, severe hypertension during pregnancy and the postpartum period. ACOG Committee Opinion No. 767. American College of Obstetricians and Gynecologists. Obstet Gynecol 2019;133:e174–80.

||Midwives who meet International Confederation of Midwives standards, such as certified nurse-midwives (CNMs) and certified midwives (CMs), and who are legally recognized to practice within the jurisdiction of the state.

¶Scope of practice for nurse anesthetists and anesthesiologist assistants may vary by state.

#Also includes physicians who have completed residency training and are eligible for board certification according to applicable board policies.

**Physically present at all times: the specific person should be onsite in the location where the perinatal care is provided, 24 hours a day, 7 days a week.

Levels of maternal care. Obstetric Care Consensus No. 9. American College of Obstetricians and Gynecologists [published erratum appears in Obstet Gynecol 2019;134:883]. Obstet Gynecol 2019;134:e41–55. doi: 10.1097/AOG.0000000000003383 https://journals.lww.com/greenjournal/Fulltext/2019/08000/Levels_of_Maternal_Care__Obstetric_Care_Consensus.44.aspx

Appendix E [48 and 70]

TABLE E-1. General Guidance Regarding Obstetric Interventions for Threatened and Imminent Periviable Birth by Best Estimate of Gestational Age*

	20 0/7 WEEKS TO 21 6/7 WEEKS	22 0/7 WEEKS TO 22 6/7 WEEKS	23 0/7 WEEKS TO 23 6/7 WEEKS	24 0/7 WEEKS TO 24 6/7 WEEKS	25 0/7 WEEKS TO 25 6/7 WEEKS
Neonatal assessment for resuscitation*	Not recommended 1A	Consider 2B	Consider 2B	Recommended 1B	Recommended 1B
Antenatal corticosteroids	Not recommended 1A	Not recommended 1A	Consider 2B	Recommended 1B	Recommended 1B
Tocolysis for preterm labor to allow for antenatal corticosteroid administration	Not recommended 1A	Not recommended 1A	Consider 2B	Recommended 1B	Recommended 1B
Magnesium sulfate for neuroprotection	Not recommended 1A	Not recommended 1A	Consider 2B	Recommended 1B	Recommended 1B
Antibiotics to prolong latency during expectant management of preterm PROM if delivery is not considered imminent	Consider 2C	Consider 2C	Consider 2B	Recommended 1B	Recommended 1B
Intrapartum antibiotics for group B streptococci prophylaxis†	Not recommended 1A	Not recommended 1A	Consider 2B	Recommended 1B	Recommended 1B
Cesarean delivery for fetal indication‡	Not recommended 1A	Not recommended 1A	Consider 2B	Consider 1B	Recommended 1B

Abbreviation: PROM, premature rupture of membranes.

*Survival of neonates born in the periviable period is dependent on resuscitation and support. Between 22 weeks and 25 weeks of gestation, there may be factors in addition to gestational age that will affect the potential for survival and the determination of viability. Importantly, some families, concordant with their values and preferences, may choose to forgo such resuscitation and support. Many of the other decisions on this table will be linked to decisions regarding resuscitation and support and should be considered in that context.

†Group B streptococci carrier, or carrier status unknown.

‡For example, persistently abnormal fetal heart rate patterns or biophysical testing, malpresentation.

Modified from Periviable birth. Obstetric Care Consensus No. 6. American College of Obstetricians and Gynecologists. Obstet Gynecol 2017;130:e187–99. doi: 10.1097/AOG.0000000000002352 https://journals.lww.com/greenjournal/Fulltext/2017/10000/Obstetric_Care_Consensus_No__6__Periviable_Birth.57.aspx

Appendix F [79 and 209-213]

TABLE F-1. Summary of Maternal Immunization Recommendations

VACCINE*	INDICATED DURING EVERY PREGNANCY	MAY BE GIVEN DURING PREGNANCY IN CRTAIN POPULATIONS	CONTRAINDICATED DURING PREGNANCY	CAN BE INITIATED POSTPARTUM OR WHEN BREASTFEEDING OR BOTH
COVID-19[†,1] (see footnote for recommendations)				
Inactivated influenza	X[‡,2,3]			X[§]
Tetanus toxoid, reduced diphtheria toxoid, and acellular pertussis (Tdap)	X[‡,4,5]			X[§]
Pneumococcal vaccines		X[‖,6]		X[‖,6]
Meningococcal conjugate (MenACWY) and meningococcal serogroup B		X[¶,7]		X[¶,7]
Hepatitis A		X[#,8]		X[#,8]
Hepatitis B		X[**,9,10]		X[**,9,10]
Human papillomavirus (HPV)**				X[††,11,12]
Measles-mumps-rubella			X[‡‡,13,14]	X[‡‡]
Varicella			X[‡‡,13,15,16]	X[‡‡]

*An "X" indicates that the vaccine can be given in this window. See the corresponding numbered footnote for details.

†COVID-19 vaccination is recommended for pregnant individuals who have not previously been vaccinated. Pregnant individuals may receive any COVID-19 vaccine product available to them; however, Moderna, Pfizer-BioNtech, and Novavax vaccines are preferred over the Johnson & Johnson/Janssen vaccine. Vaccination may occur in any trimester and emphasis should be on vaccine receipt as soon as possible to maximize maternal and fetal health. Pregnant individuals should also receive a single COVID-19 booster dose, if not received prior to pregnancy. Pregnancy alone is currently not an indication for a second booster. However, pregnant patients who meet other criteria (age, vaccine product received for primary series and booster, and immune status) may choose to receive a second booster. COVID-19 vaccination is recommended for postpartum and/or lactating individuals who were not previously vaccinated.

‡Inactivated influenza vaccination can be given in any trimester and should be given each influenza season as soon as the vaccine is available. The Tdap vaccine is given at 27–36 weeks of gestation in each pregnancy, preferably as early in the 27- to 36-week window as possible. The Tdap vaccine should be given during each pregnancy in order to boost the maternal immune response and maximize the passive antibody transfer to the newborn. If not administered during pregnancy, the Tdap vaccine should be given immediately postpartum if the woman has never received a prior dose of Tdap as an adolescent, adult, or during a previous pregnancy.[1–3]

§Vaccination during every pregnancy is preferred over vaccination during the postpartum period to ensure antibody transfer to the newborn.[3,4]

‖There are two kinds of pneumococcal vaccines in the United States: pneumococcal conjugate vaccines (PCV13, PCV15, and PCV20) and pneumococcal polysaccharide vaccine (PPSV23). Pneumococcal vaccines (PCV15, PCV20, PPSV23) may be given to pregnant individuals at high risk of severe illness from pneumococcal disease. Clinicians should refer to CDC guidance for details on conditions that put individuals at high-risk for severe pneumococcal disease.[5,6]

¶Quadrivalent conjugate meningococcal vaccine is routinely recommended for adolescents aged 11–18 years, along with individuals with HIV infection, complement component deficiency (including eculizumab use), functional or anatomic asplenia (including sickle cell disease), exposure during a meningococcal disease outbreak, travel to endemic or hyperendemic areas, or work as a microbiologist routinely exposed to *Neisseria meningitidis*. If indicated, pregnancy should not preclude vaccination. The serogroup B vaccine should be deferred in pregnant individuals, unless the person is at increased risk of serogroup B meningococcal disease[7] and, after consultation with her health care provider, the benefits of vaccination are considered to outweigh the potential risks.[7]

#Pregnant individuals with any of the conditions that increase the risk of either acquiring or having a severe outcome from hepatitis A infection (eg, international travelers, persons who use injection or noninjection drugs, persons who have occupational risk for infection, persons who anticipate close personal contact with an international adoptee, or persons experiencing homelessness) or for having a severe outcome from hepatitis A infection (eg, persons with chronic liver disease or persons with HIV infection) should be vaccinated during pregnancy if not previously vaccinated. Pregnant individuals at risk of hepatitis A infection during pregnancy should also be counseled concerning all options to prevent hepatitis A infection. Any person who wants to be protected from hepatitis A or has an indication for use may receive the vaccine during pregnancy or during the postpartum period.[8]

**Hepatitis B vaccination is recommended for all adults who have not previously been vaccinated. Importantly, Heplisav-B and PreHebrio are not recommended in pregnancy because of lack of safety data in pregnant individuals. Pregnant individuals at risk of hepatitis B infection during pregnancy should be counseled concerning other methods to prevent hepatitis B infection.[1,9]

††The HPV vaccination in pregnancy is not recommended; however, inadvertent HPV vaccination during pregnancy is not associated with adverse events for the pregnant individual or their fetus. The HPV vaccine can be given to postpartum and lactating individuals. The HPV vaccine should be administered to individuals through age 26 years who were not previously vaccinated. Vaccination timing and number of doses should follow Centers for Disease Control and Prevention and American College of Obstetricians and Gynecologists' guidance.[11,12]

‡‡Live attenuated vaccines, including measles-mumps-rubella, varicella, and live attenuated influenza vaccine, are contraindicated for pregnant individuals. If indicated (ie, among seronegative individuals), the measles-mumps-rubella vaccine and the varicella vaccine should be given during the postpartum period. Inadvertent administration during pregnancy has not been associated with congenital rubella or congenital varicella syndromes.[13–16]

Table F-1 *(continued)*

[1] American College of Obstetricians and Gynecologists. COVID-19 vaccination considerations for obstetric–gynecologic care. Practice Advisory. ACOG; 2020. Accessed July 27, 2022. https://www.acog.org/clinical/clinical-guidance/practice-advisory/articles/2020/12/covid-19-vaccination-considerations-for-obstetric-gynecologic-care.

[2] Influenza vaccination during pregnancy. ACOG Committee Opinion No. 732. American College of Obstetricians and Gynecologists. Obstet Gynecol 2018;131:e109-14. doi: 10.1097/AOG.0000000000002588.

[3] Centers for Disease Control and Prevention. Influenza (flu) vaccine and pregnancy. CDC; 2019. Accessed July 27, 2022. https://www.cdc.gov/vaccines/pregnancy/hcp-toolkit/flu-vaccine-pregnancy.html.

[4] Centers for Disease Control and Prevention. Tdap (pertussis) vaccine and pregnancy. CDC; 2017. Accessed July 27, 2022. https://www.cdc.gov/vaccines/pregnancy/hcp-toolkit/tdap-vaccine-pregnancy.html.

[5] Update on immunization and pregnancy: tetanus, diphtheria, and pertussis vaccination. Committee Opinion No. 718. American College of Obstetricians and Gynecologists. Obstet Gynecol 2017;130:e153-7. doi: 10.1097/AOG.0000000000002301.

[6] Kobayashi M, Farrar JL, Gierke R, Britton A, Childs L, Leidner AJ, et al. Use of 15-valent pneumococcal conjugate vaccine and 20-valent pneumococcal conjugate vaccine among U.S. Adults: updated recommendations of the Advisory Committee on Immunization Practices - United States, 2022. MMWR Morb Mortal Wkly Rep 2022;71:109-17. doi: 10.15585/mmwr.mm7104a1.

[7] Mbaeyi SA, Bozio CH, Duffy J, Rubin LG, Hariri S, Stephens DS, et al. Meningococcal vaccination: recommendations of the Advisory Committee on Immunization Practices, United States, 2020. MMWR Recomm Rep 2020;69(RR-9):1-41. doi: 10.15585/mmwr.rr6909a1.

[8] Nelson NP, Weng MK, Hofmeister MG, Moore KL, Doshani M, Kamili S, et al. Prevention of hepatitis A virus infection in the United States: Recommendations of the Advisory Committee on Immunization Practices, 2020 [published erratum appears in MMWR Morb Mortal Wkly Rep 2021;70:294]. MMWR Recomm Rep 2020;69(RR-5):1-38. doi: 10.15585/mmwr.rr6905a1.

[9] American College of Obstetricians and Gynecologists. Hepatitis B prevention. Practice Advisory. ACOG; 2018. Accessed July 27, 2022. https://www.acog.org/clinical/clinical-guidance/practice-advisory/articles/2018/01/hepatitis-b-prevention.

[10] Weng MK, Doshani M, Khan MA, Frey S, Ault K, Moore KL, et al. Universal hepatitis B vaccination in adults aged 19-59 years: updated recommendations of the Advisory Committee on Immunization Practices - United States, 2022. MMWR Morb Mortal Wkly Rep 2022;71:477-83. doi: 10.15585/mmwr.mm7113a1.

[11] Human papillomavirus vaccination. ACOG Committee Opinion No. 809. American College of Obstetricians and Gynecologists. Obstet Gynecol 2020;136:e15-21. doi: 10.1097/AOG.0000000000004000.

[12] Meites E, Szilagyi PG, Chesson HW, Unger ER, Romero JR, Markowitz LE. Human papillomavirus vaccination for adults: updated recommendations of the Advisory Committee on Immunization Practices. MMWR Morb Mortal Wkly Rep 2019;68:698-702. doi: 10.15585/mmwr.mm6832a3.

[13] American Academy of Pediatrics; American College of Obstetricians and Gynecologists. Guidelines for perinatal care. 8th ed. American Academy of Pediatrics; American College of Obstetricians and Gynecologists; 2017.

[14] McLean HQ, Fiebelkorn AP, Temte JL, Wallace GS. Prevention of measles, rubella, congenital rubella syndrome, and mumps, 2013: summary recommendations of the Advisory Committee on Immunization Practices (ACIP). Centers for Disease Control and Prevention [published erratum appears in MMWR Morb Mortal Wkly Rep 2015;64:259]. MMWR Recomm Rep 2013;62(RR-4):1-34.

[15] Centers for Disease Control and Prevention, (CDC). Updated recommendations for use of VariZIG--United States, 2013. MMWR Morb Mortal Wkly Rep 2013;62:574-6.

[16] Marin M, Güris D, Chaves SS, Schmid S, Seward JF. Prevention of varicella: recommendations of the Advisory Committee on Immunization Practices (ACIP). Advisory Committee on Immunization Practices, Centers for Disease Control and Prevention (CDC). MMWR Recomm Rep 2007;56(RR-4):1-40.

American College of Obstetricians and Gynecologists. Maternal immunization. Practice Advisory. ACOG;2022.

Appendix G [101 and 201-204]

TABLE G-1. Anticoagulation Regimen Definitions

ANTICOAGULATION REGIMEN	ANTICOAGULATION DOSAGE*
Prophylactic LMWH†	Enoxaparin, 40 mg SC once daily Dalteparin, 5,000 units SC once daily Tinzaparin, 4,500 units SC once daily Nadroparin, 2,850 units SC once daily
Intermediate-dose LMWH	Enoxaparin, 40 mg SC every 12 h Dalteparin, 5,000 units SC every 12 h
Adjusted-dose (therapeutic) LMWH†	Enoxaparin, 1 mg/kg every 12 h Dalteparin, 200 units/kg once daily Tinzaparin, 175 units/kg once daily Dalteparin, 100 units/kg every 12 h Target an anti-Xa level in the therapeutic range of 0.6–1.0 units/mL 4 h after last injection for twice-daily regimen; slightly higher doses may be needed for a once-daily regimen.
Prophylactic UFH	UFH, 5,000–7,500 units SC every 12 h in first trimester UFH, 7,500–10,000 units SC every 12 h in the second trimester UFH, 10,000 units SC every 12 h in the third trimester, unless the aPTT is elevated
Adjusted-dose (therapeutic) UFH‡	UFH, 10,000 units or more SC every 12 h in doses adjusted to target aPTT in the therapeutic range (1.5–2.5 × control) 6 h after injection
Postpartum anticoagulation	Prophylactic, intermediate, or adjusted-dose LMWH for 6–8 weeks as indicated. Oral anticoagulants may be considered postpartum based upon planned duration of therapy, lactation, and patient preference.
Surveillance	Clinical vigilance and appropriate objective investigation of women with symptoms suspicious of deep vein thrombosis or pulmonary embolism. VTE risk assessment should be performed prepregnancy or early in pregnancy and repeated if complications develop, particularly those necessitating hospitalization or prolonged immobility.

Abbreviations: aPTT, activated partial thromboplastin time; INR, international normalized ratio; LMWH, low-molecular-weight heparin; SC, subcutaneously; UFH, unfractionated heparin; VTE, venous thromboembolism.

*The dosages in the table were published by ACOG in 2018. For the most up-to-date dosing information, please review ACOG's guidance at acog.org.

†Although at extremes of body weight, modification of dose may be required.

‡Also referred to as weight-adjusted, full-treatment dose.

Reprinted from Thromboembolism in pregnancy. ACOG Practice Bulletin No. 196. American College of Obstetricians and Gynecologists [published erratum appears in Obstet Gynecol 2018;132:1068]. Obstet Gynecol 2018;132:e1–17. doi: 10.1097/AOG.0000000000002706 https://journals.lww.com/greenjournal/Fulltext/2018/07000/ACOG_Practice_Bulletin_No__196__Thromboembolism_in.54.aspx

Appendix H [167-171 and 214-218]

BOX H-1

Three-Tiered Information System to Aid in Reading, Communicating, and Managing Fetal Heart Rate Tracings

A. Category I (normal). Strongly predictive of normal fetal acid–base status, these FHR tracings may be followed in a routine manner and include all of the following:
- Baseline rate 110–160 beats per minute
- Moderate variability
- Absent late or variable decelerations
- Early decelerations may or may not be present
- Accelerations may or may not be present

B. Category II (indeterminate). Not predictive of abnormal fetal acid–base status but requiring evaluation, continued surveillance, and re-evaluation, taking into account the clinical context. This category includes any of the following:
- Baseline rate
  - Bradycardia not accompanied by absent baseline variability
  - Tachycardia
- Baseline FHR variability
  - Minimal baseline variability
  - Absent baseline variability not accompanied by recurrent decelerations
  - Marked baseline variability
- Accelerations
  - Absence of induced accelerations after fetal stimulation
- Periodic or episodic decelerations
  - Recurrent variable decelerations accompanied by minimal or moderate baseline variability
  - Prolonged deceleration of 2 min or more but less than 10 min
  - Recurrent late decelerations with moderate baseline variability
  - Variable decelerations with other characteristics, such as slow return to baseline, "overshoots," or "shoulders"

C. Category III (abnormal). Predictive of abnormal fetal acid–base status; requires prompt evaluation and management. Includes either of the following:
- Absent baseline FHR variability with:
  - Recurrent late decelerations
  - Recurrent variable decelerations, or
  - Bradycardia
- Sinusoidal FHR

Abbreviation: FHR, fetal heart rate.

Modified from Intrapartum fetal heart rate monitoring: nomenclature, interpretation, and general management principles. ACOG Practice Bulletin No. 106. American College of Obstetricians and Gynecologists. Obstet Gynecol 2009;114:192–202. doi: 10.1097/AOG.0b013e3181aef106 https://journals.lww.com/greenjournal/Citation/2009/07000/ACOG_Practice_Bulletin_No__106__Intrapartum_Fetal.51.aspx.

Index

NOTE: Numbers refer to questions, not pages.

NOTE: Numbers refer to questions, not pages.

NOTE: Numbers refer to questions, not pages.

NOTE: Numbers refer to questions, not pages.

NOTE: Numbers refer to questions, not pages.

PROLOG

Personal Review of Learning in Obstetrics and Gynecology

Obstetrics

NINTH EDITION

Assessment Book

ONLINE ASSESSMENT
See instructions on the inside front cover.

ACOG
American College of Obstetricians & Gynecologists

Assessment Instructions

To earn continuing medical education (CME) credits, you need to submit the assessment online. Assessment results must be 80% or higher to achieve a passing score and attain CME credit. Instructions for the electronic submission are included on this page. **Paper answer sheets are not available for this edition.**

The online assessment is included with the price of the print book of this edition of PROLOG. You can retake the online assessment as many times as needed at no cost.

Instructions for Submitting the Electronic Assessment for CME Credit

To complete the online assessment for *Obstetrics*, Ninth Edition, follow these steps:

1. Go to https://prolog.acog.org.
2. Click "GET STARTED."
3. Log in to your ACOG account.
4. After you are logged in, your browser should redirect you to the PROLOG dashboard.
5. If it does not redirect you, refresh the page or go back to https://prolog.acog.org.
6. Find the assessment for *Obstetrics*, Ninth Edition, and click "Redeem Code."
7. Enter the key code located inside the red box on the inside cover of the Critique book. Follow the instructions provided and click "Redeem Code."

You will then be taken to the online assessment.

You will receive your test results immediately after submitting the online assessment. With a passing score of 80% or higher, your CME certificate will be available as a PDF within the online assessment. You are able to take the assessment as many times as needed to achieve the passing score for CME credit.

Electronic Assessment for CME Credit

To receive the CME credits for this edition, participants must complete an online assessment. Assessment results must be 80% or higher to achieve a passing score and attain CME credit. To access the online assessment, please visit https://prolog.acog.org. Test results and the CME certificate will be available upon completion of the examination.

If you purchased a print book, use the key code located on the inside front cover of the Critique Book and follow the directions provided. If you purchased an eBook, please follow the instructions online through https://prolog.acog.org to purchase and access the assessment. **Paper answer sheets are not available for this edition.**

DIRECTIONS: Each of the questions or incomplete statements below is followed by suggested answers or completions. On the online assessment select the ONE option that is BEST in each case.

1

A 36-year-old gravida 3, para 2, presents for the initiation of prenatal care in the third trimester. She has a history of a term cesarean birth followed by a term vaginal birth. She has no other surgical history and has no medical problems. On physical examination, she has a fundal height of 36 cm. She undergoes an obstetric ultrasonographic examination. The gestational age is estimated at 36 5/7 weeks of gestation by fetal biometry. She has an anterior placenta previa. Placental lacunae are identified along with loss of the retroplacental hypoechoic zone. The retroplacental myometrium is measured at 1 mm. Excessive color Doppler flow is present in the retroplacental space. The sonographic feature exhibited in this patient's examination that has the strongest association with a placenta accreta is the

(A) excessive color Doppler flow in the retroplacental space
(B) loss of the retroplacental hypoechoic zone
(C) placental lacunae
(D) placenta previa
(E) thin retroplacental myometrium

2

A 31-year-old gravida 3, para 1, is admitted in labor at 38 weeks of gestation. Her body mass index (BMI) is 51. Her obstetric history is notable for a previous cesarean birth, and she elects to undergo a trial of labor. During labor she is diagnosed with intra-amniotic infection. Two hours later, the fetal heart rate shows tachycardia with persistent late decelerations, and cesarean birth is performed. In addition to the use of pneumatic compression devices, the best pharmacologic management to reduce the risk of venous thromboembolism (VTE) in this patient is to initiate

(A) direct oral anticoagulant
(B) low-molecular-weight heparin (LMWH)
(C) unfractionated subcutaneous heparin
(D) warfarin

3

A 32-year-old multiparous patient at 14 weeks of gestation has a positive treponemal-specific chemiluminescent immunoassay test. She reports feeling well. Human immunodeficiency virus and other sexually transmitted infection screenings are negative. She reports a penicillin allergy as a child. The best next step in the management of the positive treponemal test is

(A) ceftriaxone
(B) penicillin desensitization
(C) penicillin skin testing
(D) quantitative nontreponemal test
(E) repeat treponemal testing in 2 weeks

4

A 30-year-old transgender woman is in the process of adopting a neonate and is interested in chestfeeding. She wants to start immediately after delivery. She has done her own research and is following a lactation induction program available on the internet. In addition to taking higher doses of estrogen and progesterone, she has started using a breast pump several times daily. She also has continued androgen suppression medication because she has not yet had an orchiectomy. The most appropriate U.S. Food and Drug Administration (FDA)-approved medication to recommend to this patient in support of her chestfeeding goal is

(A) cabergoline
(B) domperidone
(C) droperidol
(D) metoclopramide
(E) spironolactone

5

A 32-year-old gravida 1 presents for her initial prenatal visit at 8 weeks of gestation. She is a vegan and has a body mass index of 36. She currently takes a vitamin B_{12} supplement and is concerned about other nutritional deficiencies. In addition to routine prenatal laboratory tests, the best additional test to screen for nutritional deficiencies is

(A) folate level
(B) iron level
(C) 25-hydroxy vitamin D level
(D) zinc level

6

A 29-year-old transgender patient at 12 weeks of gestation presents for a scheduled obstetric visit. The patient's partner recently tested positive for human immunodeficiency virus (HIV) and has started antiretroviral therapy. Previously, the couple was not using condoms but started to use them after this test result. The patient's routine prenatal screening included a negative HIV screening test 2 weeks ago. In addition to repeat HIV testing, the best next step to reduce this patient's risk of contracting HIV is to initiate

(A) dolutegravir
(B) enfuvirtide
(C) fostemsavir
(D) lamivudine and abacavir
(E) tenofovir and emtricitabine

7

A 15-year-old presents for an initial prenatal visit at 16 weeks of gestation, measured by her last menstrual period. She has a copy of her report from her ultrasonography performed 1 week ago demonstrating a crown-rump length of 87 mm. On examination today, her fundal height measures 22 cm and ultrasound biometry is consistent with 18 2/7 weeks of gestation. For the described patient, the most appropriate measurement to establish gestational age is

(A) average of both ultrasound measurements
(B) crown-rump length performed last week
(C) fundal height measurement
(D) last menstrual period
(E) ultrasound biometry performed today

8

A 30-year-old gravida 1, para 0, at 30 weeks of gestation presents to the labor and delivery unit with a fetal death. She has no significant medical, surgical, or social history. She undergoes an uncomplicated induction of labor and vaginal delivery. The fetal weight is in the 1st percentile for gestational age, and gross physical examination of the fetus is unremarkable. The patient requests an autopsy evaluation. A cytogenetic specimen of placenta is sent for chromosomal microarray analysis, and the remaining placenta is sent for pathologic examination. In addition to this placental evaluation, the next most appropriate test to determine the cause of the fetal death is

(A) antiphospholipid antibodies
(B) factor V Leiden
(C) hemoglobin A_{1c}
(D) parvovirus immunoglobulin G (IgG) or M (IgM)
(E) toxicology screen

9

A 17-year-old gravida 1, para 0, at 31 weeks of gestation was admitted to the hospital with fatigue, vomiting, and right upper quadrant pain. Her blood pressure on admission was 148/96 mm Hg, and a urine dipstick was negative for protein. Laboratory evaluation revealed the following: alanine aminotransferase, 1,038 units/L; aspartate aminotransferase, 966 units/L; creatinine, 0.6 mg/dL; platelet count, 72,000/mm^3; hemoglobin, 12.2 g/dL; hematocrit, 36%; and lactate dehydrogenase, 854 units/L. Delivery was recommended, and the patient underwent cesarean birth due to a breech presentation, with a quantitative blood loss of 1,200 mL. On the first postoperative day the patient reports minimal bleeding. Her vital signs are within normal limits, her abdomen is soft and nondistended, and the incision is dry and intact. Postoperative hemoglobin is 8.2 g/dL, and platelets are 44,000/mm^3. The best next step in the management of her postoperative laboratory findings is

(A) dexamethasone
(B) hematology consultation
(C) intravenous immunoglobulin
(D) platelet transfusion
(E) serial complete blood counts

10

A 28-year-old gravida 3, para 1, at 24 weeks of gestation presents to establish prenatal care. She reports no complications with this pregnancy. She has no contributing medical problems. Her first pregnancy was an emergency cesarean birth with low transverse hysterotomy at 27 weeks of gestation due to bradycardia after a motor vehicle collision. Her second pregnancy was an emergency cesarean birth at 37 weeks of gestation when she presented in labor and experienced a uterine rupture. Her prenatal laboratory tests are normal, and her physical examination is unremarkable. An obstetric ultrasonography examination confirms her gestational age and a fundal placenta. The most appropriate gestational age for a planned repeat cesarean birth for this patient is

(A) 30 weeks
(B) 32 weeks
(C) 34 weeks
(D) 36 weeks
(E) 38 weeks

11

A 36-year-old gravida 3, para 1, presents for prenatal care at 8 weeks of gestation. Her obstetric history is complicated by the second-trimester loss of her first pregnancy with painless cervical dilation and a 26-week delivery in her second pregnancy, in which she had a history-indicated cerclage placed at 13 weeks of gestation. To prevent preterm birth in this pregnancy, the best next step is progesterone supplementation and

(A) cervical pessary
(B) serial cervical length ultrasonography
(C) transvaginal cerclage
(D) transabdominal cerclage

12

A 28-year-old gravida 2, para 1, presents for a fetal anatomic assessment at 20 weeks of gestation. On ultrasonography, several abnormalities are noted, including fetal growth restriction, periventricular calcifications, hyperechoic bowel and liver, and a thickened placenta. She reports no recent illnesses. She is a vegetarian, has no pets, occasionally smokes marijuana, and has a young child in daycare. She is up to date on all vaccinations. The most likely fetal diagnosis is

(A) cytomegalovirus (CMV)
(B) herpes simplex virus
(C) parvovirus
(D) toxoplasmosis
(E) varicella zoster virus

13

A 36-year-old gravida 1 presents for prenatal care at 8 weeks of gestation. She is currently incarcerated. Her prenatal labs are all negative, including for human immunodeficiency virus (HIV) testing. The best next step for screening for HIV is

(A) no further HIV screening
(B) screening during the second trimester
(C) screening during the third trimester
(D) screening on admission to labor and delivery

14

A 39-year-old gravida 4, para 2, presents to labor and delivery at 33 weeks of gestation with contractions. Her history is complicated by prior preterm birth, and she received vaginal progesterone during this pregnancy. She is found to be 4-cm dilated with regular contractions. If she were to deliver in the next week, the minimum level of neonatal care required to care for her newborn is

(A) Level I
(B) Level II
(C) Level III
(D) Level IV

15

A 37-year-old gravida 3, para 2, is admitted at 41 weeks of gestation for induction of labor. Her second child developed anemia during infancy, and she is concerned about the risk in this neonate. The most appropriate method to increase iron stores in the neonate is

(A) breastfeeding
(B) delayed cord clamping
(C) early skin-to-skin contact
(D) iron supplementation

16

A patient who self-reports Southeast Asian ancestry presents at 20 weeks of gestation for a survey of fetal anatomy. Ultrasonographic findings are shown in Figure 16-1. Laboratory studies are remarkable for hemoglobin of 8.9 g/dL and mean corpuscular volume (MCV) of 74 cubic micrometers. Her noninvasive prenatal testing showed a low risk of aneuploidy. Her hemoglobin electrophoresis is normal, and serum ferritin concentration is 46 micrograms/dL. The patient declines an amniocentesis. The best next maternal test is

(A) DNA analysis of the α-globin gene
(B) DNA analysis of the β-globin gene
(C) methylenetetrahydrofolate reductase gene testing
(D) parvovirus immunoglobulin G and immunoglobulin M antibodies
(E) total iron binding capacity

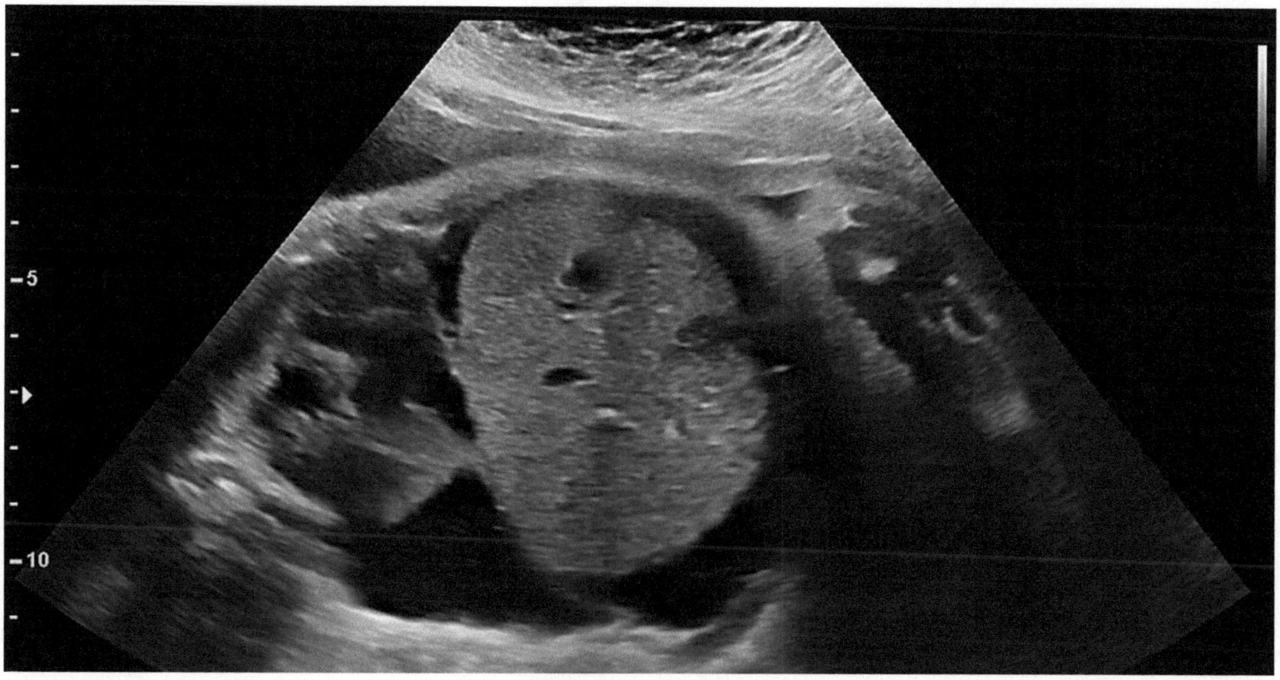

FIGURE 16-1. Described Patient's Fetal Ultrasonography

17

A patient with pregestational diabetes mellitus at 24 weeks of gestation presents with drooping of her left eyelid, increased tearing, and acute-onset decreased taste on the left side of her tongue for 2 days. She reports no other symptoms. Her distal motor examination is unremarkable, and her speech is fluent. There is obvious asymmetry at rest in the forehead and mouth and incomplete closure of the right eye. Her physical appearance is seen in Figure 17-1. Her House–Brackmann facial paralysis score is grade 5. In addition to protecting her left eye with a patch, the best next monotherapy for the patient is

(A) acyclovir
(B) azithromycin
(C) hydroxyzine
(D) immunoglobulin
(E) prednisone

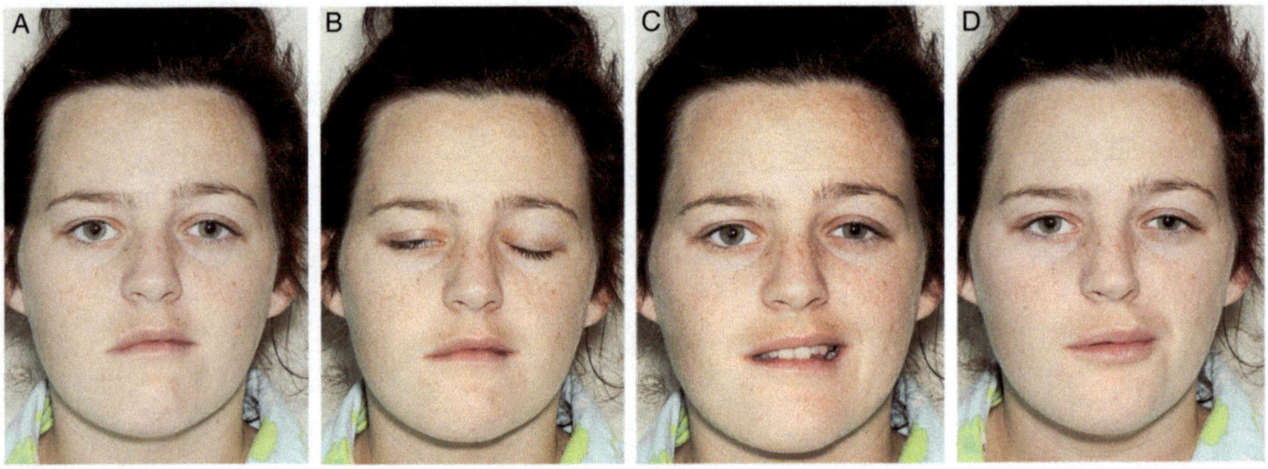

FIGURE 17-1. Described patient's facial examination findings. Patient at rest, closing her eyes, smiling, and whistling. (Reprinted from Fuller G, Morgan C. Bell's palsy syndrome: mimics and chameleons. Pract Neurol 2016;16:439–44. doi: 10.1136/practneurol-2016-001383. https://pn.bmj.com/content/16/6/439.long)

18

A 33-year-old gravida 5, para 1, with a body mass index (BMI) of 28 presents at 12 weeks of gestation for her first prenatal visit. She has experienced three first-trimester losses and is currently pregnant through intrauterine insemination. Her one live birth was delivered at 36 weeks of gestation because of fetal growth restriction. She takes hydroxychloroquine for systemic lupus erythematosus. She has no other significant health issue. The most appropriate indication for low-dose aspirin administration in this patient is

(A) assisted reproductive technology pregnancy
(B) BMI
(C) history of fetal growth restriction
(D) recurrent pregnancy losses
(E) systemic lupus erythematosus

19

A 22-year-old gravida 1 at 14 weeks of gestation is an athlete who exercises vigorously 5–6 days per week. She wants to continue her exercise regimen during pregnancy. She wears a heart rate monitor during exercise to gauge her intensity level. You advise her that vigorous exercise can be continued during pregnancy. Based on limited data on safety, it is recommended that her intensity level (as determined by percentage of her maximum heart rate) not exceed

(A) 60%
(B) 70%
(C) 80%
(D) 90%

20

A 31-year-old primigravida at 11 weeks of gestation undergoes first-trimester screening and is found to have a nuchal translucency measurement of 6 mm. Chorionic villus sampling returns 46, XY. The most likely fetal anomaly to be found on targeted ultrasonography is

(A) abdominal wall
(B) cardiac
(C) neural tube
(D) renal
(E) skeletal

21

A 32-year-old multigravida presents to establish prenatal care at 7 weeks of gestation. She reports recent heroin use and continued craving for heroin, although she wants to stop using and is interested in medication-assisted treatment. The most appropriate approach to decrease the severity of neonatal opioid withdrawal syndrome in her neonate is

(A) buprenorphine
(B) disulfiram
(C) methadone
(D) naloxone
(E) supervised withdrawal

22

A 32-year-old gravida 1, para 1, presents for a prepregnancy visit. Her previous pregnancy was significant for gestational diabetes mellitus treated with insulin. She is on levetiracetam for seizures. Her husband has no significant medical conditions and his sister's child has an open neural tube defect (ONTD). The patient's body mass index (BMI) is 31, and a recent hemoglobin A_{1C} was 5.9%. The most appropriate prepregnancy dose of folic acid to reduce the risk of an ONTD with her next pregnancy is

(A) 400 micrograms
(B) 800 micrograms
(C) 1,000 micrograms
(D) 4,000 micrograms

23

A 40-year-old gravida 3, para 2, at 39 weeks of gestation presents for a visit with 2 weeks of fatigue, edema, and increasing shortness of breath with her normal activities. She reports feeling short of breath when lying flat. On physical examination, her blood pressure is 135/80 mm Hg, respiratory rate is 22 breaths per minute, temperature is 37 °C (98.6 °F), and heart rate is 110 beats per minute. She has jugular venous distension to the angle of her right jaw, pulmonary rales bilaterally, and peripheral edema. She reports two previous uncomplicated pregnancies and no medications or medical conditions. The best next diagnostic test to order to confirm a diagnosis is

(A) computed tomography angiography
(B) duplex Doppler ultrasonography
(C) echocardiogram
(D) electrocardiogram
(E) magnetic resonance imaging

24

A 40-year-old multiparous patient had a spontaneous vaginal birth yesterday. Her pregnancy was notable for diagnosis of a deep vein thrombosis (DVT) at 34 weeks of gestation. She received a labor epidural that was removed yesterday morning after delivery. The patient plans to breastfeed. The best next step in management of her postpartum anticoagulation is initiation of

(A) antiplatelet agent
(B) direct thrombin inhibitor
(C) factor Xa inhibitor
(D) heparin
(E) vitamin K antagonist

25

A 39-year-old primiparous patient at 28 weeks of gestation presents for evaluation of hypertension, and vital signs include a blood pressure of 155/100 mm Hg, a pulse of 110 beats per minute, and brisk reflexes. Magnesium sulfate and betamethasone are initiated. Laboratory test results include creatinine of 1.2 mg/dL, aspartate aminotransferase (AST) and alanine aminotransferase (ALT) of 736 and 502 IU/L, respectively, and a platelet count of 30,000/mm^3. Ultrasonography reveals the fetus in breech presentation. The best next step in the treatment of this patient is

(A) cesarean birth
(B) intravenous dexamethasone
(C) intravenous immunoglobulin
(D) rebolus magnesium sulfate
(E) transfuse platelets

26

A 31-year-old primiparous patient presents for initial prenatal care at 28 weeks of gestation. Her laboratory studies are notable for positive hepatitis B surface antigen, positive hepatitis B core antibodies, and negative immunoglobulin M antibody to hepatitis B core antigen, and her hepatitis B DNA viral load is greater than 10^8 copies/mL. Given her test results, the best next step in reducing the risk of neonatal infection is

(A) avoidance of breastfeeding
(B) avoidance of fetal scalp electrode
(C) cesarean birth at term
(D) prenatal antiretroviral medication

27

A 30-year-old gravida 3, para 1, at 12 weeks of gestation presents for a routine prenatal visit. Her pregnancy is complicated by asthma and obesity. She uses albuterol approximately 4 days per week for wheezing. Her peak expiratory flow rate in the office is 85% of predicted, and she has no wheezing on examination. The best next step in management of her asthma is to initiate a(n)

(A) antihistamine
(B) leukotriene receptor agonist
(C) long-acting β_2-agonist
(D) low-dose inhaled corticosteroid
(E) oral corticosteroid

28

A 22-year-old gravida 1, para 1, presents 5 weeks postpartum with breast pain. The patient describes the pain as being in both nipples. The symptoms started 2 weeks ago and have progressively worsened. The pain is at its worst when her infant is nursing, with sharp pains occurring as the infant actively feeds. The pain does not improve when the breast is emptied. She has had minimal relief with use of over-the-counter analgesic medications. The patient's pregnancy was complicated by gestational diabetes mellitus. Her vital signs are normal. On physical examination, both nipples are erythematous. There is a scaly sheen overlying the areola. No fluctuance or mass is noted. A sample of breast milk is obtained by manual expression and examined under microscopy (Fig. 28-1). The most appropriate initial treatment is

(A) dicloxacillin
(B) fluconazole
(C) lanolin cream
(D) miconazole gel
(E) nonsteroidal anti-inflammatory drugs

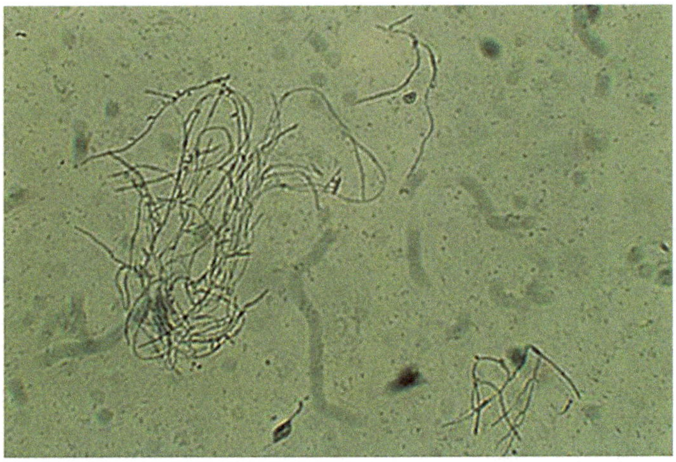

FIGURE 28-1. Breast milk cytology. (Reprinted from Sobel JD. Mucocutaneous candidiasis. In: Mandell GL, Diamond RD, editors. Atlas of infectious diseases: fungal infections. Current Medicine; 2000. p. 117–33.)

29

A 21-year-old gravida 3, para 2, presents at 27 weeks of gestation with a pregnancy complicated by Rh D alloimmunization. Her first pregnancy was uncomplicated, but her second pregnancy was affected by Rh D alloimmunization. This pregnancy has the same paternity, and the fetal antigenicity was confirmed Rh D positive with cell-free DNA testing in the second trimester. Doppler velocimetry measurements of the peak systolic velocity in the fetal middle cerebral artery have been conducted every 2 weeks for the last 2 months. The values of the Doppler measurements have ranged from 1.1 to 1.35 multiples of the mean for gestational age. Based on the current antenatal testing, delivery should be planned at a gestational age of

(A) 31 0/7 to 32 6/7 weeks
(B) 33 0/7 to 34 6/7 weeks
(C) 35 0/7 to 36 6/7 weeks
(D) 37 0/7 to 38 6/7 weeks
(E) 39 0/7 to 40 6/7 weeks

30

A 29-year-old gravida 4, para 0, presents a month after her fourth spontaneous first-trimester loss. Previously, she has had normal saline sonohysterography, maternal and paternal karyotype, and thyroid screening. She requests additional testing to evaluate the causes of her recurrent miscarriage. The most appropriate thrombophilia testing for this patient is

(A) antiphospholipid syndrome
(B) antithrombin deficiency
(C) factor V Leiden mutation
(D) methylenetetrahydrofolate reductase mutation
(E) prothrombin mutation

31

A 39-year-old gravida 3, para 0, presents for an initial prenatal visit at 13 weeks of gestation. She has a body mass index (BMI) of 26, and her medical history is significant for hypothyroidism and hypertension treated with nifedipine. She has had two first-trimester miscarriages and reports a family history of type 2 diabetes mellitus in her maternal grandmother. You recommend early diabetes screening with a 50-g, 1-hour glucose tolerance test based on her BMI and

(A) advanced maternal age
(B) chronic hypertension
(C) family history
(D) hypothyroidism
(E) recurrent pregnancy loss

32

A 27-year-old gravida 2, para 1, presents for a prenatal visit at 36 weeks of gestation. She plans to breastfeed, and she would like to discuss postpartum contraception. She previously had abnormal bleeding with the etonogestrel implant and prefers to avoid this method in the future. She wants to delay her next pregnancy for 2–3 years, and she is interested in highly effective contraception that she can start shortly after delivery. She will lose her health insurance 6 weeks after giving birth. For this patient, the contraceptive option you recommend is

(A) combined hormonal contraception
(B) depot medroxyprogesterone acetate
(C) intrauterine device (IUD) placement
(D) progesterone-only oral contraceptives

33

During an emergent cesarean birth, the surgical technologist, who is pregnant at 28 weeks of gestation, experiences an accidental needle stick. The patient had no prenatal care, and her rapid human immunodeficiency virus (HIV) test on admission to labor and delivery was positive. The best next step to decrease the risk of vertical transmission to the surgical technologist's fetus is

(A) administer zidovudine in labor
(B) await the surgical patient's fourth-generation HIV test results
(C) begin postexposure prophylaxis (PEP) immediately
(D) perform HIV testing at 36 weeks of gestation

34

A 34-year-old gravida 5, para 2, is at 39 weeks of gestation and has gestational hypertension without severe features. She delivered her first pregnancy vaginally at term, and her second was delivered at 38 weeks of gestation by cesarean birth for fetal intolerance of labor. She wants a trial of labor. Her cervix is 3-cm dilated and 50% effaced, in the anterior position, and soft, with the fetal vertex at −3 station and ballotable. The most appropriate management is

(A) dinoprostone
(B) expectant management
(C) misoprostol
(D) oxytocin
(E) transcervical balloon

35

A 38-year-old gravida 4, para 2, at 12 weeks of gestation with a dichorionic twin pregnancy desires aneuploidy testing as early as possible. On ultrasonography, one twin has no fetal heart motion and measures about 4 weeks smaller than the co-twin with fetal heart motion. The appropriate aneuploidy test is

(A) amniocentesis
(B) cell-free DNA (cfDNA) screening
(C) chorionic villus sampling
(D) first-trimester screening
(E) integrated screening

36

A 36-year-old multigravida presents at 22 weeks of gestation. She has been trying to quit smoking since early in pregnancy using cognitive behavioral techniques but has been unsuccessful. The patient is interested in additional therapy to help her quit. The best next step is to prescribe

(A) bupropion
(B) nicotine replacement therapy
(C) sertraline
(D) venlafaxine

37

A patient presents for a fetal anatomy survey. She had low-risk cell-free DNA screening but declined other genetic testing. Her ultrasonographic findings are shown in Figure 37-1. The best next genetic carrier testing to recommend is

(A) cystic fibrosis
(B) expanded carrier screening
(C) fragile X
(D) spinal muscular atrophy
(E) Tay–Sachs

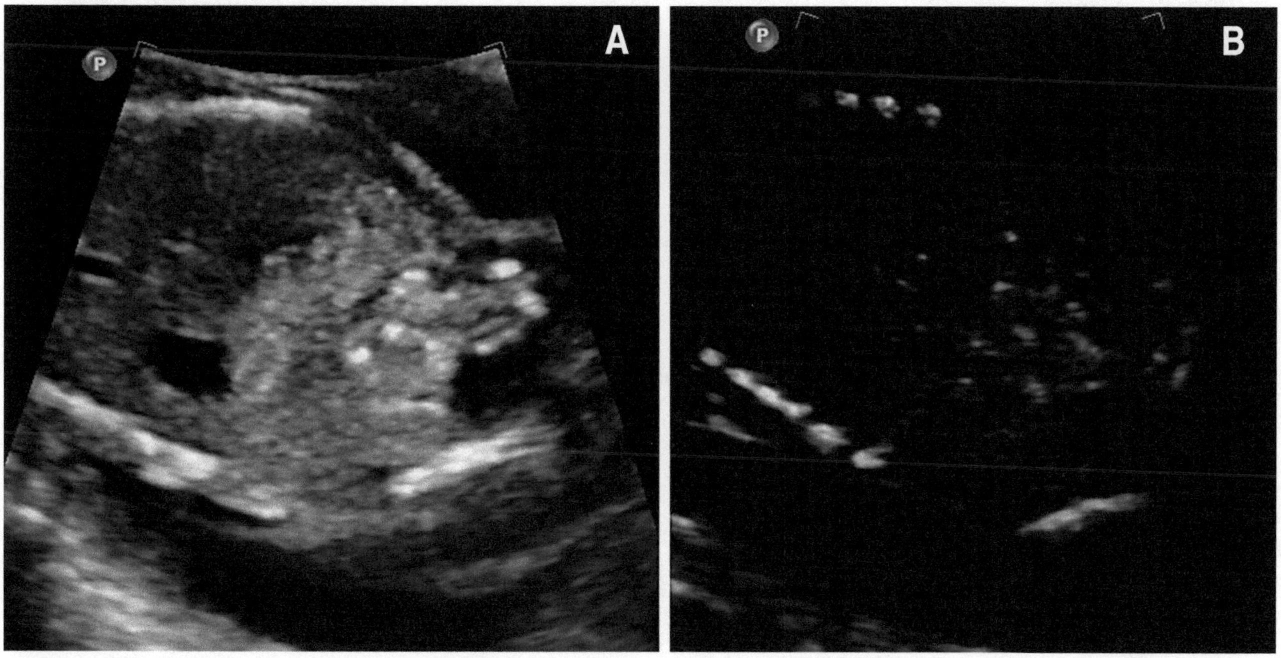

FIGURE 37-1. Ultrasonographic findings of the fetal abdomen for the described patient. Image B is the same as image A but with a modified transducer gain velocity curve.

38

A previously healthy 38-year-old gravida 1 at 35 weeks of gestation presents to the labor and delivery unit with a severe headache and nausea. Her initial blood pressure is 182/108 mm Hg, and repeat blood pressure is 174/110 mm Hg. Hydralazine is administered intravenously. Ultrasonography on presentation showed the fetus in the cephalic presentation. The fetal heart tracing was reassuring upon arrival with a baseline of 120 beats per minute, moderate variability, and accelerations. Laboratory values are pending. You are called to the room after the patient experiences a tonic-clonic seizure. She is in the left lateral decubitus position, bedrails are padded, and oxygen is being administered through a nonrebreather face mask. The fetal heart tracing is shown in Figure 38-1. The most appropriate next step is to

(A) administer diazepam
(B) administer magnesium sulfate
(C) initiate induction of labor
(D) perform imaging of the brain
(E) perform immediate cesarean delivery

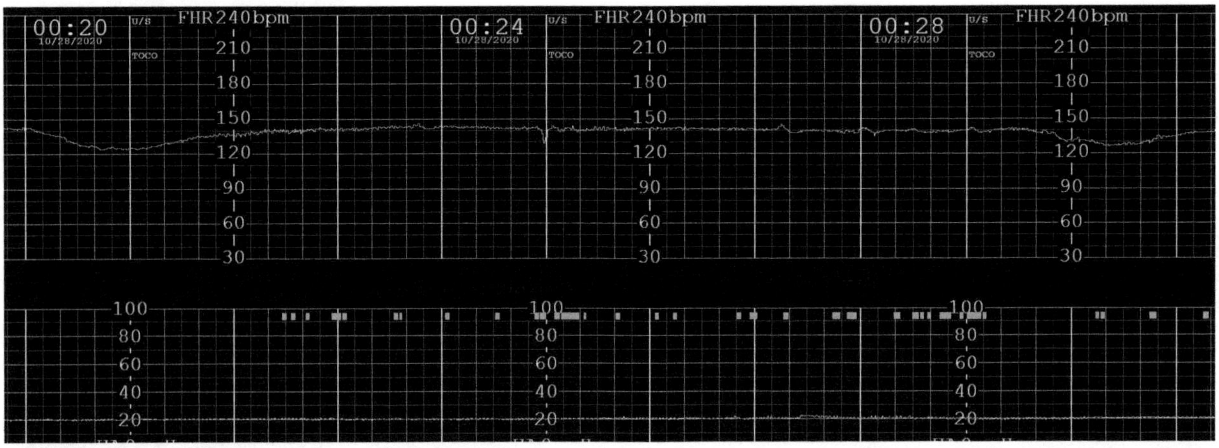

FIGURE 38-1. Fetal heart tracing after the patient experiences a tonic-clonic seizure.

39

A 34-year-old gravida 3, para 2, at 18 weeks of gestation with a history of laparoscopic cholecystectomy and Roux-en-Y gastric bypass procedure presents to the emergency department reporting nausea, vomiting, and upper abdominal pain for 3 days. You suspect internal herniation. The best imaging technique to evaluate this patient is

(A) computed tomography (CT)
(B) magnetic resonance imaging (MRI)
(C) ultrasonography
(D) X-ray

40

A 30-year-old and her husband present to the office at 24 weeks of gestation to discuss her mode of delivery. She was in your care for her two prior uncomplicated low transverse cesarean births. Her partner initially is supportive but appears less so as you review the risks and benefits of a trial of labor and another cesarean birth. She verbalizes understanding of her choices and would like a repeat cesarean birth. Her husband interrupts to say that she does not want another surgery and that he will not support her if she chooses to have a repeat cesarean birth. She turns to you and says she has changed her mind and would like a trial of labor. The best next step is to

(A) proceed with signing the consent for a trial of labor
(B) request a court order for a cesarean birth
(C) request a psychiatric consult evaluating capacity
(D) speak with the patient alone
(E) terminate the patient–physician relationship

41

A 25-year-old gravida 1 at term delivered after a prolonged second stage of labor. A second-degree laceration was repaired. A few hours later, she reports increasing vulvar pain and inability to void. An indwelling Foley catheter was placed. Her vital signs show a blood pressure of 110/70 mm Hg, a heart rate of 100 beats per minute, and a respiratory rate of 18 breaths per minute. Her fundus is firm, and she has minimal lochia. Her external examination is shown in Figure 41-1, and the area appears to be enlarging. On bimanual examination, there is no palpable lesion along the vaginal side wall. Her hemoglobin on admission was 11 g/dL and a repeat measurement was 9 g/dL with normal coagulation studies. The best next step in management is

(A) external ice pack
(B) hypogastric artery ligation
(C) incision and drainage
(D) transfusion
(E) vascular embolization

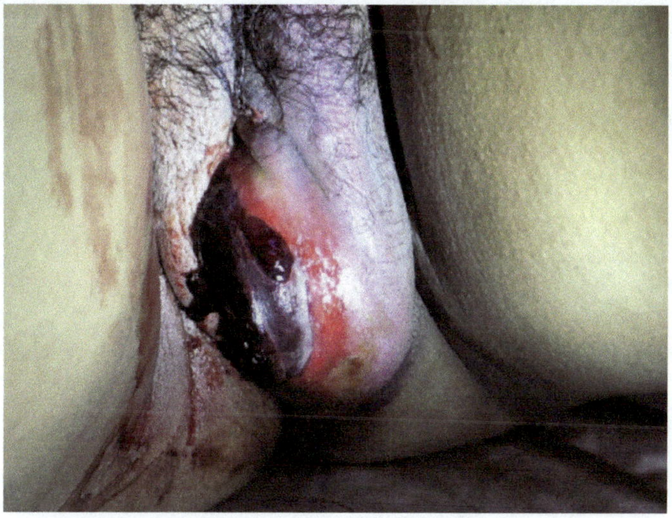

FIGURE 41-1. Left vulva hematoma with rupture and protruding blood clots. (Reprinted from Tseng JY, Lin IC, Lin JH, Chang CM, Chao WT, Wang PH. Optimal approach for management of post-partum vulva hematoma: Report of three cases. Taiwan J Obstet Gynecol 2020;59:780–3. doi: 10.1016/j.tjog.2020.07.030 https://www.sciencedirect.com/science/article/pii/S1028455920301844)

42

A 28-year-old multiparous patient with term prelabor rupture of membranes undergoes an uncomplicated cesarean birth for arrest of the active phase of labor. On postoperative day 2, she reports severe abdominal pain, fever, and chills. Her vital signs include temperature of 39.8 °C (103.8 °F), a heart rate of 138 beats per minute, and blood pressure of 80/42 mm Hg. Laboratory studies reveal leukocytosis and lactic acidosis. Antibiotics are started, and several hours later a follow-up examination reveals the finding in Figure 42-1. The best next step in her treatment is

(A) administer intravenous immunoglobulin
(B) broaden antibiotic coverage
(C) expectant management with repeat cultures
(D) surgical debridement

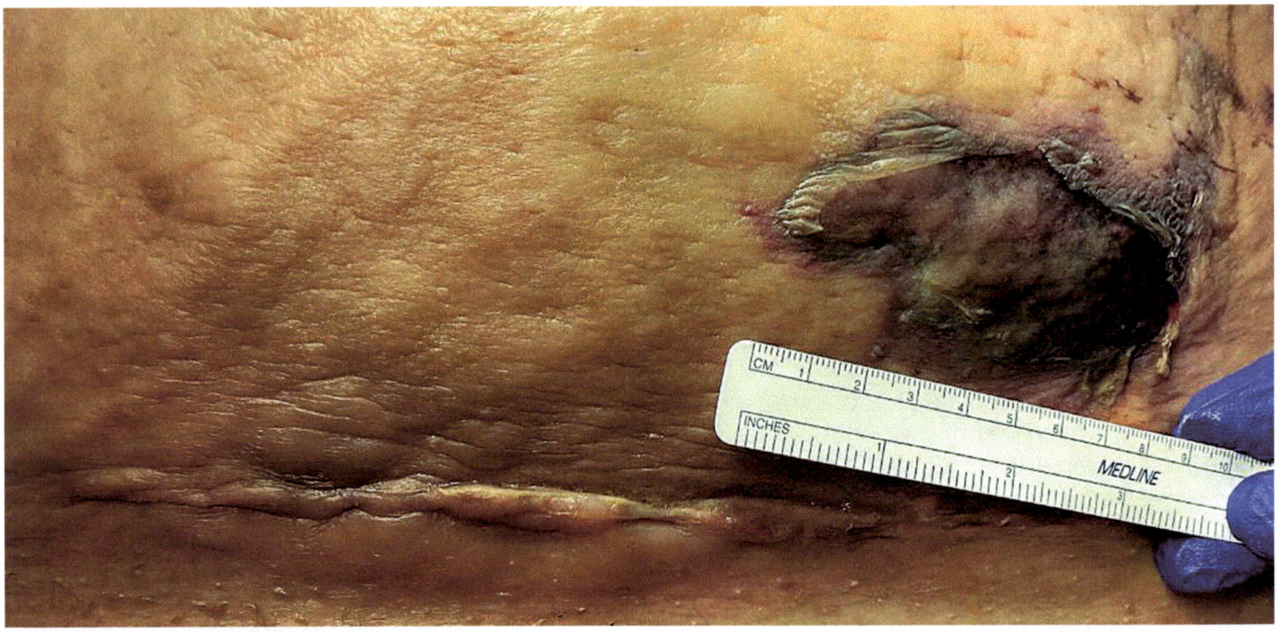

FIGURE 42-1. Maternal abdomen after cesarean birth. (Image courtesy of Rebecca Barbaresso, DO, Baystate Medical Center.)

43

A 38-year-old gravida 4, para 2, at 8 weeks of gestation presents for initial prenatal care. Her medical history includes chronic hypertension and peripartum cardiomyopathy. She is currently taking labetalol and aspirin. She reports feeling short of breath with physical activity but is otherwise asymptomatic. Her vital signs are within normal limits. A recent echocardiogram demonstrates a left ventricular ejection fraction (EF) of 25%. The best next step is to

(A) administer furosemide
(B) discuss termination of pregnancy
(C) perform exercise stress test
(D) place a left ventricular assist device
(E) refer to maternal–fetal medicine

44

A 23-year-old gravida 1, para 0, at 38 weeks of gestation presents to the labor and delivery unit in spontaneous labor. Her pregnancy has been uncomplicated. Her labor is progressing normally with a Category I fetal tracing on electronic fetal monitoring (EFM). The use of continuous EFM in this patient reduces the risk of

(A) cerebral palsy
(B) cesarean birth
(C) neonatal seizures
(D) operative vaginal delivery
(E) perinatal death

45

A 42-year-old gravida 4, para 3, presents for a routine postpartum visit. The patient is exclusively breastfeeding. Her breast examination is normal. She reports no family history of breast cancer. After counseling about breast cancer screening recommendations from various societies, the patient opts to begin screening. The most appropriate breast cancer screening option for this patient is

(A) deferment while breastfeeding
(B) magnetic resonance imaging (MRI)
(C) mammography
(D) ultrasonography

46

A 21-year-old gravida 1, para 0, presents at 33 weeks of gestation with fever and intermittent abdominal pain. The patient appears agitated and has proptosis. On physical examination, she has bilateral pedal edema and bibasilar rales. Her blood pressure is 102/60 mm Hg, heart rate is 140 beats per minute, temperature is 39.4 °C (102.9 °F), respiratory rate is 24 breaths per minute, and pulse oximetry is 96% on room air. A complete blood count is obtained, which shows a white blood cell count of 13×10^9/L. The most appropriate laboratory test to confirm the most likely diagnosis is a (an)

(A) amniotic fluid culture
(B) antinuclear antibodies test
(C) rapid human immunodeficiency virus (HIV) test
(D) thyroid-stimulating hormone (TSH) test
(E) urine drug screen

47

A 24-year-old gravida 1 is in labor at 37 weeks of gestation. Her pregnancy has been complicated by gestational diabetes mellitus, which has been managed with subcutaneous insulin therapy, and maternal obesity. Her body mass index is 44. The estimated fetal weight from an obstetric ultrasonographic examination 1 week ago was 3,600 g. Her hospital course has lasted 48 hours and included intravenous oxytocin after cervical ripening. She has effective neuraxial anesthesia in place. After 45 minutes of pushing, the head delivers and retracts against the perineum. Downward axial traction to deliver the anterior shoulder is unsuccessful. The obstetrician alerts the care team to a shoulder dystocia. Two assistants hyperflex the patient's hips and lay the patient flat while a third assistant provides suprapubic pressure, but the shoulder dystocia persists. The best next maneuver is to

(A) apply fundal pressure
(B) deliver the posterior arm
(C) fracture the anterior fetal clavicle
(D) perform an episiotomy
(E) reposition the patient to hands and knees

48

A 32-year-old gravida 4, para 3, at 23 4/7 weeks of gestation presented with preterm labor 3 days ago to a community hospital. Her cervix was 3-cm dilated, 50% effaced, and she was actively contracting. She received indomethacin tocolysis and was transferred to a hospital with a Level III neonatal intensive care unit. She received a two-dose betamethasone course and an intravenous magnesium sulfate infusion for the past 48 hours. She is now completely dilated, and delivery is imminent. After counseling with the neonatologists and considering neonatal resuscitation, the patient and her partner decline resuscitation and request palliative care for the neonate. The best next step in management is to

(A) await delivery and provide neonatal comfort care
(B) consult psychiatry
(C) inform the hospital risk-management services
(D) report the patient's decision to the local government health agency
(E) review the case with the hospital ethics committee

49

A patient at 32 weeks of gestation arrives at the emergency department trauma bay. She suffered cardiac arrest while in the ambulance 7 minutes ago. Chest compressions were started along with bag mask ventilation. Intubation before arrival was unsuccessful because of poor visualization. The obstetric emergency response team and emergency department team are present on the patient's arrival. She is positioned supine with left lateral tilt. Chest compression and bag mask ventilation are continued. A defibrillator is placed, and the maternal rhythm is asystole. In addition to intravenous epinephrine, the best next step in management is

(A) biphasic defibrillation
(B) central venous access
(C) cesarean birth
(D) endotracheal intubation
(E) transfer to the operating room

50

A healthy 32-year-old gravida 3, para 2, at 34 weeks of gestation has a dichorionic–diamniotic twin pregnancy. She has had two previous low transverse cesarean births and desires a repeat cesarean birth. Her pregnancy is uncomplicated other than her experiencing significant pelvic pain with movement, standing, or walking, and she is undergoing physical therapy for pubic symphysis laxity. You recommend delivery at a gestational age of

(A) 36 0/7 to 36 6/7 weeks
(B) 37 0/7 to 37 6/7 weeks
(C) 38 0/7 to 38 6/7 weeks
(D) 39 0/7 to 39 6/7 weeks
(E) 40 0/7 to 40 6/7 weeks

51

A 30-year-old gravida 1, para 0, at 34 weeks of gestation is undergoing induction of labor. An urgent cesarean birth is planned because of fetal heart rate decelerations, and spinal anesthesia is placed with the patient in a seated position. Shortly after the abdominal incision, the patient exhibits upper extremity weakness and difficulty breathing. She attempts to speak but is unable to form words. The most likely diagnosis is

(A) amniotic fluid embolism
(B) high neuraxial block
(C) myocardial infarction
(D) spinal hematoma
(E) stroke

52

A 24-year-old gravida 1 is diagnosed with gestational diabetes mellitus (GDM) at 26 weeks of gestation. She is following the diet recommended by her nutritionist and is exercising 30 minutes daily. She uses a continuous glucose monitor because of a needle phobia. Her blood glucose values have been consistently elevated for several weeks. She declines insulin treatment. The best next step in management of her GDM is

(A) a ketogenic diet
(B) exercise for 60 minutes daily
(C) glyburide
(D) metformin
(E) needle exposure therapy

53

A 24-year-old primigravida at 24 weeks of gestation presents to your office reporting a painful vulvar rash. On examination you note clusters of vesicles on the labia that are tender to touch. She reports no prior history of sexually transmitted infection. She undergoes confirmatory testing and treatment, and the lesions resolve. The best next step to prevent neonatal transmission is

(A) cesarean birth
(B) herpes zoster immunization
(C) imiquimod therapy
(D) valacyclovir prophylaxis

54

A 37-year-old gravida 3, para 2, at 32 weeks of gestation presents to the emergency department reporting right lower quadrant abdominal pain that has worsened over the course of the day. She also has associated nausea and vomiting. The fetal heart rate is 155 beats per minute. Ultrasonography of the abdomen is remarkable for an inflamed appendix, and the general surgeon starts intravenous antibiotics and recommends appendectomy. The best approach to assess fetal well-being around the time of surgery is to

(A) obtain fetal heart tones before and after surgery
(B) perform a nonstress test before and after surgery
(C) perform continuous fetal monitoring during surgery
(D) perform intermittent fetal monitoring during surgery

55

A 21-year-old gravida 2, para 1, at 33 weeks of gestation calls with nausea and vomiting and decreased fetal movement. Her pregnancy is complicated by sickle cell trait. She denies any sick contacts at home. In triage, she has a temperature of 38.9 °C (102 °F). Her examination is unremarkable, with a closed cervix. There is no uterine activity. The fetal heart rate tracing shows fetal tachycardia at 185 beats per minute (bpm), with minimal variability. The patient is admitted for observation, and intravenous fluids are started. Respiratory pathogen testing, serum blood tests, and urine analysis are ordered. The best next step in management is

(A) acetaminophen
(B) antibiotics
(C) betamethasone
(D) cesarean birth
(E) induction of labor

56

A 31-year-old gravida 3, para 1, underwent repeat cesarean birth. Blood loss in the operating room was 850 mL. Three hours later, she develops vaginal bleeding. Fundal massage is started. Blood and clot measuring 450 mL are expressed. The patient is asymptomatic. Her blood pressure is 115/70 mm Hg, pulse is 100 beats per minute, and her respiratory rate is 16 breaths per minute. She has had 85 mL of urine output in the last hour. An oxytocin infusion has been continuous since her transfer to the postpartum unit. The best next step is to

(A) administer additional uterotonic agent
(B) call for a critical care team
(C) initiate blood transfusion
(D) obtain coagulation studies
(E) transfer her to the operating room for further assessment

57

A patient at 8 weeks of gestation (dated by last menstrual period) presents for evaluation of vaginal spotting. Her ultrasonographic findings are shown in Figures 57-1 and 57-2. Fetal cardiac activity was not seen with M-mode or the video images obtained. She is Rh-positive, and this is a desired pregnancy. The best next step in management is to

(A) administer mifepristone and misoprostol
(B) obtain serial β-human chorionic gonadotropin (β-hCG) concentrations
(C) perform dilation and curettage
(D) repeat ultrasonography

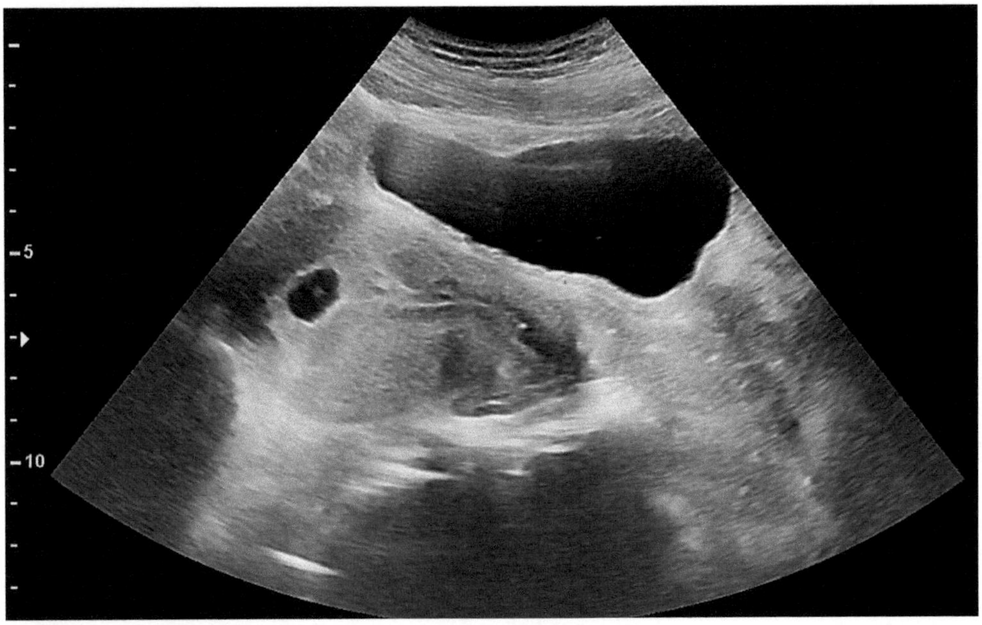

FIGURE 57-1. Described patient's abdominal ultrasonography.

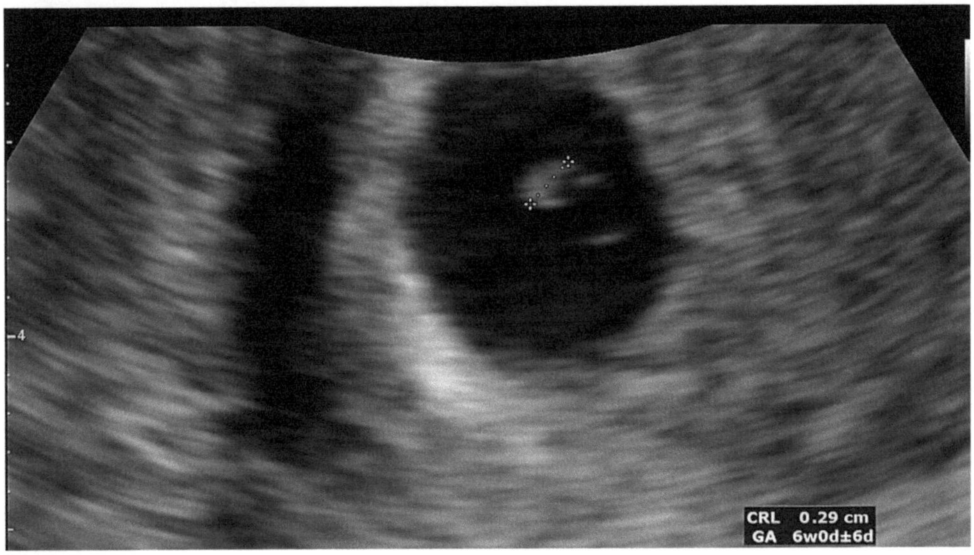

FIGURE 57-2. Described patient's transvaginal ultrasonography.

58

A patient at 18 weeks of gestation with a history of sickle cell disease presents with fever. She has chest pain, cough, and shortness of breath that have been present for 1 day. Her temperature is 38.2 °C (100.8 °F), her pulse is 115 beats per minute, and pulse oximetry is 92% on room air. She appears ill on examination with an expiratory wheeze. Her COVID-19 polymerase chain reaction test is negative. Her chest X-ray is normal, and chest computed tomography angiogram is positive for a right segmental thrombus. Electrocardiogram shows sinus tachycardia, and cardiac troponin levels are normal. In addition to pulmonary embolism, the most likely concurrent diagnosis is

(A) acute chest syndrome
(B) myocardial infarction
(C) myocarditis
(D) sickle cell pain crisis

59

A 17-year-old gravida 1 presents at 27 weeks of gestation with increased pelvic pressure and back pain for 3 days. On cervical examination, she is 3-cm dilated and 50% effaced, with an unchanged examination over 2 hours. Fetal tracing shows a normal baseline with contractions every 4 minutes on tocodynamometer. She is given penicillin, betamethasone, magnesium sulfate, and indomethacin. Ultrasonography is performed 2 days later, and the maximum vertical pocket of amniotic fluid is 1.6 cm. The medication mostly likely responsible for the ultrasonographic finding is

(A) betamethasone
(B) indomethacin
(C) magnesium
(D) penicillin

60

A 35-year-old gravida 1 at 34 weeks of gestation presents with pruritus, concentrated on the palms of her hands and soles of her feet, that keeps her awake at night. She does not have a rash or other skin lesions. Her blood pressure is normal. Her total bile acid level is 102 micromoles/L. The proposed mechanism most likely associated with an increased risk of fetal death is

(A) bile salts in the fetal liver causing cirrhosis
(B) chronic placental insufficiency
(C) fetal arrhythmia
(D) placental abruption
(E) thrombi in the placental vessels

61

A 26-year-old gravida 1 with a monochorionic–diamniotic twin pregnancy had normal nuchal translucency measurements at 13 weeks of gestation. At 20 weeks of gestation, ultrasonographic evaluation revealed normal fetal anatomical surveys for both twins, appropriate fetal growth, a transvaginal cervical length of 3.4 cm, and a fetal weight discordance of 5%. There was no evidence of twin-to-twin transfusion syndrome. She is scheduled for ultrasonographic evaluations every 2 weeks to assess amniotic fluid volume and bladder filling. At 22 weeks of gestation, the most appropriate additional evaluation is

(A) amniocentesis
(B) biophysical profiles
(C) fetal echocardiography
(D) transvaginal cervical length
(E) umbilical artery Doppler velocimetry

62

A 36-year-old gravida 1 with chronic hypertension well-controlled on medications underwent cell-free DNA screening in the first trimester. The test result indicated a low risk of aneuploidy, and her detailed fetal anatomy survey at 20 weeks of gestation showed no abnormalities. On routine ultrasonography to evaluate fetal growth at 31 0/7 weeks of gestation, estimated fetal weight was at the 4th percentile, and the umbilical artery Doppler systolic/diastolic ratio was greater than the 95th percentile for gestational age. After the ultrasonography, she received a course of antenatal corticosteroids, and weekly surveillance including umbilical artery Doppler assessment was initiated. At 32 weeks, the umbilical artery Doppler findings are shown in Figure 62-1. The best next step in management is to admit the patient to the hospital and

(A) administer rescue course of antenatal corticosteroids
(B) deliver
(C) initiate twice-weekly umbilical artery Doppler assessments
(D) schedule delivery at 37 weeks of gestation
(E) screen for TORCH (toxoplasmosis, syphilis, rubella, cytomegalovirus, and herpes simplex virus)

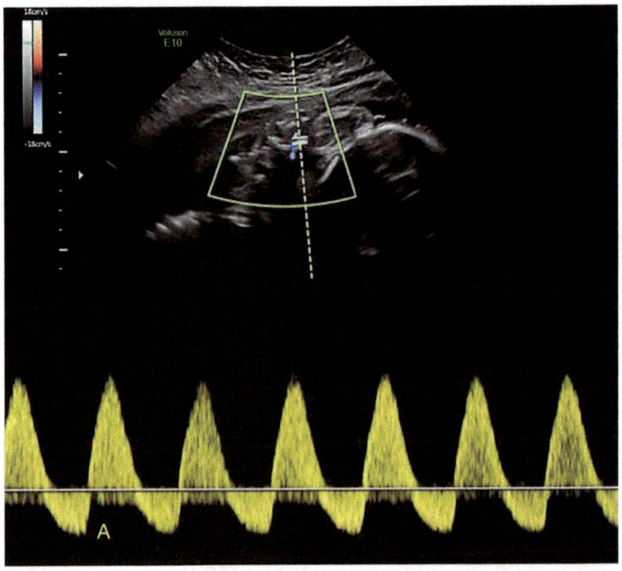

FIGURE 62-1. Ultrasonographic image of umbilical artery Doppler at 32 weeks of gestation.

63

A 33-year-old gravida 3, para 2, was diagnosed with a placenta previa earlier in her pregnancy. At 36 weeks of gestation, she presents for ultrasonographic reevaluation of the placental location. Her obstetric history includes one previous low transverse cesarean birth followed by a successful vaginal birth after cesarean. She desires a trial of labor if she is a candidate. After reviewing Figure 63-1, you determine that the best next step is to

(A) continue routine care
(B) deliver with cesarean by 37 6/7 weeks of gestation
(C) perform magnetic resonance imaging (MRI)
(D) repeat ultrasonography in 2 weeks

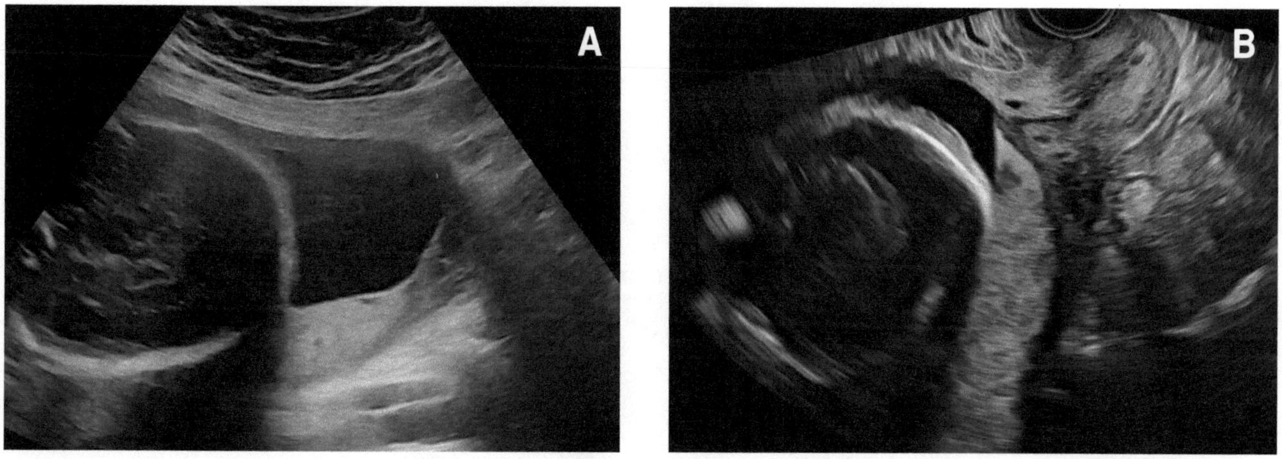

FIGURE 63-1. A. Patient's transabdominal ultrasonography. B. Patient's transvaginal ultrasonographic image.

64

A 34-year-old gravida 1 at 24 weeks of gestation presents to the emergency department with a headache with 8 out of 10 intensity, nausea, vomiting, and photophobia. She has tried acetaminophen and caffeine, which have helped her in the past, at home with no relief. She reports having this type of headache when not pregnant. Her blood pressure is 110/84 mm Hg, she has a normal complete metabolic profile, and her urinalysis is notable only for ketonuria. In addition to receiving intravenous fluids, the best next step in management of her headache is to administer

(A) dexamethasone
(B) ketorolac
(C) magnesium sulfate
(D) metoclopramide
(E) sumatriptan

65

A 34-year-old multigravida presents for prepregnancy counseling. She has a history of delivery at 36 weeks of gestation with preeclampsia with severe features, a second-trimester fetal death at 13 weeks of gestation after normal 10-week ultrasonography, and an early pregnancy loss at 6 weeks of gestation. Her mother and sister have a history of venous thromboembolism (VTE). The clinical history that most supports screening for antiphospholipid antibody syndrome (APS) is

(A) family history of vascular thrombosis
(B) history of severe preeclampsia at 36 weeks of gestation
(C) second-trimester fetal death at 13 weeks of gestation
(D) two consecutive fetal losses

66

A 28-year-old gravida 3, para 2, presents to your office at 28 weeks of gestation. Her prepregnancy body mass index (BMI) is 32. She lost weight during the first trimester, and although her weight has stabilized, her current BMI is 29. The most likely pregnancy complication associated with weight loss during pregnancy among women with obesity is

(A) fetal growth restriction
(B) preeclampsia
(C) preterm labor
(D) preterm prelabor rupture of membranes
(E) stillbirth

67

A 33-year-old patient at 29 weeks of gestation presents with burning with urination and fever. Her temperature is 39.4 °C (103 °F), pulse is 115 beats per minute, and respiratory rate is 22 respirations per minute. Her pulse oximetry is 97%, and her urine output is adequate. She has costovertebral angle tenderness, bibasilar rales, and diffuse diaphoresis. The finding in this patient that most strongly indicates a potential need for intensive care support is the

(A) bibasilar rales
(B) diaphoresis
(C) pyrexia
(D) tachycardia
(E) tachypnea

68

A gravida 2, para 1, at 36 weeks of gestation presents for her preoperative history and physical examination for her second cesarean birth. She experienced significant nausea and vomiting with her first birth. You discuss preoperative and postoperative strategies to reduce nausea. In the preoperative anesthesia care unit, she is given a scopolamine patch and ondansetron. In the operating room, after placement of a spinal anesthetic, she experiences increased nausea and hypotension. The best next intraoperative medication to treat her nausea is a

(A) dopamine antagonist
(B) gamma-aminobutyric acid analog
(C) glucocorticoid
(D) serotonin antagonist
(E) vasopressor

69

A 22-year-old primipara at 32 weeks of gestation presents with shortness of breath, fever, and cough. She has had no prenatal care. Her history reveals limited access to preventive medicine, and this visit is her first interaction with the health care system. She reports fever and malaise starting 1 week ago, followed by development of a widespread pruritic, vesicular, and painful rash (Fig. 69-1). Her COVID-19 test is negative, and a chest radiograph reveals diffuse bilateral infiltrates. The best next step in her treatment is to administer

(A) acyclovir
(B) azithromycin
(C) ceftriaxone
(D) isoniazid
(E) oseltamivir

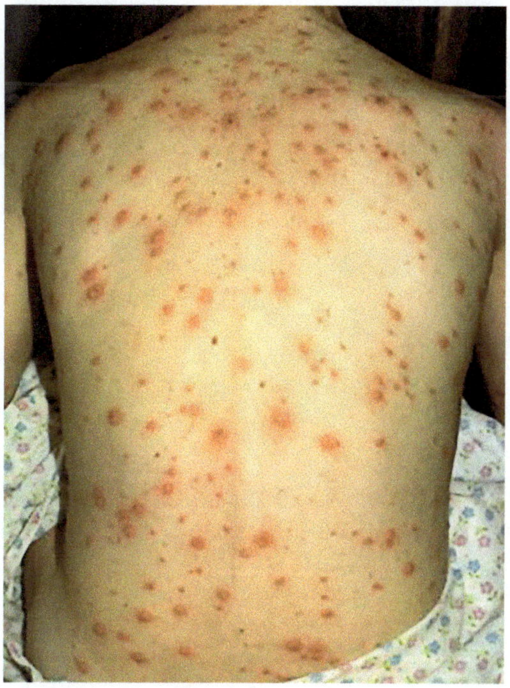

FIGURE 69-1. Varicella rash. (Reproduced with permission from American Academy of Pediatrics. Varicella-zoster virus infections. In: Kimberlin DW, Barnett ED, Lynfield R, Sawyer MH, editors. Red Book: 2021-2024 Report of the Committee on Infectious Diseases. 32nd ed. AAP; 2021. p. 831–43.)

70

A 28-year-old nulliparous patient at 22 0/7 weeks of gestation is diagnosed with preterm prelabor rupture of membranes (PPROM). Her due date was determined with first-trimester ultrasonography concordant with her last menstrual period. On examination, she is afebrile with a nontender fundus, is 2-cm dilated on speculum examination, and has a white blood cell count of 9,000. The patient and her wife are interested in pursuing potential obstetric interventions to optimize outcomes for the pregnancy. The most appropriate intervention at this gestational age is

(A) antenatal corticosteroids
(B) antibiotics
(C) cesarean birth
(D) magnesium sulfate
(E) tocolytic

71

A 32-year-old gravida 2, para 1, presents in spontaneous labor at 40 weeks of gestation. She has a history of one prior cesarean birth. She is treated with antibiotics for chorioamnionitis. She develops a persistent Category II fetal heart rate tracing unresponsive to resuscitative measures. She undergoes a repeat cesarean birth. At the time of delivery, a uterine rupture is identified. Apgar scores are 3 and 7 at 1 and 5 minutes, respectively. The umbilical cord arterial pH is 6.9 with a base excess of 11 mmol/L. The neonate is subsequently diagnosed with neonatal encephalopathy. The finding most associated with an intrapartum cause of hypoxic ischemic encephalopathy is

(A) Apgar score of 7 at 5 minutes
(B) Category II fetal heart rate tracing
(C) chorioamnionitis
(D) umbilical arterial cord pH of 6.9

72

A 35-year-old woman presents for a prenatal visit at 10 weeks of gestation. She requests a thyroid-stimulating hormone (TSH) test because of her family history of thyroid disease. Her TSH concentration is 4.3 mU/L and free thyroxine (T_4) is 0.9 ng/dL. Based on the laboratory results, the best next step in management is to

(A) initiate levothyroxine
(B) measure thyroid antibodies
(C) measure total triiodothyronine
(D) reassure the patient
(E) repeat thyroid function tests in the second trimester

73

A 25-year-old gravida 1, para 0, presents for a prenatal visit at 32 weeks of gestation. Routine third-trimester laboratory results returned a hemoglobin concentration of 9.2 g/dL, a hematocrit of 28.6%, a mean corpuscular volume (MCV) of 102.8 fL, and a platelet count of 219,000/mm^3. The patient has a history of gastric bypass, but her pregnancy is otherwise uncomplicated. The laboratory test that is most likely to determine the etiology of her anemia is a (an)

(A) ferritin level
(B) hemoglobin electrophoresis
(C) iron panel
(D) peripheral smear
(E) vitamin B_{12} level

74

A 28-year-old gravida 2, para 1, presents with a fetal death at 23 0/7 weeks of gestation. Her first pregnancy was complicated by preeclampsia with severe features requiring cesarean birth by low transverse incision at 35 weeks of gestation. She has no significant medical history. The patient's vital signs are normal. She requests delivery at this time, and she would like to hold the newborn. Her fetus is presenting as a complete breech on ultrasonographic examination, and her cervix is closed with no effacement. The most appropriate initial method of induction is oral mifepristone followed by

(A) high-dose intravenous oxytocin
(B) low-dose intravenous oxytocin
(C) transcervical mechanical dilation
(D) vaginal misoprostol
(E) vaginal prostaglandin E2

75

A 19-year-old gravida 1 at 33 weeks of gestation arrives to the obstetric triage unit by emergency medical services. She has altered sensorium and is reporting abdominal pain. Her pregnancy is complicated by type 1 diabetes mellitus. Her blood pressure is 115/80 mm Hg, her heart rate is 105 beats per minute, her respiratory rate is 25 respirations per minute, and her temperature is 37.2 °C (99.0 °F). Her blood glucose concentration is 108 mg/dL. An arterial blood gas reveals a pH of 7.15. Her anion gap is 14 mEq/L, and her serum bicarbonate is 12 mEq/L. She is placed on continuous electronic fetal monitoring with the tracing demonstrated below (Fig. 75-1). In addition to starting intravenous fluids, the most appropriate next step in management is

(A) betamethasone
(B) cesarean birth
(C) insulin
(D) oxytocin
(E) terbutaline

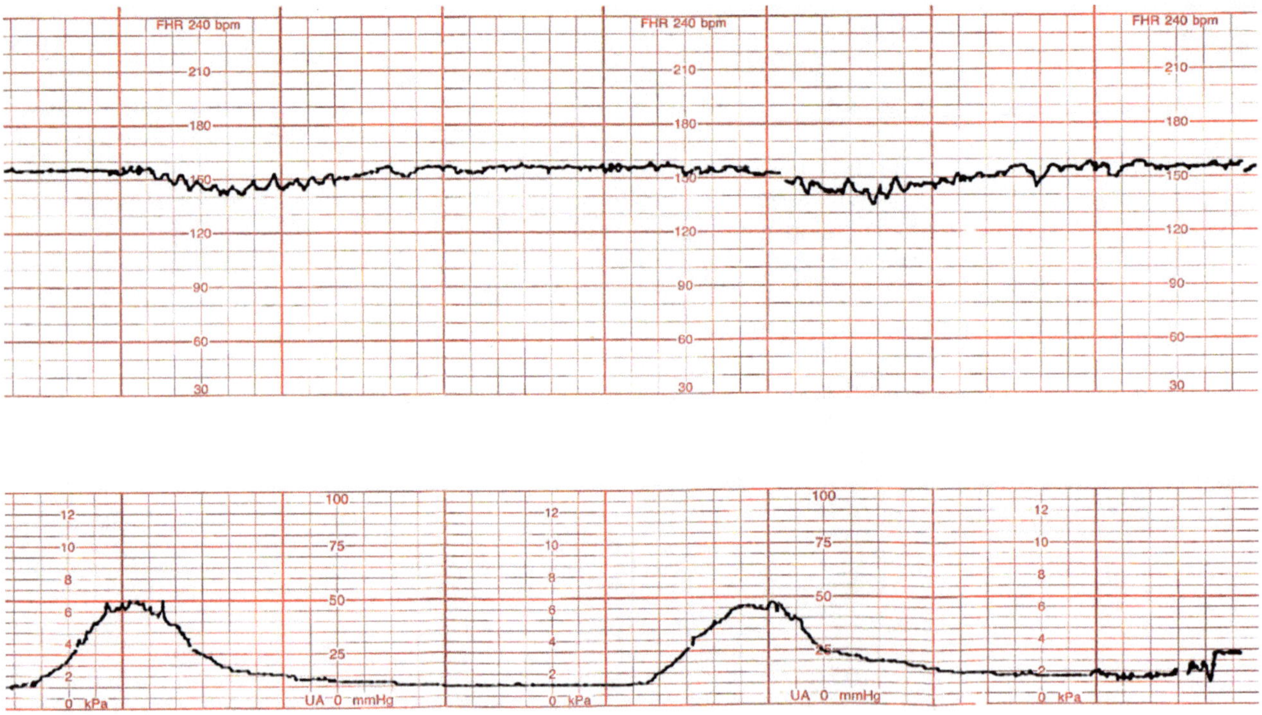

FIGURE 75-1. Patient's fetal heart rate tracing

76

A patient is having an ultrasonographic examination at 19 weeks of gestation to assess fetal anatomy and cervical length. In her last pregnancy, she delivered at 28 weeks of gestation after preterm prelabor rupture of membranes (PPROM). She is receiving vaginal progesterone supplementation for prevention of preterm labor. Her examination shows normal fetal anatomy, and her transvaginal cervical length is 22 mm. The best next step in management of her pregnancy is

(A) cervical cerclage
(B) cervical pessary
(C) fetal fibronectin
(D) repeat cervical length measurement

77

A 38-year-old gravida 1, para 1, develops heavy vaginal bleeding 4 hours after an uncomplicated primary cesarean birth of a term neonate. The uterus is massaged and uterotonics are administered, including misoprostol, oxytocin, methylergonovine, and 15-methyl prostaglandin $F_{2\alpha}$. A uterine tamponade balloon is attempted but placement is unsuccessful. The massive transfusion protocol is initiated. Her abdomen is reopened and uterine atony is identified. A B-Lynch suture is placed without a significant decrease in bleeding. Her blood pressure is 80/40 mm Hg, and her pulse is 130 beats per minute. You continue to transfuse with blood product replacement. Quantitative blood loss is 4,500 mL. The best next step is

(A) administration of tranexamic acid
(B) hysterectomy
(C) repeat administration of methylergonovine
(D) second uterine compression suture
(E) uterine artery embolization

78

A 16-year-old gravida 1 presents in the third trimester for prenatal care. She reports intense itching on her abdomen that started 2 weeks ago, followed by widespread, large red plaques with areas of blistering. On physical examination, she has papules, plaques, and vesicles on her entire abdomen and trunk, involving the periumbilical area, and spreading to the proximal extremities (Fig. 78-1). The most likely diagnosis is

(A) contact dermatitis
(B) eczema
(C) intrahepatic cholestasis of pregnancy
(D) pemphigoid gestationis
(E) polymorphic eruption of pregnancy

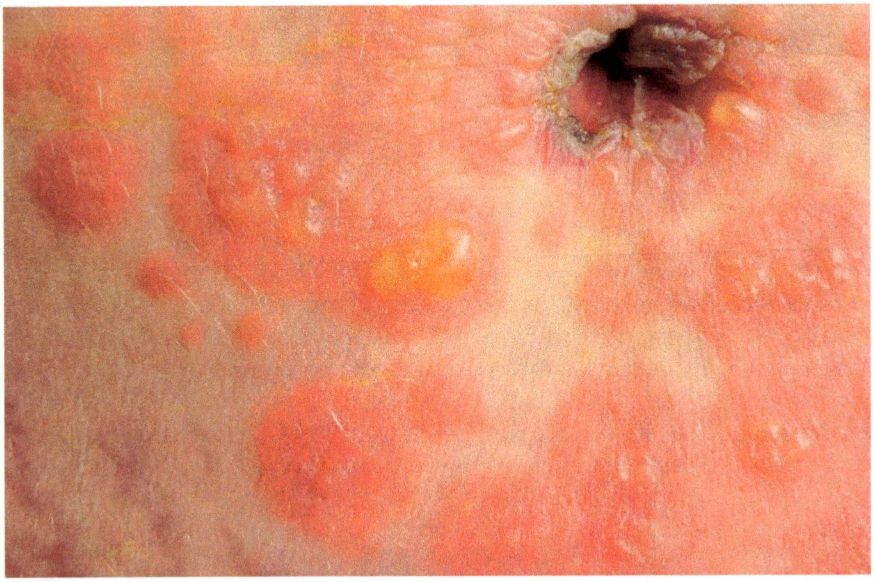

FIGURE 78-1. Periumbilical eruption. (Reprinted from Sävervall C, Sand FL, Thomsen SF. Dermatological diseases associated with pregnancy: pemphigoid gestationis, polymorphic eruption of pregnancy, intrahepatic cholestasis of pregnancy, and atopic eruption of pregnancy. Dermatol Res Pract 2015;2015:979635. doi: 10.1155/2015/979635 https://www.hindawi.com/journals/drp/2015/979635/)

79

A 27-year-old gravida 2, para 1, at 23 weeks of gestation presents for a prenatal visit in October. She has a history of mild intermittent asthma without recent exacerbation. She has received vaccination for COVID-19. She is concerned about respiratory illness in her newborn. The immunization most appropriate at this visit to decrease the risk of respiratory illness in both the woman and her newborn is

(A) influenza
(B) measles–mumps–rubella
(C) pneumococcal
(D) respiratory syncytial virus
(E) tetanus toxoid, reduced diphtheria toxoid, and acellular pertussis (Tdap)

80

A 28-year-old gravida 1, para 1, presents to your office at 5 days postpartum with a report of fever. She underwent primary cesarean birth for arrest of dilation after a labor complicated by presumed intra-amniotic infection. She received intravenous antibiotic therapy intrapartum and remained afebrile during the remainder of her hospitalization. The patient had an indwelling catheter during labor and cesarean birth that was removed on the first postoperative day. She has no dysuria, urinary frequency, or back pain. Her fever started yesterday along with incisional pain. Breastfeeding is going well, and she has no breast tenderness other than engorgement. Her vital signs are normal. On examination, the incision is intact with surrounding erythema and induration without drainage or fluctuance. Her examination is otherwise normal. The most likely diagnosis is

(A) cellulitis
(B) endometritis
(C) mastitis
(D) urinary tract infection

81

A 23-year-old primigravida at 29 weeks of gestation is admitted to labor and delivery with persistent vaginal bleeding. On admission, her blood pressure is 167/115 mm Hg, and repeat blood pressure 4 hours later was 172/112 mm Hg. She receives oral nifedipine, and her blood pressure decreases to 142/87 mm Hg. Her hematocrit is 36%, platelet count is 112×10^9/L, creatinine is 0.67 mg/dL, aspartate transaminase concentration is 31 units/L, and alanine transaminase concentration is 34 units/L. Baseline fetal heart rate is 150 beats per minute with moderate variability and accelerations. Fetal growth ultrasonography shows an estimated fetal weight at the 5th percentile, with normal umbilical artery Doppler velocimetry and placentation. The clinical finding that indicates the need for expedited delivery rather than expectant management is

(A) blood pressure greater than 160/110 mm Hg that responds to nifedipine
(B) fetal growth at the 5th percentile
(C) platelet count
(D) vaginal bleeding in the absence of placenta previa

82

A 33-year-old gravida 3, para 2, presents at 21 weeks of gestation for anatomical survey. A fetal death is noted on ultrasonography, with the composite measurements showing a fetal size of 20 weeks of gestation. She desires a dilation and evacuation (D&E). In addition to osmotic dilators, the most effective cervical preparation is

(A) mifepristone
(B) misoprostol
(C) oxytocin
(D) prostaglandin E2

83

A 29-year-old gravida 4, para 2, at 37 weeks of gestation is noted to have a fetus in breech presentation. She has a history of two prior vaginal deliveries and opts for external cephalic version (ECV). She has an anxiety disorder and poor pain tolerance, and she receives epidural anesthesia. To improve the chance of successful ECV, the most appropriate medication to administer is

(A) diazepam
(B) morphine
(C) nitroglycerin
(D) nitrous oxide
(E) terbutaline

84

A patient presents at 10 weeks of gestation with nausea and vomiting. She has been unable to tolerate food for 2 days and fluids for 1 day. She has lost 4 kg in the past week and her prepregnancy weight was 79 kg. To treat her nausea at home, she has tried ginger supplements and replaced her prenatal vitamin with a folic acid supplement. Urinalysis shows 4+ ketones. Her medical history is significant for inherited prolonged QT interval, and she is taking nadolol and has an implantable defibrillator in place. The best antiemetic to administer for immediate relief is

(A) lorazepam
(B) ondansetron
(C) promethazine
(D) scopolamine
(E) corticosteroids

85

A 38-year-old gravida 3, para 2, who has not initiated prenatal care presents to the emergency department with acute vaginal bleeding. Her last menstrual period is unknown because she has experienced intermittent vaginal bleeding for months. She reports constant abdominal pain and intermittent low back pain. She has a history of substance use and reports cocaine use during the last 36 hours. Her blood pressure is 105/75 mm Hg, heart rate is 115 beats per minute, and her temperature is 37.5 °C (99.5 °F). On physical examination, her abdomen is firm and tender, and her fundal height is 35 cm. Her cervix is visually closed with 30 cc of fresh blood in the vaginal vault and active bleeding from the cervical os. Obstetric ultrasonography is performed at the bedside. The placental location is fundal, and the fetus is in cephalic presentation. Electronic fetal heart tracing is Category III. She is contracting every 2 minutes. Her hemoglobin is 5.4 g/dL, and her fibrinogen is 150 mg/dL. In addition to initiating blood product transfusion, the best next step in management is

(A) cesarean birth
(B) fetal monitoring with intrauterine resuscitation
(C) intramuscular betamethasone
(D) intravenous magnesium sulfate
(E) nifedipine tocolysis

86

A patient presents at 24 weeks of gestation and is admitted for preeclampsia with severe features (Appendix C) and fetal growth restriction. During cesarean birth for nonreassuring fetal testing, a placental abruption is identified. Apgar scores are 4 and 6 at 1 and 5 minutes, respectively. The neonatal birth weight is 505 g. The factor most strongly associated with the risk of cerebral palsy in this neonate is

(A) Apgar scores
(B) birth weight
(C) gestational age
(D) placental abruption
(E) preeclampsia

87

A patient at 24 weeks of gestation has a fundal height of 30 cm at a routine obstetric visit. All maternal testing, including noninvasive prenatal screening and 18 weeks of gestation anatomy ultrasonography, has yielded normal results. Ultrasonography is performed and fetal growth is at the 50th percentile. Figure 87-1 represents the deepest vertical pocket. In addition to a glucose challenge, the best next step is

(A) amniocentesis with fluid reduction
(B) detailed fetal anatomic survey
(C) fetal magnetic resonance imaging (MRI)
(D) maternal cytomegalovirus (CMV) serology
(E) reassurance

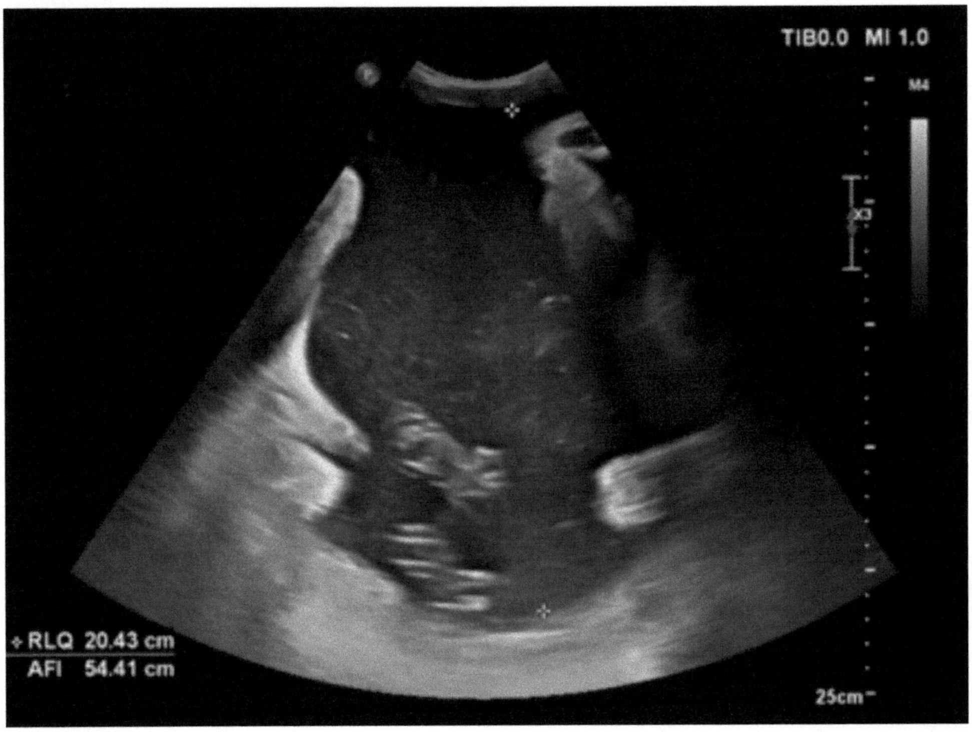

FIGURE 87-1. Maximal vertical pocket. (Image courtesy of Dr. Marcie Treadwell.)

88

A 19-year-old is seen at 12 weeks of gestation for their first prenatal visit and they report feeling well. They have been living in a homeless shelter for 6 months. The patient has a history of prior bacillus Calmette-Guérin (BCG) vaccination. In addition to routine prenatal care, the best next test in evaluation of latent tuberculosis (TB) infection is

(A) chest X-ray
(B) interferon-gamma release assay (IGRA)
(C) pulmonary function tests
(D) sputum culture
(E) tuberculin skin testing

89

A 25-year-old primigravida at 39 weeks of gestation is admitted with prelabor rupture of membranes and undergoes an induction of labor. The patient has a history of insulin-dependent diabetes mellitus and obesity. Maternal vital signs include a temperature of 39.1 °C (102.4 °F), a pulse of 138 beats per minute, and blood pressure of 118/76 mm Hg. Fetal tachycardia is noted. Ampicillin and gentamicin are initiated. After a prolonged induction of labor, she undergoes a cesarean birth. The best next step in her antibiotic therapy is to

(A) add cefazolin
(B) add clindamycin
(C) change antibiotics to piperacillin–tazobactam
(D) discontinue antibiotics

90

A 33-year-old multiparous patient at 29 weeks of gestation calls your office to report that her two young children have tested positive for influenza. She has no fever, cough, or other symptoms. She is without significant medical history and is up to date with her routine prenatal care. In addition to providing education on transmission risk reduction strategies, the best next step is to

(A) perform a physical examination
(B) perform influenza testing
(C) prescribe oseltamivir
(D) recommend peramivir
(E) recommend temperature monitoring

91

A 32-year-old gravida 1, para 0, presents at 37 weeks of gestation with decreased fetal movement. Her pregnancy has been uncomplicated. She has a reactive nonstress test, and her vital signs are within normal limits. The amniotic fluid index (AFI) is 4 cm, and the deepest vertical pocket is shown in Figure 91-1. The best next step in management is

(A) biophysical profile (BPP)
(B) contraction stress test
(C) discharge to home
(D) induction of labor
(E) prolonged fetal monitoring

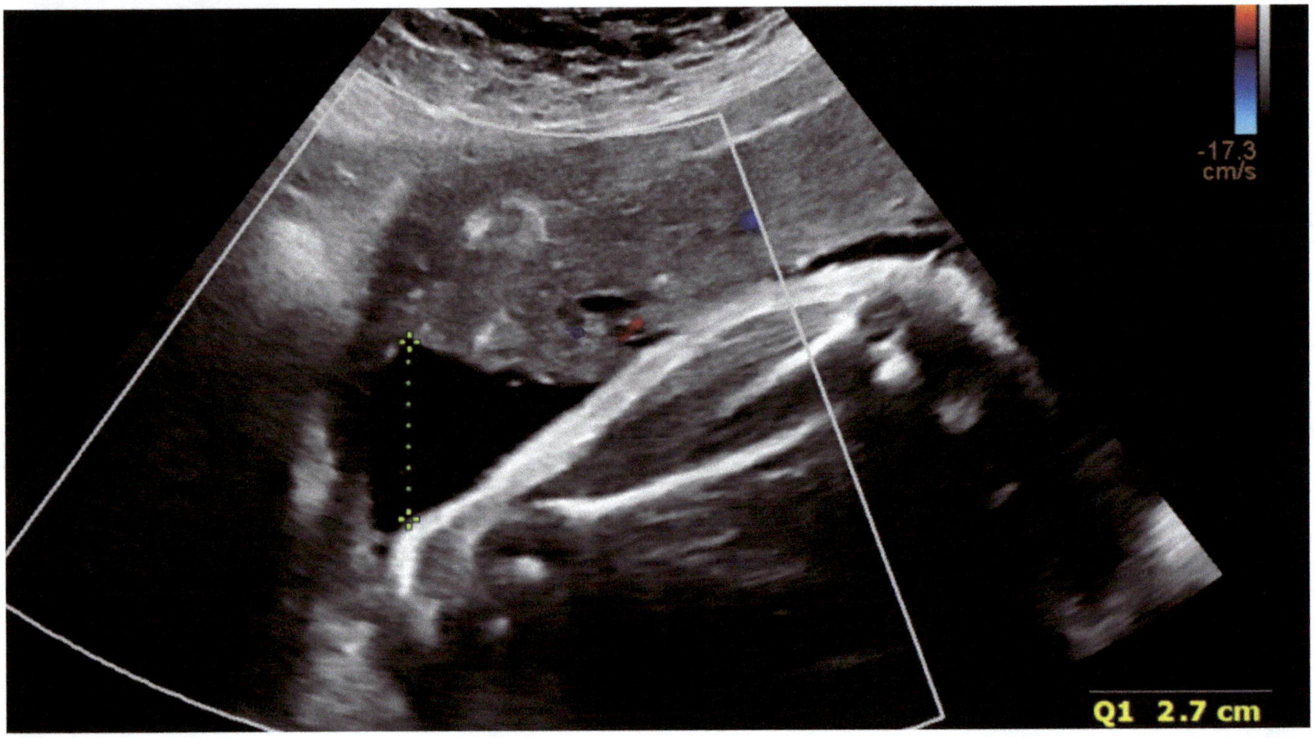

FIGURE 91-1. Deepest vertical pocket measurement.

92

A 30-year-old gravida 2, para 1, presents for her prenatal visit at 39 weeks of gestation. Her first delivery was a cesarean birth because of an arrest of active labor at 41 weeks of gestation. She requests induction of labor, preferring to avoid another cesarean birth. Her cervix is 1-cm dilated and 20% effaced. The presenting fetal part is at −3 station. The fetus has a cephalic presentation on ultrasonographic examination. The most appropriate initial step of labor induction is

(A) amniotomy
(B) dinoprostone
(C) misoprostol
(D) oxytocin
(E) transcervical Foley catheter

93

A 29-year-old presents with preterm prelabor rupture of membranes at 35 weeks of gestation. Her pregnancy had previously been uncomplicated with no hospitalizations. Her vital signs are normal. You discuss administration of antenatal corticosteroids and counsel her that the administration of late-preterm corticosteroids increases the risk of neonatal

(A) hyperbilirubinemia
(B) hypoglycemia
(C) necrotizing enterocolitis
(D) respiratory distress
(E) sepsis

94

A 39-year-old gravida 3, para 1, at 10 weeks of gestation is seen for an initial prenatal visit, during which ultrasonography is performed. The ultrasonography shows a fetus with no cardiac activity and placental tissue with multiple cystic areas. The patient undergoes dilation and suction curettage. Chromosomal evaluation of the retained fetal tissue identifies a 69,XXY karyotype. The most appropriate frequency of human chorionic gonadotropin (β-hCG) monitoring for this patient is

(A) monthly until negative
(B) weekly until negative for three consecutive tests
(C) weekly until negative, then confirmed 1 month later
(D) weekly until negative, then monthly for 6 months

95

A 34-year-old gravida 2, para 0, is undergoing primary cesarean birth for arrest of dilation in labor. Her prenatal course was complicated by class III obesity, with a prepregnant body mass index (BMI) of 51. She received preoperative antibiotics at an appropriate dose for her weight. The surgical team replaces their sterile gloves after hysterotomy closure. The intervention at surgical closure that is most likely to decrease the risk of postoperative infectious morbidity is use of

(A) delayed absorbable braided suture to close the fascial layer
(B) irrigation of the subcutaneous layer
(C) negative pressure wound dressing
(D) subcutaneous drain
(E) suture approximation of the subcutaneous layer

96

A 40-year-old gravida 1 at 12 weeks of gestation presents for counseling on aneuploidy screening. She had multiple previous unsuccessful in vitro fertilization cycles, and after careful counseling and shared decision making, two embryos were transferred after preimplantation genetic screening for aneuploidy was performed. She has a dichorionic pregnancy following in vitro fertilization. The best next step in aneuploidy screening is

(A) cell-free DNA (cfDNA) screening
(B) fetal anatomic survey
(C) first-trimester screening
(D) no further screening
(E) nuchal translucency

97

A 37-year-old gravida 7, para 6, presents at 38 weeks of gestation in active labor. Her pulse is 98 beats per minute (bpm), and her blood pressure is 104/68 mm Hg. She delivers within 1 hour of admission, and oxytocin is administered after delivery of the fetus. Continued bleeding due to uterine atony is noted after placental delivery. Her intravenous fluids are increased, and tranexamic acid and methylergonovine are given. You have emptied her bladder and are preparing to insert an intrauterine balloon tamponade because of continued hemorrhage. You have estimated the blood loss to be 1,100 mL. The patient's heart rate is 130 bpm, her blood pressure is 90/54 mm Hg, and she has had no urine output in the past 15 minutes. The nurse notifies you that the quantitative blood loss is 2,440 mL. Laboratory studies are obtained, and you note that the phlebotomy site is bleeding significantly. The most appropriate method to estimate this patient's blood loss in preparation for a massive transfusion protocol is the

(A) hematocrit
(B) qualitative blood loss
(C) quantitative blood loss
(D) vital signs with urine output

98

A 23-year-old gravida 1, para 1, presents 6 weeks after delivery for an office visit. Her pregnancy was complicated by systemic lupus erythematosus (SLE), Sjögren syndrome type A (Ro or SS-A) antibodies, and intrapartum preeclampsia with thrombocytopenia. She cannot tolerate hydroxychloroquine and is currently taking azathioprine and low-dose prednisone to control lupus flares. She delivered a small-for-gestational-age neonate at 37 weeks of gestation and is currently breastfeeding. Her blood pressure is 120/68 mm Hg. She talks with you about a skin rash her infant has had on the head and neck for the past month (Fig. 98-1). The most likely maternal cause of the infant's rash is

(A) azathioprine
(B) corticosteroids
(C) preeclampsia
(D) SS-A antibodies

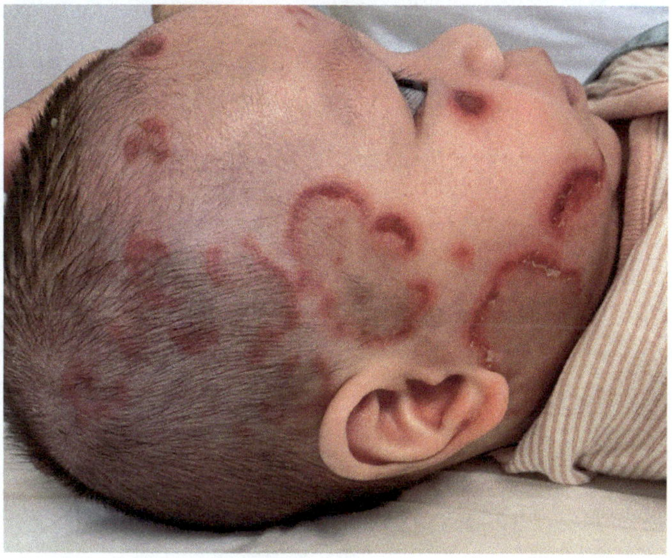

FIGURE 98-1. Neonatal rash. (Reprinted from Wu J, Berk-Krauss J, Glick SA. Neonatal lupus erythematosus. JAMA Dermatol 2021;157:590. doi: 10.1001/jamadermatol.2021.0041 https://jamanetwork.com/journals/jamadermatology/article-abstract/2777663)

99

A 26-year-old gravida 1 with a history of epilepsy presents to the emergency department after experiencing a tonic-clonic seizure. She is at 7 weeks of gestation. She discontinued her antiepileptic medication therapy 6 months ago for financial reasons. Since her epilepsy diagnosis 10 years ago, she has been on numerous antiepileptic medications, including carbamazepine, levetiracetam, phenytoin, topiramate, and valproic acid, all of which have been effective in managing her seizures. Of the antiepileptic medications that she has previously taken, you recommend that she restart

(A) carbamazepine
(B) levetiracetam
(C) phenytoin
(D) topiramate
(E) valproic acid

100

A 33-year-old gravida 2, para 1, presents at 15 1/7 weeks of gestation for follow-up imaging of a right adnexal mass incidentally noted on ultrasonographic evaluation at 8 weeks of gestation. The right adnexa was visualized (Fig. 100-1). The most likely diagnosis is

(A) endometrioma
(B) hydrosalpinx
(C) mature cystic teratoma
(D) serous cystadenoma
(E) theca lutein cyst

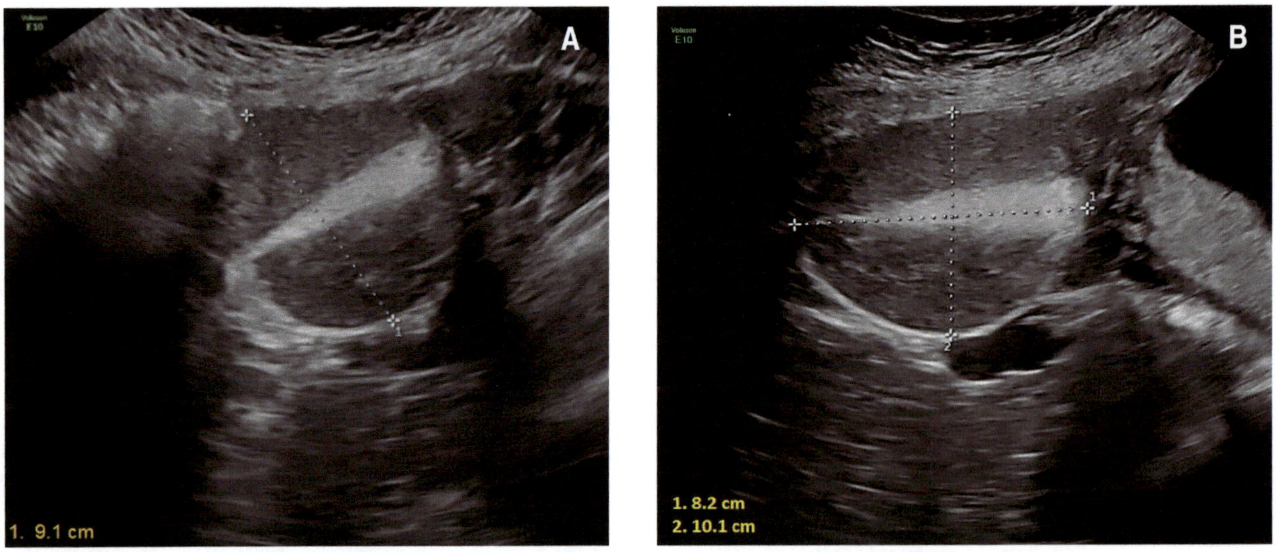

FIGURE 100-1. A and B. Ultrasonographic images of patient's right adnexa showing measurements in two orthogonal planes.

101

A 38-year-old gravida 1 has been prescribed low-molecular-weight heparin daily during her pregnancy because her mother experienced a deep vein thrombosis during pregnancy, and she and her mother are heterozygous for factor V Leiden mutation. She is scheduled for induction of labor at 39 weeks of gestation and desires an epidural for pain management during labor. The most appropriate timing for discontinuation of this patient's anticoagulation before epidural placement is

(A) 6 hours
(B) 12 hours
(C) 24 hours
(D) 48 hours

102

A 38-year-old gravida 3, para 1, with a previous cesarean birth at 38 weeks of gestation presents to labor and delivery with a report of leaking fluid. She reports that her first cesarean birth was performed for breech presentation at term. Ruptured membranes are confirmed. The cervix is 4-cm dilated, 50% effaced, with fetal station at −2. Fetal heart rate tracing shows a baseline of 135 beats per minute, moderate variability, the presence of accelerations, and the absence of decelerations. She had planned to deliver at a hospital 30 miles away. With regard to delivery planning, the most appropriate next step is to

(A) offer a trial of labor
(B) perform immediate repeat cesarean birth
(C) perform ultrasonographic evaluation of the lower uterine segment
(D) transfer the patient to her primary obstetrician

103

A 39-year-old primigravida at 14 weeks of gestation presents to the emergency department with intractable nausea and vomiting. This is her third presentation for nausea and vomiting. The patient reports that she has self-treated with marijuana. She has been treated with doxylamine, pyridoxine, and ondansetron with no improvement in her symptoms. She mentions that the only thing that seems to be helping is frequent hot showers. On presentation, she is afebrile, her blood pressure is 100/62 mm Hg, and her heart rate is 110 beats per minute. Her weight is decreased to 65 kg from 76 kg before pregnancy. She is hospitalized for intravenous hydration and optimization of antiemetic therapy. The best next step to resolve her nausea and vomiting is

(A) cessation of marijuana use
(B) methylprednisolone taper
(C) metoclopramide
(D) psychotherapy

104

A 27-year-old gravida 1, para 0, will be undergoing primary cesarean birth for breech presentation following an unsuccessful external cephalic version. She reports that she is allergic to penicillin and states that her allergic reaction was a rash after treatment with amoxicillin as a child. Rectovaginal culture at 37 weeks of gestation is positive for group B streptococcus (GBS), which is sensitive to ampicillin, clindamycin, and erythromycin. The most appropriate antibiotic surgical prophylaxis for this patient is

(A) ampicillin and sulbactam
(B) azithromycin
(C) cefazolin
(D) clindamycin and gentamicin
(E) vancomycin

105

A 34-year-old gravida 3, para 2, presents at 36 weeks of gestation for her third cesarean birth. Her pregnancy is complicated by placenta previa. Placenta accreta is suspected at the time of delivery, requiring immediate hysterectomy, which is complicated by adhesive disease and heavy intraoperative bleeding. Massive transfusion protocol is initiated. Total quantitative blood loss is 6,350 mL. She is intubated and transferred to the intensive care unit for monitoring. Her temperature is 37.1 °C (98.8 °F), her blood pressure is 122/70 mm Hg, and she is ventilated with pressure support only. She is sedated, but otherwise her physical examination is normal. Telemetry shows peaked T-waves and wide QRS interval (Fig. 105-1). The most likely massive transfusion complication is

(A) electrolyte derangement
(B) febrile hemolytic reaction
(C) transfusion-associated circulatory overload (TACO)
(D) transfusion-related acute lung injury (TRALI)

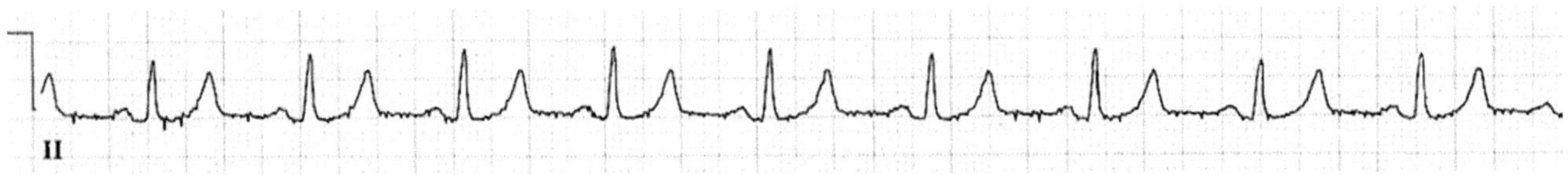

FIGURE 105-1. Postoperative electrocardiogram. (Image courtesy of Baystate Medical Center Division of Nephrology.)

106

A 42-year-old gravida 2, para 2, presents for her routine 6-week postpartum visit. On breast examination, you palpate a 4-cm mass in the upper outer quadrant of her right breast. She reports that it has been present for about 1 month. It is nontender and is not erythematous. She has not had any fevers or chills. The best next step is to

(A) apply warm compresses and massage the area
(B) obtain breast ultrasonography
(C) perform an incision and drainage
(D) prescribe dicloxacillin
(E) reevaluate the breast in 4 weeks

107

A 38-year-old patient with a normal body mass index (BMI) presents for a prenatal visit and genetic testing. She and her partner have an unremarkable genetic history in their families. She decided to have cell-free DNA (cfDNA) screening with a microdeletion panel. The results indicate that the fetus has a high risk of 22q11 deletion syndrome. The most likely cause of a false-positive screening test for this condition in this patient is

(A) advanced maternal age
(B) BMI
(C) family history
(D) low disease incidence
(E) low fetal fraction

108–112

Match the genetic disorder (108–112) to the appropriate patient pedigree (A–C):

(A) Pedigree A

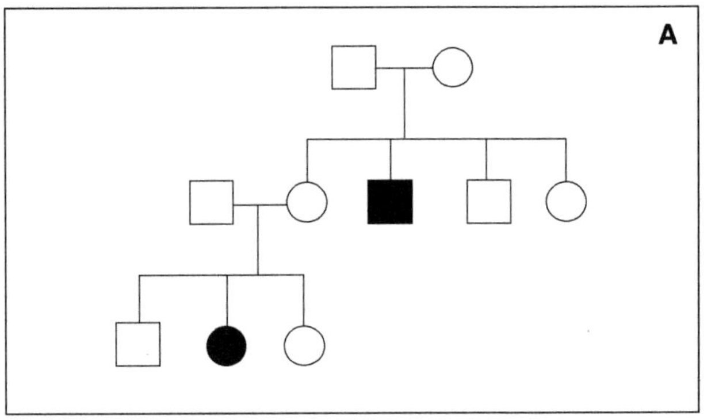

(B) Pedigree B

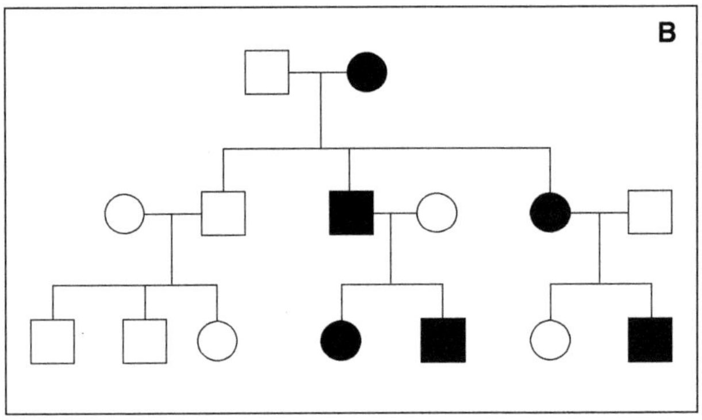

(C) Pedigree C

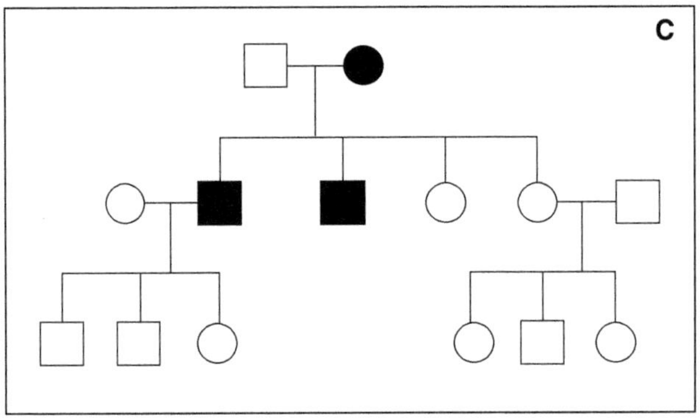

108. Spinal muscular atrophy

109. Hemophilia A

110. Cystic fibrosis (CF)

111. Neurofibromatosis

112. Marfan syndrome

113–115

For each clinical scenario (113–115), choose the best next step (A–D).

(A) Administer caffeine
(B) Order computed tomography (CT) imaging
(C) Order magnetic resonance arteriogram and venogram
(D) Place a blood patch

113. A 45-year-old at 38 weeks of gestation presents with acute onset of blurry vision, an unsteady gait, and a diffuse, severe headache. She has no history of headaches. Her blood pressure is 100/60 mm Hg, papilledema is noted on fundoscopic examination, and laboratory results are normal.

114. A 31-year-old who is 2 weeks postpartum presents with a new, sudden, painful headache that woke her from sleep this morning. The headache did not respond to acetaminophen or ibuprofen. Her blood pressure was 165/100 mm Hg on admission. Liver function and platelets are normal, and a protein/creatinine ratio is 1.0. The next morning, the headache returns despite use of magnesium sulfate, antihypertensives, and analgesics. Magnetic resonance imaging reveals no pathology.

115. A 20-year-old on postpartum day 1 has a frontal headache that is worse when she is sitting or standing but resolves when she lies supine. Her labor was uncomplicated, with use of epidural analgesia.

116–119

For each clinical scenario (116–119), choose the optimal contraceptive method (A–E).

(A) Copper intrauterine device (IUD)
(B) Etonogestrel implant
(C) Levonorgestrel IUD
(D) Oral estrogen and progestogen combination pills
(E) Progestin-only pills

116. A 23-year-old gravida 3, para 2, is admitted for a repeat cesarean birth. She is planning on breastfeeding and requests the longest-lasting reversible contraceptive option.

117. A 38-year-old gravida 2, para 2, presents for a 4-week postpartum visit and requests contraception. They are a current smoker, and they are breastfeeding. They decline inserting anything in their body or any injections for contraception.

118. A 28-year-old gravida 3, para 3, presents 3 months after giving birth. She is breastfeeding. She reports worsening acne and would like a contraceptive method to reduce this.

119. A 29-year-old gravida 2, para 2, on postpartum day 1 requests long-acting reversible contraception before her discharge from the hospital.

120–124

For each ultrasound finding (120–124), choose the most likely maternal condition(s) (A–E) that contributed to the increased risk of congenital malformation(s).

(A) Generalized seizure disorder
(B) Severe refractory bipolar disorder
(C) Autoimmune hepatitis with recent liver transplant
(D) Mechanical heart valve
(E) Chronic hypertension and insulin-requiring diabetes mellitus

120. Spina bifida, craniofacial and cardiovascular anomalies

121. Ebstein anomaly, polyhydramnios, diabetes insipidus

122. Absent nasal bone, limb hypoplasia with stippled epiphyses, ventral midline dysplasia

123. Oligohydramnios, fetal lung hypoplasia, skeletal malformations

124. Cleft lip and ear, and eye abnormalities

125–128

For each of the following clinical scenarios (125–128), select the most appropriate type of forceps (A–D) to assist in a vaginal delivery.

(A) Tucker–McLane forceps
(B) Simpson–Luikart forceps
(C) Piper forceps
(D) Kielland forceps

125. A nulliparous patient at term with a prolonged second stage of labor.

126. A nulliparous patient at term in labor with nonreassuring tracing and a left occiput transverse presentation.

127. A multiparous patient at term with maternal cardiac disease necessitating a passive second stage of labor.

128. A multiparous patient at term with diamniotic-dichorionic twins. The second twin is delivered by breech extraction, and additional assistance is needed with the aftercoming head.

129–133

Match each clinical scenario (129–133) with the most likely diagnosis (A–E).

(A) Acute fatty liver of pregnancy
(B) Gestational thrombocytopenia
(C) Immune thrombocytopenia (ITP)
(D) Preeclampsia with severe features
(E) Thrombotic thrombocytopenic purpura (TTP)

129. A nulliparous patient presents at 7 weeks of gestation. She has no significant medical history. Her platelet count is 35,000/mm^3.

130. A nulliparous patient at 32 weeks of gestation presents with nausea and abdominal pain. Examination reveals a blood pressure of 150/100 mm Hg and evidence of jaundice. Laboratory test results include an ammonia level of 60 micromoles/L and platelet count of 68,000/mm^3.

131. A multiparous patient at 30 weeks of gestation has a routine third-trimester platelet count of 105,000/mm^3 and normal blood pressure.

132. A nulliparous patient at 18 weeks of gestation presents with headache, abdominal pain, fever, and decreased fetal movement. On examination, she is noted to have petechiae and a fetal death. Laboratory testing reveals a hematocrit of 24%, platelet count of 10,000/mm^3, and proteinuria.

133. A nulliparous patient at 34 weeks of gestation presents with a headache and epigastric pain. On examination, she is found to have new-onset hypertension. Laboratory testing reveals an aspartate aminotransferase of 220 IU/L, alanine aminotransferase of 250 IU/L, and a platelet count of 98,000/mm^3.

134–138

For each clinical scenario (134–138), choose the most appropriate next step for preterm birth prevention (A–C).

(A) Cerclage
(B) Cervical length screening
(C) Expectant management

134. A 23-year-old gravida 2, para 1, presents for fetal anatomy ultrasonography at 19 weeks of gestation. She has no history of preterm birth. Her cervical length on examination is 4 mm, and the cervix is dilated 5 mm.

135. A 33-year-old gravida 2, para 1, presents for fetal anatomy ultrasonography at 19 weeks of gestation. She has a history of spontaneous preterm delivery at 30 weeks of gestation. Her cervical length is 26 mm, and the cervix is closed on examination.

136. A 28-year-old gravida 2, para 1, presents for initiation of prenatal care at 12 weeks of gestation. She has a history of asymptomatic cervical dilation, requiring cerclage placement at 20 weeks in her last pregnancy.

137. A 30-year-old gravida 2, para 1, presents for transvaginal ultrasonography at 16 weeks of gestation because of a history of spontaneous preterm birth at 28 weeks of gestation. Her cervical length is 20 mm, and the cervix is closed on examination.

138. A 25-year-old gravida 3, para 2, presents for her anatomy ultrasonography at 19 weeks of gestation. She has no history of preterm birth. Her cervical length is 29 mm, and the cervix is closed on examination.

139–143

For each clinical scenario (139–143), choose the recommended intrapartum group B streptococcus (GBS) prophylaxis strategy (A–E).

(A) Cefazolin
(B) Clindamycin
(C) Penicillin
(D) Prophylaxis not indicated
(E) Vancomycin

139. A 26-year-old gravida 2, para 1, presents in spontaneous labor at 38 weeks of gestation. Current GBS status is unknown, but she was a GBS carrier in her prior pregnancy. She has no allergies to medications.

140. A 30-year-old gravida 3, para 2, presents for scheduled induction of labor at 39 weeks of gestation. Earlier in the pregnancy, she had a urine culture positive for GBS at 10^2 colony-forming units/mL. She has a history of a mild rash after taking penicillin as a young child.

141. A 39-year-old gravida 1, para 0, at 37 weeks of gestation is being induced for chronic hypertension. Her amniotic membranes have been ruptured for 24 hours, she is 3-cm dilated, and she is continuing to labor. A GBS screening culture was negative at 36 weeks of gestation. She has no allergies to medications.

142. A 20-year-old gravida 1, para 0, presents in spontaneous preterm labor at 37 weeks of gestation. Her intrapartum nucleic acid amplification test (NAAT) GBS screening was negative. Amniotic membranes have been ruptured greater than 18 hours, and on cervical examination she is 6-cm dilated. She has a history of hives with penicillin.

143. A 33-year-old gravida 2, para 1, is in spontaneous preterm labor at 36 weeks of gestation. A GBS culture was negative at 28 weeks of gestation when she was admitted for a prior episode of preterm labor. She has no allergies to medications.

144–147

For each ultrasound image (Figs. 144–147) choose the likely diagnosis (A–F).

(A) Ascites
(B) Bowel obstruction
(C) Echogenic bowel
(D) Gastroschisis
(E) Hydronephrosis
(F) Omphalocele

144.

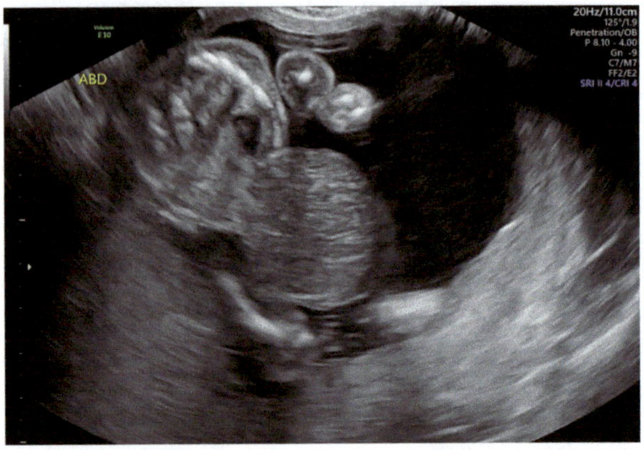

145.

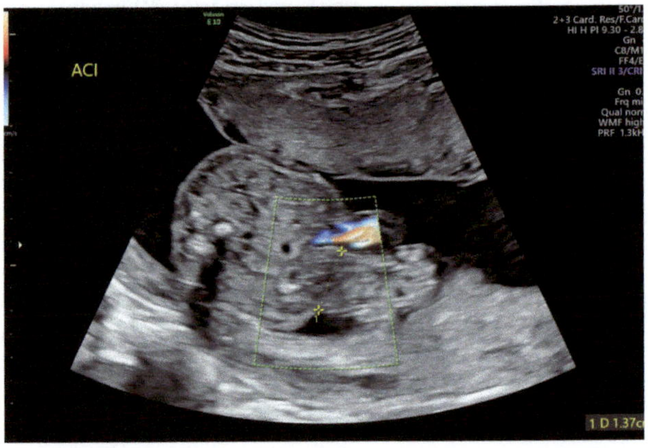

146.

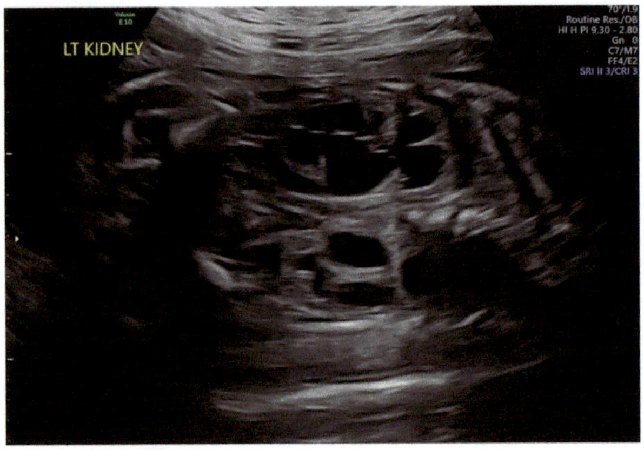

147.

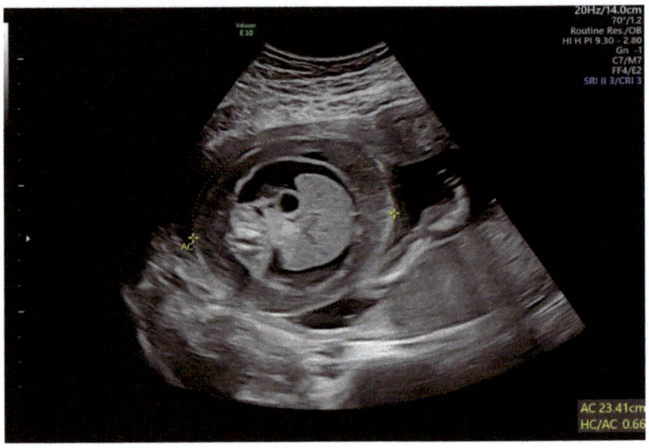

148–151

For each clinical scenario (148–151), choose the best diagnosis (A–E).

(A) Arrest of dilation
(B) Protracted dilation
(C) Arrest of descent
(D) Unsuccessful induction
(E) Normal labor

148. A gravida 2, para 0, at term presented with prelabor rupture of membranes 24 hours ago. She has received oxytocin for 18 hours with no cervical change.

149. A gravida 2, para 1, at term presented in latent labor and progressed to a cervical dilation of 7 cm. Her cervix has remained unchanged for the past 6 hours despite oxytocin administration and ruptured membranes.

150. A gravida 1, para 0, at term presented in spontaneous labor, received an epidural, and progressed to complete dilation. After 4 hours of pushing, the fetal head remains at +2 station.

151. A gravida 1, para 0, at term presented in spontaneous latent labor 14 hours ago. Membranes remain intact, and cervical dilation has progressed from 2 cm on admission to 5 cm.

152–156

For each hepatitis B virus testing result (152–156), choose the most likely status (A–E).

(A) Acutely infected
(B) Chronically infected
(C) Immune because of hepatitis B vaccination
(D) Immune because of natural infection
(E) Susceptible to infection

152.	HBsAg	Negative
	IgG anti-HBc	Negative
	IgG anti-HBs	Negative
153.	HBsAg	Positive
	IgG anti-HBc	Positive
	IgM anti-HBc	Negative
	IgG anti-HBs	Negative
154.	HBsAg	Positive
	IgG anti-HBc	Positive
	IgM anti-HBc	Positive
	IgG anti-HBs	Negative
155.	HBsAg	Negative
	IgG anti-HBc	Positive
	IgG anti-HBs	Positive
156.	HBsAg	Negative
	IgG anti-HBc	Negative
	IgG anti-HBs	Positive

157–161

For each clinical scenario 157–161, choose the minimum level of maternal care necessary given the resources anticipated (A–E).

(A) Birth center
(B) Level I
(C) Level II
(D) Level III
(E) Level IV

157. Uncomplicated diamniotic-dichorionic twin pregnancy at term

158. Anterior placenta with three previous cesarean births and ultrasound findings suspicious for a placenta accreta

159. Severe maternal pulmonary hypertension

160. Placenta previa and no previous uterine surgery

161. Uncomplicated antenatal course and a singleton vertex fetus in labor at 41 weeks of gestation

162–166

For each term neonate (162–166), choose the correct Apgar score (A–E).

(A) 4
(B) 5
(C) 6
(D) 7
(E) 8

162. A neonate, precipitously delivered, has blue feet and hands. The heart rate is 95 beats per minute. The neonate is crying, with active movement and good respiratory effort.

163. A neonate, delivered by forceps, is pale and has a weak cry. The heart rate is 90 beats per minute. The neonate grimaces with weak flexion.

164. A neonate, delivered by breech extraction (twin B), has blue feet and hands. The heart rate has increased to 110 beats per minute. When stimulated, the infant grimaces, with some flexion, and has begun crying loudly.

165. A neonate was delivered by cesarean birth after an unsuccessful vacuum delivery. The infant is pale and demonstrates a weak cry. The heart rate is 105 beats per minute. There is some flexion and a grimace to stimulation.

166. A neonate who was delivered by cesarean birth for breech is acrocyanotic, and the heart rate is 110 beats per minute. The infant grimaces and has weak flexion. The infant demonstrates a weak cry.

167–171

For each clinical scenario (167–171), choose the most appropriate *Eunice Kennedy Shriver* National Institute of Child Health and Human Development (NICHD) fetal heart rate tracing classification or fetal testing interpretation (A–E).

(A) Category I
(B) Category II
(C) Category III
(D) Nonreactive nonstress test (NST)
(E) Reactive NST

167. A 38-year-old gravida 3, para 2, at 35 weeks of gestation with hypertension and gestational diabetes mellitus presents for scheduled prenatal testing (Fig. 167–171-1).

168. A 17-year-old gravida 1, para 0, in triage with abdominal pain at 37 weeks of gestation is having regular uterine contractions. Her cervix is 6-cm dilated and fully effaced (Fig. 167–171-2).

169. A 28-year-old gravida 1, para 0, at 36 weeks of gestation and with type 1 diabetes mellitus presents for an office visit with scheduled fetal testing (Fig. 167–171-3).

170. A 30-year-old gravida 2, para 1, at 36 weeks of gestation presents to triage for evaluation after a low-speed motor vehicle collision. She is contracting painfully every 1–2 minutes (Fig. 167–171-4).

171. A 23-year-old gravida 3, para 0, is admitted in early labor with spontaneously ruptured membranes (Fig. 167–171-5).

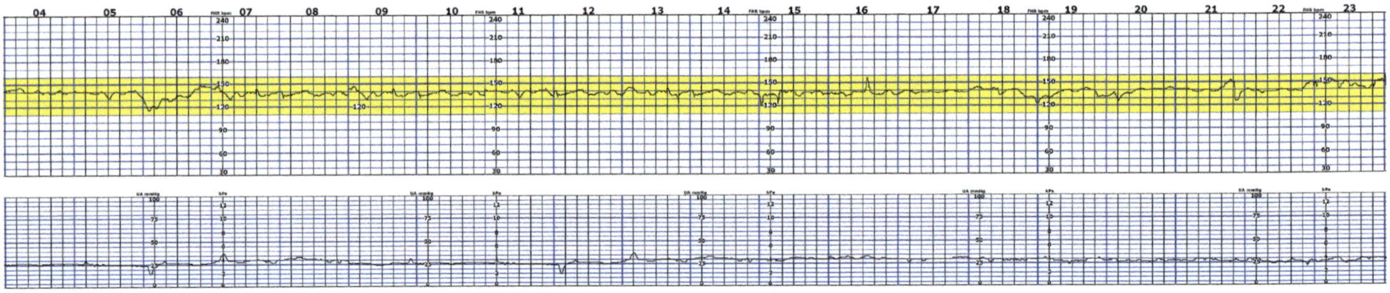

FIGURE 167–171-1. Patient's fetal heart rate tracing. (Image courtesy of James Woods, MD, and periFACTS OB/GYN Academy.)

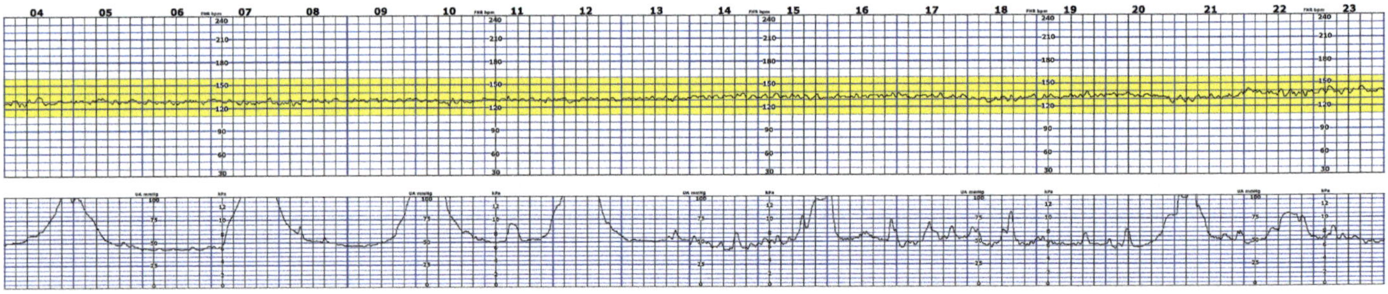

FIGURE 167–171-2. Patient's fetal heart rate tracing. (Image courtesy of James Woods, MD, and periFACTS OB/GYN Academy.)

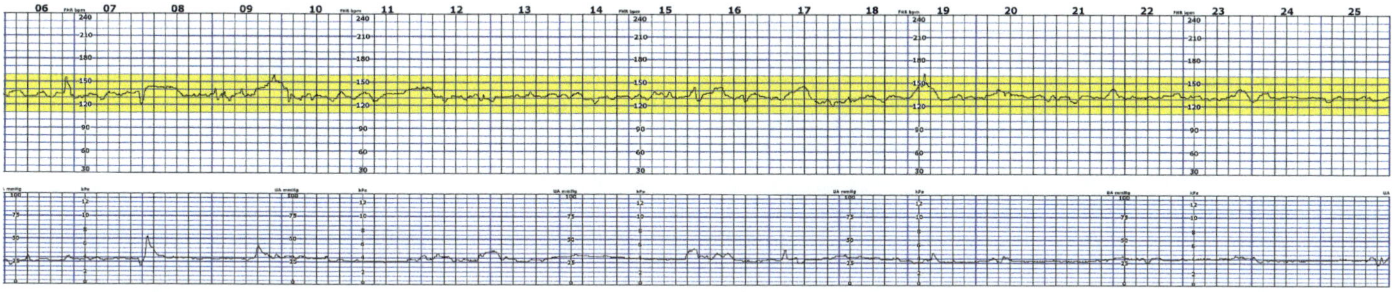

FIGURE 167-171-3. Patient's fetal heart rate tracing. (Image courtesy of James Woods, MD, and periFACTS OB/GYN Academy.)

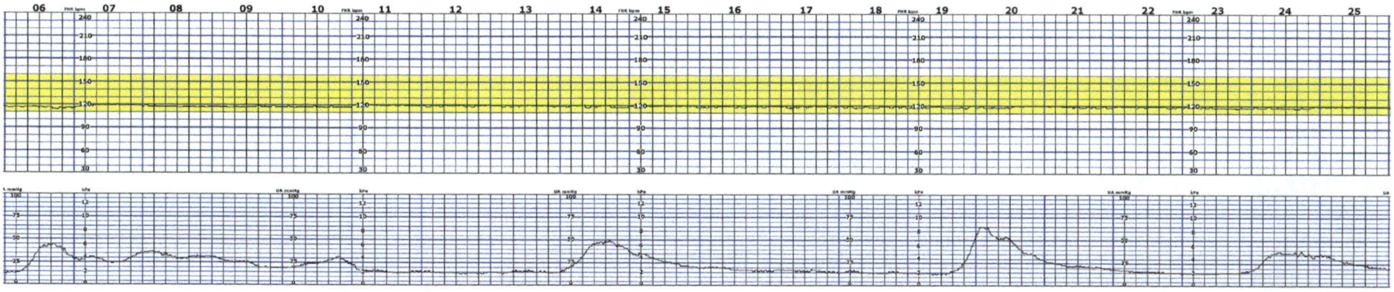

FIGURE 167-171-4. Patient's fetal heart rate tracing. (Image courtesy of James Woods, MD, and periFACTS OB/GYN Academy.)

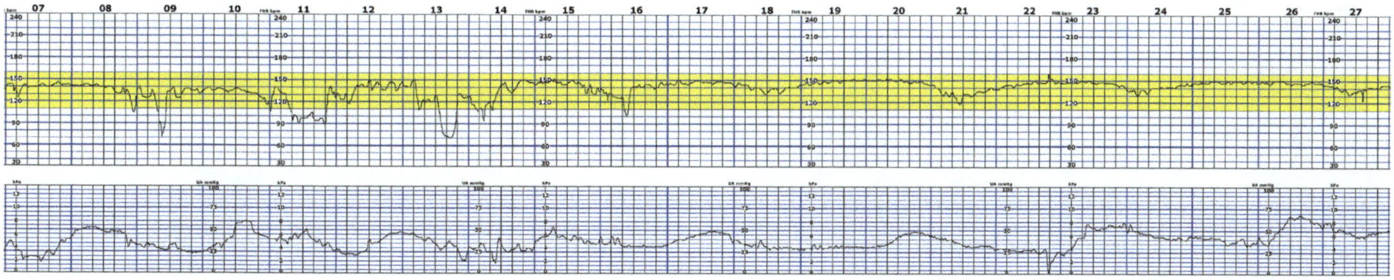

FIGURE 167-171-5. Patient's fetal heart rate tracing. (Image courtesy of James Woods, MD, and periFACTS OB/GYN Academy.)

172–175

A 33-year-old gravida 3, para 2, is admitted at 34 weeks of gestation with preterm prelabor rupture of membranes (PPROM). Both of her previous births were vaginal deliveries. The biophysical profile is 10/10. The patient is not experiencing contractions or vaginal bleeding. She is afebrile, and there is no uterine tenderness. She expresses concern regarding neonatal intensive care unit admission. Continued expectant management until 37 weeks could have the following effect (A–C) on the listed morbidities (172–175).

(A) Increased
(B) Decreased
(C) Unchanged

172. Maternal hemorrhage

173. Neonatal respiratory distress

174. Neonatal sepsis

175. Maternal infection

176–179

For each of the following diagnoses (176–179), choose whether the diagnosis prevalence decreased, increased, or was unchanged (A–C) during the first year of the COVID-19 pandemic.

(A) Decreased
(B) Increased
(C) Unchanged

176. Influenza

177. Opioid overdose

178. Stillbirth

179. Postpartum depression

180–184

For each of the following clinical scenarios (180–184), choose the most likely diagnosis (A–E).

(A) Acute fatty liver of pregnancy
(B) COVID-19
(C) HELLP (hemolysis, elevated liver enzymes, and low platelet count) syndrome
(D) Preeclampsia with severe features
(E) Systemic lupus erythematosus (SLE) flare

180. A primigravida presents for a routine prenatal visit at 41 weeks of gestation. She has noticed increased fatigue and severe headache over the past 2 days. On physical examination, she has bilateral lower-extremity pitting edema and clonus. Her blood pressure is 160/105 mm Hg. Laboratory studies show a white blood cell count of 10.4×10^9/L, platelet count of 52,000/mm^3, hemoglobin of 9.6 mg/dL, creatinine of 1.0 mg/dL, serum alanine aminotransferase of 88 units/L, lactate dehydrogenase of 722 units/L, and total urine protein–creatinine ratio of 0.25.

181. A patient at 29 weeks of gestation presents to the emergency department with malaise for 3 days, headache, and cough. She is lethargic and has difficulty breathing. Vital signs are a temperature of 38.4 °C (101.1 °F), blood pressure of 130/90 mm Hg, pulse of 130 beats per minute, and respiratory rate of 24 breaths per minute. Her pulse oximetry is 92% on room air. Chest X-ray shows bilateral opacities. Laboratory studies show a white blood cell count of 12.0×10^9/L, platelet count of 110,000/mm^3, hemoglobin of 8.2 mg/dL, creatinine of 1.2 mg/dL, and serum alanine aminotransferase of 62 units/L.

182. A multigravida at 37 weeks of gestation presents with malaise, nausea, and decreased fetal movement for 24 hours. She appears ill. Her temperature is normal, blood pressure is 140/80 mm Hg, and pulse is 114 bpm. She has right upper quadrant pain with scleral icterus. Laboratory studies show a white blood cell count of 14.3×10^9/L, platelet count of 120,000/mm^3, creatinine of 1.3 mg/dL, glucose of 49 mg/dL, and serum alanine aminotransferase of 450 units/L. The urine protein–creatinine ratio is 0.32. Fetal cardiac activity is absent on ultrasonography.

183. A primigravida at 29 weeks of gestation presents with an unrelenting headache and difficulty breathing. Her temperature is 36.8 °C (98.2 °F), blood pressure is 180/110 mm Hg, respiratory rate is 23 breaths per minute, and pulse oximetry is 95% on room air. She has bilateral crackles on her pulmonary examination. Laboratory studies show a white blood cell count of 12.4×10^9/L, platelet count of 95,000/mm^3, hemoglobin of 13.2 mg/dL, creatinine of 1.1 mg/dL, serum alanine aminotransferase of 24 units/L, lactate dehydrogenase of 450 units/L, and urine protein–creatinine ratio of 0.5. Chest X-ray shows pulmonary edema with bilateral pleural effusions.

184. A 23-year-old gravida 4, para 0, at 21 weeks of gestation presents with severe headache and confusion. Her temperature is 37.0 °C (98.6 °F), and blood pressure is 150/94 mm Hg. On physical examination, there is lower-extremity pitting edema to the hips. Computed tomography of the head is negative for thrombus or mass. Laboratory studies show white blood cell count of 4.5×10^9/L, platelets count of 87,000/mm^3, hemoglobin of 11.4 mg/dL, creatinine of 1.9 mg/dL, serum aspartate aminotransferase of 30 units/L, and urine protein–creatinine ratio of 4.6. Urinalysis shows 4+ protein, erythrocytes 6/HPF, and granular and hyaline casts. Serial laboratory tests and symptoms are stable over 24 hours.

185–188

For each second-trimester fetal ultrasound finding (185–188), choose the most likely abnormal fetal karyotype (A–D).

(A) 69,XXY
(B) 45,X
(C) 47,XY (+21)
(D) 47,XX (+18)

185. Cystic hygroma

186. Large cystic placenta

187. Omphalocele

188. Thickened nuchal fold

189–192

For each clinical scenario (189–192), choose the most appropriate timing of antepartum fetal surveillance with nonstress test or biophysical profile (A–D).

(A) No ongoing surveillance
(B) Once weekly
(C) Twice weekly
(D) Once weekly plus once-weekly umbilical artery Doppler assessment

189. A 26-year-old gravida 1 at 34 weeks of gestation was found to have a maximum vertical pocket of amniotic fluid of 8.5 cm and amniotic fluid index of 26 cm on ultrasonographic evaluation. She has had an otherwise uncomplicated pregnancy.

190. A 29-year-old gravida 1 at 33 weeks of gestation underwent ultrasonographic evaluation for the finding of a fundal height of 29 cm. The estimated fetal weight was at the 12th percentile, and the abdominal circumference was at the 5th percentile.

191. A 36-year-old gravida 2, para 1, is at 33 weeks of gestation and has a history of chronic hypertension. She has no other pregnancy complications and her blood pressure has been well controlled on labetalol.

192. A 23-year-old gravida 2, para 1, at 31 weeks of gestation has been diagnosed with preeclampsia without severe features. An ultrasonographic evaluation of the fetus showed an estimated fetal weight of 1,650 grams (33rd percentile).

193–196

For each scenario of racial and ethnic disparity in obstetrics (193–196), choose the underlying cause (A–D).

(A) Health inequity
(B) Implicit bias
(C) Social determinants of health
(D) Structural racism

193. The lack of diversity among physicians perpetuates a system of decreased quality of care for marginalized populations.

194. Seventy-three percent of a group of medical students falsely believe that there are biological differences in pain among people of different races.

195. Lack of transportation is associated with fewer prenatal visits and increased rate of preeclampsia.

196. Racial and ethnic minorities tend to receive lower quality of health care than nonminorities, even when controlling for access factors, such as insurance status and income.

197–200

A 28-year-old primigravida at 16 weeks of gestation with a history of Marfan syndrome undergoes maternal echocardiogram and is found to have an aortic root that is dilated to 52 mm. She is considered World Health Organization Class IV with extremely high risk of maternal morbidity or mortality, and pregnancy is contraindicated. For this patient scenario, match the possible next steps in 197–200 to the ethical principles they represent (A–D).

(A) Autonomy
(B) Beneficence
(C) Conscientious refusal
(D) Fiduciary responsibility

197. Provide continued pregnancy care according to her wishes after informed consent.

198. Advise the patient that you recommend termination of pregnancy and perform the procedure after informed consent.

199. Decline to perform pregnancy termination because you are morally opposed to pregnancy termination.

200. Refer the patient to a different physician because you are morally opposed to pregnancy termination.

201–204

For each clinical scenario (201–204), choose the most appropriate anticoagulation recommendation (A–C).

(A) Prophylactic anticoagulation
(B) Surveillance without coagulation
(C) Therapeutic (adjusted dose) anticoagulation

201. A 35-year-old gravida 4, para 2, presents at 12 1/7 weeks of gestation with a body mass index (BMI) of 42 experienced a deep vein thrombosis (DVT) 3 years ago after knee surgery. She was prescribed and completed 3 months of anticoagulation therapy. Testing was negative for factor V Leiden, prothrombin gene mutation, and deficiencies in antithrombin, Protein S, and Protein C.

202. A 38-year-old gravida 2, para 1, at 8 2/7 weeks of gestation has a history of two previous DVTs, one after a long airplane flight, and the second after foot surgery. Testing reveals that she is heterozygous for factor V Leiden and the prothrombin G20210A mutation. Testing for deficiencies in antithrombin, Protein S, and Protein C was negative. After her second DVT, she was started on rivaroxaban, an anti-Xa inhibitor.

203. A 21-year-old gravida 1 with a BMI of 31 underwent an uncomplicated cesarean birth. She is heterozygous for the factor V Leiden mutation. She has no personal history of a venous thromboembolism (VTE). Her mother experienced a DVT at age 45.

204. A 25-year-old gravida 1 underwent a full-term vaginal delivery. She smokes one-half pack of cigarettes daily, and her BMI is 24. She has no personal history of VTE. Her maternal aunt was diagnosed with a pulmonary embolism after a surgical procedure at age 54 years.

205–208

For each clinical scenario (205–208), choose the type of intimate partner violence (A–D).

(A) Physical violence
(B) Psychologic aggression
(C) Reproductive coercion
(D) Sexual violence

205. A pregnant patient presents after falling down the stairs. With questioning, she reveals she was shoved by her partner.

206. A pregnant patient reports that her partner shares suggestive photographs of her on social media without her consent or knowledge.

207. A patient informs you that her partner repeatedly threatens to hurt her children.

208. A patient has an unplanned pregnancy, and she reports that her partner threatens to hurt her if she seeks pregnancy termination.

209–213

For each vaccine (209–213), choose the appropriate recommendation for administration during pregnancy (A–C).

(A) Contraindicated during pregnancy
(B) Indicated during every pregnancy
(C) May be given during pregnancy in indicated persons

209. Hepatitis A

210. Tetanus toxoid, reduced diphtheria toxoid, and acellular pertussis (Tdap)

211. Varicella

212. Measles-mumps-rubella

213. Inactivated influenza

214–218

For each clinical scenario (214–218), choose the best next management option.

(A) Amnioinfusion
(B) Cesarean birth
(C) Decrease of oxytocin
(D) Expectant management
(E) Operative vaginal delivery

214. A 24-year-old gravida 1, para 0, is undergoing induction of labor with oxytocin at 41 weeks of gestation. Vaginal examination reveals the cervix to be 6 cm, 100% effaced, soft and anterior, with the fetal vertex at +2 station (Fig. 214–218-1).

215. A 22-year-old gravida 2, para 0, is admitted at 37 weeks of gestation with prelabor rupture of membranes. Oxytocin is initiated. Vaginal examination reveals the cervix to be 4-cm dilated, 80% effaced, soft and anterior, with the fetal vertex at 0 station (Fig. 214–218-2).

216. A 31-year-old gravida 3, para 2, has a history of two previous cesarean births and elects to undergo a trial of labor. She is admitted at 41 weeks of gestation with ruptured membranes. Oxytocin is initiated. She receives epidural anesthesia. Several hours later, she reports increased lower abdominal pain. Vaginal examination reveals the cervix to be 7-cm dilated with the fetal vertex at −4 station and significant vaginal bleeding (Fig. 214–218-3).

217. A 38-year-old gravida 4, para 3, is admitted for spontaneous rupture of membranes at 39 weeks of gestation. She is admitted for expectant management. Several hours later, her cervix is 5-cm dilated, 50% effaced, and −2 station (Fig. 214–218-4).

218. A 37-year-old gravida 7, para 6, presents to labor and delivery in active labor at 36 weeks of gestation. She has a history of cesarean birth at 32 weeks of gestation for her second child and has since had four vaginal deliveries. She requires oxytocin augmentation after placement of an epidural. Vaginal examination reveals the cervix to be 10-cm dilated and fully effaced, with the fetal vertex at +3 station in the occiput anterior position (Fig. 214–218-5).

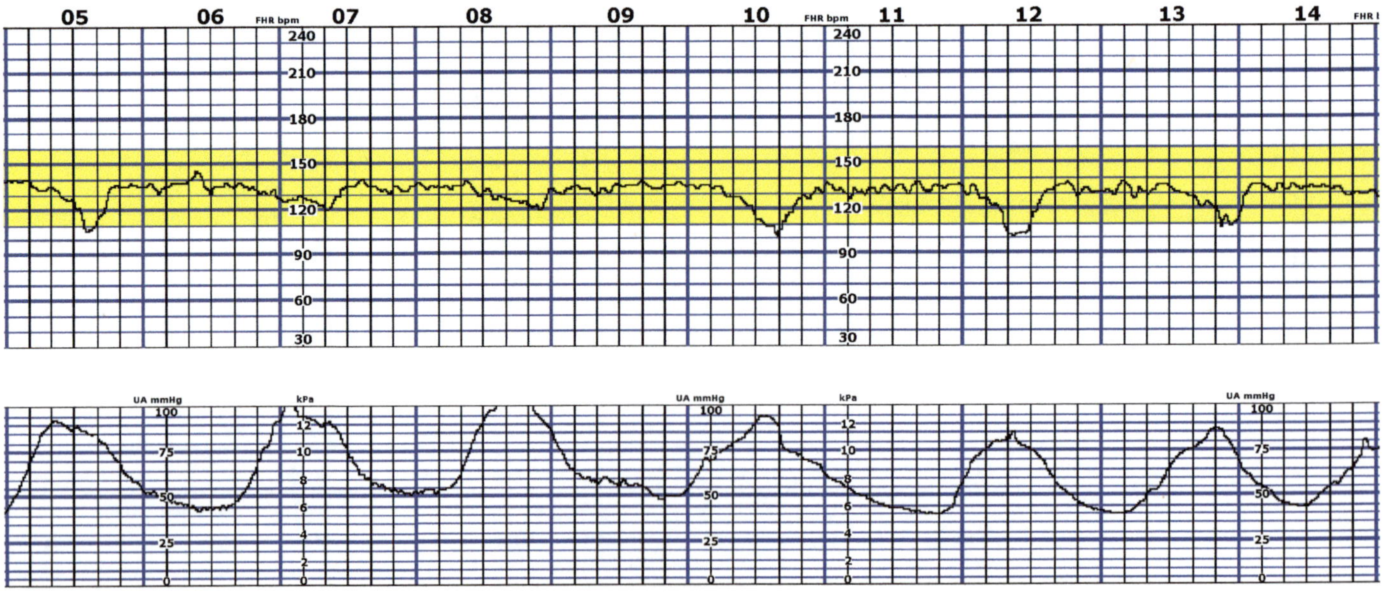

FIGURE 214-218-1. Fetal heart tracing in patient 214. (Image courtesy of James Woods, MD, and periFacts OB/GYN Academy.)

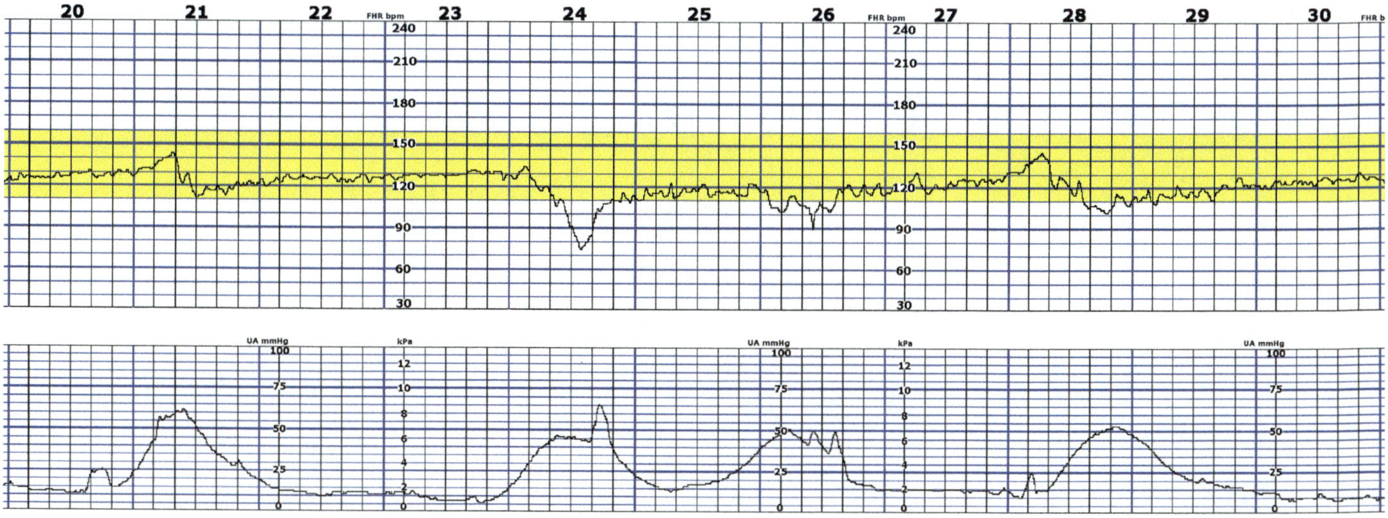

FIGURE 214-218-2. Fetal heart tracing in patient 215. (Image courtesy of James Woods, MD, and periFacts OB/GYN Academy.)

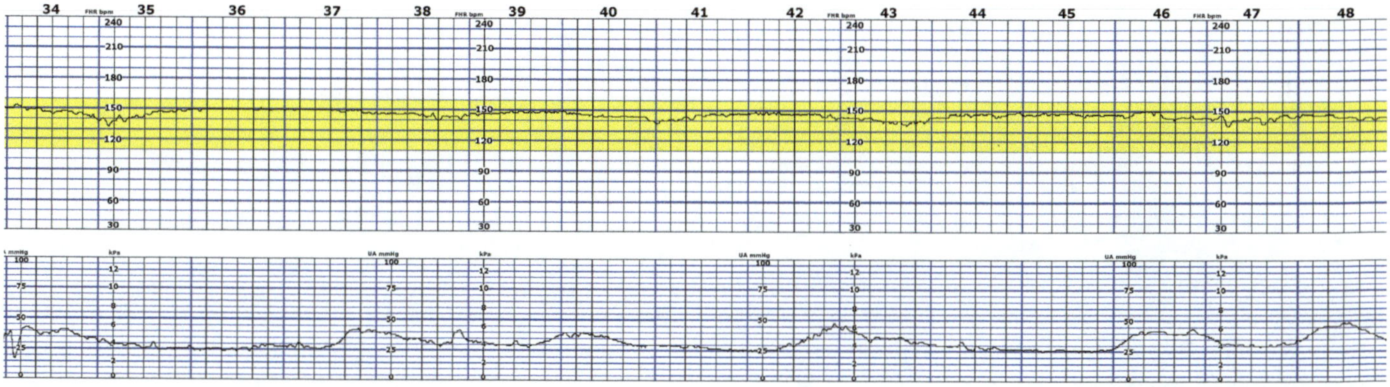

FIGURE 214-218-3. Fetal heart tracing in patient 216. (Image courtesy of James Woods, MD, and periFacts OB/GYN Academy.)

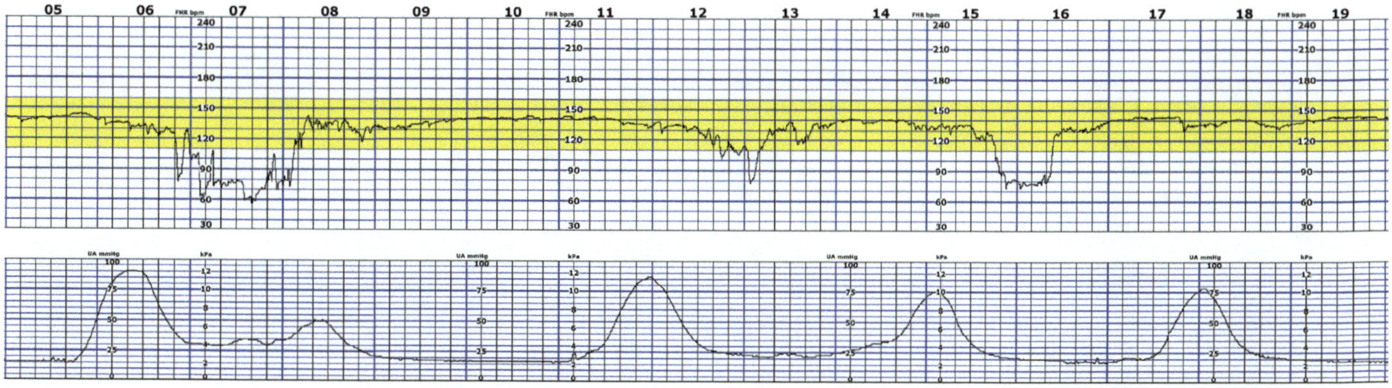

FIGURE 214-218-4. Fetal heart tracing in patient 217.

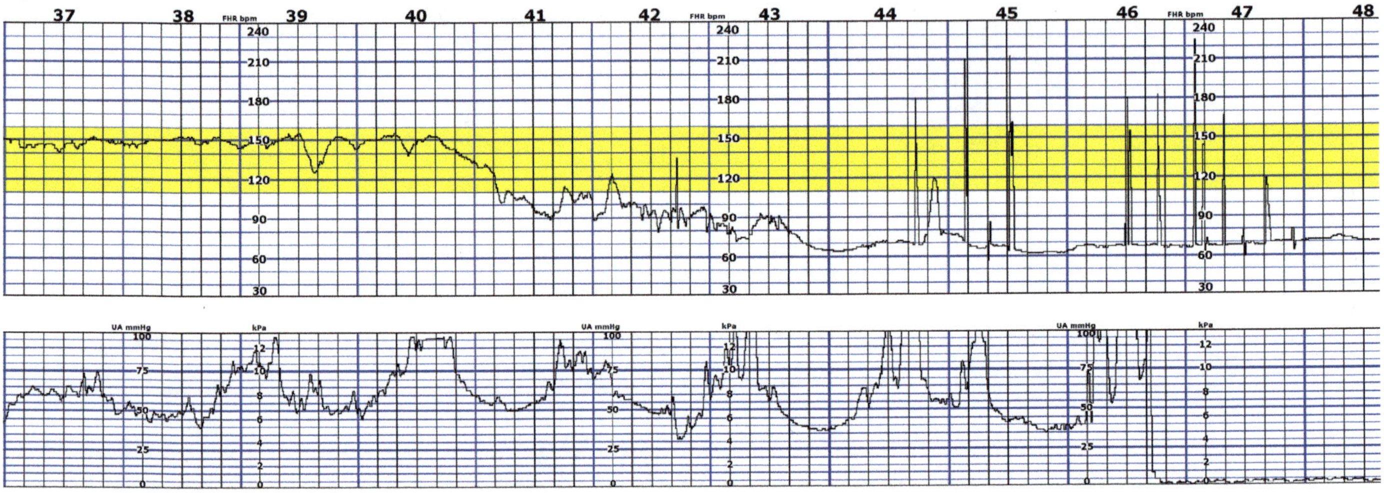

FIGURE 214-218-5. Fetal heart tracing in patient 218. (Image courtesy of James Woods, MD, and periFacts OB/GYN Academy.)